Sepsis and Septic Shock

Sepsis and Septic Shock

Edited by **Scarlett Beckinsale**

hayle medical

New York

Published by Hayle Medical,
30 West, 37th Street, Suite 612,
New York, NY 10018, USA
www.haylemedical.com

Sepsis and Septic Shock
Edited by Scarlett Beckinsale

International Standard Book Number: 978-1-63241-353-6 (Hardback)

Printed in China.

Contents

Preface

This is a comprehensive book which provides up-to-date detailed information regarding sepsis and septic shock. Even though extensive progress in the handling of severe sepsis and septic shock has been made, it is still one of the foremost causes of deaths around the world. Certain experts regard it as one of the most challenging issues due to its varied presentations and diverse complexities. Dedicated researchers from around the globe have contributed important information on this lethal condition. It is hoped that the hard work put in by the researchers will lead to the compilation of a useful source of guidance for continuing the intense work and interest in patient-care.

Significant researches are present in this book. Intensive efforts have been employed by authors to make this book an outstanding discourse. This book contains the enlightening chapters which have been written on the basis of significant researches done by the experts.

Finally, I would also like to thank all the members involved in this book for being a team and meeting all the deadlines for the submission of their respective works. I would also like to thank my friends and family for being supportive in my efforts.

Editor

Part 1

Definition and Epidemiology

1

Epidemiology of Severe Sepsis and Septic Shock

Arturo Artero[1], Rafael Zaragoza[2] and José Miguel Nogueira[3]
[1]*Departments of Internal Medicine*
[2]*Intensive Care*
[3]*Clinical Microbiology*
Hospital Universitario Dr. Peset, Valencia
Departaments of Medicine and Microbiology, Universitat de València
Spain

1. Introduction

Sepsis is defined as the combination of pathologic infection and physiological changes known collectively as the systemic inflammatory response syndrome (Martin, 2003). This response results in physiological alterations that occur at the capillary endothelial level. In the early stages, the clinical manifestations of this process are unspecific and it is often underappreciated in clinical practice. However, early recognition of this syndrome is vital to reducing mortality in sepsis.

From clinical studies sepsis can be seen as a continuum of severity that begins with an infection, followed in some cases by sepsis, severe sepsis - with organ dysfunction - and septic shock. There has been a substantial increase in the incidence of sepsis during the last decades, and it appears to be rising over time, with an increasing number of deaths occurring despite a decline in overall in-hospital mortality (Bone, 1992). Advanced age, underlying comorbidities and number of organ dysfunction are factors which are consistently associated with higher mortality in severe sepsis and septic shock.

In this chapter we are going to review the definitions of sepsis syndromes, the factors that have contributed to the widening of physicians' awareness of sepsis, severe sepsis and septic shock; the incidence of severe sepsis and septic shock; the epidemiological data of patients with severe sepsis and septic shock in the emergency departments and intensive care units; the causative microorganisms, and the changes observed over recent years.

2. Definitions

The concept of sepsis syndrome originated during the time of Hippocrates. But it was not until the nineteenth century when Sir William Osler recognized that "except on few occasions, the patient appears to die from the body's response to infection rather than to the infection" (Hodgkin, 2008). During a long period of time great confusion existed as to the description of systemic inflammatory response to infection, and several terms were used interchangeably: septicemia, sepsis, sepsis syndrome and septic shock. In clinical practice sepsis is the most confusing term used to describe the body's systemic response to infection, and to many clinicians sepsis implies a life-threatening state.

Bacteremia	The presence of viable bacteria in the blood
SIRS	The systemic inflammatory response to a variety of severe clinical insults which is manifested by two or more of the following conditions: (1) temperature >38°C or <36°C (2) heart rate >90 beats per minute (3) respiratory rate >20 breaths per minute or $PaCO_2$ <32 mm Hg (4) white blood cell count >12,000/cu mm, <4,000/cu mm, or >10% immature (band) forms
Sepsis	The systemic inflammatory response (SIRS) as a result of infection
Severe Sepsis	Sepsis associated with organ dysfunction, hypoperfusion, or hypotension. Hypoperfusion and perfusion abnormalities may include, but are not limited to lactic acidosis, oliguria, or an acute alteration in mental status
Septic Shock	Sepsis-induced with hypotension despite adequate fluid resuscitation along with the presence of perfusion abnormalities that may include, but are not limited to, lactic acidosis, oliguria, or an acute alteration in mental status. Patients who are receiving inotropic or vasopressor agents may not be hypotensive at the time that perfusion abnormalities are measured.

Table 1. Definition of bacteremia, SIRS, sepsis, severe sepsis and septic shock.

In 1991, the American College of Chest Physicians and the Society of Critical Care Medicine convened a Consensus Conference and the definitions of sepsis syndromes were published in order to clarify the terminology used to describe the body's systemic responses to infection (Bone, 1992). These definitions are easy to use, based on clinical data of the patients, and describe a clinical continuum response to infection.

In the opinion of the authors of this chapter these definitions have not only been widely used in practice and clinical trials of therapeutic interventions but they have greatly contributed to the recognition of these syndromes. Before analyzing the epidemiology of severe sepsis and septic shock the reader should be familiarized with all these terms. The definitions of bacteremia, systemic inflammatory response syndrome (SIRS), sepsis, severe sepsis and septic shock are shown in **table 1**, and the relationships between infection, systemic inflammatory response syndrome (SIRS) and septic syndromes are shown in **figure 1**.

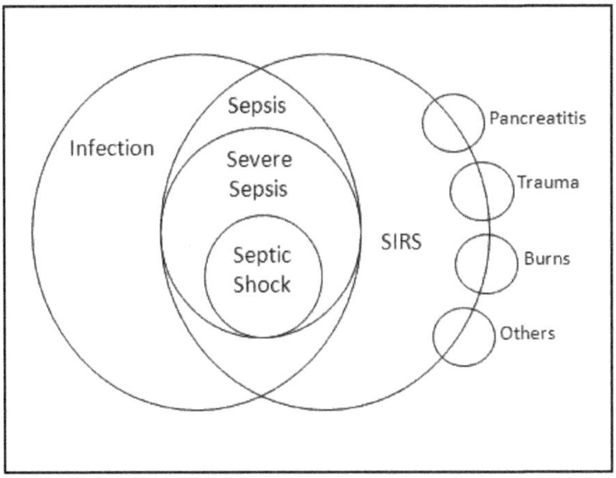

Fig. 1. The relationship between infection, systemic inflammatory response syndrome (SIRS) and sepsis syndromes.

In 2001, an International Sepsis Definitions Conference (Levy, 2003; Dunne, 2003) was sponsored by the Society of Critical Care Medicine (SCCM), the European Society of Intensive Care Medicine (ESICM), the American College of Chest Physicians (ACCP), the American Thoracic Society (ATS), and the Surgical Infection Society (SIS) to revisit the 1992 sepsis guidelines. Based on this conference a consensus document was developed, concluding that there was not enough evidence to support a change to the previous definitions. This document expanded the list of signs and symptoms of sepsis to reflect clinical bedside experience. Besides, the document developed a classification scheme for sepsis, called PIRO (Predisposition, Insult infection, Response, Organ dysfunction), that will stratify patients on the basis of their predisposing conditions, the nature and extent of the insult (in the case of sepsis, infection), the nature and magnitude of the host response, and the degree of concomitant organ dysfunction. This has provided a basis for introducing PIRO as a hypothesis-generating model for future research.

Predisposition (P) was the new element which was added to the IRO model proposed by John Marshall and based on the TNM system used in oncology patients. Factors that predispose patients to outcome in sepsis include genetic factors, environment, cultural factors and pre-existing diseases.

Infections (I) have four categories with a significant impact on outcome: The site, extent, source (hospital vs. community-acquired, etc) and type of organism. Besides, the immune status of a patient is related with opportunistic infections, which are associated with worse prognosis.

Response (R) is affected by several factors, such as: age, type of invading microorganism, genotype and co-morbidities. The use of biomarkers to stratify the degree of response is one of the most promising elements for diagnosis and risk assessment in the future. Given the complexity of the immune response in sepsis a single static measurement of a biomarker (pro-calcitonin or any other biomarker) may not be as important as a dynamic assessment of change over time.

The level of organ dysfunction is similar to the presence of metastatic disease in cancer. The evaluation of organ dysfunction has evolved from describing it in all-or-nothing terms to use organ failures scores to describe the degree of organ dysfunction developing over the course of critical illness.

The participants in this conference gave priority to the facilitation of bedside diagnosis over standardized sepsis entry criteria for clinical trials. The conclusions of this conference can be summarized as: 1) The current concepts of sepsis, severe sepsis, and septic shock seem to be robust definitions and should remain as described 10 yrs ago. 2) Current definitions do not allow for precise staging of the host response to infection. 3) Signs and symptoms of sepsis are more varied than the initial criteria established in 1991. 4) A list of these signs and symptoms, for the diagnosis of sepsis is presented. 5) The future lies in developing a staging system that will characterize progression of sepsis. A new system, PIRO, is proposed for characterizing and staging the host response to infection.

The diagnostic criteria for sepsis in adults are shown in **table 2**. The definition of Systemic Inflammatory Response Syndrome (SIRS) in pediatrics is defined as: "The presence of two or more of the following criteria, one of which must be abnormal temperature or leukocyte count: a) Core temperature of > 38.5°C *or* < 36°C. b) Tachycardia, defined as a mean heart

Documented o suspected Infection and some of the folloging:	
- General variables	Fever (core temperature >38.3°C) Hypothermia (core temperature <36°C) Heart rate >90 min Tachypnea Altered mental status Significant edema or positive fluid balance (>20 mL/kg over 24 hrs) Hyperglycemia (plasma glucose >120 mg/dL or 7.7 mmol/L) in the absence of diabetes
- Inflammatory variables	Leukocytosis (WBC count >12,000 μL^{-1}) Leukopenia (WBC count <4000 μL^{-1}) Normal WBC count with >10% immature forms Plasma C-reactive protein>2 SD above the normal value Plasma procalcitonin >2 SD above the normal value
- Hemodynamic variables	Arterial hypotension (SBP <90 mm Hg, MAP <70, or an SBP decrease >40 mm Hg SvO2 >70% Cardiac index >3.5 $L{\cdot}min^{-1}{\cdot}M^{-23}$
- Organ dysfunction variables	Arterial hypoxemia (PaO2/FIO2 <300) Acute oliguria (urine output <0.5 mL·kg-1·hr-1 or 45 mmol/L for at least 2 hrs) Creatinine increase >0.5 mg/dL Coagulation abnormalities (INR >1.5 or aPTT >60 secs) Ileus (absent bowel sounds) Thrombocytopenia (platelet count <100,000 μL^{-1}) Hyperbilirubinemia (plasma total bilirubin >4 mg/dL or 70 mmol/L)
- Tissue perfusion variables	Hyperlactatemia (>1 mmol/L) Decreased capillary refill or mottling

Table 2. Diagnostic criteria for sepsis in aduts

rate > 2 sd above normal for age in the absence of external stimulus, chronic drugs, or painful stimuli; or otherwise unexplained persistent elevation over a 0.5- to 4-hour time period *or* for children < 1 year old: Bradycardia, defined as a mean heart rate < 10th percentile for age in the absence of external vagal stimulus, beta-blocker drugs, or congenital heart disease; or otherwise unexplained persistent depression over a 0.5-hour time period. c) Mean respiratory rate > 2 sd above normal for age or mechanical ventilation for an acute process not related to underlying neuromuscular disease or the receipt of general anesthesia. d) Leukocyte count elevated or depressed for age (not secondary to chemotherapy-induced leukopenia) or > 10% immature neutrophils.

Criteria for sepsis in the pediatric population are different: arterial hypotension is defined as <2 SD below normal for age; neither SvO2 >70% nor cardiac index >3.5 $L{\cdot}min^{-1}{\cdot}M^{-2}$[3] should be used as signs of sepsis in newborns or children. Diagnostic criteria for sepsis in the pediatric population are signs and symptoms of inflammation plus infection with rectal temperature >38.5 or <35°C, tachycardia (may be absent in hypothermic patients), and at least one of the following indications of altered organ function: altered mental status, hypoxemia, increased serum lactate level, or bounding pulses.

A bedside diagnosis of sepsis is not frequently base only on these criteria. Instead, experienced clinicians consider some physical and laboratory finding that prompt them to conclude that an infected patient "looks septic". These findings include general variables (altered mental status, significant edema ...), inflammatory variables (plasma C-reactive protein, plasma procalcitonin ...), hemodynamic variables (arterial hypotension, SvO2 ...), organ dysfunction variables (arterial hypoxemia, acute oliguria, coagulation abnormalities ...), and tissue perfusion variables (decreased capillary refill or mottling, hyperlactatemia).

In summary, the definitions of sepsis, severe sepsis and septic shock established in 1992 are useful to clinicians and researchers. However they are not precise tools to predict the outcomes of these syndromes, so the inclusion of clinical, microbiological and biological factors in clinical practice may aid to better characterize the prognosis of sepsis. Further evidence is needed to support changes in the current definitions of sepsis.

3. Incidence of severe sepsis and septic shock

The epidemiology of sepsis, severe sepsis and septic shock is not well known due to the absence of population base prospective cohort studies, and to the fact that most of the studies on the epidemiology of sepsis are based on hospital discharge diagnoses which do not use the consensus definitions. The incidence of severe sepsis and septic shock has notably increased in recent years, and appears to be rising over time (**figure 2**).

A comparison of population incidence and hospital prevalence of severe sepsis reported from several studies is shown in **table 3**.

In 1990, the Centers for Disease Control (CDC), based on data from the National Hospital Discharge Survey, estimated that there were 450,000 cases of sepsis per year in the United States (CDC, 1990). Angus, using ICD-9-CM codes, in a large observational cohort study (n=6,621,559) in the United States in 1995, identified 192,980 cases of severe sepsis which represents an estimated incidence of 3.0 cases per 1,000 population, 2.26 cases per 100 hospital discharges, and 11 percent of all admissions to the ICU (Angus, 2001). However, the accuracy of ICD-9-CM coding for the identification of specific medical conditions remains controversial, and Martin (Martin, 2003) suggested that Angus's estimates may overstate the incidence of severe sepsis by as much as a factor of two to four.

Martin et al. (Martin, 2003) identified 10,319,418 cases of sepsis from an estimated 750 million hospitalizations in the United States over a 22-yr period, with an increase in frequency from 82.7 cases per 100,000 population in 1979 to 240.4 cases per 100,000 population in 2000, therefore there was an annualized increase in the incidence of sepsis of 8.7 percent.

Country	Author, yr	Prevalence in hospital per 100 admissions	Prevalence in ICUs per 100 ICU admissions	Estimated incidence per 100,000 population
Australia	Sundarajan, 2005	4.3	NR	76
Australia & N.Zeland	Finfer, 2004	-	11.8	77
Europe	Alberti, 2001	-	15.5	-
Europe	Vincet, 2006	-	30.0	-
Finland	Karlsson, 2007	-	10.5	69
France	Brun-Buisson, 1995	2.9	11.9	-
France	Episepsis, 2004	-	14.6	95
Germany	Engel, 2006	-	11.0	76
Netherlands	Van Gestel, 2004	-	11.0	54
Norway	Flaatten, 2004	3	-	48
United Kingdom	Padkin, 2003	-	27.1	51
Spain	Esteban, 2007	12.4	-	104
USA	Angus, 2001	2.6	11	300
USA	Martin, 2003	4.7	-	81

Table 3. Prevalence of severe sepsis in several studies around the world. (Adapted from Brun-Buisson C. Impact of Sepsis on Public Health. In: Dellinger P, Carlet J, editors. Sepsis handbook. 1st ed. Marcy l'Etoile: Editons Biomerieux;2009. p. 8-17).

In a recent prospective, observational study in Iceland, the incidence of severe sepsis and septic shock was 0.48 per 1,000 inhabitants ≥18 years of age per year [95% confidence intervals (CI) 0.42-0.55] (Vesteinsdottir, 2011).

The Italian SEPSIS study found that in 99 ICUs the prevalence of SIRS, sepsis, severe sepsis and septic shock in patients admitted to ICUs were 58%, 16%, 5% and 6%, respectively (Salvo, 1995). These and other results provide evidence of how the progression from sepsis to septic shock follows a continuum.

In an international multicenter cohort study on sepsis and infection in intensive care unit patients (Artigas 2002), infections had a crude incidence of 21.1%. Among 3,034 infectious episodes 24% were associated with severe sepsis and 30% with septic shock. The frequency of septic shock is increasing with more multiresistant strains. Annane et al analyzed the epidemiology of septic shock from 100,554 intensive care unit admissions and found that the frequency of septic shock increased from 7.0 per 100 admissions in 1993 to 9.7 per 100 admissions in 2000 (Annane, 2003).

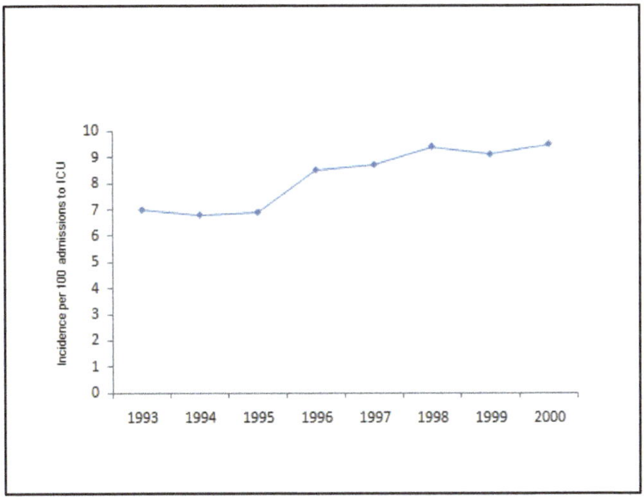

Fig. 2. Incidence of septic shock. Data collected over an 8-year period from 22 hospitals (adapted from Annane et al Am J Respir Crit Care Med 2003; 168:165-72).

Using the Emergency Department data of 2001-2004 from the National Hospital Ambulatory Medical Care Survey, and applying the 2003 international consensus criteria, Wang et al (Wang 2007) estimated the burden of severe sepsis in Emergency Departments as more than 500,000 adult patients per year, with individual patients spending an average of almost 5 hrs in the Emergency Department. Due to limitations of the study, such as not having access to data of respiratory rate, the true number of cases may be even higher.

Most cases of severe sepsis occur in patients who are already hospitalized for other reasons. In a series of 166 patients with bloodstream infections admitted to an intensive care unit we found that 82.5% of patients had nosocomial acquired infections, and the nosocomial origin of the bacteremia was associated with inadequate empirical antimicrobial treatment (Zaragoza, 2003).

Dombrovskiy et al. used the NIS to show that from 1993 to 2003, the age-adjusted rate of hospitalization for severe sepsis increased from 66.8 to 132.0 cases per 100,000 persons (Dombrovskiy, 2007).

Sepsis remains a significant cause of morbidity and mortality in pediatric population. Watson et al (Watson, 2003) using 1995 hospital discharge and population data from seven states analyzed the incidence of severe sepsis in children in the United States (see **figure 3**). The incidence was highest in infants (5.16 cases per 1000) and over 20% were low birth weight neonates. The respiratory tract (37%) and primary bloodstream infections (25%) were the most common sources of infection.

Sepsis is an important source of postoperative morbidity and mortality. Recently, Bateman et al studied the temporal trends in the epidemiology of severe postoperative sepsis after elective surgery in patients aged 18 years or older for any of the 20 most common primary procedure types who had a length of stay more than 3 days from the NIS dataset for the years 1997-2006, and found that the rate of severe sepsis increased from 0.3% in 1997 to 0.9% in 2006. This trend persisted after adjusting for relevant covariables—the adjusted odds ratio of severe sepsis per year increase in the study period was 1.12 (95% CI, 1.11-1.13; *P* _ 0.001) (Bateman, 2010). Abdominal surgery has been described as the most prevalent class of surgical procedure in severe postoperative sepsis. The reasons for the increased rate of severe postoperative sepsis are unknown, but possible causes are an increase in the proportion of infections caused by resistant microorganisms and an increase in the comorbidities that predispose to sepsis.

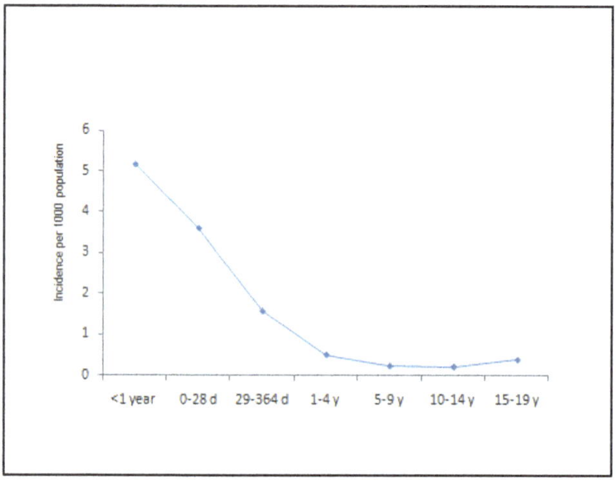

Fig. 3. Annual incidence of severe sepsis by age in the pediatric population of the United States (Modified from Watson RS et al. The epidemiology of severe sepsis in children in the United States. Am J Respir Crit Care Med 2003;167:695-701).

4. Epidemiological data of patients

Age

There is a direct relationship between advanced age and the incidence of severe sepsis y septic shock, with a sharp increase in incidence in elderly people (Wang, 2007; Angus, 2001). The incidence of severe sepsis in infants is also elevated, with an annual rate of 5.3 cases per 1,000 population (Angus, 2001).

The median age of patients with severe sepsis in most studies is between 60 to 65 years, and when the patients are stratified at the age of 65, the relative risk for sepsis was 13 times higher for patients aged 65 and above. Martin et al (Martin, 2006) found that the incidence rates of sepsis increased 20.4% faster among older patients 65 years of age or older than among younger patients from 1979 to 2002 (mean increase per year, 11.5% versus 9.5%; P<.001). Epidemiological studies analyzing data from the 1990s found an increased incidence of severe sepsis in young people, especially men in their thirties, which could be attributed to patients with human immunodeficiency virus related conditions. However, the better control of the HIV epidemic in developed countries is changing this trend.

Gram-negative microorganisms are more frequent in older patients than in younger patients. *Escherichia coli* has found to be the most common microorganism in patients older than 65 years, whereas *Staphylococcus aureus* was the most frequent microorganism in younger patients with community acquired bacteremia (Diekema, 2002). Likewise, the source of infection has also been different among older patients with sepsis than among younger patients. Urinary tract infection is more frequently the source of sepsis in older patients than in younger patients.

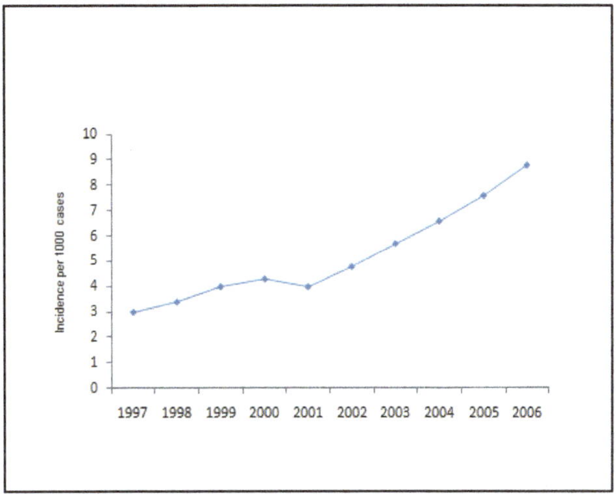

Fig. 4. Rate of severe postoperative sepsis after elective surgery by year (adapted from Bateman, Anesthesiology 2010).

The relationship between age and incidence of severe sepsis and septic shock in a series of 455 adult patients with these disorders admitted to an ICU at the Hospital Universitario Dr. Peset, in Valencia (Spain) is shown in **figure 5**.

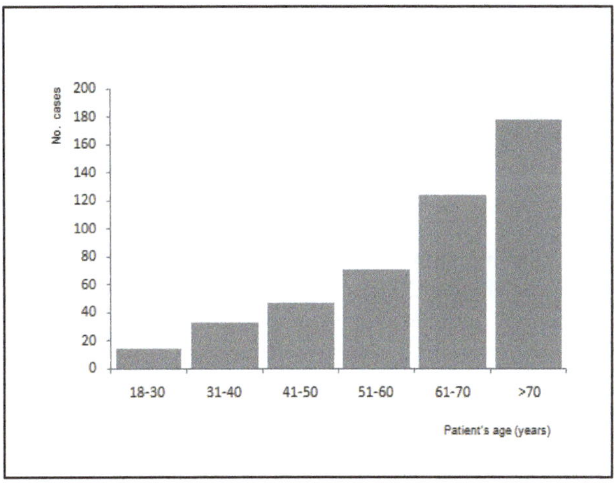

Fig. 5. Relationship between the incidence of severe sepsis and septic shock and patient's age in a series of 455 cases with these disorders admitted to ICU at the Hospital Universitario Dr. Peset, Valencia, Spain.

Race

Epidemiologic studies have shown a higher incidence of severe sepsis and septic shock in black people, suggesting a possible genetic predisposition. Alternatively, a higher prevalence of renal disease and diabetes in the black population might explain the higher incidence of these syndromes (Mayr 2010; Martin 2003).
Besides, a higher incidence of severe sepsis and septic shock in black people could be related to the higher percentage of black people living in poverty. Otherwise, the mean age of black people has been found to be lower in black people than in white people.
A higher infection rate and a higher risk of acute organ dysfunction in black as compared to white individuals could explain racial differences in severe sepsis (Mayr 2010). Lastly, race specific genetic polymorphisms in the host response to infection may predispose certain racial groups to increased incidence or worse outcomes with sepsis (Berkowitz 2007).

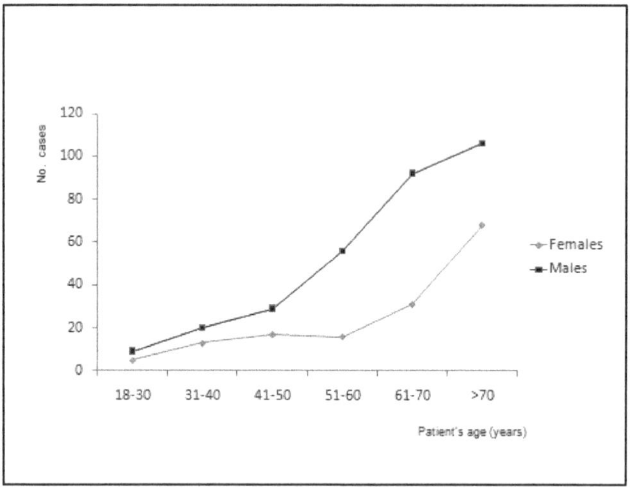

Fig. 6. Relationship between gender and the incidence of severe sepsis and septic shock according to the patient's age in a series of 455 cases with these disorders admitted to ICU (see text).

Sex

Men are more likely than women to develop sepsis, with a mean annual relative risk of 1.28 (95% CI 1.24-1.32) (Martin, 2003). However, it is not clear whether this difference could be due to a higher prevalence of comorbidities in men, or whether women are protected against the inflammatory changes that occur in severe sepsis and septic shock (Angus, 2001).
2001; Martin, 2003). Female gender has been found to substantially decrease the risk for developing severe sepsis, independent of other patient and surgical risk factors, after elective surgery (Bateman, 2010).
In **figures 5** and **6** are shown the distribution of severe sepsis and septic shock according to gender and age in a series of 455 patients with these disorders admitted to an ICU at the Hospital Universitario Dr. Peset in Valencia (Spain).

The absence of a link between the incidence of severe sepsis and menopause argues against the gender differences being solely mediated through sex hormones. Also, women appear to have a lower rate of age-adjusted severe sepsis as a consequence of fewer episodes of respiratory origin (Angus 2001).

The sources of infections in severe sepsis are different between genders. Women are more likely than men to have genitourinary infections urinary tract infections, whereas men are more likely to have respiratory infections, but other sources of sepsis appears to have a similar distribution.

Comorbidities

Patients with severe sepsis and septic shock frequently have underlying comorbidities which predispose them to infections and may have an additive contribution to mortality. McCabe classification has been widely used for assessing the severity of underlying diseases in patients with severe sepsis and septic shock.

McCabe Class	Frequency
0 = No underlying disease	27%
1 = Non-fatal disease or expected death within >5 years	33%
2 = Ultimately fatal disease or expected death within 1-5 years	30%
3 = Rapidily fatal disease or expected death within <1 year	10%

Table 4. Frequency of underlying diseases according to MaCabe classification among patients with severe sepsis (adapted from Brun-Buisson et al, Care Med 2004).

Angus et al in a large observational study on severe sepsis (n=192,980) found that any underlying comorbidity occurred in 55.5% of cases, and the most prevalent coexisting conditions were chronic obstructive pulmonary disease (12.3%) and nonmetastatic neoplasm (11.6%) (Angus, 2001). Annane et al analyzed 8,251 cases of septic shock from 22 intensive care units and found a high proportion of patients having underlying disease with presumably reduced life expectancy (Annane, 2003). In this series the most common comorbidities were: Immune deficiency (21.9%), chronic pulmonary disease (9.2%) and hematologic malignancy (8.4%). Martin et al over a 22-year period identified 10,319,418 cases of sepsis with a proportion of organ failure in 33.6 percent of patients during the most recent subperiod, resulting in the identification of 184,060 cases of severe sepsis in 1995 and 256,033 in 2000. In this series the most frequent comorbidities were diabetes (12.2-18,7%), hypertension (7.0-18.6%), cancer (14.5-18.0%) and congestive heart failure (8.6-15.2%).

The coexisting conditions represented in observational studies (Zaragoza 2003 and Artero 2010) are probably more representative of those in all patients with severe sepsis and septic shock than are the conditions documented in participants in clinical trials, from which patients with certain medical conditions (e.g., HIV infection, or cancer) may be excluded. In our series of 455 patients with severe sepsis and septic shock admitted to ICU diabetes mellitus was the most prevalent comorbity, followed by chronic heart failure and CPOD (See **table 5**).

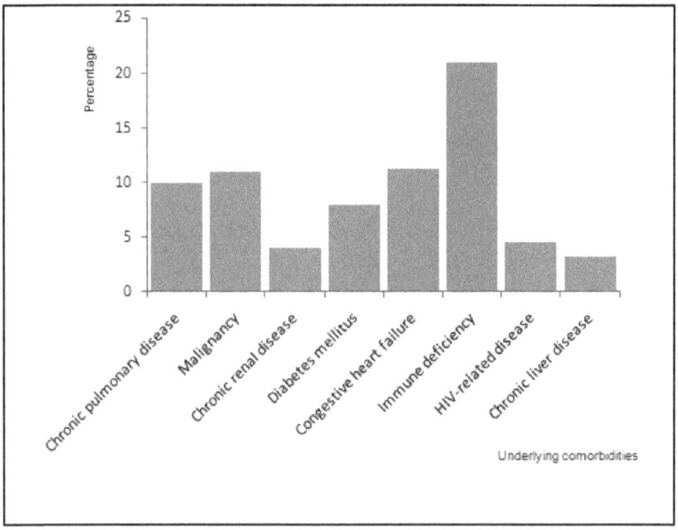

Fig. 7. Coexistent conditions in patients with severe sepsis and septic shock (adapted from several large observational studies).

5. Sources of severe sepsis and septic shock

The lung is the primary source of infection both in severe sepsis and in septic shock, followed by the abdomen, the urinary tract, soft tissues and primary blood stream infection (Annane 2003, Blanco 2008, Kumar 2010). The sites of infection in a series of 4,662 patients with septic shock is shown in **figure 8**, and the sites of infection in a cohort study of 192,980 cases of severe sepsis is shown in **figure 9**.

Comorbidities	Number	Percentage
Diabetes mellitus	102	22.4
COPD	81	17.8
Heart failure	99	21.7
Alcoholism	49	10.7
Malignancy	51	11.2
Liver cirrhosis	26	5.6
Chronic renal insufficiency	39	8.5
HIV	17	3.7

Table 5. Underlying comorbidities in 455 adult patients with severe sepsis and septic shock in an ICU.

Intra-abdominal and respiratory sources of sepsis have been considered as risk foci of infection, because these foci were associated with a higher mortality than other sources of sepsis. These foci have also been related to inadequate empirical antimicrobial treatment (Zaragoza, 2003).

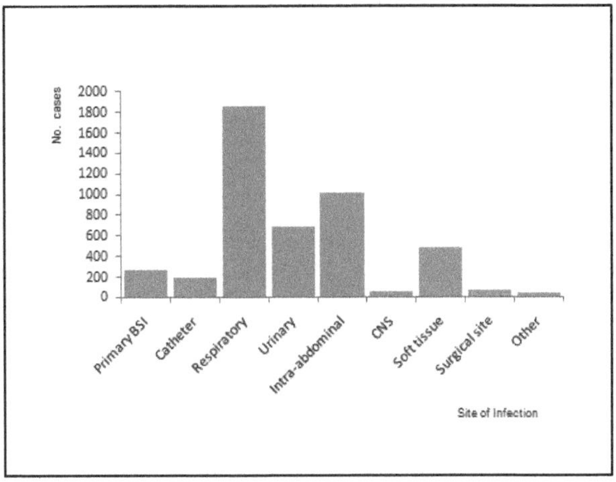

Fig. 8. Sources of septic shock (adapted from Kumar et al, Crit Care Med 2010; 38:1773–85).

6. Microorganisms that cause severe sepsis and septic shock

The proportion of severe sepsis and septic shock with unidentified pathogen is about one third. In some studies the infection was not documented in 40% of cases, possibly due to the increase in empiric antibiotic treatment (Guidet 2005). The percentage of positive blood culture increases with the severity of the sepsis syndrome.

Traditionally, Gram-negative bacilli - mostly represented by *Escherichia coli, Pseudomonas aeruginosa, Klebsiella pneumonia* - were more prevalent than Gram-positive cocci - *Staphylococcus aureus, Streptococcus pneumonia, Enterococcus* spp. - . However, Gram-positive microorganisms have become the most common microorganisms isolated in the more recent

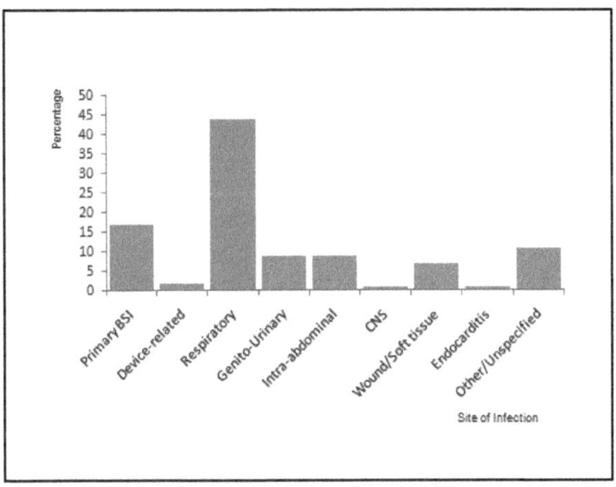

Fig. 9. Sources of severe sepsis (adapted from Angus et al, Crit Care Med 2001; 29:1303–10).

studies (Guidet, 2005). The percentage of polymicrobial infection as well as the proportion of multiresistant bacteria like *Pseudomonas* and methicillin-resistant *Staphylococci,* has significantly increased over time (Annane 2003). The incidence of fungi has also been reported to be increasing in recent years.

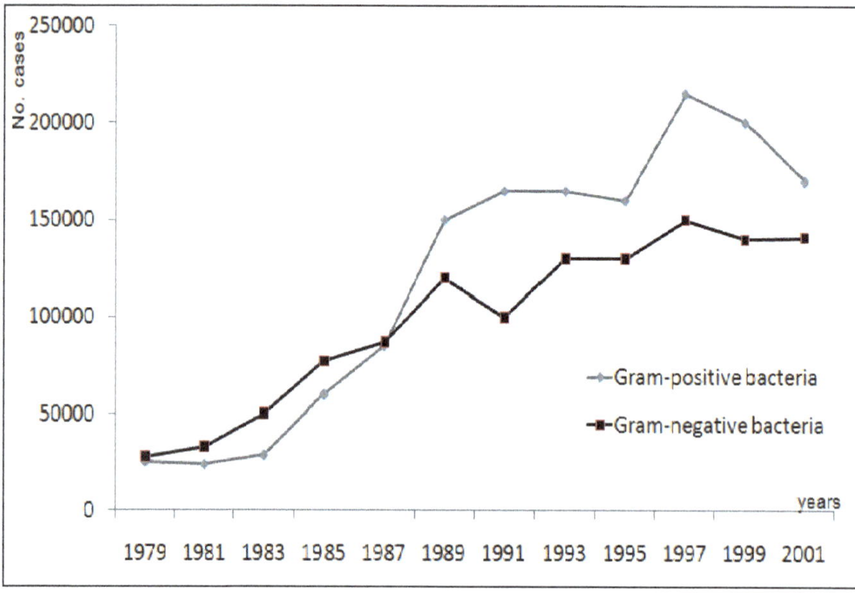

Fig. 10. Cases of severe sepsis according to the causative origin (adapted from Martin et al New Engl J Med 2003;348:1546-1554).

Age influence the etiology of severe sepsis and septic shock in the pediatric population. During the neonatal period the most frequent microorganisms isolated are group B streptococci and enteric bacilli, such as *Escherichia coli. Listeria monocytogenes,* enterococci, *Haemophilus influenzae,* and *Streptococcus pneumoniae* are less common pathogens isolated. The incidence of coagulase-negative staphylococci, *Staphylococcus aureus,* gram-negative bacilli, and fungi are increasing in the pediatric population as a consequence of the advances in neonatology. *S. pneumoniae, Neisseria meningitidis,*and *H. influenzae* type B are common pathogenes beyond the neonatal period.

Immunodeficiency predispose children to some specific microorganisms, such as gram-negative bacteria, alpha-hemolytic streptococci, Viridans group streptococci and cytomegalovirus in neutropenic patients; *Streptococcus pneumoniae,P. aeruginosa, Staphylococcus aureus,* and *Haemophilus influenza type B* in patients with acquired immunodeficiency virus; and *Streptococcus pneumoniae, Salmonella* spp., *Haemophilus influenza type B,* and *N. meningitides* in patients with asplenia.

7. Morbidity

Half of severe sepsis survivors are readmitted to hospital within a year, and their quality of life is comparable with survivors of polytrauma. Jagodič et al studied the long-term survival and quality of life of patients treated in a surgical ICU because of sepsis or trauma, and found that the quality of life (assessed after 2 years following ICU admission using the EuroQol 5D questionnaire) was reduced to the same level in both groups (see figure 12), and

82% of patients reported a problem (moderate or extreme) in at least one dimension of EuroQol 5D (Jagodič, 2006).

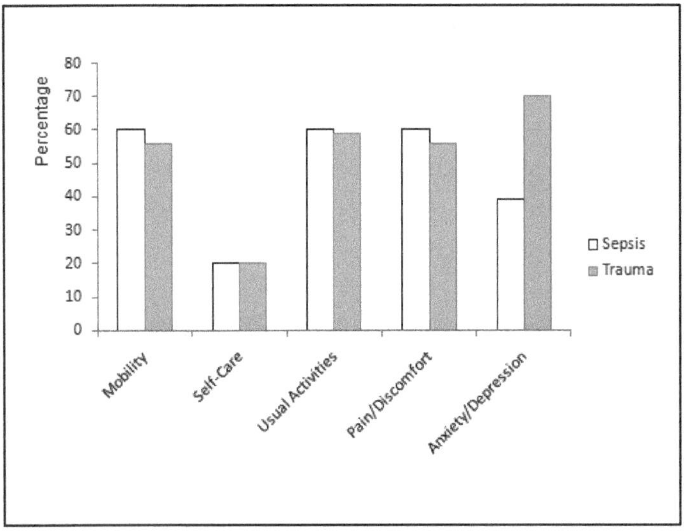

Fig. 11. Quality of life of 164 patients with sepsis or trauma after 2 years following ICU admission using the EuroQol 5D questionnaire (Jagodič et al, Crit Care 2006).

Acute respiratory distress syndrome, myocardial dysfunction, acute renal failure and chronic dysfunction, disseminated intravascular coagulation (DIC), and liver failure are all significant sequels of severe sepsis and septic shock. Furthermore, recent evidence shows that septic shock in elderly persons leads to significant long-term cognitive and functional disability as a consequence of prolonged tissue hypoperfusion (Iwashyna 2010).

8. Mortality

The Centers for Disease Control and Prevention has estimated that sepsis is the tenth leading cause of death overall in the United States (Hoyert 2001). Severe sepsis is considered to be the most common cause of death in noncoronary critical care units. The deaths related to severe sepsis exceed the numbers of persons with other diseases that attract higher public awareness, such as breast cancer and AIDS (Moss 2005). The mortality rates of severe sepsis and septic shock are 25 to 30% and 40 to 70%, respectively.

The mortality rate according to sepsis diagnostic criteria in shown in **figure 12**.

In this picture the global in-hospital mortality rate in 624 patients with sepsis syndromes admitted to the ICU in our hospital was 37.7%, 55.9% and 66.2% in sepsis, severe sepsis and septic shock, respectively. However the related mortality to infection was quite a few lower (7.7%, 16.7% and 30.1% in sepsis, severe sepsis and septic shock, respectively).

The crude mortality rate of septic shock is decreasing, but patients with septic shock still have a high excess risk of death than critically ill patients who are nonseptic. Annane et al in an epidemiological study analyzed 100,554 intensive care unit admissions on the Collège des Utilisateurs de Bases de données en Réanimation (CUB-Re´a) database, collected from

22 hospitals over a 8-year period, 1993 to 2000, and found an overall frequency of septic shock of 8.2 per 100 admissions, and a crude mortality of 60.1% and declined from 62.1% (in 1993) to 55.9 (in 2000) ($p < 0.001$). As compared with matched intensive care unit admissions without sepsis, the excess risk of death due to septic shock was 25.7 (95% confidence interval, 24.0–27.3) and the matched odds ratio of death was 3.9 (95% confidence interval, 3.5–4.3) (Annane, 2003).

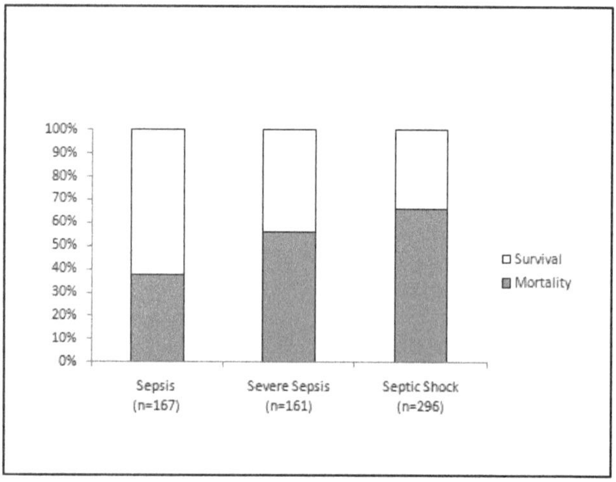

Fig. 12. Mortality rate according to sepsis diagnostic criteria.

The severity of severe sepsis and septic shock do not markedly depend on the source of infection or on its causative microorganism. On the contrary, mortality is directly related to the occurrence of organ failure in sepsis, and this relationship has remained consistent among patients of different races and sexes. However, organ failure scores may have difficulty quantifying the contribution that preexisting organ dysfunction adds to risk.

The patient's underlying comorbidities are directly related to mortality in several studies. The index of McCabe and Jackson is one of the most useful scores used in epidemiological and clinical studies to quantify underlying consitions. APACHE II, Simplified Acute Physiology Score (SAPS II) and the sequential organ failure assessments (SOFA) are prognostic scores based on bedside evaluation which are widely used to predict the prognosis of severe sepsis and septic shock.

The hospital mortality of severe sepsis is about 30% according to several studies, but this rate has been found much lower in children and previously healthy adults. Mirzanejad et al found that mortality from pneumococcal bacteremia varied from 3.2% in children to 43% in the elderly (Mirzanejad, 1996). This fact suggest attributable mortality of sepsis may be much less than the commonly observed 30% and that the mechanism by which sepsis causes death is highly dependent on individual patient factors, many of which may not be reversible by single antisepsis agents (Angus, 2001).

Patients with sepsis who had any organ failure have higher mortality. Besides, organ failure has a cumulative effect on outcomes: mortality in patients without organ failure is approximately 15 percent, whereas it reaches 70 percent in patients with three or more failing organs (classified as having severe sepsis and septic shock). The organs that failed most frequently in patients with sepsis are shown in **figure 13**.

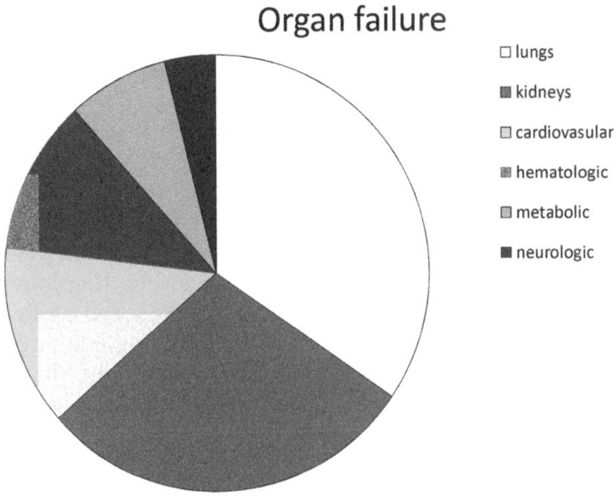

Fig. 13. Organs that fail most frequently in patients with sepsis.

Predictors of mortality in severe sepsis and septic shock in community acquired blood stream infectios are shown in **table 3**. In this study (Artero 2010) the global mortality rate was 41.9%, 44.5% in community acquired septic shock and 34.4% in severe sepsis, and by univariate analysis, age, Acute Physiology and Chronic Health Evaluation II score, at least 3 organ dysfunctions, and albumin differed significantly between survivors and nonsurvivors. Acute Physiology and Chronic Health Evaluation II (odds ratio, 1.13; 95% confidence interval, 1.06-1.21) and albumin (odds ratio, 0.34; 95% confidence interval, 0.15-0.76) were independent predictors of global mortality in logistic regression analysis.

	Total (n=112)	Hospital Survivors (n=65)	Hospital Nonsurvivors (n=47)	OR (95%CI)	P
Mean age, y	63.5	61.0	67.1	1.02 (1.00-1.05)	.047
COPD	19	7	12	2.84 (1.02-7.89)	.045
Mean APACHE II	22.0	18.7	26.5	1.16 (1.08-1.23)	<.001
≥3 organ dysfunctions	56	19	37	3.70 (2.04-6.68)	<.001
Unknown source	15	5	10	3.24(1.02-10.23)	.045
Albumin <20g/L	27	10	17	2.85 (1.11-7.33)	.026

Table 6. Predictors of mortality in severe sepsis and septic shock in community acquired blood stream infections (Adapted from Artero et al, J Crit Care 2010).

Recent antibiotic exposure has been associated with increased hospital mortality in Gram-negative bacteremia complicated by severe sepsis or septic shock (Johnson, 2011). A likely explanation for the association between hospital mortality and prior antibiotic exposure is the greater degree of antimicrobial resistance in the causative pathogen(s) of patients receiving prior antibiotics. Clinicians caring for patients with severe sepsis or septic shock should consider recent antibiotic exposure when formulating empiric antimicrobial regimens for suspected Gram-negative bacterial infection.

Boussekey et al in a five-year observational study in an ICU identified six independent mortality risk factors in septic shock: mechanical ventilation (OR = 4.97), Simplify Acute Physiology Score (SAPS) II > 60 (OR = 4.28), chronic alcoholism (OR = 3.38), age >65 years (OR = 2.65), prothrombin ratio <40% (OR = 2.37), and PaO_2/FiO_2 ratio <150 (OR = 1.91). The identification of these risk factors recovered in the multivariate analysis can easily be available on admission and allow screening immediately a group of patients with a high mortality risk in septic shock (Boussekey, 2010).

Mortality of sepsis appears to be higher in ICU-acquired sepsis than in community-acquired sepsis. Vincet et al described a direct relationship between intensive care unit mortality rates for all patients and frequency of sepsis in various European countries (Vincent, 2006).

Winters et al performed a systematic review of studies reporting long-term mortality and quality-of-life data (>3 months) in patients with severe sepsis and septic shock using defined search criteria and found that patients with sepsis showed ongoing mortality up to 2 yrs and beyond after the standard 28-day inhospital mortality end point. Patients with sepsis also had decrements in quality-of-life measures after hospital discharge (Winters, 2010).

9. Cost of care

The information on the cost of care of patients with severe sepsis and septic shock is quite scarce. The cost of care for patients with sepsis has been related to their length of stay in the intensive care unit and hospital. However, several studies have found that many patients with sepsis did not receive intensive care unit care. The length of stay for patients with severe sepsis has been reported to be twice higher than in sepsis (Brun-Buisson, 2004). The average total cost per intensive care unit day is estimated at approximately 1200 Euro for countries with a highly developed healthcare system (based on various studies conducted between 1989 and 2001 and converted at 2003 currency rates). US cost-of-illness studies focusing on direct costs per sepsis patient have yielded estimates of 34,000 Euro, whereas European studies have given lower cost estimates, ranging from 23,000 Euro to 29,000 Euro (Burchardi, 2004).

The introduction of new biotechnology products to treat patients with severe sepsis and septic shock should also be considered in cost analysis. In order to achieve the greatest benefits from these drugs they should be used in selected patients.

Indirect costs associated with severe sepsis account for 70-80% of costs and arise mainly from productivity losses due to mortality. Sepsis is an acute disease and so most studies of sepsis have been done in the hospital environment. However, other important factor related to the cost of care is the long-term sequels of sepsis, which unfortunately is not usually taken into account.

The cost of care of patients with sepsis presents notable variation among hospitals, and there is not good correlation between cost and mortality. Recently, Lagu et al in a large multicenter study analyzed data from 166,931 patients with sepsis found that hospital spending and adjusted mortality rates for patients with sepsis vary substantially, and higher hospital expenditures are not associated with better survival (Lagu, 2011).

10. Conclusion

Severe sepsis and septic shock have a significant and increasing impact on public health, and are one of the leading causes of mortality. Studies done in the last decades have shown that the incidence of these syndromes has increased over the last thirty years, with an increasing number of deaths occurring despite a decline in overall in-hospital mortality.

The definitions of sepsis syndromes established in 1992 and 2001 have contributed to improve not only epidemiological research, but also bedside diagnosis. Severe sepsis is defined as the presence of sepsis (systemic inflammatory response + probable or confirmed infection); severe sepsis defined as sepsis + acute organ dysfunction, hypoperfusion abnormality, or transient hypotension, independent of other cause than sepsis; and septic shock is defined as sepsis + hypotension persisting for more than 1 hour despite adequate fluid resuscitation. The syndromes of sepsis can be seen as a continuum of severity that starts with an infection and can progress to septic shock. However, these definitions are not good enough tools to predict outcomes.

The epidemiology of severe sepsis and septic shock is not well known mainly due to the absence of population base prospective cohort studies. Reported rates of severe sepsis from different studies ranged from 50 to 104 per 100.000 population, with an incidence of 300/100.000 in a single study from the United States (Angus, 2001). However, the incidence of severe sepsis in this last study could have been overstated due to the authors used ICD-9-CM coding for the identification of the syndromes. The prevalence of severe sepsis and septic shock in patients admitted to intensive care units is 11-30% and 6-10%, respectively. Studies using data from admissions to emergency departments and intensive care units have also found increasing rates of severe sepsis and septic shock in the last decades.

The increasing aging of the population and the increased prevalence of underlying comorbidities in developed countries are the main variables influencing the incidence of severe sepsis and septic shock. The relative risk for sepsis is thirteen times higher for patients aged 65 and above than in younger patients. *Escherichia coli* has been found to be the most frequent microorganism in patients older than 65 years, and urinary tract infection the most frequent source of infection in older population. Patients with severe sepsis and septic shock frequently have coexisting conditions, such as chronic pulmonary diseases, immune deficiency, malignancy or diabetes mellitus. McCabe classification has been widely used in epidemiological studies to assess comorbidities which predispose patients to infections and may have an additive contribution to mortality.

Black people have a higher incidence of severe sepsis and septic shock than white people, and the age of black population with these disorders is lower than the age of white people. There is no consensus about whether the worse outcomes of black people with severe sepsis and septic shock is due to genetic factors or a higher prevalence of subjacent comorbidities in black population.

Men have a higher prevalence of severe sepsis and septic shock than women. The fact that this lower rate of sepsis syndromes observed in women is present over all range of age argues against the gender differences being solely mediated through sex hormones.

Respiratory infections are the major source of severe sepsis and septic shock, which is more prevalent in men than in women, followed by intra-abdominal infections, urinary tract infections and primary bloodstream infections. Respiratory infections and abdominal infections appear to have a worse prognosis than other foci.

Gram-positive cocci have become the most common microorganisms over the past decades, taking precedence over Gram-negative bacilli. The proportion of fungi and multiresistant bacteria (multiresistant *Pseudomonas* spp, methicillin-resistant *Staphylococci* ...) has significantly increased over the last few years, which has contributed to increase the rates of inappropriate empirical antimicrobial treatment.

The mortality rates of severe sepsis and septic shock are 25 to 30% and 40 to 70%, respectively. Sepsis is the tenth leading cause of overall death in the United States and severe sepsis is the most common cause of death in noncoronary critical care units. There are several independent risk factors of mortality of severe sepsis and septic shock. Among these, the number of organ failures (commonly assessed by SOFA), the underlying comorbidities and the severity of acute illness (APACHE II) are the most constantly identified in epidemiological studies. The quality of life of survival patients of sepsis assessed after 2 years from admission to intensive care unit is markedly reduced, with more than 80% of patients reporting a problem.

The direct cost of care for patients with severe sepsis is about 30,000 Euro, with notable variations among hospitals and without good relationship between cost and mortality. The length of stay in intensive care unit and hospital are the major determinants of cost. However, 75% of the global cost is dependent of indirect cost, which is mainly caused by productivity losses due to mortality. Besides, the cost of long-term sequels is not usually included in cost-effectiveness analysis of severe sepsis and septic shock.

11. References

Angus DC, Linde-Zwirble WT; Lidicker J, Clermont G, Carcillo J,& Pinsky MR. Epidemiology of severe sepsis in the United States: Analysis of incidence, outcome, and associated costs of care. *Crit Care Med* 2001; 29 (7):1303–10.

Annane D, Aegerter P, Jars-Guincestre MC,& Guidet B. Current epidemiology of septic shock: the CUB-Rea Network. Am *J Respir Crit Care Med* 2003;168 (2):165-72.

Artero A, Zaragoza R, Camarena JJ, Sancho S, González R,& Nogueira JM. Prognostic factors of mortality in patients with community-acquired bloodstream infection with severe sepsis and septic shock. *Journal of Critical Care* 2010; 25 (2): 276–81.

Artigas A, Sicignano A, Palazzo M, Moreno S, Boulmé R, Lepage E,& Le Gall JR. Epidemiology of sepsis and infection in ICU patients from an international multicentre cohort study. *Intensive Care Med* 2002; 28 (4):108-21.

Bateman BT, Schmidt U, Berman MF,& Bittner EA. Temporal Trends in the Epidemiology of Severe Postoperative Sepsis after Elective Surgery. *Anesthesiology* 2010; 112 (4):917-25.

Bernard GR, Vincent JL, Laterre PF, LaRosa SP, Dhainaut JF, Lopez-Rodriguez A, Steingrub JS, Garber GE, Helterbrand JD, Ely EW, Fisher CJ Jr,& Recombinant human protein C Worldwide Evaluation in Severe Sepsis (PROWESS) study group. Efficacy and safety of recombinant human activated protein C for severe sepsis. *N Engl J Med* 2001; 344 (10):699-709.

Bone RC, Balk RA, Cerra FB, Dellinger RP, Fein AM, Knaus WA, Schein RM,& Sibbald WJ. Definitions for sepsis and organ failure and guidelines for the use of innovative therapies in sepsis. *Chest* 1992; 101 (6):1644-55.

Boussekey N, Cantrel J, Dorchin Debrabant L, Langlois J, Devos P, Meybeck A, Chiche A, Georges H, Leroy O. Epidemiology, prognosis, and evolution of management of septic shock in a French intensive care unit: a five years survey. *Crit Care Res Pract* 2010; 2010:436427. Epub 2010 Jun 17

Brun-Buison C, Meshaka P, Pinton P,& Vallet B. EPISEPSIS: a reappraisal of the epidemiology and outcome of severe sepsis in French intensive care units. *Intensive Care Med* 2004; 30 (4):580-588.

Brun-Buisson C. (2009) Impact of Sepsis on Public Health, In:. *Sepsis handbook.* Dellinger P, Carlet J, pp. 8-17, Editons Biomerieux, Marcy l'Etoile.

Burchardi H,& Schneider H. Economic aspects of severe sepsis: a review of intensive care unit costs, cost of illness and cost effectiveness of therapy. *Pharmacoeconomics* 2004; 22 (12):793-813.

Centers for Disease Control. Increase in national hospital discharge survey rates for septicemia — United States, 1979–1987. *JAMA* 1990; 263 (7):937–38

Dellinger RP, Levy MM, Carlet JM Bion J, Parker MM, Jaeschke R, Reinhart K, Angus DC, Brun-Buisson C, Beale R, Calandra T, Dhainaut JF, Gerlach H, Harvey M, Marini JJ, Marshall J, Ranieri M, Ramsay G, Sevransky J, Thompson BT, Townsend S, Vender JS, Zimmerman JL, Vincent JL; International Surviving Sepsis Campaign Guidelines Committee; American Association of Critical-Care Nurses; American College of Chest Physicians; American College of Emergency Physicians; Canadian Critical Care Society; European Society of Clinical Microbiology and Infectious Diseases; European Society of Intensive Care Medicine; European Respiratory Society; International Sepsis Forum; Japanese Association for Acute Medicine; Japanese Society of Intensive Care Medicine; Society of Critical Care Medicine; Society of Hospital Medicine; Surgical Infection Society;& World Federation of Societies of Intensive and Critical Care Medicine. International guidelines for management of severe sepsis and septic shock: 2008. Crit Care Med 2008; 36 (1):296-327.

Diekema DJ, Pfaller MA, Jones RN,& SENTRY Participants Group.. Age-related trends in pathogen frequency and antimicrobial susceptibility of bloodstream isolates in North America: SENTRY Antimicrobial Surveillance Program, 1997–2000. *Int J Antimicrob Agents* 2002; 20 (6): 412–418.

Dombrovskiy VY, Martin AA, Sunderram J, Paz HL: Rapid increase in hospitalization and mortality rates for severe sepsis in the United States: A trend analysis from 1993 to 2003. *Crit Care Med* 2007; 35 (5):1244 -1250.

Girard TD, Ely E W, Bacteremia and Sepsis in Older Adults. Clin Geriatr Med 2007; 23 (3): 633–647.

Martin GS, Mannino DM, Eaton S, Moss M. The epidemiology of sepsis in the United States from 1979 through 2000. *N Engl J Med* 2003; 348 (16):1546-1554.

Hodgkin KE, Moss M. The epidemiology of sepsis. *Curr Pharm Des* 2008; 14 (19):1833-1839.

Hoyert DL, Arias E, Smith BL, Murphy SL, Kochanek KD. Deaths: final data for 1999. *Natl Vital Stat Rep* 2001; 49 (8):1–113.

Iwashyna TJ, Ely EW, Smith DM, Langa KM. Long-term cognitive impairment and functional disability among survivors of severe sepsis. *JAMA* 27 2010; 304 (16):1787-1794.

Jagodič KH, Jagodič K, Podbregar M. Long-term outcome and quality of life of patients treated in surgical intensive care: a comparison between sepsis and trauma. *Crit Care* 2006; 10 (5): R134.

Johnson MT, Reichley R, Hoppe-Bauer J. Impact of previous antibiotic therapy on outcome of Gram-negative severe sepsis. *Crit Care Med* 2011; 39 (8):1859 -1865.

Kumar A, Zarychanski R, Light B, Parrillo J, Maki D, Simon D, Laporta D, Lapinsky S, Ellis P, Mirzanejad Y, Martinka G, Keenan S, Wood G, Arabi Y, Feinstein D, Kumar A, Dodek P, Kravetsky L, Doucette S,& Cooperative Antimicrobial Therapy of Septic Shock (CATSS) Database Research Group. Early combination antibiotic therapy yields improved survival compared with monotherapy in septic shock: a propensity-matched analysis. *Crit Care Med.* 2010; 38 (9):1773-1785.

Lagu T, Rothberg MB, Nathanson BH, Pekow PS, Steingrub JS,& Lindenauer PK. The relationship between hospital spending and mortality in patients with sepsis. *Arch Intern Med* 2011 28; 171 (4):292-299.

Levy MM, Fink MP, Marshall JC, Abraham E, Angus D, Cook D, Cohen J, Opal SM, Vincent JL, Ramsay G,& SCCM/ESICM/ACCP/ATS/SIS. 2001SCCM/ESICM/ACCP/ATS/SIS International Sepsis Definitions Conference. *Crit Care Med* 2003; 31 (4):1250–1256.

Martin GS, Mannino DM, Moss M. The effect of age on the development and outcome of adult sepsis. *Crit Care Med* 2006; 34 (1): 15-21.

Mayr FB, Yende S, Linde-Zwirble WT, Peck-Palmer OM, Barnato AE, Weissfeld LA, Angus DC. Infection Rate and Acute Organ Dysfunction Risk as Explanations for Racial Differences in Severe Sepsis. *JAMA*. 2010; 303 (24):2495-503.

Mirzanejad Y, Roman S, Talbot J, Nicolle L. Pneumococcal bacteremia in two tertiary care hospitals in Winnipeg, Canada. Pneumococcal Bacteremia Study Group. *Chest* 1996; 109 (1):173-178.

Moss M. Epidemiology of Sepsis: Race, Sex, and Chronic Alcohol Abuse. *Clin Infect Dis* 2005; 41 (Suppl 7):S490-S497.

Salvo I, de Cian W, Musicco M, Langer M, Piadena R, Wolfler A, Montani C, Magni E. The Italian SEPSIS study: preliminary results on the incidence and evolution of SIRS, sepsis, severe sepsis, and septic shock. *Intensive Care Med* 1995; 21 (Suppl 2):S244-S249.

Vesteinsdottir E, Karason S, Sigurdsson SE, Gottfredsson M, Sigurdsson GH. Severe sepsis and septic shock: a prospective population-based study in Icelandic intensive care units. *Acta Anaesthesiol Scand* 2011; 55 (6):722-31. doi: 10.1111/j.1399-6576.2011.02437.x. Epub 2011 Apr 11.

Vincent JL, Sakr Y, Sprung CL, Ranieri VM, Reinhart K, Gerlach H, Moreno R, Carlet J, Le Gall JR, Payen D,& Sepsis Occurrence in Acutely Ill Patients Investigators. Sepsis in European intensive care units: results of the SOAP study. *Crit Care Med*. 2006; 34 (2):344-353.

Wang HE, Shapiro NI, Angus DC, Yealy DM. National estimates of severe sepsis in United States emergency departments. *Crit Care Med*. 2007; 35 (8):1928-36.

Zaragoza R, Artero A, Camarena JJ, Sancho S, González R, Nogueira JM. The influence of inadequate empirical antimicrobial treatment on patients with bloodstream infections in an intensive care unit. *Clin Microbiol Infect* 2003; 9 (5):1-7.

Part 2

Etiology

2

Transfusion-Associated Bacterial Sepsis

Jolanta Korsak
Military Institute of Medicine
Poland

1. Introduction

Transfusion-associated bacterial sepsis (TABS) is caused by bacteria present in blood components. It is one of the earliest recognized adverse transfusion-associated reactions. Blood components most often become contaminated while blood is being collected from a donor; more seldom in the case of asymptomatic bacteremia or erroneous blood processing procedures (1). Although the risk for transfusion-associated bacterial sepsis has diminished considerably since the introduction of new methods of bacteria detection and of increasingly better means of skin disinfection, reappearing reports about severe or fatal reactions after contaminated blood component transfusions prove that the problem is still very serious. Most often bacterial contamination affects red blood cell concentrates and platelet concentrates. There have been cases reported of bacterially contaminated plasma or cryoprecipitate, although bacteria do not proliferate in these components when they are stored (1,2). Of note, bacterial sepsis is an adverse reaction not only after allogenic transfusions but also after autologous ones.

Bacteria are very rarely transmitted during blood component transfusion, but if they are, they usually cause severe, life-threatening adverse reactions, with the mortality rate of 20 - 30%. In USA, bacteria transmission during transfusion is the second (just after "administrative error") most common cause of fatal transfusion-associated reactions. It is estimated that every year 100 - 150 patients undergoing blood component transfusion die because of that (1). This number is probably underestimated. There are a few causes of this situation. Tests which can confirm or exclude the infectious background of adverse reactions occurring during or right after transfusion are not always performed. Besides, the organism's response to infection may be misinterpreted as a manifestation of the underlying disease or another non-infectious transfusion-associated reaction. That is why the estimated prevalence of fatal adverse reactions may be overestimated because the adverse reactions that have the most severe course are predominantly reported to the relevant registering centers.

The risk for transfusion-associated bacterial sepsis results from the nature of pathogens themselves and from determinants connected with blood donors and recipients.

From the transfusiology point of view, the characteristic features of infectious agents include their biology, the course of infection, the degree of infectivity, and how harmful they are for the recipient if transfusion-associated bacterial infection occurs. The crucial issues are whether:

- An infectious agent is present in blood in the course of infection, how long it has been there, at what concentration;

- An infectious agent is transmitted via transfusion. Can its transfusion infectiveness be limited and how?
- In a particular population, an infectious agent is highly prevalent or not. Consequently, how many recipients are infected with it via other ways than blood component transfusions? How prevalent this infection is among donors and whether identifying uninfected donors is possible and feasible.
- An infectious agent causes a severe disease if it is transmitted with blood. Is the disease potentially lethal? What are the possibilities of treating the recipient who has acquired the disease?

The infectious agents important from the transfusiology point of view are those which are asymptomatic enough so that a donor would not report them before donation.

Infectious agents can be present only in some blood components. There are bacteria that are observed in the free form in plasma. An important parameter is also how infectious agents behave in the conditions at which blood is stored. These conditions differ for various blood components. The whole blood, its cellular components, plasma or plasma-derived preparations are stored in different forms, e.g. liquid or frozen at -25°C to +24°C. Most bacteria are able to proliferate in the components stored. There are also such that are very sensitive and quickly die once they are outside the host's organism. They include *Treponema pallidum*, which cannot survive longer than 72 hours at +4°C. The fact that bacteria have been transmitted with blood does not necessarily mean that the recipient will fall ill. To a large extent, it depends on the amount of the infectious agent, i.e. how much of the blood component has been transfused and how big concentration of the pathogen was in the component. Whether a recipient will fall ill depends on the recipient's immune condition and the possibility to control the infection (3,4,). Table 1 itemizes what promotes transfusion-associated bacterial sepsis development.

• Volume of blood component transfused
• Bacteria concentration in blood component
• Immune and general conditions of recipient
• Extent of surgery, type of invasive diagnostic procedures
• Intensity of recipient monitoring
• Mode of treatment (antibiotics)

Table 1. Parameters promoting sepsis development following transfusion of bacteria contaminated blood components (5).

2. Causes of transfusion-associated bacterial sepsis

The sources of bacterial infections may be endogenous or exogenous. Bacteremia in a donor may be an endogenous source of blood sample contamination. Chronic bacteremia is observed in syphilis. Being a carrier of *Borrelia burgdorferi*, responsible for borreliosis, a tick-derived disease, or *Brucella abortus*, may also be associated with risk. Bacteremia accompanying alimentary tract infections and alimentary toxicosis in donors is caused by such bacteria as *Salmonella* but is very rare. In order to exclude them, it is important to take a comprehensive history of the donor.

Another cause of bacterial contamination of the blood collected may be by bacteria present on the donor's skin when a needle is inserted into a vein or contamination during blood collection or processing of blood components.

The risk an infection is transmitted with a blood component depends mainly on the conditions and time a component has been stored before it is transfused to a patient. It is much higher when platelet concentrates are used than in the case of red blood cell concentrates, mainly due to the storage temperature. The risk exists when it is stored in a temperature which is suitable for bacterial survival and proliferation. Platelets are the component that is stored in the conditions which promote bacterial proliferation (room temperature). Red blood cells, stored at +4°C, are much less dangerous, and in the case of plasma or cryoprecipitate transfusion, the risk for bacterial complications is almost nil. Plasma is frozen, after it is processed at -30°C or lower, which practically eliminates the possibility for bacteria to survive. Table 2 presents possible causes of blood component bacterial contamination.

- Asymptomatic bacteremia in donor
- Inadequate disinfection of venopuncture site
- Donor's skin fragment placed in blood container (via needle)
- Contaminated blood sampling kit or anticoagulant
  - Faulty sterilization
  - Wrong storing

Table 2. Causes of bacterial contamination of blood components

Bacterial proliferation in a blood sample is limited considerably by antibacterial features of blood itself. Bacteria are destroyed by the complement and phagocytized by blood leukocytes. The risk of donor-derived infection is lower after the leukocytes which have phagocytized bacteria in blood have been removed.

The severity of adverse transfusion-associated bacterial reactions which may occur in a recipient after a contaminated blood component has been transfused depends on many factors, which are presented in Table 3.

- Number of bacteria (dose)
- Types of bacteria (Gram-positive, Gram-negative)
- Virulence of bacteria – production of exotoxins and endotoxins
- Recipient's general condition (immune system functioning, underlying disease)
- Recipient undergoing antibiotic therapy

Table 3. Factors influencing the severity of transfusion-associated adverse infectious reactions in recipients

Certain regularity is the fact that the risk for transfusion-associated septic reactions is directly proportional to the duration and temperature at which blood and its components are stored. Some bacteria die or cannot proliferate in the temperature at which blood components are stored. Yet such cryophilic bacteria as *Yersinia enterocolitica* survive in red blood concentrates because low temperatures do not act destructively on them. Platelet concentrates, which are stored in room temperature, are a more friendly environment for bacteria to survive and proliferate although some, more sensitive ones, die at 20 - 24°C. Most Gram-positive and Gram-negative bacteria are able to survive and proliferate in platelet concentrates.

In most reported cases of transfusion-associated bacterial sepsis, the sources of blood component contaminations were not identified. Yet the type of bacteria responsible for the complications enabled the probable cause of sepsis and hypothetical source of pathogenic bacteria to be established. For example, coagulase-negative *Staphylococci* or *Corynebacteria* in platelet concentrates suggest the epidermal origin, but *Streptococcus viridans* in blood most likely originates from a donor undergoing dentistry procedures.

2.1 Bacterial infections transmitted with red blood cell concentrates

Red blood cell concentrate is a blood component, which is transfused most frequently. It does not contain only red blood cells but also various amounts of platelets and leukocytes. Transfusion-associated bacterial sepsis resulting from transfusing a bacterially contaminated red blood cell concentrate is rather uncommon. Different reports estimate its rate at 1:250,000 transfusions; the relevant sepsis mortality rate ranges 58 - 70% (5). During nine years, FDA registered 25 fatalities due to transfusion of contaminated red blood cell concentrate (6). Thus, the mortality risk is estimated at 13:1,000,000 red blood cell concentrate transfusions (7). On the other hand, the Dana Farber Cancer Institute studies have found the infection prevalence at 1:38,000 transfused red blood cell concentrate units (8,9).

The bacterium most commonly responsible for sepsis associated with red blood cell concentrate transfusion is *Yersinia enterocolitica*. The prevalence of sepsis associated with *Y. enterocolitica* transmitted with blood varies. In New Zealand, it is 1:65,000 transfusions, with the sepsis fatality rate estimated at 1:104,000 transfused red blood cell concentrate units (4). In USA, 20 cases were reported of *Yersinia* being transmitted with blood components in 1987 - 1996. Twelve of them died before the 37th day following the transfusion of contaminated red blood cell concentrate. The mean time between transfusion and recipient's death is 25 hours (10). *Yersinia enterocolitica* is a Gram-negative bacterium, responsible for diarrheal diseases; it may also temporarily colonize the alimentary tract of asymptomatic people. The feature characteristic of *Yersinia* bacteria is their ability to survive and proliferate in temperatures in which red blood cell concentrates are stored, i.e. +2 - +6 °C. For their own metabolism they also use citrate as the source of carbon, which is an additional factor conducive for bacterial proliferation. Citrate compounds are included in commonly used anticoagulants. *Yersinia* bacteria present in a blood component are a typical example of endogenous contamination resulting from asymptomatic donor's bacteremia. A study has shown that around 2/3 of donors, in whom *Yersinia enterocolitica* was detected, had complained of gastrointestinal disorders in the time preceding blood donation. Most often these ailments had a mild course (9,11,12,13,14). *Yersinia* may remain in the circulation, inside leukocytes, even for a few days after intestinal complaints subside. This bacterium is also resistant to the action of complement components and to phagocytosis due to the presence of Yersinia outer proteins (Yops) (15,16).

The likelihood of transmitting bacteria via red blood cell transfusion is directly associated with the duration of their storing. Tests of red blood cell concentrates that had been contaminated with *Yersinia* showed that in the 38th day after blood donation, the number of bacteria reached 10^8 - 10^9 CFU/ml. Between the 21st and 34th days, bacteria very quickly proliferated and released endotoxin, whose concentration reached around 315 μg/ml (17).

Except for *Yersinia enterocolitica,* the bacteria which may contaminate red blood cell concentrates and potentially cause an endotoxic shock, are *Pseudomonas* spp., *Serratia* spp., *Enterobacter* spp., *Campylobacter* spp. and *Escherichia coli* (15).
Pseudomonades are Gram-negative bacteria commonly found in water and soil. They can proliferate in temperature 4°C. They often contribute to red blood cell concentrate contamination during concentrate preparation (18). *Serratia marcescens* was a causative factor in transfusion-associated sepsis reported in Denmark and Sweden, where bacterially contaminated containers were used at blood donations (19).
Serratia is also a Gram-negative bacterium, which proliferates easily in poor environment at +4 - +22°C. The bacteria were isolated from both red blood cell concentrates and platelets concentrates. Transmitting *Serratia,* especially *Serratia liquefaciens,* causes transfusion-associate sepsis, most often fatal (1,20).
A prospective analysis of bacterial cultures from whole blood and red blood cell concentrates has shown that bacterial contamination is much more common in blood components, i.e. 2 - 4 per 4,000 units. The bacteria most often cultured were *Staphylococcus* and *Propionibacterium* spp. They very rarely cause sepsis in recipients because they do not proliferate at +2 - +6 °C, and red blood cells are stored just at this temperature range. Table 4 shows bacteria found in red blood cell concentrates.

Blood component	Bacteria	Prevalence of bacteria detected that caused complications
Red blood cell concentrate	*Yersinia enterocolitica*	51.0%
	Pseudomonas fluorescens	26.5%
	Pseudomonas putida	4.1%
	Treponema pallidum	4.1%
	Other bacteria	14.3%

Table 4. Bacteria detected in red blood cell concentrates

There have been also two fatal cases of transfusion-associated sepsis described caused by *Pantoeae agglomerans,* which used to be known as *Enterobacter agglomerans* (21). That bacterium possesses plasmid-associated factors, which make it resistant to phagocytosis (22,23).
Autologous blood is also a source of severe transfusion-associated sepsis. There are cases reported in the literature describing transmitting *Y.enterocolitica* infection following autologous transfusion (12,23). In Japanese studies, a common bacterium contaminating blood from autologous transfusions was coagulase-negative *Staphylococcus* (24,25).

2.2 Bacterial infections transmitted by contaminated platelet concentrate

The risk for being infected with bacteria in transfused platelets is 50 to 250 times higher than that associated with red blood cell transfusions (26).
In platelet concentrate transfusion-associated sepsis, bacteria belonging to the donor's skin flora are the main infectious factor. Thus, they are typical exogenous infections resulting from badly disinfected skin in the site of needle insertion. The bacteria most commonly contaminating platelet concentrates are *Staphylococcus epidermidis,* which constitutes over 50% of all bacteria detected and *Bacillus cereus,* which belong to the physiological skin flora (27,28). These bacteria do not proliferate at 0°C, but are able to proliferate in the temperature

at which platelets are stored, i.e. 20 - 24°C. If the course of the infection associated with platelet transfusion is rapid, mainly Gram-negative bacteria are to blame. There have been cases reported of fatal transfusion-associated sepsis caused by *Staphylococcus aureus* and *Clostridium perfringens*. The source of *Clostridium difficile* was a donor, who frequently changed nappies of his newborn baby. Platelet concentrates can also contain other *cocci*, *Corynebacterium pseudodiphtheriticum*, also Gram-negative fermentative bacteria of the *Pseudomonas* genus. Recently, *Listeria monocytogenes* was isolated from an apheresis platelet concentrate (29). Although there have been no cases reported of isolating *Listeria monocytogenes* from other blood components, it must be remembered that iron, which is present in blood, e.g. in red blood cells, is conductive to the growth and virulence of this bacterium T(29).

Most bacteria are able to proliferate at 20°C - 24°C, but different bacteria have different growth dynamicity. In the case of *S.aureus* and *Pseudomonas*, after the first two days they start proliferating very quickly, whereas *Enterococcus faecalis* typically grows slowly and steadily. Transfusion-associated sepsis has been reported following transfusing platelet concentrates contaminated with Gram-positive bacteria (30).

Sepsis caused by transfusing bacterially contaminated platelet concentrates is most common. Platelets are stored at room temperature and are a perfect medium for bacterial proliferation. The prevalence of symptomatic platelet transfusion-associated infections is 1:5,000 in the case of pooled concentrates, and the relevant mortality rate ranges from 1:70,000 to 1:100,000 transfusions (31,32). Table 5 shows bacteria most often detected in platelet concentrates.

Blood component	Bacteria	Prevalence of detected bacteria that caused complications
Platelet concentrate	*Staphylococcus epidermidis*	25 %
	Salmonella choleraesuis	13.5 %
	Serratia marcescens	9.6 %
	Staphylococcus aureus	9.6 %
	Bacillus cereus	3.8 %
	Streptococcus viridans	5.8 %
	Other bacteria	36.5 %

Table 5. Bacteria and their prevalence in platelet concentrates

Transfusion-associated bacterial sepsis usually manifests immediately after or still during transfusion. There have been seven cases reported of sepsis caused by *Salmonella* in platelet concentrate recipients, which manifested 5 - 12 days after transfusion (33). All the platelet units had been collected from the same donor who was later diagnosed with chronic ostitis.

Bacteria contaminating blood components can be neutralized by such bacteriostatic factors as complement and phagocytosing cells. Yet, for many bacterial types, a concentration as small as 1 CFU/ml may be sufficient to proliferate (34). After an initial 2 - 3 day latency phase, bacteria rapidly proliferate to reach a concentration of 10^8 - 10^9 CFU/ml in the 2nd - 5th day of storing.

Haemovigilance studies carried out in many countries focus on severe adverse transfusion-associated reactions caused by bacteria. Table 6 presents a summing-up of these studies.

Study	Time of study	Number of cases of blood component contamination	Kind of blood component	Number of deaths from transfusion-associated sepsis
SHOT	1996-1998	4	1 red blood cell concentrate 3 platelet concentrates	0 1
French Hemovigilance	1994-1999	185	113 red blood cell concentrates 89 platelet concentrates	8 10
Bacthem	1996-1998	41	25 red blood cell concentrates 16 platelet concentrates	6 2
BaCon	1998-2000	34	5 red blood cell concentrates 29 platelet concentrates	3 6

Table 6. Findings of studies on bacterial contamination of blood components (35)

The UK Serious Hazards of Transfusion (SHOT) study collects and analyzes all cases of transfusion-associated adverse reactions. In 1996 - 1998, there were 366 cases in all of adverse reactions registered within SHOT, four of which were transmitted by transfusing bacterial infection (36). Transfusion-associated sepsis developed after transfusing 1 unit of red blood cell concentrate contaminated with *Serratia liquefaciens* and three units of platelet concentrate which were contaminated with *Escherichia coli, Bacillus cereus* and *Staphylococcus aureus*. Transfusion-associated sepsis caused by *S.aureus* resulted in the patient's death (36). In the French Hemovigilance Study carried out in 1994 - 1999, there were 730 transfusion-associated bacterial infection events, out of which 185 were qualified in the end (89 following red blood cell concentrate transfusions and 113 after platelet concentrate transfusions) (37). Eighteen recipients died after developing transfusion-associated bacterial sepsis. The risk for transfusion-associated bacterial reactions was estimated at 12.6:1,000,000 blood component units. Bacteria isolated from red blood cell concentrates were Gram-positive *cocci* (58%), mainly *Staphylococcus* spp and *Streptococcus* spp, and Gram-negative bacteria found in 32% of units. The both types of bacteria were found in 10% of cases. In platelet concentrates, Gram-negative bacteria were found in 36% of units, Gram-positive *cocci* in 42%, and other bacteria in 22% (37). Another French study (Bacthem) focused on years 1996 - 1998. During that time, there were 41 transfusion-associated cases analyzed. 25 cases following transfusing red blood cell concentrates (4 deaths) and 16 cases following transfusing platelet concentrates (2 deaths). The bacteria contaminating the red blood cell concentrates in that study were mainly Gram-negative (52%) in contrast to 37% detected in the platelet concentrates. The risk for transfusion-associated sepsis was three times higher when platelet concentrates were transfused and 12 times higher when transfusing pooled platelet concentrates. Moreover, the risk for transfusion-associated bacterial sepsis was

higher when platelets had been stored longer than 1 day, and red blood cells for longer than eight days (38). One of the conclusions drawn from the study was that there is a strict correlation between the kind of blood component, duration of storing it and the risk for transfusion-associated bacterial sepsis (38).
The American BaCon Study assessed the prevalence of transfusion-associated bacterial adverse reactions, kinds of bacterial contamination of blood components and risk factors for transfusion-associated bacterial sepsis occurrence. The study was conducted in 1998 - 2000 (7). In that time, 34 cases of bacterial adverse reactions were assessed, nine of which were fatal. As the cause of transfusion-associated sepsis, the following bacteria were identified - Gram-positive: *Staphylococcus epidermis* (8 cases), *S.aureus* (4 cases), and Gram-negative: *Escherichia coli* (5 cases) and five cases where *Serratia* were identified (3 - *S.marcescens*, 2 - *S.liquefasciens*) (7). The course of transfusion-associated bacterial sepsis was more rapid in patients who had been transfused blood components contaminated with Gram-negative bacteria than in those in whom the component transfused was contaminated with Gram-positive bacteria. The researchers showed that transfusion-associated bacterial sepsis was developed five times more often after pooled platelet concentrates were transfused than after transfusing platelets from aphaeresis. In the BaCon study, there were 4 deaths resultant from sepsis following transfusion of aphaeresis platelet concentrates, i.e from one donor, and two deaths after transfusing pooled platelet concentrates (7,39).

3. Sources of blood components bacterial contamination

The most probable sources of blood component bacterial contamination are donor's bacteremia, blood collection and processing procedures. Table 7 presents possible sources of bacterial contamination.

Contamination source	Contamination mechanism
Blood donor	Latent bacteremia Respiratory system flora Nasopharyngeal flora
Blood collection procedures	Normal skin flora Pathological, transient skin flora Practice of and equipment for blood collection
Blood processing procedures	Contaminated containers Open systems Infected enriching fluids

Table 7. Sources and mechanisms of bacterial contamination of blood components

Blood donors suffering from asymptomatic bacteremia or recovering from bacterial infections are a source of blood component bacterial contamination. *Yersinia enterocolitica*, a Gram-negative bacterium, can cause intestinitis with diarrhea of various intensity, increased temperature and abdominal pain. Yet, the infection is asymptomatic in most cases. Thus, such donors are a potential source of blood component contamination (40,41). Transfusion associated bacterial sepsis may be caused by other intestinal pathogens, such as *Campylobacter jejuni* and *Salmonella Heidelberg*, which induce donor's bacteremia (18). They damage the intestinal mucosa and move into blood. In some people, only after they donated blood were internal latent foci of infection detected. They were asymptomatic, yet they caused low-level bacteremia. There have been cases reported of sepsis after transfusing concentrate of platelets taken from donors who were during the incubation of bacterial infections of the respiratory tract and endocarditis (41). A donor can develop a short-time bacteremia after dentistry procedures. *Staphylococcus aureus* was detected in a platelet concentrate collected from a donor two hours after his tooth was treated conservatively (18). *Staphylococcus aureus* is not the only bacterium that can be the source of blood component contamination. There have been two cases reported where bacterial toxins were detected in the bags after transfused platelet concentrates. Recipients of this component developed manifestations of septic shock 15 and 20 minutes after their respective transfusions were begun (42).

The procedures of collecting blood and its components are a source of platelet concentrate contamination mainly. Most bacteria detected in laboratory tests and reported as the cause of transfusion-associated sepsis are those which constitute the normal skin flora or those which transiently are present at the venopuncture site. An example of blood components being contaminated with bacteria that happened to be in the venopuncture site is a case of sepsis caused by *Salmonella enterica*. During an epidemiological investigation, it was found that the bacteria had originated form a platelet donor who had a snake. The bacteria were cultured from the recipient's blood, form the bag where the blood component had been stored and the snake's excrements, but *Salmonella enterica* was not cultured in the donor's blood. The bacteria, most probably, was on the donor's skin while platelet concentrate was collected by apheresis (43).

There are known cases of severe transfusion-associated bacterial sepsis caused by red blood cell concentrates contaminated with *Pseudomonas fluorescens* originating from swabs used as cooling compresses on the venopuncture site in donors with low pain tolerance (44).

Yet most blood components become contaminated because the venopuncture site has been disinfected insufficiently or because disinfectants were contaminated. There has been a case reported of red blood cell concentrate being contaminated with *Burkholderia cepacia*, because the chlorhexidine used for disinfecting the venopuncture was contaminated with this bacterium (45).

Since disposable, sterile closed plastic systems for blood collection, processing and storage were introduced, there have been very uncommon situations when lack of adequate sterilization of a blood collection kit or contamination during blood processing resulted in contaminating a blood component. A practically invisible crack in a bag for blood or blood components can result in their contamination (10).

4. Clinical picture

Diagnosing transfusion-associated bacterial sepsis is difficult when the diagnosis is to be based only on clinical manifestations. That is why the criteria to diagnose this complication have been worked out and are presented in Table 8 (4).

Transfusion-associated bacterial sepsis always manifests clinically in a very dramatic manner. The first symptoms (fever, shivering), which confirm the presence of bacteria in the recipient's circulation usually appear within 2 hours following the start of the transfusion. The symptoms to follow are blood pressure drop, nausea, vomiting, diarrhea, and shock. Other symptoms, such as dyspnea or bleeding, result from bacteria inducing endotoxins. Delayed manifestations, which appear later than one day after transfusion, have been reported following transfusing bacterially contaminated platelet concentrates (46). Transfusion-associated bacterial sepsis diagnosed too late is the most common cause of death. Early symptoms of sepsis may be diagnosed as non-infectious transfusion-associated adverse reactions, especially in neoplastic disease patients under immunosuppression, who have undergone numerous blood component transfusions.

Within around 90 minutes after transfusion was started, one of the following symptoms appears: 1. Fever ≥39°C or increase in body temperature by 2°C 2. Shivering 3. Tachycardia (≥120 beats per minute or increase by ≥40 bpm) 4. Changes in systolic pressure (increase by ≥30 mmHg or decrease in comparison to baseline values)

Table 8. Criteria to diagnose transfusion-associated bacterial sepsis

The initial number of bacteria that is transfused in contaminated blood components is not large; it rarely exceeds 10 CFU/ml. That is why transfusing blood or its components within the first two days following donation is associated with a minimal risk for infectious transfusion-associated complications. Yet, a unique group of recipients constitute patients under immunosuppression, for whom even a very small number of bacteria are very dangerous. In most transfusion-associated bacterial reactions, the level of contamination in containers was at 10^6 - 10^8 CFU/ml. Such levels were found in platelet concentrates stored for 3 - 5 days, and red blood cell concentrates stored for at least three weeks.

Severe sepsis with a rapid disease course is mostly caused by Gram-negative bacteria releasing an endotoxin which activates the immune system very strongly. Such bacteria are predominantly found in contaminated red blood cell concentrates and claim a very high mortality rate.

Bacterial endotoxins - lipopolysaccharide (LPS) - are in the Gram-negative bacterial cellular wall and penetrate the environment after a bacterium disintegrates, and in a small amount, when a bacterium proliferates because then its cellular wall becomes less dense. They stimulate macrophages to secrete such inflammatory cytokines as TNFα, IL-1ß, IL-6, IL-8, which are responsible for numerous systemic reactions associated with septic shock. Patients who had been transfused red blood cell concentrate contaminated with Gram-negative bacteria had high plasma concentrations of these cytokines. Septic shock observed in recipients of contaminated concentrates must have resulted mainly from a massive release of cytokines rather than from the bacterial proliferation in the recipient's organism (47).

Bacterial strains responsible for severe transfusion-associated reactions may have certain features, such as resistance to phagocytosis or ability to activate complement, which enable them to proliferate in blood components. Asymptomatic, Gram-negative bacteremia in a blood donor is a phenomenon that accompanies alimentary tract infections and alimentary toxicosis. In the case of intestinal motility disorders, bacteria that are present on the surface of mucosa are able to penetrate into deeper tissue and blood. Bacteremia resultant from translocation usually does not pose a serious threat to donors whose immune system functions normally. Bacteria are eliminated from the circulation and sepsis does not develop. On the other hand, the consequences of transfusing a bacterially contaminated blood component may be very severe when the number of bacteria is very large or the recipient is a patient with low immunity.

The mortality rate is high and depends on the blood component, kind and amount of contaminating bacteria and patient's clinical condition (including comorbidities). Other factors affecting the mortality rate are the ability to respond adequately to the infection and the kind of diagnostic and therapeutic procedures. Studies show that sepsis caused by transfusing contaminated red blood cell concentrates is particularly lethal (48). The factors that primarily negatively affect the defense against infections include chronic pulmonary diseases, neutropenia, immunosuppression, senility, and poor nutrition.

5. Differentiating

Differential diagnosis of transfusion-associated bacterial sepsis includes hemolytic reactions, febrile non-hemolytic reactions, TRALI, and sepsis unassociated with blood component transfusion. The diagnosis is based on culturing patient's blood and a unit of the component transfused. The bacterial background of the transfusion-associated reaction is confirmed when the same bacterium is cultured from a container with the blood component and from patient's blood. The similarity of the bacteria cultured from both sources is based on the bacterial DNA structure established with one of the methods for genetic typing (most often it is pulsed field gel electrophoresis - PFGE).

6. Treating transfusion-associated bacterial sepsis

The basic principles in treating transfusion-associated bacterial sepsis include early clinical suspicion, rigorous implementation of diagnostic procedures, appropriate causal therapy, inhibiting generalized inflammatory reactions predisposing to complications.
When a fast growing fever appears, the transfusion should be discontinued, the container with the accompanying drains secured, and a blood sample taken from the patient so that microbiological tests can be done. The blood sample for culturing should be taken from another vein than the one into which the blood component has been transfused.
Before microbiological tests findings are available, empiric therapy should be introduced. Antibiotic therapy should include such broad spectrum antibiotics as ß-lactams and aminoglycosides. When bacterially contaminated red blood cell concentrate transfusion-associated sepsis is suspected, an antibiotic with anti-*Pseudomonas* activity should be introduced. Then targeted antibiotic therapy should be started. When a septic shock occurs, shock-controlling procedures should include monitoring hemodynamics, respiratory efficiency and kidney function. In fluid resuscitation, crystalloids and natural or artificial colloid solutions are used. The first transfusion consists of 500 - 1000 ml of crystalloids or 300 - 500 ml of colloids during 30 minutes, and is repeated depending on such parameters as blood pressure, diuresis, and possibly volume overload.

7. Prevention

There are no absolutely reliable methods which can enable bacterial contamination of blood components to be detected effectively before transfusion. The methods used at present include four categories: (1) avoiding bacterial infections, (2) bacteriological testing of blood components, (3) inhibiting bacterial growth, and (4) techniques of pathogen inactivation.
A method to prevent platelet transfusion-associated bacterial sepsis may be using platelets from one donor collected by apheresis instead of pooled. The findings of a 12-year study,

where adverse septic reactions after platelet transfusions were analyzed, showed that an increase in transfusing apheresis platelet concentrates was accompanied by a decrease in such reactions (39). Other studies have confirmed these observations pointing to the fact that bacterial contamination of pooled red blood cell concentrates is higher than in those collected from one donor (40). Yet, the findings of another paper described more bacterial contaminations in apheresis concentrates (49).

7.1 Lowering the risk of donor's asymptomatic bacteremia

7.1.1 Avoiding bacterial infections

Most people infected develop clinical manifestations of infection, which naturally disqualifies them as blood donors. The problem appears when a donor has an asymptomatic infection with bacteria in blood or transient, asymptomatic, bacteremia, e.g. after dental treatment or some diagnostic procedures. A key prophylactic action is to perform a thorough epidemiologic interview in the form of a questionnaire. The questionnaire should cover the largest possible number of situations which carry the risk for infection contracting and transmitting. Yet, even a best designed questionnaire is not always able to detect asymptomatic bacteremia in a donor and to prevent transfusing contaminated blood. Studies performed by CDC (Centers for Disease Control and Prevention) have shown that out of 6,000 people asked if they had experienced any alimentary tract disorders in the previous 30 days, 13% answered positively (50). Other studies showed that 1/3 of the donors in whose blood *Yersinia enterocolitica* was found had not complained of any gastro-intestinal disorders (12).

7.1.2 Lowering the risk for contaminating collected blood with donor's skin flora

The skin is richly colonized with bacterial flora, which is present in the superficial layer, on the epidermis, and in the deeper layers colonizing sebaceous glands, sudoriferous glands, and hair follicles. Even when the venopuncture site is prepared properly, not always is it possible to avoid contaminating the blood collected with the skin flora. Contamination with coagulase-negative *Staphylococcus* species is very common. Another commensal bacterium prevalent in the deeper skin layers and frequently contaminating blood taken is *Propionibacterium*. It is a bacterium that grows slowly in a low-oxygen environment (10). A few studies have shown that blood collected became contaminated with such bacteria as *S.epidermidis*, *Pseudomonas fluorescens*, *Pseudomonas putida*, despite the fact that skin bacteriological cultures harvested from the venopuncture site were aseptic (10).

Skin disinfection at the venopuncture site is a specific way to prevent blood contamination; what is particularly important is not only using proper disinfectants but mainly disinfecting correctly and making sure the duration of particular stages of the disinfection process (time when a disinfectant is active) is as it should be.

A venopuncture site is disinfected most effectively with iodine solutions. Yet, a large number of skin allergic reactions have resulted in iodine being replaced by chlorhexidine and isopropyl alcohol (51,52). Table 9 presents the effectiveness of different disinfectants.

There should be at least two stages in the disinfection procedure with disinfectants whose manufacturers recommend the contact with the skin must be at least 30 seconds long. In practice, this means disinfectants must be used in the same manner they are used during preparations to surgery.

What significantly diminishes the risk for contaminating collected blood with a donor's skin flora is diversing the initial aliquot (around 20 - 30 ml) of the blood taken. This blood is used for standard laboratory tests. Some authors claim such a practice may reduce the initial amount of bacteria in the blood taken even by 70 - 90%, but it does not eliminate the risk for its being contaminated (53,54,55).

Number of bacterial colonies / dish	Povidone iodine (% donors)	Isopropyl alcohol and iodine solution (% donors)	Chlorhexidine (% donors)	Green soap and isopropyl alcohol (% donors)
0	34 - 49%	63%	60%	0%
1 - 10	35 - 43%	34%	25%	17%
12 - 100	10 - 14%	2%	12%	47%
> 100	0 - 13%	1%	3%	36%
P (compared to povidone)		< 0.001	> 0.001	< 0.001

Table 9. Comparison of disinfectants efficacy (Goldman et al.) (46)

7.2 Bacteriological testing of blood components

Blood components are always tested bacteriologically in two situations:

1. During an epidemiologic investigation; when sepsis signs occurred in a recipient during or after transfusion and it is suspected that an infectious agent has been transfused;
2. Randomly, as a control study within the prophylaxis against transfusion-associated adverse reactions.

The presence of bacteria in blood and its components can be detected with methods that are fast but not sensitive and have low specificity, e.g. macroscopic assessment, pH measurement, glucose concentration; or by using methods much more sensitive and specific, but requiring special equipment and highly qualified personnel. Table 10 presents different methods used to detect bacteria in blood components.

1. Macroscopic assessment of blood components
a) Red blood cell concentrate changes color
b) Hemolisis in red blood cell concentrate
c) Swirling phenomenon assessment in platelet concentrate
2. Microscopic assessment of blood and its components (Gram staining, fluorescence microscopy)
3. Measuring glucose concentration, pCO_2, pO_2 and pH while blood components are being stored
4. Detecting bacteria endotoxins
5. Microbiological testing
6. Detecting bacterial genetic material
7. Using flow cytometry to detect bacteria

Table 10. Methods used to detect bacteria in blood components

In bacterially contaminated red blood cell concentrates, some features of red blood cells are changed. While blood components were being assessed macroscopically, hemolisis and a dark color have been observed in the concentrate with high levels of *Yersinia enterocolitica*, *Enterobacter* spp. and other Gram-negative bacteria (56,57,58). This phenomenon may result from bacteria using up the oxygen bound with hemoglobin in red blood cells. In contaminated blood components, methemoglobin concentration was found to be 2 - 4 times higher than in "healthy" components. In bacterially contaminated red blood cell concentrates, pH was found to be lower.

Similar changes have been observed in platelet concentrates. Bacterial proliferation uses up glucose in the environment and, consequently, lowers pH (58). Oxygen concentration is observed to decrease and that of CO_2 to increase (35,58). Yet, changes in these parameters do not necessarily mean there are bacteria present, because leukocytes and platelets also take up glucose and oxygen form the environment. The metabolism of platelets in stored concentrates is very vivid. That is why simple and direct measurement of these parameters does not indicate unambiguously bacteria are present. The sensitivity of the macroscopic assessment of blood components is around 10^8 CFU/ml. One of the studies on bacterial contamination of blood components showed the method was more sensitive. Bacterial contamination of 1.8×10^4 to 1.6×10^9 CFU/ml was found in the whole blood which earlier at macroscopic assessment was suspected of being contaminated (57).

In bacterially contaminated platelet concentrates, the "swirling" phenomenon is observed, i.e. platelet blinking or twinkling. When platelets are seen in a light beam going through blood, they swirl and reflect light and thus the swirling phenomenon is produced. This phenomenon disappears or is attenuated when there are bacteria in platelet concentrate, which lower pH (35).

Blood components are assessed microscopically for detecting bacteria in both red blood cell concentrates and platelet concentrates. The assessment is based on Gram staining. Unfortunately, this method's sensitivity is very low. It is possible to detect bacteria when their concentration is 10^5 - 10^6 CFU/ml (59). When the two methods of detecting bacteria in blood were compared (culturing on bacteriological medium and microscopic assessment), more than half of the samples where bacteria were cultured were negative microscopically (60). The use of acridine orange to detect bacteria in blood components has also been reported (61).

Genetic methods, which detect bacterial genetic material, are of a very high sensitivity. Methods based on the polymerase chain reaction (PCR) detect the genetic material of *S.aureus*, *E.coli*, *B.cereus* and *K.pneumoniae* in platelet concentrates with the sensitivity of 10 CFU/container (62). Other genetic methods use probes directed at a precisely defined bacterial DNA fragment, mainly 16SrDNA. They enable many different bacteria to be detected in blood components (63). The presence of marked probes is detected with chemiluminescence or electroluminescence. The test lasts a few hours, so theoretically it might be performed before each transfusion, and then the duration of storing blood components could be more "flexible" (10). The advantage of genetic methods is their speed and high sensitivity. Their disadvantage is the fact that they detect bacteria both alive and non-viable.

Flow cytometry is a method of the speed and sensitivity similar to those of genetic methods. Moreover, it differentiates bacteria which are alive from those which are dead.

At present, bacteria in blood components can be detected routinely with the method of marking them with fluorescence dyes and found on a special membrane (after filtration). The principle of this method is used in an automatic system where bacteria can be detected within 30 - 72 hours since blood collection. The time of the test is short, around 90 minutes, and detects bacterial contamination at 105 CFU/ml (64).

The present "gold standard" in detecting bacteria in blood and its components is considered to be a method based on measuring CO_2 concentration in a bag with biological medium with an appropriate amount of the platelet concentrate tested. An increase in pCO_2 is detected (as a marker of bacterial presence) by the calorimetric index (10).
None of the methods described above is able to detect bacterial contamination of blood components if its concentration is very low. Donor's subclinical bacteremia in its initial phase has bacterial concentration at ≤10 CFU/ml and is undetectable. That is why blood components are tested for bacterial contamination 24 hours after blood was collected. Although this practice delays obtaining the result of the test, it allows the cause of the contamination to be found and transfusion-associated bacterial sepsis to be avoided. Because of an increased risk for platelet concentrate transfusion-associated adverse reactions, in March 2004 FDA ruled that in the USA all platelet concentrates which are to be transfused have to be tested first (65). Similar regulations are in effect in some European countries.

7.3 Modifying the conditions of storing blood components

Platelet concentrate is a blood component in which bacteria have good conditions to survive. Lowering the temperature at which platelet concentrate is stored would inhibit bacterial proliferation and reduce the risk for transfusion-associated sepsis (4 - 6°C), but it would also affect negatively platelet haemostatic features and their survival in the circulation. This mechanism became known only recently (66). Short-time exposure of platelets to cold results in platelets clustering glycosylated protein GP1B on the surface of the chilled platelets. The aggregation process is induced by the binding of glycoprotein with receptors on macrophages, which immobilizes platelets. The phenomenon is transitional if platelets are not stored in the cold for longer than two hours. If platelet concentrate is stored in the cold for longer than 48 hours, platelet functions are distorted by competitive blockade of the asialo receptors, which results in platelet survival time in the circulation becoming shorter (66). Routinely, platelet concentrates are stored at 20 - 24 °C for up to 5 days, but after each unit is tested bacteriologically, the storing period may be prolonged to 7 days. There are opinions heard universally that the present guidelines should be changed and the duration of blood component storage should be shortened (10).
Most severe cases of transfusion-associated bacterial sepsis have been reported after transfusing red blood cell concentrates stored for over 2 weeks, because at the temperature of 2 - 6°C bacterial growth and metabolism are either inhibited or considerably slower. The temperature of 4°C does not stop *Yersinia, Pseudomonas* and *Serratia* from growing. A few centers have introduced "a preceding period" to red blood cell concentrate storage. The idea was to leave red blood cells in room temperature for 5 - 7 hours, and then perform a bacteriological test. It turned out that a longer time of incubation (about 7 hours) at room temperature improved detection of *Yersinia enterocolitica,* whereas such bacteria as *Enterococcus* or *Klebsiella* were much more numerous after 4 hours of incubation (67,68).
The temperature of 2 to 6°C is an inhibiting factor not only for bacteria. Cellular activity and the activity of immune system factors in fresh blood are inhibited too. That is why it is beneficial to leave the blood collected at room temperature for 2 - 4 hours so that natural mechanisms could act and destroy bacteria (12).

7.4 Inactivation of bacteria contaminating blood components

The techniques used to reduce bacteria contaminating blood components are new methods able to limit the risk for transfusion-associated bacterial sepsis. These methods are effective both when well-known infectious agents are encountered and also when the agents have so far been neglected from the transfusiology point of view, or even those which have not been discovered yet. They should possess the following features:

- They should inactivate a broad spectrum of bacteria;
- They should not change the therapeutic properties of a blood component;
- Reagents and photoproducts, whose traces may remain after the reduction process is finished, must not be toxic to recipients;
- The costs of implementation should be proportional to their effectiveness (69,70)

The effectiveness assessment is based on comparing the number of model bacteria added to blood components before and after inactivation. The method is believed to be effective if the number of bacteria is diminished by 5 – 6 $\log_{10}$ in reference to the baseline values (71, 72).

In *in vitro* studies, the parameter defining the effectiveness of the method is the reduction index (R), which is a negative logarithm (Y) of the ratio between the number of bacteria in the baseline material to the number of bacteria after reduction plus/minus 1:

$$R = - \log (Y) \pm 1$$

The reduction index is dependent on many factors. The most important are: baseline bacterial concentration, their type and kind of blood component.

Naturally, it is not enough to establish that a particular method of pathogen reduction is effective. It is necessary to carry out *in vitro* tests of particular blood components before and after reduction (69). Such tests aim to establish to what extent blood components change their functional and metabolic properties during storing. The methods of bacterial reduction must not distort biochemical metabolic transformations of red blood cells and platelets. If a method is to be applied clinically, a blood component after pathogen reduction with a particular method should be safe, therapeutically effective and must not cause adverse reactions (69).

The methods used in order to limit transmitting bacteria by contaminated blood components can be divided into two groups. In the first group, there are those procedures which inactivate bacteria. Inactivation destroys their capsules or damages their DNA/RNA, which prevents their proliferation. One of such methods is the Solvent/detergent method used mainly to reduce pathogens in the capsule.

The second group of methods focuses on eliminating the infectious factor completely or on lowering its amount so that it would not be infectious any longer. They are methods of photoinactivation with visual or UV radiation and such radiosensitive compounds as psolarens, as well as filtration. They are used to reduce pathogens in platelet and red blood cell concentrates (73).

The methods of inactivation with riboflavin are being clinically tested. The methods used for red blood cell concentrates must not need light exposure because light is absorbed by hemoglobin.

Clinical tests in the form of transfusing platelet concentrates inactivated with psolarens have shown lack of toxicity and their photoproducts. Photoinactivation with psolarens proves to be an effective method that inactivates a broad spectrum of both Gram-negative and Gram-positive bacteria. Platelets inactivated in this way have been proved sterile for the whole time of storage and the metabolic functions of these blood cells were preserved even in the 7th day of storing. Yet, what has to be considered as negative is an approximate 10% loss in the number of platelets after the process of inactivation (71).

The methods of pathogen reduction in blood components have been recommended as priorities to be applied and further studied so that the safety of blood and its components will improve (74,75).

Filtration, used to limit bacterial contamination in blood components, results in the removal of leukocytes together with bacteria inside them. Bacteria may adhere to leukocytes on the filter too. Free forms of bacteria can be also removed by direct adhesion to the filter material. Several *in vitro* studies have shown that filters which reduce the number of leukocytes are able to rid contaminated red blood cell concentrates or whole blood of bacteria (38,49,76). The blood units, into which *Y.enterocolitica* bacteria were added a few hours after collection, and which underwent filtering so that leukocytes would be removed, contained fewer bacteria than those which had not been filtered. On the other hand, diminishing the number of leukocytes by filtering them out is less effective in removing bacteria from platelet concentrates (76). The number of bacteria grew slower in low-leukocyte platelet concentrates, but after one day the concentration of bacteria contaminating this blood component did not differ significantly from others. Similarly, molecular studies of bacterial RNA showed the same growth rate of bacteria in platelet concentrates contaminated with *S.epidermidis* (77). Filters which reduce the number of leukocytes can catch bacteria directly, which is illustrated by the fact that *Staphylococcus xylosus* can be removed from blood components which were filtered previously (77). Yet, other studies have proved that filtering blood is able to reduce the number of bacteria in blood components, but it is never able to filter out the contamination fully (78). Filtering out leukocytes from blood components can also eliminate phagocytized bacteria inside them (76). If granulocytes disintegrate before bacteria are destroyed, they can get into the blood again. The optimal time to perform filtration is probably 2 to 12 hours following blood collection. It is the time for phagocytosis and reduction of leukocytes before viable bacteria are released from them (77). This mechanism has been used to explain why bacteria are found in the blood components which were previously considered uncontaminated. The interests of the haemovigilance study program included the benefits resulting from leukocyte reduction in blood components. The results revealed that the percentage of bacterially contaminated blood components had been considerably lowered (3.8% before filtering vs 1.7% after filtering) and the number of transfusion-associated bacterial sepsis cases significantly reduced (71% vs 24%) (54).

8. Summing-up

Bacterial contamination of blood components is a cause of transfusion-associated sepsis. The components which most often become contaminated are those of red blood cells and of platelets. Blood components often become bacterially infected during blood collection from a donor; more seldom in the case of asymptomatic bacteremia or faulty blood processing. The methods used currently, which are based on culturing, visual assessment of a component, appropriate selection of donors, venopuncture site disinfection techniques, more often than not are able to prevent transfusion-associated bacterial sepsis. The techniques of pathogen inactivation may turn out to be promising in preventing bacterial infections.

9. References

[1] Brecher ME., Hay SN.: Bacterial contamination of blood components. Clin Microbiol Rev 2005;18:195-204.

[2] Goldman M., Lee JH., Blajchman M.: Skin antisepsis and initial aliquot diversion. In Brecher ME. (ed): Bacterial and parasitic contamination of blood components. Bethesda, AABB Press 2003:31-56.

[3] Seghatchian J.: Bacterial contamination of blood components. Transfus Apher Sci 2001;25:147-150.

[4] Hillyer CD., Josephson CD., Blachman MA. et al: Bacterial contamination of blood components: risks, strategies, and regulation. Hematology 2003;1:575-589.

[5] Blajchman MA., Backers EAM., Dickmeiss E. et al: Bacterial detection of platelets: Current problems and possible resolutions. Transfus Med Rev 2005;19:259-272.

[6] Niu MT., Knippen M., Simmons L. et al: Transfusion-transmitted *Klebsiella pneumonia* fatalities, 1995 to 2004. Transfus Med Rev 2006;20:49-57.

[7] Kuchnert MJ., Roth VR., Haley NR. et al: Transfusion-transmitted bacterial infection in the United States, 1998 through 2000. Transfusion 2001;41:1493-1499.

[8] Barrett BB., Anderson JW., Anderson KC.: Strategies for the avoidance of bacterial contamination of blood components. Transfusion 1993;33:228-233.

[9] Dzieczkowski JS., Barret BB., Nester D. et al: Characterization of reactions after exclusive transfusion of white cell-reduced cellular blood components. Transfusion 1995;35:20-25.

[10] Park YA., Brecher ME.: Bacterial contamination of Blood Products. In: Simon TL., Snyder L., Sdheim BG. et al (eds) Rossi's Principles of Transfusion Medicine. Bethesda, MD: AABB Press, 2009:773-790

[11] Benavides S., Nicol K., Koranyi K. et al: *Yersinia* septic shock following an autologous transfusion in a paediatric patient. Transfus Apher Sci 2003;28:19-23.

[12] US Dept. of Health and Human Services. Red blood cell transfusions contaminated with *Yersinia enterocolitica* - United States, 1991-1996 and initiation of a national study to detect bacteria-associated transfusion reactions. MMWR Morb Mortal Whly Rep 1997;46:553-555.

[13] Theakston EP., Morris AJ., Streat SJ. et al: Transfusion transmitted *Yersinia enterocolitica* infection in New Zealand. Aust NZ J Med 1997;127:62-67.

[14] Beresford AM.: Transfusion reaction due to *Yersinia enterocolitica* and review of other reported cases. Pathology 1995;27:133-135.

[15] Yomtovian R., Palavecino E.: Bacterial contamination of blood components: History and epidemiology. In: Brecher ME, et al: Bacterial and parasitic contamination of blood components. Bethesda, MD: AABB Press, 2003:1-30.

[16] Leclercg A., Martin L., Vergues ML. et al: Fatal *Yersinia enterocolitica* biotype 4 serovar 0:3 sepsis after red blood cell transfusion. Transfusion 2005;45:814-818.

[17] Arduino MJ., Bland LA., Tipple MA. et al: Growth and endotoxin production of *Yersinia enterocolitica* and *Enterobacter agglomerans* in packed erythrocytes. J Clin Microbiol 1989;27:1483-1485.

[18] Ramirez-Arcos S., Goldman M., Blajchman MA.: Bacterial contamination. In: Popovsky MA (ed): Transfusion Reactions AABB Press, Bethesda. MD. 2007:163-206.

[19] Heltberg O., Show F., Gerner-Smidt P. et. al: Nosocomial epidemic of *Serratia marcescens* septicaemia ascribed to contaminated blood transfusion bags. Transfusion 1993;33:221-227.

[20] Roth VR., Arduino MJ., Nobiletti SC. et al: Transfusion -related sepsis due to *Serratia liquefaciens* in the United States. Transfusion 2000;40:931-935.

[21] Benfell C: Unusual bacteria blamed for blood transfusion death. Circulator 2004; Fall: 2 [http://chapters.redeross.org/ca/norcal/phys/pdf/Cireulator_Oct2004.pdf].
[22] Gibb AP., Martin KM., Davidson GA. et al: Modeling the growth of *Yersinia enterocolitica* in donated blood. Transfusion 1994;34:304-310.
[23] Högman CF., Engstrand L.: Factors affecting growth of *Yersinia enterocolitica* in cellular blood products. Transfus Med Rev 1996;10:259-275.
[24] Richard C., Kolinas J., Trinidade CD.: Autologous transfusion - transmission of Yersinia - enterocolitica. JAMA 1992;268:1541-1542.
[25] Sugai Y., Sugai K., Fuse A.: Current status of bacterial contamination of autologous blood for transfusion. Transfusion Apheresis Sci 2001;24:255-259.
[26] Depcik-Smith ND., Hay SM., Brecher ME: Bacterial contamination of blood products: factors, options, and insights. J Clin Apheresis 2001;16:192-201.
[27] Klein HG.,Dodd RY., Ness PM. et al: Current status of microbial contamination of blood complements: Summary of a conference. Transfusion 1997;37:95-101.
[28] Halpin TJ., Kilker S., Epstein J. et al: Bacterial contamination of platelet pools-Ohio, 1991. MMWR Morb Mortal Whly Rep 1992;41:36-37.
[29] Guevara RE., Tormey MP., Nguyen DM. et al.: *Listeria monocytogenes* in platelets: A case report. Transfusion 2006;46:305-309.
[30] Holness L., Jones P., Knippen M. et al: 19-year review of fatalities due to contaminated blood and blood components. FDA Science, 2006 [http:// www.cfsan.fola.gov/~frf/forum06].
[31] Benjamin RJ., Mintz PD.: Bacterial detection and extended platelet storage: The next step forward. Transfusion 2005;45:1832-1835.
[32] Fang CT., Chambers LA., Kennedy J. et al: Detection of bacterial contamination in apheresis platelet products: American Red Cross experience, 2004. Transfusion 2005;45:1845-1852.
[33] Rhame FS., Root RK., MacLowry JD. et. al: Salmonella septicaemia from platelet transfusions: Study of an outbreak traced to a hematogeneous carrier of *Salmonella choleraesius*. Ann Intern Med 1973;78:633-641.
[34] Wagner SJ., Moroff G., Katz AJ. et al.: Comparison of bacteria growth in single and pooled platelet concentrates after deliberate inoculation and storage. Transfusion 1995;35:298-302.
[35] Smith LA., Wright-Kanuth MS.: Bacterial contamination of blood components. Clin Lab Scien 2003;16:230-239.
[36] Williamson LM., Lowe S., Lowe EM. et al.: Serious hazards of transfusion (SHOT) initiative: analysis of the first two annual reports. BMJ 1999;319:16-19.
[37] Andren G., Morel P., Forestier F. et al.: Hemovigilance network in France: organization and analysis of immediate transfusion incident reports from 1994 to 1998. Transfusion 2002;42:1356-1364.
[38] Perez P., Salmi LR., Follea G. et al: Determinants of transfusion-associated bacterial contamination: results of the French BACTHEM case-control study. Transfusion 2001;41:862-872.
[39] Ness P., Braine H., King K. et al.: Single-donor platelets reduce the risk of septic platelet transfusion reaction. Transfusion 2001;41:857-861.

[40] Brecher ME., Holland PU., Pineda AA. et al.: Growth of bacteria in inoculated platelets: implications for bacteria detection and the extension of platelet storage. Transfusion 2000;40:1308-1312.

[41] Engelfriet CP., Reesink HW., Blajchman MA. et al: Bacterial contamination of blood components. Vox Sang 2000;78:59-67.

[42] 42. Perpoint T., Lina G., Poyart C. et al.: Two cases of fatal shock after transfusion of platelets contaminated by *Staphylococcus aureus*: Role of superantigenic toxins. Clin Infect Dis 2004;39: e106-109.

[43] 43. Jafari M., Forsberg J., Gilcher RO. et al.: Salmonella sepsis caused by a platelet transfusion from a donor with a pet snake. N Engl J Med 2002;347:1075-1078.

[44] 44. Chaffin DJ: *Pseudomonas fluorescens*-related septic transfusion reaction resulting from contaminated cold cloths (abstract). Transfusion 2002;42:41S.

[45] 45. Garcia-Free JA., Grasa JM., Solano VM. Et al.: Bacterial contamination of blood components due to *Burkholderia cepacie* contamination of chlorhexidine battles. Vox Sang 2002;81:70-71.

[46] 46. Goldman M., Blajchman MA.: Blood product associated bacterial sepsis. Transfus Med Rev 1991;5:73-83.

[47] 47. Robertson D., Davenport MD.: Management of Transfusion Reactions. In: Mintz PD. (ed): Transfusion Therapy Clinical Principles and Practice. AABB Press, Bethesda, Maryland 2005;526-528.

[48] 48. Walther-Wenke G.: Incidence of bacterial transfusion and transfusion reactions by blood components. Clin Chem Lab Med 2008;46:919.

[49] 49. Goldman M., Sher G., Blajchman M.: Bacterial contamination of cellular blood products: the Canadian perspective. Transfusion Sci 2000;23:17-19.

[50] Grossman BJ., Kollins P., Lan PM., et al: Screening blood donors for gastrointestinal illness. A strategy to eliminate carriers of *Yersinia enterocolitica*. Transfusion 1991;31:500-501.

[51] Mc Donald CP., Lowe P., Roy A. et al: Evaluation of donor arm disinfection techniques. Vox Sang 2001;80:135-141.

[52] Goldman M., Roy G., Frechette N. et al: Evaluation of donor skin disinfection methods. Transfusion 1997;37:309-312.

[53] Bruneau C., Perez P., Chassaingue M. et al: Efficacy of a new collection procedure for preventing bacterial contamination of whole-blood donations. Transfusion 2001;41:74-81.

[54] De Korte D., Marcellis JH., Verhoeven AJ. et al: Diversion of first blood volume results in a reduction of bacterial contamination for whole-blood collection. Vox Sang 2002;83:13-16.

[55] Eder AF., Kennedy JM., Dy BA. et al.: Limiting and detecting bacterial contamination of apheresis platelets: inlet-line diversion and increased culture volume improve component safety. Transfusion 2009;49:1554-1563.

[56] Bradley RM., Gander RM., Patel SK. et al: Inhibitory effect of 0°C storage on the proliferation of *Yersinia enterocolitica* in donated blood. Transfusion 1992;37:691-695.

[57] Pichard C., Herschel L., Seery P. et al: Visual identification of bacterially contaminated red blood cells (abstract). Transfusion 1998;38 :125.

[58] Brecher ME., Foster M., Mair D.: Glucose and haemolysis as a rapid screen for contamination of red blood cells with Yersinia and Serratia. Vox Sang 2001;81:126-138.
[59] Kim DM., Brecher ME., Bland LA. et al: Visual identification of bacterially contaminated red cells. Transfusion 1992;32:221-225.
[60] Barrett BB., Anderson JW., Anderson KC.: Strategies for the avoidance of bacterial contamination of blood components. Transfusion 1993;33:228-233.
[61] Kim DM. Brecher ME., Bland LA. et al: Prostorage removal of *Yersinia enterocolitica* from red cells with white cell-reduction filters. Transfusion 1992;32:658-662.
[62] Schmidt M., Hourfar MK., Nico SB. et al: A comparison of three rapid bacterial detection methods under simulated real-life conditions. Transfusion 2006;46:1367-1373.
[63] Mohammadi T., Pietersz ANI., Vandenbroucke-Granls C. et al: Detection of bacteria in platelet concentrates: Comparison of broad-range real-time 16S rDNA polymerase chain reaction and automated culturing. Transfusion 2005;45:731-736.
[64] Brecher ME., Wong ECC., Chen SE. et al.: Antibiotic-labeled probes and microvolume fluorimetry for the rapid detection of bacterial contamination in platelet components: a preliminary report. Transfusion 2000;40:411-413.
[65] Silva MA. (ed).: Standards for blood banks and transfusiology. AABB Press. Bethesda, MD:2006.
[66] Rumjantseva V., Grewal PK., Wandall HH. et al.: Dual roles for hepatic lectin receptors in the clearance of chilled platelets. Nat Med 2009;15:1273-80.
[67] Weinberg JA., Mc Gwin G.Jr, Margues MB. et al.: Transfusion in the less severely injured: does age of transfused blood affect autcomes ? J Trauma 2008;65:794-798.
[68] Rawn J.: The silent risks of blood transfusion. Curr Opin Anaesthesiol 2008;21:664-668.
[69] Solheim BG.: Pathogen reduction of blood components. Transfus Apher Sci 2008;39:75-82.
[70] Solheim BG., Flesland O., Seghatchian J. et al.: Clinical implications of red blood cell and platelet storage lesions: an overview. Transfus Apher Sci 2004;31:185-189.
[71] Lin L., Dikeman R., Molini B. et. al: Photochemical treatment of platelet concentrates with amotosalen and long-wavelength ultraviolet light inactivates a broad spectrum of pathogenic bacteria. Transfusion 2004;44:1496-1504.
[72] Ruane PH., Edrich R., Grampp D. et al.: Photochemical inactivation of selected viruses and bacteria in platelet concentrates using riboflavin and light. Transfusion 2004;44:877-885.
[73] Pelletier JP., Tramsue S., Snyder EL.: Pathogen inactivation techniques. Best Pract Res Clin Haematol 2006;19:205-242.
[74] 96th Blood Products Advisory Committee Meeting, November 2009. Available at: http://www.fda.gov/AdvisoryCommitteeMeetingMaterials/BloodVaccinesandOtherBiologics/default.htm. AccessedMarch 17,2010.
[75] Klein HG., Glynn SA., Ness PM. et al.: Research opportunities for pathogen reduction / inactivation of blood components: summary of an NHLBI workshop. Transfusion 2009;49:1262-1268.
[76] Siblini L., Lafenillade B., Ros A. et al.: Reduction of *Yersinia enterocolitica* load in deliberately inoculated blood: the effects of blood prestorage temperature and WBC filtration. Transfusion 2002;42:422-427.

[77] Miller JP.: Leucocyte-Reduced and Cytomegalovirus-Reduced Risk Blood Components. In: Mintz PD. (ed): Transfusion Therapy Clinical Principles and Practice. AABB Press, Bethesda MD, 2005:541-578.
[78] Holden F., Foley M., Devin G. et al.: Coagulase-negative staphylococcal contamination of whole blood and its components: the effects of WBC reduction. Transfusion 2000;40:1508-1513.

3

Septic Shock by Gram-Negative Infections: Role of Outer Membrane Proteins

Marilena Galdiero[1], Marco Cantisani[2], Rossella Tarallo[2], Annarita Falanga[2] and Stefania Galdiero[2]
[1]*Second University of Naples, Naples*
[2]*University of Naples "Federico II", Naples*
Italy

1. Introduction

The magnitude of septic shock as a clinical problem is often understated. Despite advances in our ability to diagnose and treat infectious diseases, severe sepsis leading to shock due to gram-negative infections remains one of the leading causes of mortality worldwide. Septic shock develops because of a disregulation in the host response, and the mechanisms initially recruited to fight infection produce life-threatening tissue damage and death. Recent research has witnessed a significant increase in our understanding of host-pathogen interactions, particularly in the area of innate immunity and the molecular recognition of gram-positive and gram-negative bacteria. Important new mediators of sepsis and novel mechanisms of host-cell toxicity have been identified and, together with clinical trials targeting pathways considered central to sepsis pathogenesis, provide new insight into the molecular and cellular basis of sepsis for the formulation of new strategies of intervention.

Research on septic shock pathogenesis by gram-negative bacteria is mainly focused on the understanding of the molecular and cellular role played by lipopolysaccharide (LPS). Strong experimental evidence and clinical observations suggest that the release of proinflammatory cytokine mediators by LPS-responsive cells (mainly macrophages, endothelial cells and neutrophils) in response to toxic products sets in motion the genetic and physiologic program that manifests as shock. The best characterized of these toxic components is LPS, which is considered as a paradigm for other less well-characterized toxic microbial molecules. The immune protection stimulated by highly purified LPS in animals does not resolve the symptomatology of septic shock, while LPS mixed to outer membrane proteins shows a better protective activity. Several studies evidence the major role played by outer membrane proteins in the molecular interaction between the host cell and the gram-negative bacteria. Endotoxin-associated proteins consist of a complex of several major proteins that are intimately associated with the LPS. Very little is known about release of non-LPS gram-negative outer membrane components such as OMPs in sepsis. Among the OMPs, porins have been shown to play an important role in pathogenesis of bacterial infections. Porins were pyrogenic in rabbits and elicited a localized reaction when used as the sensiting and eliciting agent. Porins were also shown to kill D-galactosamine sensitized LPS-responsive and LPS-unresponsive mice. Treatment of Human Umbilical Vein Endothelial Cells: (HUVEC) with porins increased the transmigration of different leukocyte populations, in particular of neutrophils. Porins by several gram-negative bacteria induce cytokine release by human leukocytes as well as enhancement of cytokine gene expression. Also, other components of the bacterial envelope are important in the induction and pathogenesis of septic shock such as bacterial lipoproteins (LP). As anti-LPS therapies does not seem to improve by the addition of proteins from the outer membrane or small fragments of these proteins, a great alternative to existing strategies will involve the blockage of signal transduction pathways, cytokine and inflammatory mechanisms.

2. The outer membrane of gram-negative bacteria

Bacteria in order to face unpredictable and often hostile environment have evolved a sophisticated and complex cell envelope that protects them while allowing selective passage of nutrients from the outside and waste products from the inside. There are three principal layers in the envelope: the outer membrane (OM), the peptidoglycan cell wall, and the inner membrane (IM). The two membrane layers delimit an aqueous cellular compartment called periplasm. The OM is a characteristic feature of Gram-negative bacteria, and in fact Gram-positive bacteria lack this structure. The OM is a lipid bilayer intercalated with proteins, superficially resembling the plasma membrane. The OM does contain phospholipids but they are confined to the inner leaflet of this membrane. The outer leaflet is composed of glycolipids, mainly lipopolysaccharide (LPS).

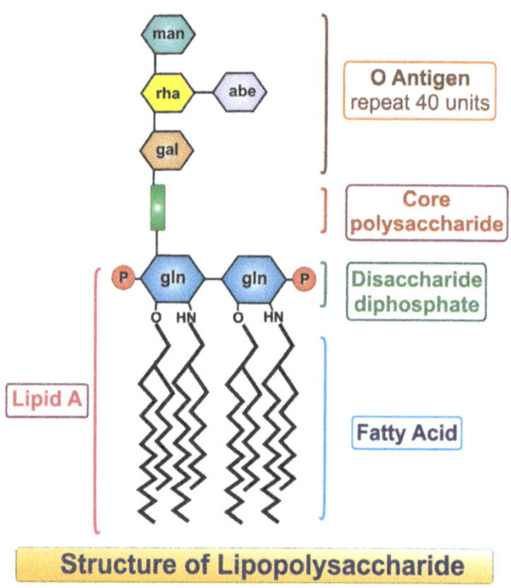

Fig. 1. Schematic representation of the structure of lipopolysaccharide (LPS).

LPS is a complex glycolipid exclusively present in the outer leaflet of the OM of gram-negative bacteria. LPS is one of the molecules responsible for the endotoxic shock associated with the septicemia, and is a sure indicator of infection as the human innate system is sensitized to this molecule. LPS molecules consist of a bisphosphorylated lipid (lipid A) forming the hydrophilic region of the outermost membrane leaflet which is stabilized by divalent cations and a hydrophilic polysaccharide (PS), extending outward from the bacterium. A schematic structure for LPS from *Escherichia coli* together with the chemical structure of lipid A (Figure 1) reveals its key features. The LPS consists generally of two distinct regions, a core oligosaccharide chain of repeating units, the O-specific chain, which constitutes the major anti-LPS immune response. The core is covalently bound to the lipid A through an acidic sugar, the 3-deoxy-D-manno-oct-2-ulopyranosonic acid (Kdo). The outer core region consists of neutral or amino hexoses such as D-glucose, D-galactose, D-glucosamine, D-galactosamine or N-acetyl derivatives, while the inner core also contains heptose residues which are often substituted by phosphate, pyrophosphate or diphosphoethanolamine. Kdo represent a covalent bridge between lipid A and heptose units joined by diester phosphate linkages. The general pattern of the lipid A from diverse gram-negative bacteria is highly conserved. The lipid A from *E. coli* has a β-1,6-linked D-glucosamine disaccharide phosphorylated in positions 1 and 4′. Lipid A often contains up to four moles of (R)-3-hydroxytetradecanoic acids symmetrically distributed on the two glucosamine residues of the backbone. The hydroxyl in position 6′ is linked to Kdo (Figure 1). The core oligosaccharide is very variable among bacterial species; so different species can express uniquely modified types of LPS. The O-antigen, if present, is the most variable part of LPS and shows even a high degree of variability between different strains of the same species.

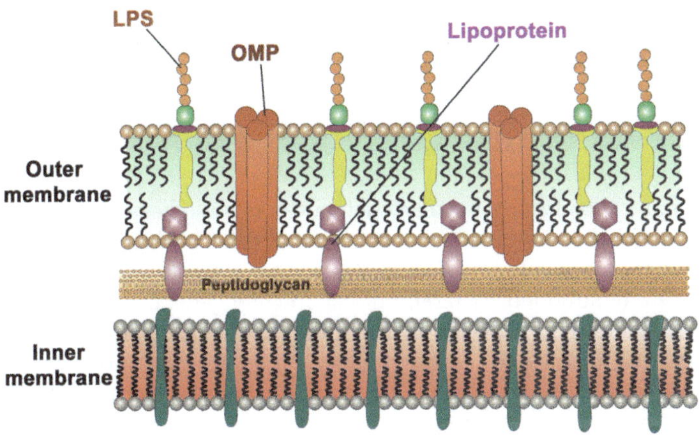

Fig. 2. Schematic representation of the inner and outer bacterial membrane.

With few exceptions, the proteins intercalated in the OM can be divided into two classes, proteins that traverse the membrane and assume a β-barrel structure and lipoproteins, anchoring the outer membrane to the underlying peptidoglycan stratum (Figure 2). Lipoproteins contain lipid moieties that are attached to an amino-terminal cysteine residue. It is generally thought that these lipid moieties embed lipoproteins in the inner leaflet of the OM, and are thus not supposed to be transmembrane proteins. Lipoproteins are low molecular weight proteins and are considered to be the most abundant proteins in the *E. coli* cell on the basis of molecular members. Lipoproteins are generally covalently linked to the peptidoglycan, but may also be present without covalent bonds.

The outer membrane proteins (OMPs) of gram-negative bacteria have been well characterized; they assume a β-barrel conformation. The OMPs serve as a molecular filter for hydrophilic substances, and mediate the transport of nutrients and ions across the membrane into the periplasm. The OMPs can be divided into three classes (Nikaido, 2003): porins, substrate specific transporters and active transporters. Porins are a group of trimeric proteins that form pores of a fixed diameter through the lipid bilayer of the membrane. They constitute the major component of the OM and are thus indicated as "major outer membrane proteins" of high molecular weight.

Porins form passive pores that do not bind their substrates; they form trimeric, water-filled pores, through which relatively small (<600 Da) solutes diffuse, driven by their concentration gradient. For nutrients that are present at low concentrations in the extracellular environment, passive diffusion is no longer efficient and transport occurs via substrate-specific (substrate specific porins and transporters) and active transporters (Galdiero, 2007). The active transporters (FepA and FhuA) bind their substrates with high affinity and transport them against a concentration gradient. This process requires energy, which is provided by the inner membrane protein Ton B. The substrate-specific porins and transporters contain low affinity substrate saturable binding sites that allow efficient diffusion of substrates at very low concentration gradients. Among the substrate specific porins are LamB (maltose and maltodextrins) and SerY (sucrose); among the substrate specific transporters are Tsx and FadL, while among auto-transporters are NaLP and Hia.

Whereas the composition, structure and function of the OM are well known, its assembly in the absence of energy sources has remained largely enigmatic. All the components of the OM are synthesized in the cytoplasm or at the cytoplasmic face of the IM, and they have to be transported across the IM and through the periplasm to reach their destination and to assemble into the OM.

3. The porins

The most abundant proteins of the bacterial outer membrane are porins which form channels with various degrees of selectivity (Schulz, 2002). Porins form β-barrels and their structures typically contain 14, 16 or 18 β-sheets. The majority of porins studied so far belong to the 16 or 18 stranded bacterial porins; and the general motif of their structural architecture is the closure of the barrel by pairing of the first and last β-strand in an antiparallel way. All strands are connected by eight or nine long loops, facing the extracellular side, with seven or eight small turns in the periplasmic space. In all porins, the constriction at the barrel center is formed by an inserted long loop L3, which is not exposed to the cell surface but folds back into the barrel, forming a constriction zone at half the height of the channel and contributing significantly to the permeability of the pore. Another feature is the presence of aromatic girdles with tyrosine and phenylalanine residues located at the outer and inner membrane boundaries. Residues located between these girdles and facing the hydrophobic lipid environment are mainly leucine, valine and isoleucine residues. At the very C-terminus almost all porins have a phenylalanine residue that is fundamental for proper import and folding in the outer membrane.

Porins made of 16 strands are called general or non-specific porins and form pores allowing the diffusion of hydrophilic molecules, showing no particular substrate specificity, despite some selectivity for either cations or anions; while 18 strands porins are substrate specific porins. Porins are passive diffusion channels with a pore diameter ranging from 15 Å for the general porins to 6 Å for the highly selective porins. Larger pores usually contain charged residues at opposite sides that form a local transversal electric field at the pore eyelet. This field constitutes an energy barrier for low-polarity solutes so that the bacterium can exclude unwanted nonpolar molecules such as antibiotics while presenting a spacious eyelet for collecting large polar molecules such as sugars. A systematic study changing the pore properties by point mutations showed a strong correlation between the eyelet cross section and diffusion rate. Charge reversals affect selectivity and voltage gating. Interesting results were obtained with mutations at loop L3, for example the specificity of the sucrose porin was changed toward that of the maltoporin.

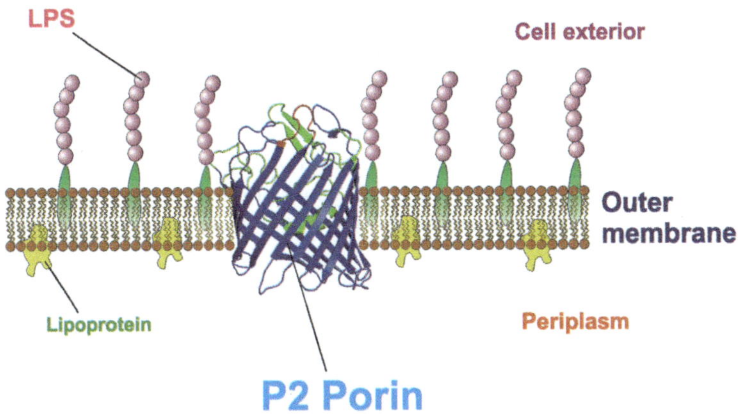

Fig. 3. Three dimensional model of the P2 monomer from *Haemophilus influenzae* type b. Surface loops are shown in green except L7 that is red. The extracellular space is located at the top of the figure and the periplasmic space is at the bottom. The position of the membrane bilayer is shown.

All porins form homotrimers in the OM; each subunit produces a channel and the trimer therefore contains three channels. For most porins, loops L1, L2 and L4 are important for monomer-monomer interactions within the porin trimer; loop L3 is internal; loops L5, L6 and L7 are superficial; loop L8 folds back into the barrel interior, contributing to the formation of the channel opening at the external side (Figure 3). Data from the literature indicate that peptide sequences corresponding to superficial loops are responsible for most of the biological activity of porins. In particular, loop L7 of porin OMPK36 from *Klebsiella pneumoniae* is involved in the interaction with C1q (Alberti, 1995); loops L5, L6 and L7 of porin P2 from *Haemophilus influenzae* activate JNK and p38 mitogen-activated protein kinase (MAPK) pathways (Galdiero, 2003) and induce the release of TNF-α and IL-6 (Galdiero, 2006); most functional antibodies raised to NTHI are directed to loop L5, which is thought to contain strain-specific and immunodominant epitopes (Yi, 1997); antibodies to loop L6 of NTHI showed complement-dependent bactericidal activity (Haase, 1994); the surface exposed loop regions are immunodominant as shown by immunizing mice with whole bacterial cells (Neary, 2001); synthetic peptides representing epitopes of outer membrane protein F of *Pseudomonas aeruginosa* elicit antibodies reactive with whole cells of heterologous immunotype strains of *Pseudomonas aeruginosa* (Hughes, 1992); major immunogenic epitopes of PorA and FetA of *meningococci* correspond to contiguous peptide sequences located in putative surface-exposed loops of those proteins (Maiden, 1991; Thompson, 2003).

4. Lipoproteins

Lipoproteins are a major component of the outer membrane of bacteria, with low molecular weights (about 7000 Da). Lipid modification of bacterial proteins enables the anchoring of hydrophilic proteins to hydrophobic surfaces through the hydrophobic interaction of the attached acyl groups to the cell wall phospholipids, allowing the protein to function effectively in the aqueous environment (Kamalakkannan, 2004). Lipoproteins can localize in various places of the cell. *E. coli* has more than 90 lipoproteins, the majority of which is located at the periplasmic face of the OM, with some present at the periplasmic face of the IM (Narita, 2004). Although all the known lipoproteins in *E. coli* face the periplasm, in some gram-negative bacteria, lipoproteins are also present on the outer leaflet of the OM. However, little is known about the exact mechanism of how they translocate across the OM whether they are exposed or not to the outside surface of the outer membrane. Moreover, in those *E. coli* strains that have defects in LPS structure, the lipoproteins seem to react with antilipoprotein serum.
Lipoproteins are low molecular weight proteins lacking histidine, tryptophan, glycine, proline and phenylalanine. They are linked by the ε-amino group of their C-terminal lysine to the carboxyl group of every tenth to twelfth meso-diaminopimelic acid residue of the peptidoglycan. The N-terminal portion of the lipoprotein consists of glycerylcysteine to which two fatty acids are linked by two ether linkages and one fatty acid by an amide linkage. The amide-linked fatty acid consists of 65% palmitate, with the rest being mainly monosaturated fatty acids. The fatty acid bound as esters are similar to the fatty acids found in the phospholipids of the inner layer of the membrane. Lipoproteins exist in the membrane also as free form without covalent bonds to the peptidoglycan. There are about 2.4×10^5 molecules of the bound form per cell, and about twice as much of the free form. The total free and bound lipoprotein molecules 7.2×10^5 make lipoproteins the numerically most abundant protein in the membrane. Lipoproteins are required for virulence and play a variety of roles in host-pathogen interactions, from surface adhesion to initiation of inflammatory processes (Kovacs-Simon, 2011).

5. Outer membrane blebbing

Extracellular secretion is the major mechanism by which gram-negative pathogens communicate with and damage host cells. Vesicles released from the envelope of the growing bacteria serve as secretory vehicles for protein and lipids of gram-negative bacteria. Vesicles production occurs in infected tissues and is influenced by environmental factors. Vesicles play an important role in colonization, carrying and transmitting virulence factors into host cells and modulating host defense and immune response. Gram-negative bacteria release membrane vesicles of average diameter 10-300 nm into the environment during all stages of normal growth as well as in a variety of growth environments such as infected tissues. The amount of released vesicles is increased several folds during periods of bacterial stress such as exposure of microorganisms to antibiotics or human serum. The vesicles are formed by protrusions of the bacterial outer membrane that are released into the environment (Ellis, 2010). Outer membrane vesicles (OMVs) are formed by blebbing and pinching off segments of the bacterial outer membrane (Kulp, 2010). These vesicles contain the main components of the outer membrane such as LPS, OMPs and fractions of the underlying bacterial periplasm. Importantly, OMVs are not a product of cell death since they are produced without concomitant bacterial lysis and newly synthesized proteins are present. Active concentrations of both LPS and porins are often accumulated at infection sites from either gram-negative bacteria outer membrane blebbing or bacterial lysis. Gram-negative bacteria contain about 10^5 molecules of porin per cell (molecular mass, about 36kDa) and about 3.4 x 10^6 molecules of LPS (molecular mass, about 4,5KDa), therefore, 10^6 to 10^9 bacterial cells are enough to reach a concentration of 500 ng/ml to 20 μg/ml (about 0.02 to 0.8 μM) for porin or a concentration of 100 ng/ml to 10 μg/ml (about 0.05 to 5 μM) for LPS.

OMVs from pathogenic bacteria contribute to the pathogenicity in vivo (Ellis, 2010). Thus, OMVs are likely a key factor in effecting an inflammatory response to pathogens, being immunogenic and capable of eliciting proinflammatory responses. Immunization with *Vibrio cholera* OMVs induces protection in mice (Schild, 2008); the OMVs immunized mice were protected against *Salmonella* infections (Alaniz, 2007). Furthermore, OMVs influence inflammation and disease in vivo; it was shown that, in response to *Helicobacter pylori* and *Pseudomonas aeruginosa* OMVs (Bauman, 2006), epithelial cells produce interleukin-8, a cytokine that plays a fundamental role in neutrophil and monocyte recruitment.

Septic shock has been associated with an early excessive inflammatory response to LPS and other bacterial components, among which OMPs and lipoproteins. During sepsis and septic shock large quantities of OMVs are released into serum and tissues. In particular, fragments containing LPS, OMPA and a protein of 17kDa, were affinity purified from filtrate of human serum incubated with *Salmonella enterica* serovar *Abortus equi* using O-chain-specific anti-LPS IgG (Freudenberg, 1992); similarly, complexes containing LPS and at least three OMPs, with molecular masses of 35, 18 and 5-9 kDa were affinity purified from filtrates of normal human serum incubated with *Escherichia coli* cells, using O-chain-specific anti-LPS IgG (Hellman, 2000). These molecules or macromolecular complexes have been shown to derive from the OMVs formed by the blebbing of bacterial cells.

6. OMPs and endothelial cells

Bacteria or bacterial products may constitute important inducers of surface molecule expression on endothelial cells (Rawadi, 1996). The microvascular endothelium plays an important role in regulating the exchange of fluids, macromolecules and cells between the blood and the extravascular tissues. The endothelium is a pervasive organ covering a surface area of 4000-7000 m^2. Endothelial cells are highly active, constantly responding to alteration in the local extracellular environment, as might occur in the setting of transient bacteremia or other important stress such as septic invasion. Endothelial cell activation occurs as a normal adaptative response, the nature and duration of which depends on the type of stimulus. Endothelial cell injury contributes significantly to the pathophysiology of bacterial sepsis and endotoxic shock. Components of the bacterial surface activate pattern recognition receptors on the surface of the endothelium. Gram-negative bacteria contain several surface molecules interacting with endothelial cells. The role of LPS is well known while the roles of other surface molecules of gram-negative bacteria are less understood. Several studies have recently shown the activity of major outer membrane proteins on endothelial cells. The bacterial surface contains a wide assortment of molecules that interfere with the complex network regulating the leucocyte traffic. The initial adhesion of circulating leukocyte to vascular endothelium is induced by interaction of constitutively functional leukocyte homing receptors with regulated endothelial cell ligands or counter receptors. Leukocyte-endothelial cell interactions both in vivo and in vitro are active multistep processes, as clearly demonstrated in studies of neutrophil interactions with inflamed sites (Von Andrian, 1991). During sepsis a dramatic increase of endothelial cell surface molecules expression occurs that facilitate adhesion of blood leukocytes. These kinds of interactions have been mainly studied in brain microvascular endothelial cells (BMEC).

The crossing of the blood-barrier by circulating bacteria is a complex process, requiring several bacterial and host factors and their interactions, such as a high degree of bacteremia, binding to and invasion of BMEC, BMEC actin cytoskeleton rearrangements and related signaling pathways. Among *E. coli* structures necessary for crossing of the blood-brain barrier in vitro and in vivo, outer membrane protein A (OmpA) contributes to *E. coli* K1 invasion of BMEC (Kim, 2002). OmpA has been implicated as an important virulence factor in several gram-negative bacterial infections such as *E. coli* K1, a leading cause of neonatal meningitis associated with significant mortality and morbidity (Mittal, 2011). *E. coli* K1 OMPA interacts with a gp96 protein on human BMEC. Purified OMPA as well as gp96 and gp96 antibody inhibited *E. coli* K1 invasion of human BMEC in a dose dependent fashion. OMPA is a major outer membrane protein of *E. coli*; it is present as an 8-stranded and anti-parallel β-barrel structure in the membrane, connected by large hydrophilic surface exposed loops and short periplasmic turns (Smith, 2007). Although OMPA's role in pathogenesis has been demonstrated, the exact role of individual loops is still to be determined (Maruvada, 2011). In particular, the synthetic peptides representing a part of the first loop and the tip of the second loop of OMPA have been shown to inhibit *E. coli* adhesion to BMEC (Prasadarao, 1996). The first and second loops are shown to be the sites for the interaction with the carbohydrate epitope of the BMEC receptor glycoprotein. OmpA extracellular loops play a fundamental role in the pathogenesis of meningitis and may help in designing effective preventive strategies against this deadly disease (Mittal, 2011). Loop regions 1 and 2 play an important role in the survival of *E. coli* K1 inside neutrophils and dendritic cells, and loop regions 1 and 3 are needed for survival in macrophages. Mutations in loop 4 of OmpA enhance the severity of the pathogenesis by allowing the pathogen to survive better in circulation and to produce high bacteremia levels. Loop 2 appears to be involved in the majority of the interactions and represents an interesting target for immunization.

Among the major surface proteins, the 34K and 36K porins from *Salmonella typhimurium* modulate leukocyte migration by acting on endothelial cells and leukocytes. The transmigration increase was dose-dependent and optimal endothelial activation occurred after 4-6 hours using porin as stimulus, after 2-4 hours using LPS. Stimulation of leukocytes with either porins or LPS slightly increased their transmigration through porin-non-activated endothelial cells. The simultaneous stimulation in vitro of HUVEC with IL-1β and either porins or LPS causes overlapping effects leading to a very high migration index (Galdiero, 1999). In natural inflammatory process the combination of several stimuli induces high endothelial permeability of vessels to migrating cells. The main adhesion molecules of endothelial cells are activated by porins. Neutrophil transmigration through HUVEC cells treated with porins was partially inhibited by MoAbs binding to E-selectin; the transmigration of lymphocytes and monocytes was partially inhibited by MoAb anti-VCAM-1; the transmigration of neutrophils, lymphocytes and monocytes was partially inhibited by MoAb anti ICAM-1. Soluble E-selectin and ICAM-1 were found in the supernatants from IL-1 and TNF-α activated endothelial cells. Also porins were able to stimulate the release of soluble E-selectin and soluble ICAM-1. Protein H from *Pasteurella multocida* in vitro induces neutrophil adhesion and transmigration through bovine endothelial cells (Galdiero, 2000). An increase of the expression of the vascular cell adhesion molecule 1 on the aortic endothelium has been reported in rabbit experimentally infected with *Pasteurella multocida* (Galdiero, 2000). These results evidence a local and systemic microcirculatory dysfunction that is considered central in the development of multiple organ dysfunction syndromes in septic shock.

7. OMPs and host-cells

Among surface components, porins and LPS may be important inducers of biological activity in host-interactions. Several studies have been carried out to dissect the immunobiological activities of *Salmonella enterica* or *typhimurium* porins, showing that these proteins have important effects on macrophage viability and functions; in particular, porins inhibit their phagocytic activity in a dose dependent fashion by activating the adenylate cyclase system (Di Donato, 1986). Porins induce the activation of the complement system by acting both on the classic pathway and on the alternative pathway (Galdiero, 1984), acting as mitogens for B lymphocytes. Furthermore, in rats they increase the toxicity of cardio-toxic molecules (Galdiero, 1986) and damage renal tubules (Tufano, 1987). Porins are clearly endowed with pro-inflammatory activity; when injected into the rat paw induce dose-dependent edema with long-lasting effects. The inflammation induced by porins is sensitive to both steroid (dexamethasone) and non-steroid (indomethacin) anti-inflammatory drugs. The in vitro studies carried out on peritoneal cells of the rat show that porins are able to induce the release of histamine and also of prostacyclin. Porin-induced inflammation may depend on the release of histamine, even though the arachidonic acid metabolites may also participate. In fact, in vitro results exclude an increase of 6-keto-prostaglandin and subsequent prostacyclin release, whereas in vivo results confirm both the prolonged duration of porin-induced edema and its marked inhibition by indomethacin. Porin-induced inflammation was also observed in decomplemented animals; therefore, it is unlikely that the activation of the complement system plays a major role in the inflammation induced by porins (Galdiero, 1984). Porins isolated from *S. typhimurium* are lethal at the dose of 100 ng to both LPS-responder (BALB/cByS) and non responder (C3H/HeJ) mice sensitized with D-galactosamine. The lethal action could be prevented by anti-TNF-α serum. Porins were also pyrogenic to rabbits and elicited a Shwartzman reaction when used as the sensitizing and eliciting agent (Galdiero, 1994). *Haemophilus influenza* type b (Hib) porin also induces the early release of cytokines in central nervous system cells, amplifying the inflammatory response. Hib porin inserted into the fourth ventricle of the brain elicited the appearance of serum proteins and the development of brain edema. These modifications were followed by increase in the number of neutrophils both in cerebrospinal fluid and in the tissue sections around the porin inoculation site. IL-1α, TNF-α and MIP-2 mRNA appeared quickly in the tissue near the inoculation site (Galdiero, 2001a).

Activation of the coagulation and fibrinolytic systems is an important manifestation of the systemic inflammatory response of the host to infection. The in vivo effect of a synthetic peptide corresponding to loop L7 from *Haemophilus influenzae* type b (Hib) porin was compared with the effect of the entire protein to evaluate its role on the coagulative/fibrinolytic cascade and the circulating markers of endothelial injury (Vitiello,

2008). Plasma was obtained from rats injected intravenously with the peptide and tested for fragment 1+2 (F1+2), tissue-type plasminogen activator (tPA), plasminogen activator inhibitor type I (PAI-1) antigen, von Willebrand factor (vWF) and soluble E-selectin (sE-selectin). The coagulative/fibrinolytic cascade was impaired as determined by the increased level of PAI-1. Concomitantly, E-selectin, a marker of endothelial injury, was also significantly elevated. In addition either loop L7 or Hib porin injection induced hyperglycaemia and inflammatory cytokine production. The data were correlated with hemodynamic functions (significant reduction of blood pressure and increase of heart rate). The results indicated that, in that experimental model, the loop L7 plays an essential role in the pathophysiologic events observed during gram-negative infection.

OMPA from *E. coli* K1 plays a fundamental role in pathogenesis and great importance are correlated with the host signaling events underlying its entry into host cells. OMPA contributes to endothelial cells activation through a ligand- receptor interaction. OMPA activates PI3K but exhibited no effect on RhoA activation. The RhoA and PI3K host cell signaling pathways involvement in *E. coli* K1 invasion of human BMEC was further supported by the treatment of human BMEC with Rho kinase inhibitor (Y27632) and PI3K inhibitor (LY294002) which resulted in significant greater inhibition of *E. coli* K1 invasion compared to individual inhibitors alone.

The properties of Lipid-A associated proteins (LAP) have been extensively reviewed by Hitchcock and Morris (Hitchcock, 1984). Preparations of LAP from *S. typhimurium* have IL-1 like properties. LAP from *Actinobacillus actinomycetemcomitans,* an aquaporin associated with various forms of inflammatory periodontal disease, stimulate the release of IL-1β and IL-6 from human monocytes or human gingival fibroblast. LAP from *Porphyromonas gingivalis,* one of the causative organisms of peridontitis, are potent stimulators of IL-6 release from human gingivalis fibroblasts (Reddi, 1995).

8. Activation of eukaryotic cell signaling and transcriptional activation induced by OMPs

The molecular mechanisms during the interaction of gram-negative bacteria with macrophages are well understood, but the mechanisms used by porins to activate cells is not well characterized. LPS, porins or other OMPs probably activate cells through similar but not identical mechanisms (Galdiero, 2003b). A variety of extracellular factors, such as growth factors or bacterial surface components, induce a complex cellular signaling by binding specific transmembrane receptors on the host cell membrane. The intracellular signaling pathways are complex networks of biochemical events that culminate in specific patterns of nuclear gene expression mediated by transcription factors. Signal transduction pathways and transcriptional activation known to occur during immune cell activation have been investigated by numerous authors and protein tyrosine phosphorylation plays a central role in transduction mediated by bacteria or LPS or toxins (Evans, 1998; Rosenshine, 1992; Weinstein, 1992). Cytoplasmic signal transduction is regulated by several enzymatic pathways among which the mitogen-activated protein kinase (MAPK) pathway is especially activated during the adhesion and penetration of bacteria into the host cell (Evans, 1998; Rosenshine, 1992) and when stimulating the cell with products of bacterial origin (Weinstein, 1992).

MAPK/extracellular signal-regulated kinases are serine/threonine protein kinase members of sequential protein phosphorylation pathways involving c-Jun N-terminal kinases (JNKs) and ERKs (Davis, 2000). The MAPK pathway activates a number of transcription factors such as activating protein-1 (AP-1) and nuclear factor-kappa B (NFκB). The contribution of AP-1 family members to transcriptional regulation is controlled by a number of well characterized mechanisms (Karin, 1997). AP-1 is a ubiquitous class of gene regulatory factors and AP-1 proteins form either Jun-Jun homodimers comprised of members of the Jun family (c-Jun, JunD, and JunB) or Fos-Jun heterodimers derived from the various Fos family members. The AP-1 family members differ in their abilities to transactivate or repress transcription (Karin, 1997). NF-κB is a dimeric transcription factor and has multiple functions in immunity and is also critical for development and cellular survival. Mammalian cells contain five NF-κB subunits (p65, c-Rel, RelB, p50and p52) which form various hetero- and homodimers. NF-κB is present in the cytoplasm of resting cells bound to its inhibitor IκBα. The activation of NF-κB requires sequential phosphorylation, ubiquitination, and degradation of IκB. Multiple kinases have been shown to phosphorylate IκB at specific amino-terminal serine residues. In response to a large spectrum of chemically diverse agents and cellular stress conditions including LPS and porins, microbial and viral pathogens, cytokines and growth factors, NF-κB translocates in the nucleus, activating expression of target genes mainly involved in inflammatory and immunological responses (Caamano, 2002).

Several studies have addressed the mechanism by which porins stimulate cells. *S. enterica* serovar typhimurium porins induce signal transduction in mouse macrophages (Gupta, 1999). Porin activation of macrophages results in increased inositol triphosphate and intracellular Ca^{2+} mobilization, translocation of protein kinase C (PKC) to the membrane, NO release within the macrophages and increased binding of infected macrophages resulting in macrophage activation and triggering of specific signaling pathways. *S. enterica* serovar typhimurium, *Mannheimia haemolytica*, and *Haemophilus influenzae* (Hib) porins induce tyrosine phosphorylation in THP-1 cells and in C3H/HeJ mouse macrophages (Galdiero, 2001), with Hib porin being the most powerful stimulator. Incubation of porins with either THP-1 or macrophages from C3H/HeJ mice resulted in tyrosine phosphorylation of specific host cell proteins with the appearance of tyrosine-phosphorylated proteins in the soluble cytoplasmic fraction, in the membrane fraction and in the insoluble protein fraction. The pattern of phosphorylation observed following LPS or porin stimulation is essentially similar, but a difference can be observed in the cytoplasmic fraction bands of 50-60 kDa, which are more evident after treatment with LPS, and in the insoluble fraction band of 80kDa and the cytoplasmic fraction band of 250kDa, which are more evident after porin treatment.

Among the most prominent tyrosine-phosphorylated bands in porin-stimulated cells, a number of proteins with a molecular mass that is similar to that of the family of tyrosine/serine/threonine protein kinases were observed. *S. enterica* serovar typhimurium porins induce tyrosine phosphorylation of ERK1-2. Porins of *S. enterica* serovar typhimurium were also able to stimulate protein kinase A (PKA), PKC and protein-tyrosine kinase (NT-PTKs) in U937 cells. In the cells pretreated with tyrphostin, a specific PTK inhibitor, or with H-89, a specific PKA inhibitor, or calphostin C, a specific PKC inhibitor, decrease of the relevant activity was observed (Galdiero, 2003a).

Neisserial porins induce protein tyrosine phosphorylation and alter the surface expression of the co-stimulatory molecule B7-2 (Massari, 2003). Recent evidence suggests that the Raf-1-MEK1/2-MAPK pathways are included among the proteins which are phosphorylated following porin stimulation (Galdiero, 2002). The use of some specific inhibitors of phosphorylation pathways such as SB-203580 (p38 inhibitor), PD-098059 (MEK/ERK kinase inhibitor) and forskolin (Raf-1 inhibitor) demonstrated that they modulate in a different way cytokine mRNA expression in cells stimulated with porins. Neisserial porins induce nuclear translocation of the transcription factor NF-κB in B cells and dendritic cells that was maximal by 3 h of stimulation (Massari, 2003). *S. enterica* serovar typhimurium porins also activate AP-1 and NF-κB in U937 cells involving the Raf-1-MEK1/2-MAPK pathways (Galdiero, 2002); pretreatment with PD-098059 and with SB-203580 markedly affected the activation, indicating that the p38 signaling pathway is mainly involved in AP-1 and NF-κB activation. In contrast, forskolin pretreatment did not block transcription factor activation by porins, suggesting that a Raf-1-independent pathway may also be involved following porin stimulation. Electrophoresis mobility shift assays, using antibodies to specific transcription factor protein subunits, showed that in U937 cells the AP-1 complex contains Jun-D and c-Fos heterodimers and probably no other homodimers or heterodimers. In U937 cells treated with LPS, AP-1 complexes containing Jun-D, c-Fos and c-Jun appeared, while stimulation by porins induces AP-1 complexes containing fra-2 in addition to the other subunits. The formation of a different complex represents a further difference between stimulation with LPS and stimulation with porins. This may be added to past observations where mRNA

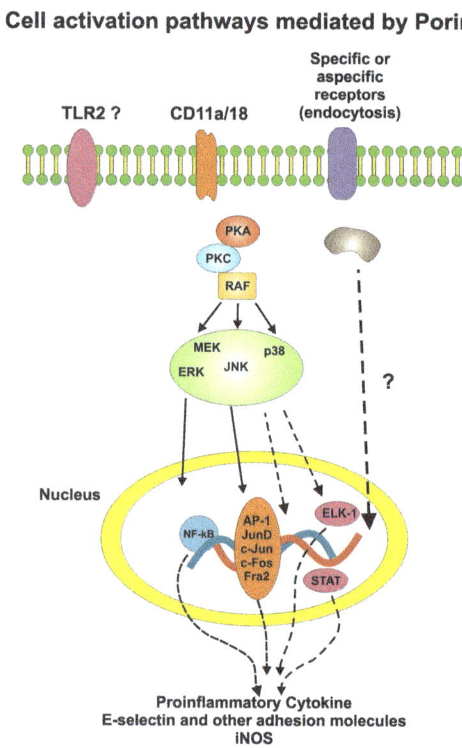

Fig. 4. Speculative scheme of porin signal transduction pathways. Putative porin-specific receptors are shown to be transmembrane. The solid arrows indicate the known association between superficial porin receptors and activation of several transcription factors; dotted arrows indicate hypothetical events.

cytokine expression after stimulation with porin begins after 120 min and continues for 5-6 h, while following LPS stimulation begins after 30 min and decreases at 120 min. Forskolin did not block NF-κB translocation after porin stimulation. Raf-1 induces the dissociation of cytoplasmic NF-κB-IκB complexes (Li, 1993), suggesting that a Raf-1-dependent pathway may be involved in NF-κB activation. However, it is known that PKC triggers the activation of several kinases suggesting that MEK/ERK pathways may also participate in NF-κB activation by enhancing an AP-1-NF-κB cross-coupling mechanism. The porin P2 from *Hib*, like porins from *S. enterica* serovar typhimurium, activates mainly but not exclusively the JNK and p38 pathways. Synthetic peptides, corresponding to the amino acid sequences of variable loop regions facing the cell exterior and thus more probably involved in the initial interaction with the host cell, proved to be able to activate the MEK1-MEK2/MAPK pathways similarly to the entire protein. In contrast, peptides modelled on internal β-strands were ineffective in inducing phosphorylation of such pathways (Galdiero, 2003c).
A speculative scheme of signal transduction pathways involved in porin-mediated responses is depicted in Figure 4. Accumulating evidence has suggested that the regulation of transcriptional factors and the subunit composition by porin stimulation may affect the adaptive immune mechanism to modulate the production of biologically active proteins or peptides. The engagement of multiple pathways during signal transmission makes the possible use of molecular inhibitors as therapeutic agents very difficult; although recent findings show that peptides complementary to loop regions have a certain ability to block the activity of the porin (Cantisani, 2011).

9. OMPs and septic shock

Septic shock is a major cause of death in the world. Gram-negative infection frequently results in systemic manifestations of sepsis and septic shock. The systemic syndrome is caused by the host response to gram-negative surface components. This response may set in motion a cascade of pathophysiologic consequences that result in multiple organ systemic failure and death. The host response to gram-negative bacterial infection is complex and multifaceted. Strong experimental evidence and clinical observations suggest that the release of proinflammatory cytokine mediators in response to toxic bacterial products set in motion an uncontrolled pathophysiologic program that manifests as sepsis or septic shock. The best characterized and most important of these toxic products is gram-negative endotoxin. For the general scientific public, the terms endotoxin and LPS are interchangeable. The term lipopolysaccharide (LPS) obtained by using the Westphal extraction procedure (Westphal, 1952), should be reserved for purified bacterial LPS extracts which are free of detectable contaminants, particularly proteins. In contrast, the term endotoxin should be used to refer to macromolecular complexes of LPS, protein and phospholipid normally obtained by extraction of bacteria with trichloroacetic acid, butanol and EDTA. Endotoxin associated protein consist of complex of four or five major proteins that range in size from 10 to 35 kDa. Originally considered to be a superfluous carrier of LPS, endotoxin associated proteins are now recognized to have potent biological activities (Mangan, 1992). Endotoxin associated proteins are powerful mitogen for C3H/HeJ mice, which are hyporesponsive to LPS. Techniques previously used in the extraction of stable LPS from the endotoxin had greatly favored the study of this portion of the molecule, ignoring the denaturable protein fraction, allowing the identification of most of the effects of endotoxin with those of LPS. Subsequent extraction techniques for membrane proteins (in their native form) then allowed the study of the protein fraction, which was extracted globally in the endotoxin (Hindennach, 1975). Although much is known about the role of LPS in septic shock, little is known about the role of the proteic components. Approximately 50% of the dry mass of the outer membrane of the gram-negative bacteria consists of proteins and more than 20 immunochemically distinct proteins (OMPs) have been identified in *E. coli*. Several OMPs have been shown to be potent inducers of cytokine synthesis. The most abundant of OMPs are porins. Porins isolated from *Salmonella enterica* serovar typhimurium, *Yersimia enterocolitica,* and *Mannheimia haemolytica* have been shown to stimulate the release of a range of proinflammatory and immunomodulating cytokines including IL-1, IL-4, Il-6, IL-8, TNF-α and INN-γ by monocytes and lymphocytes. Porins stimulate also the release of granulocyte-monocyte colony stimulating factor (GM-CSF), soluble intercellular adhesion molecule-1 (ICAM-1) and soluble E-selectin (SE-selectin) in a dose-dependent fashion by HUVEC cells (Donnarumma, 1996).

In vitro and in vivo experiments supported the involvement of porins in the septic shock pathogenesis. The administration of porin to animals affects their hemodynamics, body temperature, blood clotting, cellular and humoral immunities proliferation of B lymphocytes and macrophages, and release of various endogenous mediators. The role played by porins and in general by OMPs in sepsis has been further supported by conflicting results obtained with the immunotherapy. The notion that the core regions of most strains of gram-negative bacterial LPS were quite similar, supported the development of a broadly effective immunotherapy for gram-negative sepsis using antibodies raised against LPS, through the use of a bacterial strain with an outer membrane that features no side chains, while bearing only the conserved core elements of LPS. The strain selected was the J5 mutant of *E. coli* O111:B4, whose LPS contains only the core determinants, primarily lipid A. Although it has generally been assumed that immunoglobulins to rough mutant *E. coli* J5 protect by binding to LPS, it has been demonstrated that IgG in those antisera bind only weakly to LPS from heterologous gram-negative strains. Also anti-lipid A monoclonal antibodies did not induce the expected results (Siber, 1985). Recently, it has been demonstrated that IgG in polyclonal antiserum raised to heat-killed *E. coli* J5 binds to three conserved gram-negative bacterial outer-membrane proteins. (5-9, 18, and 35 kDa). These OMPs are exposed on the surface of bacterial cells and are released into human serum in complexes that also contain LPS (Binkley, 1945). The role of porins in pathogenesis is also confirmed by studies on the development of an effective vaccine against serogroup B *Neisseria meningitides*. The nonimmunogenicity of serogroup B capsular polysaccharide has led to the development of outer membrane vesicle (OMV) vaccines, based on the presence of PorB (Jolley, 2001; Wright, 2002). The porin proteins adopt a β-sheet structure within the outer membrane with surface exposed loops (Van der Ley, 1991). OMPs epitopes mainly involved in the interaction with the host cells are those on the surface. The wide antigenic variability of gram-negative bacteria is due also to the great sequence amino acid variability of surface exposed loops. Although, cross-reactivity of the major OMPs of *Enterobacteriacae* has been reported by several investigators (Hofstra 1979, Hofstra, 1980), their role in the pathogenesis of sepsis and shock has not been fully dissected.

Bacterial lipoproteins are important in the induction and pathogenesis of septic shock; in fact, they induce proinflammatory cytokine production in macrophages and lethal shock in LPS-responsive and nonresponsive mice. Lipoproteins are released from growing bacteria and released lipoproteins may play an important role in the induction of cytokine production and pathologic changes associated with gram-negative bacterial infections; treatment of bacteria with antibiotics significantly enhances lipoprotein release.

Lipoproteins activate macrophages; induce lethal shock in mice, and act synergistically with LPS to induce these responses (Zhang, 1997). Some gram-negative microorganisms have the ability to secrete lipoproteins to the extracellular environment; among those peptidoglycan-associated lipoproteins, Pal is released into the bloodstream during infection, and this process contributes to the development of septic shock (Hellman, 2002; Liang, 2005). Lipoproteins play an important role in septic shock induced by bacteria; moreover, they act synergistically with LPS to induce lethal shock which suggest that they activate cells through different mechanisms. Bacterial lipoproteins have been shown to affect both the innate and acquired immune system via TLR2 signaling and generation of cytotoxic T lymphocytes and bactericidal antibodies (Masignani, 2003).

10. Novel perspectives for therapies

Gram-negative sepsis remains a significant cause of morbidity and mortality in site of the ongoing development of new antimicrobial agents (Lazaron, 1999); the reason may be attributed to the failure of antimicrobial therapy to address the described pathogenetic mechanism involved in the systemic inflammatory response due to gram-negative bacteria. The systemic syndrome is caused by the host response to gram-negative infection; which sets in motion a cascade of pathophysiologic consequences that result in dysregulation of hemodynamics, oxygen use, and intermediate metabolism, and often results in multiple organ failure with further increased morbidity and mortality; these may happen also after apparent eradication of the original infection. The immunotherapy in the treatment of sepsis and shock did not produce the expected results. In fact, polyclonal *E. coli* J5 antiserum is not suitable for commercial development, especially for the viability of antiserum activity. The mass production of IgM monoclonal antibodies allowed the obtainment of an antibody E5 binding more specifically to Lipid A. E5 monoclonal antiserum, tested in two randomized placebo-controlled clinical trials demonstrated no clinical benefit to patients with gram-negative sepsis (Greenman, 1991). Also a human hybrid monoclonal antibody, HA-1A has been problematic. Anti-LPS core directed antibodies have not shown a survival benefit in clinical trials. The sometimes protective results observed using polyclonal *E. coli* J5 antiserum, may be attributed to the presence of antibodies against surface epitopes of OMPs. The great variability of surface loops of OMPs makes it rather difficult the preparation of specific antiserum that could be used for all gram-negative infections. As death by septic shock has been derived by an early excessive inflammatory response, therapeutic strategies have been designed to block the cytokines and other mediators involved into pathogenesis. However, the sepsis and septic shock are not restricted only to the activation of the inflammatory response, but also to compensatory anti-inflammatory mechanism usually leading to immunosuppression. Patients in this state have a poor prognosis; in fact, the majority of deaths occur in patients with sepsis who are immunosuppressed (Adib-Conquy, 2009).

11. Acknowledgment

This work was supported by MIUR (FIRB Prot. RBRN07BMCT)

12. References

Adib-Conquy, M. & Cavaillon, J.M. (2009). Compensatory anti-inflammatory response syndrome. *Journal of Thrombosis and Haemostasis*, Vol.101, No.1, pp.36-47.

Alaniz, R.C., Deatherage, B.L., Lara, J.C. & Cookson, B.T. (2007). Membrane vesicles are immunogenic facsimiles of Salmonella typhimurium that potently activate dendritic cells, prime B and T cell responses, and stimulate protective immunity in vivo. *Journal of Immunology*, Vol.179, No.11, pp.7692-701.

Alberti, S., Rodriquez-Quinones, F., Schirmer, T., Rummel, G., Tomas, J. M., Rosenbusch, J. P. & Benedi, V. J. (1995). A porin from Klebsiella pneumoniae: sequence homology, three-dimensional model, and complement binding. *Infection and Immunity*, Vol.63, No.3, pp.903-910.

Bauman, S.J. & Kuehn, M.J. (2006). Purification of outer membrane vesicles from Pseudomonas aeruginosa and their activation of an IL-8 response. *Microbes and Infection*, Vol.8, No.9-10, pp. 2400-2408.

Binkley, F., Goebel, W.F., & Perlman, E. (1945). Studies in the Flexner group of dysentery bacilli. II. The chemical degradation of the specific antigen of type Z Shigella paradysenteiae (Flexner). *Journal Experimental Medicine*, Vol.81, No.4, pp.331-341.

Caamano, J. & Hunter, C.A. (2002) NF-UB family of transcription factors: central regulators of innate and adaptive immune functions. *Clinical Microbiology Reviews*, Vol.15, No.3, pp.419-429.

Cantisani, M., Vitiello, M., Falanga, A., Finamore, E., Pedone, C., Galdiero, M. & Galdiero, S. (2011) Peptides complementary to the active loop of porin P2 from Haemophilus influenzae modulate its activity, unpublished data

Davis, R.J. (2000) Signal transduction by the JNK group of MAP kinases. *Cell*, Vol.103, No.2, pp.239-252.

Di Donato, A., Draetta, G.F., Illiano, G., Tufano, M.A., Sommese, L. & Galdiero, F. (1986) Do porins inhibit the macrophage phagocyting activity? *Journal of Cyclic Nucleotide and Protein Phosphorylation Research* Vol.11, No.2, pp.87-97.

Donnarumma, G., Brancaccio, F., Cipollaro de l'Ero, G., Folgore, A., Marcatili, A. & Galdiero, M. (1996) Release of GM-CSF, sE-Selectin, and sICAM-1 by human vascular endothelium stimulated with gram-negative and gram-positive bacterial components. *Endothelium* Vol.4, pp.11-22.

Ellis, T.N. & Kuehn, M.J. (2010) Virulence and immunomodulatory roles of bacterial outer membrane vesicles. *Microbiology Molecular Biology Review* Vol.74, No.1, pp.81-94.

Evans, D.J., Frank, D.W., Finck-Barbancon, V., Wu, C. & Fleiszig, S.M. (1998) Pseudomonas aeruginosa invasion and cytotoxicity are independent events, both of which involve protein tyrosine kinase activity. *Infection and Immunity*, Vol.66, No.4, pp.1453-1459.

Freudenberg, M. A., Meier-Dieter, U., Staehelin, T. & Galanos, C. (1991) Analysis of LPS released from Salmonella abortus equi in human serum. *Microbial Pathogenesis*, Vol.10, No.2, pp.93–104.

Galdiero, F., Tufano, M.A., Sommese, L., Folgore, A. & Tedesco, F. (1984) Activation of complement system by porins extracted from Salmonella typhimurium. *Infection and Immunity* Vol.46, No.2, pp.559–563.

Galdiero, F., Tufano, M.A., Rossi, F., Filippelli, W., De Santis, D., Matera, C., Berrino, L. & Marmo, E. (1986) Effect of Salmonella typhimurium porins on the cardiovascular and renal apparatus. *Journal of Medicine*. Vol.17, No.5-6, pp.285–297.

Galdiero, F., Sommese, L., Scarfogliero, P. & Galdiero, M. (1994) Biological activities-lethality, Shwartzman reaction and pyrogenicity- of salmonella typhimurium porins. *Microbial Pathogenesis* Vol.16, No.2, pp.111-119.

Galdiero, M., Folgore, A., Molitierno, M. & Greco, R. (1999) Porins and lipopolysaccharide (LPS) from Salmonella typhimurium induce leucocyte transmigration through human endothelial cells in vitro. *Clinical and Experimental Immunology*, Vol. 116, No.3, pp.453-461.

Galdiero, M., Folgore, A., Nuzzo, I. & Galdiero, E. (2000) Neutrophil adhesion and transmigration through Bovine endothelial cells in vitro by protein H and LPS of Pasteurella multocida. *Immunobiology*, Vol.202, No.3, pp. 226-238.

Galdiero, M., D'Amico, M., Gorga, F., Di Filippo, C., D'Isanto, M., Vitiello, M., Longanella, A. & Tortora, A. (2001a) Haemophilus influenzae porin contributes to signaling of the inflammatory cascade in rat brain. *Infection and Immunity*, Vol.69, No.1, pp.221-227.

Galdiero, M., Vitiello, M., D'Isanto, M., Peluso, L. & Galdiero, M. (2001b) Induction of tyrosine phosphorylated proteins in THP-1 cells by Salmonella typhimurium, Pasteurella haemolytica and Haemophilus influenzae porins. *FEMS Immunology and Medical Microbiology*, Vol.31, No.2, pp.121-130.

Galdiero, M., Vitiello, M., Sanzari, E., D'Isanto, M., Tortora, A., Longanella, A. & Galdiero, S. (2002) Porins from Salmonella enterica serovar Typhimurium activate the transcription factors activating protein 1 and NF-kappaB through the Raf-1-mitogen-activated protein kinase cascade. *Infection and Immunity*, Vol.70, No.2, pp.558-568.

Galdiero, M., D'Isanto, M., Vitiello, M., Finamore, E., Peluso, L. & Galdiero, M. (2003a) Monocyte activation of protein-tyrosine-kinase, protein kinase A and protein kinase C induced by porins isolated from Salmonella enterica serovar Typhimurium. *Journal of Infection*, Vol.46, pp.111-119.

Galdiero, M., Vitiello, M. & Galdiero S. (2003b) Eukaryotic cell signaling and transcriptional activation induced by bacterial porins. *FEMS Microbiology Letters*, Vol.226, No.1, pp.57-64.

Galdiero, S., Capasso, D., Vitiello, M., D'Isanto, M., Pedone, C. & Galdiero, M. (2003c) Role of surface-exposed loops of Haemophilus influenzae protein P2 in the mitogen-activated protein kinase cascade. *Infection and Immunity*, Vol.71, No.5, pp.2798-2809.

Galdiero, S., Vitello, M., Amodeo, P., D'Isanto, M., Cantisani, M., Pedone, C. & Galdiero, M. (2006) Structural requirements for proinflammatory activity of porin P2 Loop 7 from Haemophilus influenzae. *Biochemistry*, Vol.45, No.14, pp.4491- 4501.

Galdiero, S., Galdiero, M. & Pedone C. (2007). β-barrel membrane bacterial proteins: structure, function, assembly and interaction with lipids. *Current Protein & Peptide Science*, Vol.8, (No.1) pp.63-82.

Greenman, R.L., Schein, R.M., Martin, M.A., Wenzel, R.P., MacIntyre, N.R., Emmanuel, G., Chmel, H., Kohler, R.B., McCarthy, M., Plouffe, J., et al. (1991) A controlled clinical trial of E5 murine monoclonal IgM antibody to endotoxin in the treatment of gram-negative sepsis. The XOMA Sepsis Study Group. *JAMA*, Vol.266, No.8, pp.1097-1102.

Gupta, S., Kumar, D., Vohra, H. & Ganguly, N.K. (1999) Involvement of signal transduction pathways in Salmonella typhimurium porin activated gut macrophages. *Molecular and Cellular Biochemistry*, Vol.194, No.1-2, pp.235-243.

Haase, E. M., Yi, K., Morse, G. D. & Murphy, T. F. (1994) Mapping of bactericidal epitopes on the P2 porin protein of nontypeable Haemophilus influenzae. *Infection and Immunity*, Vol.62, No.9, pp.3712-3722.

Hellman, J., Loiselle, P.M., Tehan, M.M., Allaire, J.E., Boyle, L.A., Kurnick, J.T., Andrews, Sik, D.M., Kim, K. & Warren, H.S. (2000) Outer membrane protein A, peptidoglycan-associated lipoprotein, and murein lipoprotein are released by Escherichia coli bacteria into serum. *Infection and Immunity*, Vol.68, No.5, pp.2566-2572.

Hellman, J., Roberts, J.D., Tehan, M.M. Allaire, J.E. & Warren, H.S. (2002) Bacterial peptidoglycan-associated lipoprotein is released into the bloodstream in gram-negative sepsis and causes inflammation and death in mice. *The Journal of Biological Chemistry*, Vol. 277, No.16, pp. 14274-14280.

Hindennach, I. & Henning, U. (1975) The major proteins of Escherichia coli outer cell envelope membrane preparative isolation of all major membrane proteins. *European Journal of Biochemistry*, Vol.59, No.1, pp.207-213.

Hitchcock, P. J., & Morrison, D. C. (1984) The protein component of bacterial endotoxins, pp. 339-374. In E. T. Rietschel (ed.), Handbook of endotoxin, vol. 1. Chemistry of endotoxin. Elsevier/North-Holland Publishing Co., Amsterdam.

Hofstra, H. & Dankert, J. (1979) Antigenic cross-reactivity of major outer membrane proteins in Enterobacteriaceae species. *Journal General Microbiology*, Vol.111, No.2, pp.293-302.

Hofstra, H., Van Tol, M.J.D. & Dankert, J. (1980) Cross-reactivity of major outer membrane proteins of Enterobacteriaceae, studied by crossed immunoelectrophoresis. *Journal of Bacteriology*, Vol.143, No.1, pp.328-337.

Hughes, E.E., Gilleland, L.B. & Gilleland, H.E.jr (1992) Synthetic peptides representing epitopes of outer membrane protein F of Pseudomonas aeruginosa that elicit antibodies reactive with whole cells of heterologous immunotype strains of P. aeruginosa. *Infection and Immunity*, Vol. 60, No.9, pp.3497-3503.

Jolley, K.A., Appleby, L., Wright, J.C., Christodoulides, M. & Heckels, J.E. (2001) Immunization with recombinant Opc outer membrane protein from Neisseria meningitides: influence of sequence variation and levels of expression on the bactericidal immune response against meningococci. *Infection and Immunity*, Vol.69, No.6, pp.3809-3916.

Kamalakkannan, S., Murugan, V., Jagannadham, M.V., Nagaraj, R. & Sankaran, K. (2004) Bacterial lipid modification of proteins for novel protein engineering applications. *Protein Engineering Design Selection*, Vol.17, No.10, pp.721-729.

Karin, M., Liu, Z. & Zandi, E. (1997) AP-1 function and regulation. *Current Opinion Cell Biology*, Vol.9, No.2, pp.240-246.

Kim, K.S. (2002) Strategy of Escherichia coli for crossing the blood-brain barrier. *The Journal of Infection Disease*, Vol.186, Suppl 2, pp.S220-224.

Kovacs-Simon, A., Titball, R.W., Michell, S.L. (2011) Lipoproteins of bacterial pathogens. *Infection and Immunity*, Vol79, No.2, pp548-561.

Kulp, A. & Kuehn, M.J. (2010) Biological functions and biogenesis of secreted bacterial outer membrane vesicles. *Annual Review Microbiology*, Vol.64, pp.163-84.

Lazaron, V. & Barke, R.A. (1999) Gram-negative bacterial sepsis and the sepsis syndrome. *Urologic Clinics of North America*, Vol.26, No.4, pp.687-699.

Li, S., & Sedivy, J.M. (1993) Raf-1 protein kinase activates the NFkappa B transcription factor by dissociating the cytoplasmic NFkappa B-I kappa B complex. *Proceedings of the National Academy of Sciences USA*, Vol.90, pp.9247-9251.

Liang, M.D., Bagchi, A., Warren, H. S. Tehan M.M., Trigilio J.A., Beasley-Topliffe L.K., Tesini B.L., Lazzaroni J.C., Fenton M.J. & Hellman J. (2005) Bacterial peptidoglycan-associated lipoprotein: a naturally occurring toll-like receptor 2 agonist that is shed into serum and has synergy with lipolysacchardide. The *Journal of Infectious Disease*, Vol.191, No.6, pp.939-948.

Maiden, M.C.S., Suker, J., Mekema, A.S., Buggraves, J.A. & Feavers, I.M. (1991) Comparison of the class 1 outer membrane proteins of eight serological reference strains of Neisseria meningitidis *Molecular Microbiology* Vol.5 , No.3, pp.727-736.

Mangan, D.F., Wahl, S.M., Sultzer, B.M. & Mergenhagen, S.E. (1992) Stimulation of Human monocytes by endotoxin-associated protein: inhibition of programmed cell death (apoptosis) and potential significance in adjuvanticity. *Infection and Immunity* Vol.60, No.4, pp.1684-1686.

Maruvada, R. & Kim, K. S. (2011) Extracellular loops of the Escherichia coli outer membrane protein A contribute to the pathogenesis of meningitis. *The Journal of Infectious Diseases*, Vol. 203, No.1, pp.131-140.

Masignani, V., Comanducci, M., Giuliani, M.M., Bambini, S., Adu-Bobie, J., Arico, B., Brunelli, A., Pieri, A., Santini, L., Savino, S., Serruto, D., Litt, D., Kroll, S., Welsch, J.A., Granoff, D.M., Rappuoli, R. & Pizza, M. (2003) Vaccination against Neisseria meningitidis using three variants of the lipoprotein GNA1870. *Journal Experimental Medicine*, Vol. 197, No.6, pp.789-799.

Massari, P., Ram, S., Macleod, H., & Wetzler, L.M. (2003) The role of porins in neisserial pathogenesis and immunity. *Trends Microbiology*, Vol.11, No.2, pp.87-93.

Mittal, R., Krishnan, S., Gonzalez-Gomez, I. & Prasadarao, N.V. (2011) Deciphering the roles of outer membrane protein A extracellular loops in the pathogenesis of Escherichia coli K1 meningitis. *Journal of Biological Chemistry*, Vol.286, No.3, pp.2183-2193.

Narita, S., Matsuyama, S. & Tokuda, H. 2004. Lipoprotein trafficking in Escherichia coli. *Archives Microbiology*, Vol.182, No.1, pp.1-6.

Neary, J. M., Yi, K., Karalus, R. J. & Murphy, T. F. (2001) Antibodies to loop 6 of the P2 porin protein of nontypeable Haemophilus influenzae are bactericidal against multiple strains. *Infection and Immunity*, Vol.69, No.2, pp.773-778.

Nikaido H. (2003) Molecular basis of bacterial outer membrane permeability revisited. *Microbiology and Molecular Biology Reviews*, Vol.67, No.4, pp.593-656.

Prasadarao, N.V., Wass, C.A., Weiser, J.N., Stins, M.F., Huang, S.H. & Kim, K.S. (1996) Outer membrane protein A of Escherichia coli contributes to invasion of brain microvascular endothelial cells. *Infection and Immunity*, Vol.64, No.1, pp.146-153.

Rawadi, G. & Roman-Roman, S. (1996) Mycoplasma membrane lipoproteins induced proinflammatory cytokines by a mechanism distinct from that of lipopolysaccharide. *Infection and Immunity*, Vol.64, No.2, pp.637-643.

Reddi, K., Poole, S., Nair, S., Meghji, S., Henderson, B. & Wilson, M. (1995) Lipid A-associated proteins from periodontopathogenic bacteria induce interleukin-6 production by human gingival fibroblasts and monocytes. *FEMS Microbiology Immunology*, Vol.11, No.2, pp.137–144.

Rosenshine, I., Donnenberg, M.S., Kaper, J.B. & Finlay, B.B. (1992) Signal transduction between enteropathogenic Escherichia coli (EPEC) and epithelial cells: EPEC induces tyrosine phosphorylation of host cell proteins to initiate cytoskeletal rearrangement and bacterial uptake. *EMBO Journal*, Vol.11, No.10, pp.3551-3560.

Schild, S., Nelson, E.J. & Camilli, A. (2008) Immunization with Vibrio cholerae outer membrane vesicles induces protective immunity in mice. *Infection and Immunity*, Vol.76, No.10, pp.4554-63.

Schulz, G.E. (2002) The structure of bacterial outer membrane proteins. *Biochimica Biophysica Acta*, Vol.1565, No.2, pp.308-17.

Siber, G.R., Kania, S.A. & Warren, H.S. (1985) Cross-reactivity of rabbit antibodies to lipopolysaccharides of Escherichia coli J5 and other gram-negative bacteria. *Journal of Infectious Disease*, Vol.152, No.5, pp.954-64.

Smith, S.G.J., Mahon, V., Lambert, M.A. & Fagan, R.P. (2007) A molecular Swiss army knife: OmpA structure, function and expression. *FEMS Microbiology Letters*, Vol.273, No.1, pp.1-11.

Thompson, E.A., Feavers, I.M. & Maiden, M.C. (2003) Antigenic diversity of meningococcal enterobactin receptor FetA, a vaccine component. *Microbiology*, Vol.149, No.7, pp.1849-1858.

Tufano, M.A., Capasso, G., Anastasio, P., Giordano, D.R., Giordano, D., Galdiero, E., Sommese, L. & De Santo, N.G. (1987) Clearance studies on the renal action of porins extracted from Salmonella typhimurium. *International Journal Pediatric Nephrology*, Vol.8, No.4, pp.193–198.

Van der Ley, P., Heckels, J.E., Virji, M., Hoogerhout, P. & Poolman, J.T. (1991) Topology of outer membrane porins in pathogenic Neisseria spp. *Infection and Immunity*, Vol.59, No.9, pp.2963-2971.

Vitiello, M., Galdiero, S., D'Isanto, M., D'Amico, M., Di Filippo, C., Cantisani, M., Galdiero, M. & Pedone, C. (2008) Pathophysiological changes of gram-negative bacterial infection can be reproduced by a synthetic peptide mimicking loop L7 sequence of Haemophilus influenzae porin. *Microbes and Infections*, Vol.10, No.6, pp.657-663.

Von Andrian, U.H., Chambers, J.D., McEvoy, L., Bargatze, R.F., arfors, K.E. & Butcher, E. C. (1991) A two step model of leukocyte-endothelial cell interaction in inflammation: distinct roles for LECAM-1 and the leukocyte b2 integrins in vivo. *Proceedings of the National Academy of Sciences USA*, Vol.88, No.17, pp.7538-7542.

Weinstein, S.L., Sanghera, J.S., Lemke, K., DeFranco, A.L. & Pelech, S.L. (1992) Bacterial lipopolysaccharide induces tyrosine phosphorylation and activation of mitogen-activated protein kinases in macrophages. *Journal Biological Chemistry*, Vol.267, No.21, pp.14955-14962.

Westphal, O., Luderitz, O. & Bister, F. (1952) Uber die extraktion von bacterien mit phenol/wasser. *Naturforsch,* Vol.7, pp.148–156.

Wright, J.C., Williams, J.N., Christodoulides, M. & Heckels, J.E. (2002) Immunization with recombinant PorB outer membrane protein induces a bactericidal immune response against Neisseria meningitides. *Infection and Immunity,* Vol.70, No.8, pp.4028-4034.

Yi, K. & Murphy, T. F. (1997) Importance of an immunodominant surface-exposed loop on outer membrane protein P2 of nontypeable Haemophilus influenzae. *Infection and Immunity*, Vol.65, No.1, pp.150-155.

Zhang, H., Peterson, J.W., Niesel, D.W. &Klimpel, G.R. (1997) Bacterial lipoprotein and lipopolysaccharide act synergistically to induce lethal shock and proinflammatory cytokine production. *Journal of Immunology*, Vol.159, No.10, pp.4868-78.

Part 3

Pathological Findings

4

The Autopsy Pathology of Sepsis-Related Death

Sebastian Lucas
Dept of Histopathology
KCL School of Medicine
St Thomas' Hospital
London
UK

1. Introduction

Sepsis is defined as infection plus systemic manifestations of infection (Dellinger.R.P. et al. 2008). Thus it is more than just the local organ pathology damage, and indicates malfunction of one or more other critical organs. There are few systematic reviews of what autopsy can contribute to sepsis studies, so this chapter attempts to summarise the main pathological concepts around sepsis with particular focus on diagnostic features - gross and histopathological - and differential diagnosis. The focus is information for practising pathologists. Currently, detailed non-forensic autopsy practice seems to have fewer enthusiasts than heretofore, and the case is made that in sepsis-related fatality, there is much to observe and learn. This chapter is a revision of an article on the autopsy and sepsis published in 2007 (Lucas 2007).

Autopsy pathologists not infrequently use the term 'septicaemia' (implying blood infection) as the final process causing death, implying that there was bacteraemia - hopefully proven but sometimes assumed - associated with one or more organ failures. This is an uneasy combination of clinical, laboratory and gross pathological features, because:

1. there are no specific morbid anatomical features of 'septicaemia'
    - the historical 'diffluent' or 'septic' spleen is a debatable gross entity (Arismendi-Morrillo et al. 2004)
    - 'shock lung' and 'acute tubular necrosis' are difficult to diagnose on gross examination alone
2. the interpretation of pre-mortem, let alone post-mortem, blood cultures is not easy (Morris, Harrison, & Partridge 2006)
3. there are no standard histopathological features that reliably point to 'septicaemia'
4. there is no agreed case definition of 'septicaemia'.

It is more logical to consider 'sepsis': its local origins, systemic consequences, and degrees of severity.

Within intensive care units (ICU), where most patients with severe sepsis are cared for (Dellinger et al. 2004), autopsy analysis still reveals previously unknown diagnoses that could, if treated differently, have altered the outcome; and this despite the panoply of investigative procedures now available to modern ICU medicine. From the 21st century, a USA study (Roosen et al. 2000) found 16% Goldman class 1 discrepancies (ie missed opportunity to change therapy and prolong survival (Goldman et al. 1983)), and fungal infections were notably under-diagnosed pre-mortem. In a recent French study (Combes et al. 2004) 32% of autopsies showed Goldman class 1 or 2 discrepancies, particularly among the immuno-compromised patients. The diseases missed included cancer, stroke, myocardial infarction, endocarditis, and pulmonary embolism. A British study (Perkins et al. 2003) noted that only 7.7% of ICU deaths underwent autopsy, and found similar discrepancy patterns to the French study. What few of these studies address is the precise contribution of sepsis and its management to death, although severe sepsis is noted to be both under- and over-diagnosed pre-mortem (Blosser, Zimmerman, & Stauffer 1998) (Perkins, McAuley, Davies, & Gao 2003).

1.1 The role of the autopsy in sepsis

What can autopsy pathology - and pre-mortem cellular pathology - contribute to improving the care and outcomes of sepsis patients? There are three main categories of positive contribution:

1. assisting in diagnosis pre-mortem, through tissue examination (histopathology and cytopathology (Schnadig, Molina, & Aronson 2007))
2. evaluating dead patients for actual clinico-pathological outcomes
    - confirming or refuting pre-mortem diagnoses
    - including potential complications of intensive care
    - identifying co-morbidities that affected recovery
3. providing this information back to clinicians and IC units as monitoring and audit in order to feed into improving future managements

The 2008 revision of the clinical Recommendations for Surviving Sepsis Campaign (Dellinger.R.P., Levy, Carlet, & et al 2008) can be scrutinized against possible contributions of pathology. For several of the Recommendations, autopsy pathology investigations can contribute nothing specifically:

1. Initial Resuscitation
2. Glucose Control
3. Renal Replacement
4. Bicarbonate Therapy
5. Selective Digestive Tract Decontamination
6. Consideration of Limitation of Support

But for the other Recommendations, autopsy pathology can contribute significantly to the evaluation in their efficacy and complications:

1. Diagnosis - of infections and co-morbidities
2. Antibiotic Therapy - effectiveness of therapy, and potential toxic complications of therapy
3. Source Control - as with Diagnosis of infections
4. Fluid Therapy - overload, underperfusion
5. Vasopressors & Inotrope Therapies - complications such as cardio-toxicity
6. Corticosteroids - complications including opportunistic infections6
7. Recombinant Activated Protein C - haemorrhagic complications
8. Blood Product Administration - identification of Transfusion Associated Lung Injury (TRALI)
9. Mechanical Ventilation of acute lung injury - the impact of tidal volume and O2 concentration on alveolar membranes

10. Extracorporeal Membrane Oxygenation (ECMO) - its contribution to lung pathology (eg aspergillosis)
11. Sedation - the issue of possible morphine toxicity
12. Deep Vein Thrombosis Prophylaxis - its efficacy
13. Gastric Stress Prophylaxis - its efficacy

2. Epidemiology

Epidemiologically, the incidence of severe sepsis (as defined below) in industrialised countries is 50-95 cases per 100,000 population and is rising by up to 9% each year, for reasons still unexplained. It accounts for 2% of hospital admissions in the USA, affecting about 700,000 people per year, causing death in 210,000; and is the tenth leading cause of death (Annane, Bellisant, & Cavaillon 2005) (Riederman, Guo, & Ward 2003) (Danai & Martin 2005) (Lever & Mackenzie 2007).

3. Clinical case definitions

As a result of consensus meetings in the early 1990s- intended to improve not only patient management but also the comparability of clinical trials in intensive care unit settings (ICU) - there are agreed clinical case definitions of sepsis, including severity and organ syndromes (see Table 1) (Riederman, Guo, & Ward 2003) (Levy & et al 1992). The recognition of the systemic inflammatory response syndrome (SIRS) is central to the definitions.

Diagnosis	Definition
SIRS (systemic inflammatory response syndrome)	Temperature >38 deg C or <36 deg C Heart rate >90/min Systolic blood pressure <90mmHg Respiratory rate >20/min or $PaCO_2$ <32mmHg Blood white cell count >$12x10^9$/L or <$4x10^9$/L, or >10% immature band forms.
Sepsis	Systemic response to infection, as manifested by two of more of the above list (ie SIRS + infection).
Severe sepsis	Sepsis with associated organ dysfunction, hypoperfusion, or hypotension including lactic acidosis, oliguria, or acute alteration in mental state.
Septic shock	Sepsis-induced hypotension despite adequate fluid resuscitation, along with presence of severe sepsis.
MODS (Multiple organ dysfunction syndrome)	The presence of altered organ function in an acutely ill patient such that homeostasis cannot be maintained without intervention.

Table 1. Clinical definitions of sepsis

The six most common sites of infection associated with sepsis are pneumonia, blood stream infections (including infective endocarditis), intravascular catheter-related sepsis, intra-abdominal infections, urological sepsis, and surgical wound infections. Florid septic shock syndromes also arise post-delivery, from necrotising fasciitis, and menstrual toxic shock syndrome (see Table 2).

Syndrome	Clinical features
Meningococcal (*Neisseria meningitidis*) bacteraemic shock	Disseminated intravascular coagulation prominent Haemorrhagic rash (see Figs 2 & 3) Mortality = 10-20%
Staphylococcal (*S.aureus*) toxic shock syndrome	Menstrual (tampon-related) Non-menstrual Skin wounds, surgical wounds Pneumonia Catheter infections Mortality = 5%
Streptococcal (group A) toxic shock syndrome	Deep seated infections Necrotising fasciitis Surgical operation sites Puerperal sepsis Mortality = 50%

Table 2. The three most severe fulminant and toxic shock syndromes (TSS) and some of their characteristics (Munford 2005) (Moreillon, Que, & Glauser 2005) (Bisno & Stevens 2005).

The staphylococcal and streptococcal TSS have a rapid onset because the bacteria secrete superantigens which directly activate T-cells, with release of much TNFα, and a rapid cytokine storm.

Further consensus meetings have arrived at agreed organ-specific case definitions, with emphasis on the stringency of the clinical characteristics and the microbiological investigations (Calandra, Cohen, & et al 2005). Table 3 indicates that for pneumonia.

4. Infections causing sepsis

The spectrum of infections has changed. In the 1970-80s, gram-negative bacteria predominated. But in the 21st century, the in-hospital case pattern is (Annane, Bellisant, & Cavaillon 2005) (van der Poll.T & Opal 2008):

- 25-30% gram-negative infections
- 30-50% gram-positive infections
- 25% polymicrobial infections
- 25% multi-drug resistant organisms (eg MRSA and fungi)
- 2-4% viral and parasitic infections (but probably underestimated) including malaria
    - eg HHV8/HIV co-infection (Fowler et al. 2006)
- ~30% negative cultures: community-acquired sepsis treated with antibiotics before admission; and higher rates of negative cultures reported in neutropaenic sepsis.
- *Mycobacterium tuberculosis*, particularly when it is anergic pattern due to host immunosuppression (see Figs 12 & 13).

Level of Certainty	Definition
Microbiologically confirmed (ie definite)	• New or progressive radiological infiltrate • Clinical suspicion of pneumonia, or a Clinical Pulmonary Infection Score (CPIS) =>6; this six-feature scale includes identification of bacteria on gram stain of lower respiratory tract samples. • Identification of a pathogen - one or more of the following categories: a. Uncontaminated sample (blood, pleural fluid, transthoracic or transtracheal aspirate b. Respiratory secretions, not a pathogen that colonises the upper airways a. A likely pathogen using quantitative cultures of lower respiratory tract samples b. Positive infection serology
Probable	Clinically as above, but the identification of a pathogen is a. Below the diagnostic threshold, or b. Negative within 72 hours of starting a new antibiotic regime
Possible	Abnormal chest radiograph of uncertain cause in a patient with moderate or low suspicion of pneumonia, but with microbiological or serological evidence of definite or probable pneumonia (as defined above).

Table 3. Pneumonia case definitions

The purpose of detailing these clinical case definitions is to contrast them with the morbid anatomical features of sepsis, which are less well depicted. Pathologists can assist clinical colleagues in evaluating patients dying of known or suspected sepsis, proving sepsis or identifying the differential diagnoses. They could thereby more usefully contribute to audit and the evaluation of novel therapies in sepsis.

5. Pathogenesis of the sepsis syndromes

SIRS is characterised as 'an abnormal generalised inflammatory reaction in organs remote from the initial insult' (Munford 2005). SIRS can result from non-infective causes, such as trauma, pancreatitis and cardiac-bypass procedures, and the pathologist needs to bear this in mind when evaluating deaths presented as '?sepsis'.

Enormous research has gone into identifying the pathogenesis of the remote organ damage that characterises severe sepsis; three recent reviews (Munford 2005) (Calandra, Cohen, & et al 2005) (Annane, Bellisant, & Cavaillon 2005) (van der Poll.T & Opal 2008) (Lever & Mackenzie 2007) emphasise how much we do not understand.

In brief, infections trigger a cytokine cascade via Toll-like receptors on inflammatory cells, with the excess secretion of many pro-inflammatory mediators including IL-1, TNFα, IL-6, nitric oxide (NO), platelet activating factor (PAF) (Mitchell 2005). Systemically, these affect organ function via damage to epithelia and endothelial cells (with abnormal microcirculation), inflammatory cell infiltration, initiation of the coagulation system, endocrine stimulation, and activation of the autonomic nervous system. The microbial triggers include endotoxin (lipopolysaccharide) in gram-negative bacilli and superantigens in gram-positive cocci. The cholinergic nervous system appears to be important in that it suppresses the production of pro-inflammatory cytokines (van der Poll.T & Opal 2008).

Modern thinking is that in the early phase of SIRS, the response is balanced and with elimination of the infection, there can be full recovery. But if the response is unbalanced, with over-production of inflammatory cytokines, the outcome is less good: acute organ dysfunction can result in early death; and if the lymphopaenia phase is associated with immune suppression (see below), then opportunistic infections contribute to the worsening mortality rates.

Two underlying processes have been more recently highlighted in severe sepsis:

i. there is apoptosis of lymphocytes in the spleen and gut (Hotchkiss et al. 1999). It is hypothesised that this leads to impairment of immune responses in sepsis, following the acute phase (van der Poll.T & Opal 2008).
ii. organ failure is not always from observable necrosis and/or fibrosis (ie structural) but is functional. There is reduction in cellular mitochondrial activity, and this 'hibernation' may be a protective response (Singer et al. 2004) (Levy et al. 2005).

There are significant controversies, including:

1. the significance of bacteraemia: does this trigger severe sepsis, or is it a transient leakage phenomenon, and contribute little, per se, to outcome?
2. the continuum of the sepsis syndromes: is this a true final common path, independent of the actual initiating infection? Or do different infection-host interactions produce severe sepsis and septic shock through different mechanisms? (Munford 2005).
3. the concept that a major determining factor in patient outcome, for any given aetiology and set of co-morbidities, is not the particular therapy in ICU but the individual's genetic make up (Annane, Bellisant, & Cavaillon 2005) (Villar et al. 2004)?
4. The contribution of virulence factors in outcomes of sepsis (van der Poll.T & Opal 2008)
5. it is not always evident grossly and histologically why patients with sepsis have died. A new paradigm is needed (Hotchkiss, Swanson, Freeman, & et al 1999).

6. Autopsy protocols

In the UK, >95% of adult autopsies are performed for a coroner, or (in Scotland) a procurator fiscal, under medico-legal conditions. Since the basic remit of the medico-legal autopsy is to exclude unnatural or violent death, and, if possible, to avoid having an inquest (National Confidential Enquiry into Patient Outcome and Death 2006), the level of detail of examination of cases that may have a sepsis syndrome is varied. Often the autopsy does not address the questions raised by the clinical course of the patient with sepsis. In this brief review, there is no attempt to address the requirements of what coroners might want from pathologists in '?sepsis' cases.

7. Microbiology sampling

One of the problems in the septic autopsy is the lack of agreed methods of sampling blood, tissues and other fluids so that

- Contamination from other organs is minimised
- The consequences of the post-mortem spread of gut flora bacteria into the blood and tissues is minimised (Morris, Harrison, & Partridge 2006)

Also there are no agreed strategies of what to sample for each clinico-pathological-microbiological scenario. In all cases, doing the sampling as soon after death as logistically feasible reduces the problems in the interpretation of bacterial culture results. See Table 4 for interim recommended practice.

Tissue	Sampling method
Cerebrospinal fluid	With syringe and needle through alcohol-cleaned skin, through either or both of: • Cisternal puncture (posterior neck below the occipital protruberance; aim anteriorly for the eyes) • Lumbar puncture (between L4-5)
Urine	Syringe and needle through cleaned suprapubic skin
Blood	Cardiac puncture blood, through the left 4th intercostals space, or peripheral venous blood • Subclavian vein (above clavicle), or • once the body is opened and before any organs opened or removed (particularly the intestines), tie off an iliac vein proximally, insert syringe needle pointing distally and withdraw 10 ml blood. Inoculate 5 ml into each of aerobe and anaerobe blood culture bottles.
Cardiac vegetations	Divide between a sterile bottle for culture and histopathology.
Lung tissue	Attempts to sterilise the outer surface are probably futile. A compromise is to cut the lung with a clean organ-slicing blade on a clean surface and sample the relevant areas with a sterile scalpel blade.

Table 4. Sampling autopsy tissues for microbiological culture

7.1 Interpretation of bacteriological cultures

In all cases, the microbiology department must be advised what range of organisms is being sought; culture set-ups and molecular diagnostic techniques vary accordingly. Interpretation of positive results is often difficult, and consultation with an experienced microbiologist is critical. In cultures, confidence that the identified organism is significant is appropriate if there is *Mycobacterium tuberculosis, Streptococcus* group A (pyogenes), *Streptococcus pneumoniae,* or *Neisseria meningitides* since these are most unlikely to be present incidentally or from contamination.

The introduction of the new molecular sepsis assay technologies for the rapid, sensitive and specific identification of bacterial species in blood and other samples may change much of this (Tissari et al. 2010). They have yet to be introduced into autopsy-related practice, and it will be important to determine whether they make simpler or more complicated the interpretation of post-mortem blood cultures.

8. Non-microbiological means of identifying severe sepsis

In many cases at autopsy, the need to confirm or exclude sepsis happens without positive microbiology, either because all attempts (including pre-mortem) were negative (perhaps due to anti-microbial chemotherapy), or because samples were not taken at all. Where histological evidence of pyogenic infection with definite bacteria or fungi is present, this can indicate the organ-site of the sepsis.

If no infection is identified, there is an immunocytochemical technique that may assist. In SIRS, endothelial cells are upregulated, and express cell more adhesion molecules such as ICAM-1 (intercellular adhesion molecule-1; CD54) and E-selectin (CD62E). It is possible to immunostain for these (Fig 1) and at least one author holds that positive ICAM-1 staining of alveolar capillary endothelial cells indicates septic shock with high sensitivity and specificity (Tsokos 2003).

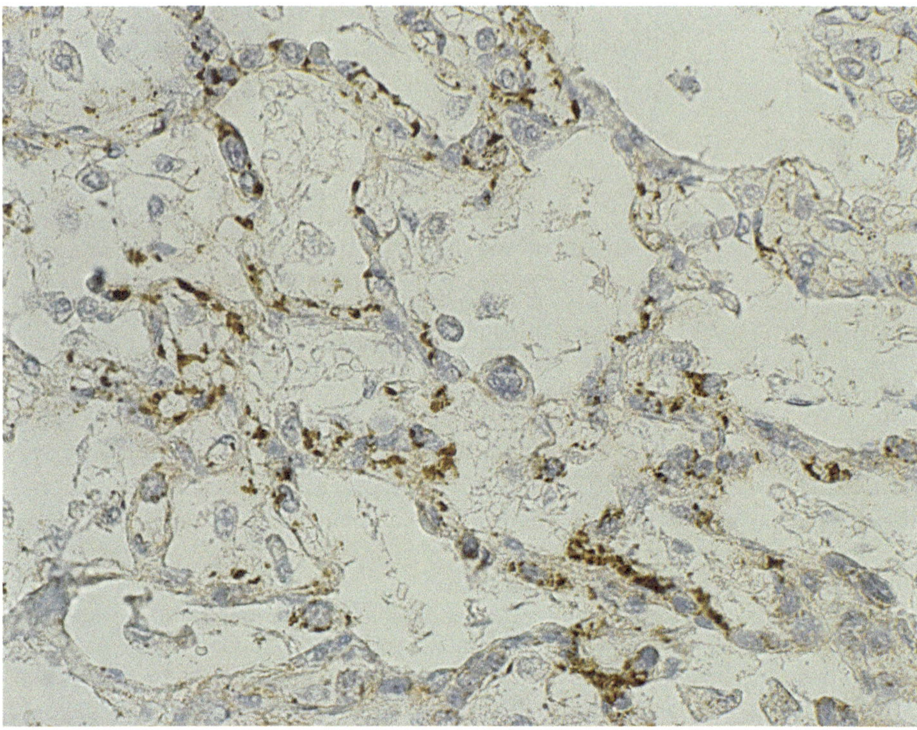

Fig. 1. Lung in septic shock, stained for CD54, showing endothelial cell (EC) upregulation (normal lung ECs do not stain).

There are suggestive reports on the estimation of post-mortem serum endotoxin level as an indicator of sepsis (Zhu et al. 2005).

9. Simulators of septic shock

Patients with clinical manifestations similar to those of septic shock come to ICU and die despite empirical therapy. The differential diagnosis includes

- Disseminated cancer, including carcinoma and lymphoma. For example, pulmonary micro-emboli from an occult carcinoma can obstruct pulmonary arterioles and cause cardio-respiratory failure (Hirata et al. 1988).

- Haemophagocytic syndrome
- HHV8-associated multicentric Castleman disease syndrome in HIV-infected persons (Stebbing et al. 2011)
- Thrombotic microangiopathy syndromes
- Other conditions that mimic SIRS, but not considered in more detail (Munford 2005)
  - Multi-organ atherosclerosis, NO expression being a common factor
  - Burns
  - Adrenal insufficiency
  - Thyroid storm
  - Major trauma
  - Pancreatitis
  - Cardio-pulmonary bypass
  - Drug hypersensitivity reaction and acute anaphylaxis
  - Malignant hyperthermia and heat stroke

10. Specific organs at autopsy

The organ pathology of sepsis comprises gross and histopathological lesions. The histopathological lesions can often identify a specific infection, or at least point to a limited range of possible infectious agents (Table 5). 'Pathology' is, essentially, the study of host reaction to injury. Thus in the diagnosis of sepsis there are the two complementary pathways for evaluating infectious disease:

1. the gross pathology
2. the microscopic pathology (histopathology and cytopathology), which is subdivided into:
   - identification and quantification of infectious agents
   - categorising the host inflammatory reaction, or absence of reaction

Considering acute host inflammatory reactions, they can be considered as shown in Table 5.

10.1 Heart

The syndrome of sepsis-related myocardial dysfunction includes reduced left and right ejection fractions and elevated heart rate (Table 6) (Munford 2005). There is evidence of apoptotic damage to cardiac myofibres in the rodent model of sepsis (Ha et al. 2006). But the clinical experience of patients surviving sepsis is that there is no evidence of persistent cardiac defects attributable to such a process. Presumably, the dysfunction is cytokine driven and reversible (Levy, Piel, ACton, & et al 2005). The heart in autopsied non-survivors shows prominent interstitial mononuclear cells - this is not myocarditis but mainly enlargement of capillary endothelial cells, as part of the generalised endothelial up-regulation phenomenon.

Given the generally old age of patients admitted to ICU with sepsis, many will have coronary artery disease, with or without previous myocardial infarction, at autopsy. The extent to which this contributes (if at all) to death needs to be carefully considered in the context of the whole case. The Davies scale of certainty for ischaemic heart disease death (although designed for sudden cardiac death in the community) is a bench-mark from which to work (Royal College of Pathologists 2005). Nothing irritates ICU clinicians more than to be told that the cause of death was 'ischaemic heart disease' in a complex case of

Pattern of inflammation	**Quantity of infectious agent**	**Example**
Haemorrhage only	- to +++	Anthrax, streptococcal skin rash
Minimal inflammation	+++	Neutropaenic sepsis (many bacteria types, including anergic tuberculosis)
Usual acute inflammation	- to +++	Pneumococcus, other streptococci, gram-ve bacilli, anergic tuberculosis
No inflammation; vasculopathy and necrosis	+++	*Pseudomonas* vasculitis, toxoplasmosis
Necrosis and inclusion bodies (intranuclear and/or intracytoplasmic)	+ to +++	Virus infections: herpes, Ebola
Mixed granulomatous and acute inflamation	- to +++	Melioidosis, tularaemia, typhoid
Chronic inflammation	- to +	Chagas' disease
Necrosis, no inflammation	+++	*Strep.pyogenes* (necrotising fasciitis), *Clostridium perfringens*, leptospirosis
Vasculitis and thrombosis	+ to +++	Pseudomonas, meningococcus (Fig 2,3)
Botryomycosis	+++	*Staphylococcus aureus*
No inflammation, parasites in vessels	+ to +++	Malaria

Table 5. Some consistent patterns of inflammation associated with particular infections

multi-organ failure and sepsis. If the patient was part of a therapeutic protocol trial, it is even more unfortunate, as the aspects of apparent therapy failure will be mis-apportioned.

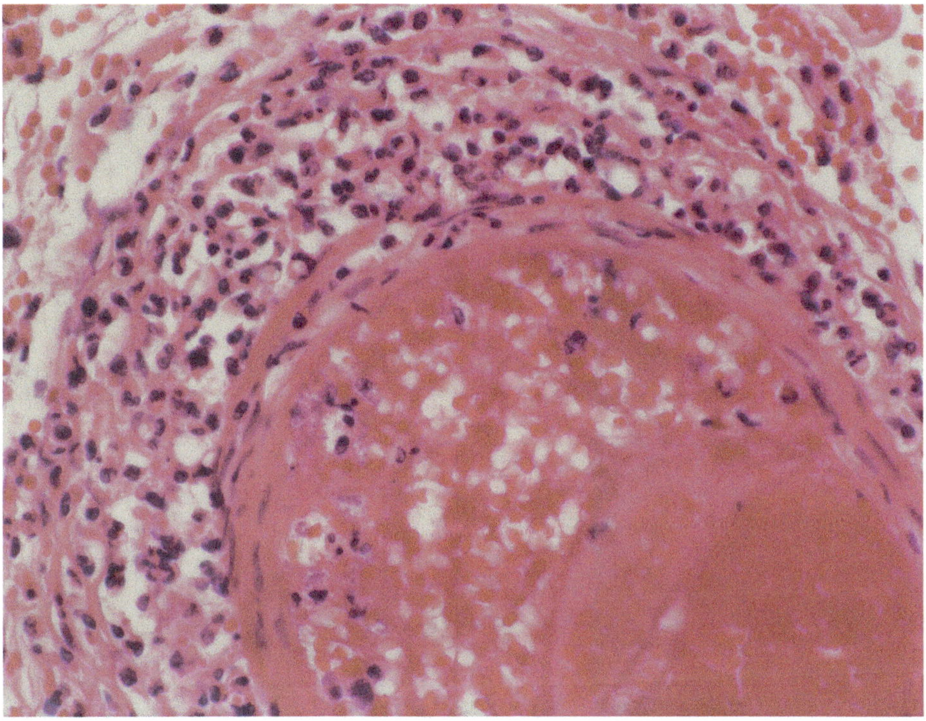

Fig. 2. Skin in a fatal case of meningococcal sepsis. The artery is vasculitic and thrombosed (H&E)

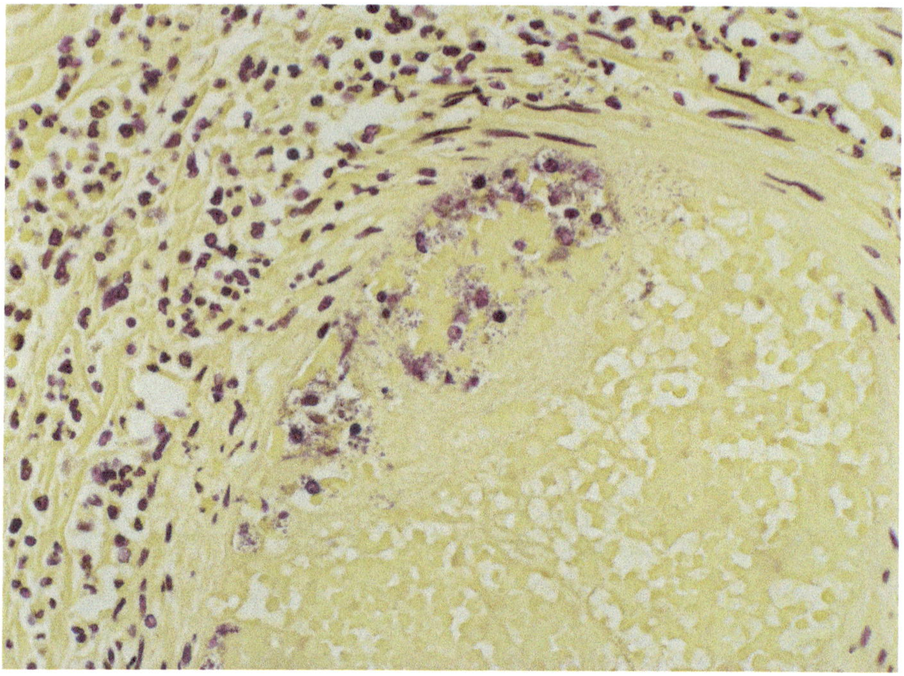

Fig. 3. Same vessel as in Fig 2, stained with Brown-Hopps gram stain, to demonstrate gram-ve cocci in the lumen and endothelium

	Ischaemic Necrosis (atonic fibres)	Contraction band necrosis (hyper-contracted fibres)	Interstitial inflammation	Myocarditis	Interstitial haemorrhage
Myocardial Infarction	+	-	-	-	+
Re-perfusion Injury	+	+	-	-	+
Inotropes & cocaine	+	+	-	-	-
Sepsis	+/-	-	+	+/-	+
Infective endocarditis	+/-	-	+	+	-
Cardio-pulmonary resuscitation	+	+	-	-	+

Table 6. Cardiac pathologies encountered in ICU patients and sepsis syndromes (Baroldi 2006) ; (Nishida et al. 2006)

10.1.1 Heart examination

Given the subtle nature of cardiac lesions in sepsis and its treatment, there is an argument for proper histopathological examination of a complete horizontal slice, with a minimum of 5 blocks taken: 2 from the right ventricle in one block, and one full thickness section from each left ventricular quadrant (Royal College of Pathologists 2005).

10.2 Brain

At the gross and standard microscopic level, the brain is not directly affected by sepsis and septic shock. This matches the lack of imaging-detected damage despite the common clinical cognitive and performance deficiencies (Munford 2005), and is presumably a transient cytokine-based phenomenon. However, certain cerebral pathologies are associated with sepsis syndromes for more tangible reasons, including:

- Cerebral infarction from thrombo-embolisation
- Hypoxic-ischaemic encephalopathy (HIE) following temporary cessation of blood and/or oxygen supply during a crisis
- Metastatic cerebral abscess and/or meningitis from a remote focus of sepsis
- Microinfarction from thrombotic microangiopathy affecting all areas of the brain

In the case of HIE, post-mortem pathology does not form part of the case definition, which is solely clinical, neurophysiological and radiological. The most sensitive zones of the brain for such damage are the cerebellar nuclei and the hippocampus, followed by the cerebral cortex in the watershed areas at the junctions of the cerebral artery supply zones. It is useful to sample these to confirm HIE, and to be aware of the problem with artefacts (Whitwell 2005)

10.3 Lung

Lung dysfunction at the commencement of severe sepsis is present in about 20% of such patients (Munford 2005).The clinical diagnosis of acute lung injury is made when there arterial hypoxaemia ($PaO2/FiO2<300mmHg$) and bilateral chest pulmonary infiltrates on chest X ray, in the absence of pneumonia or heart failure. It becomes acute respiratory distress syndrome (ARDS) when hypoxaemia is more severe ($PaO2/FiO2<200mmHg$). Ventilation/perfusion mismatch (effectively right-to-left shunting) of blood flow occurs, exacerbating the hypoxaemia.

Pathologically, the process is diffuse alveolar damage (DAD). This is not specific to the sepsis syndromes as it also occurs in inhalational injury (smoke, toxic gases, oxygen in high concentration), aspiration of gastric contents, and X-irradiation damage; these represent direct damage to the lung tissue. DAD also follows from remote injury as part of SIRS, the pathogenesis being mediators in the blood stream; the causes include cytotoxic drug therapy, pancreatitis, cardio-pulmonary bypass, blood transfusion reaction, fat embolism, paraquat poisoning, and systemic shock from any cause (Corrin & Nicholson 2011). Reduction of surfactant through epithelial cell damage is a key event, which leads to further alveolar and alveolar duct damage.

DAD goes through stages termed the exudative, regenerative, and repair phases.

The exudative phase lasts up to a week, and grossly the lungs are dark red and heavy. The early stage histologically comprises:

- Alveolar wall congestion and expansion
- Variable neutrophils in the interstitium (usually not)
- Oedema and red cells in the alveolae

- Type 1 epithelial cell and alveolar capillary endothelial cell damage (but this is difficult to identify on light microscopy)

The later exudative phase is the classic and, histologically, readily identifiable stage often termed 'shock lung' (Fig 4):

- Alveolar collapse, haemorrhage and oedema
- Hyaline membrane formation on the epithelial surface of respiratory bronchioles and alveolar ducts: this comprises fibrin and necrotic epithelial cells
- Variable neutrophil accumulation in alveolar capillaries

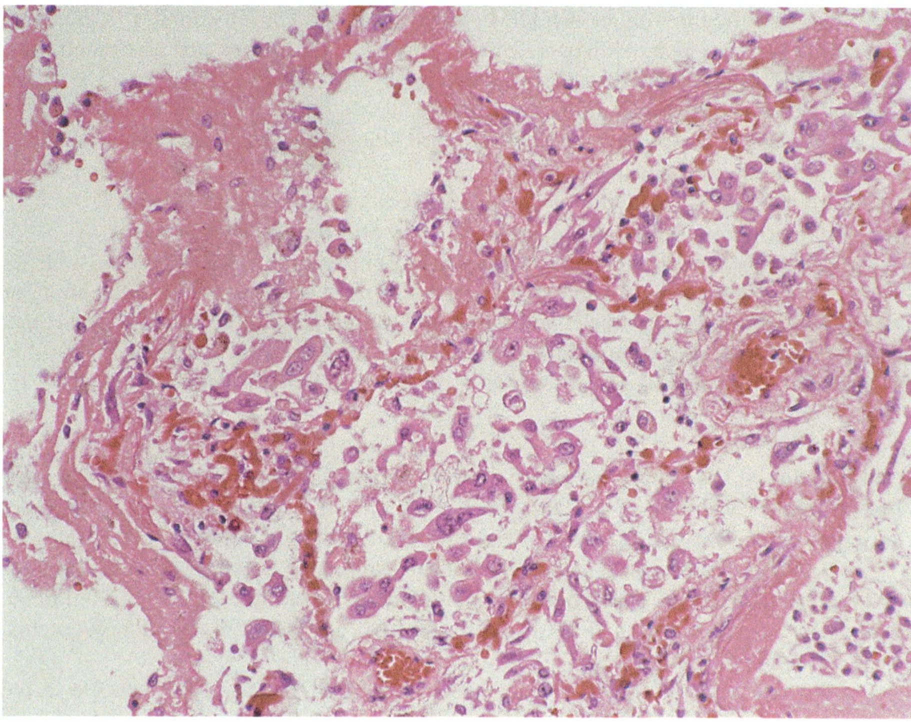

Fig. 4. Hyaline membrane disease in the lung alveoli in septic shock; the pink membranes are partly fibrin exudates and partly necrotic epithelium (H&E)

The regenerative phase permits healing and recovery of the lung to normal structure or progresses to fibrosis via the repair phase. Type 2 epithelial cells proliferate to replace the denuded epithelium; they may be large and elongated, resembling macrophages in the airways. The epithelium may regrow beneath the hyaline membrane, which is sloughed off; or over the membrane, in which case it becomes incorporated into the alveolar wall and is a mechanism for interstitial fibrosis. In the capillaries, the endothelial repair may be accompanied by local thrombosis, organisation and local vascular remodelling.

The repair phase occurs in those whose DAD has not resolved through regeneration. As well as the progressive interstitial thickening from incorporation of hyaline membranes and the ingress of fibroblasts into this tissue, the alveolar exudates organise. There are granulation tissue buds in the alveoli, as seen in organising pneumonias. This fibrosis can happen within a few weeks, if the patient is maintained and alive (Vincent & Singer 2010).

In practice, if patients survive long periods in ICU with episodes of severe sepsis and infective pneumonia and have been mechanically ventilated for long periods, the resulting lung tissue at autopsy can show a varied pattern with some areas of nearly normal tissue, organising pneumonia and interstitial fibrosis separately and combined: it can be difficult if not impossible to ascribe specific aetio-pathogeneses to this end-stage lung fibrosis (Fig 5).

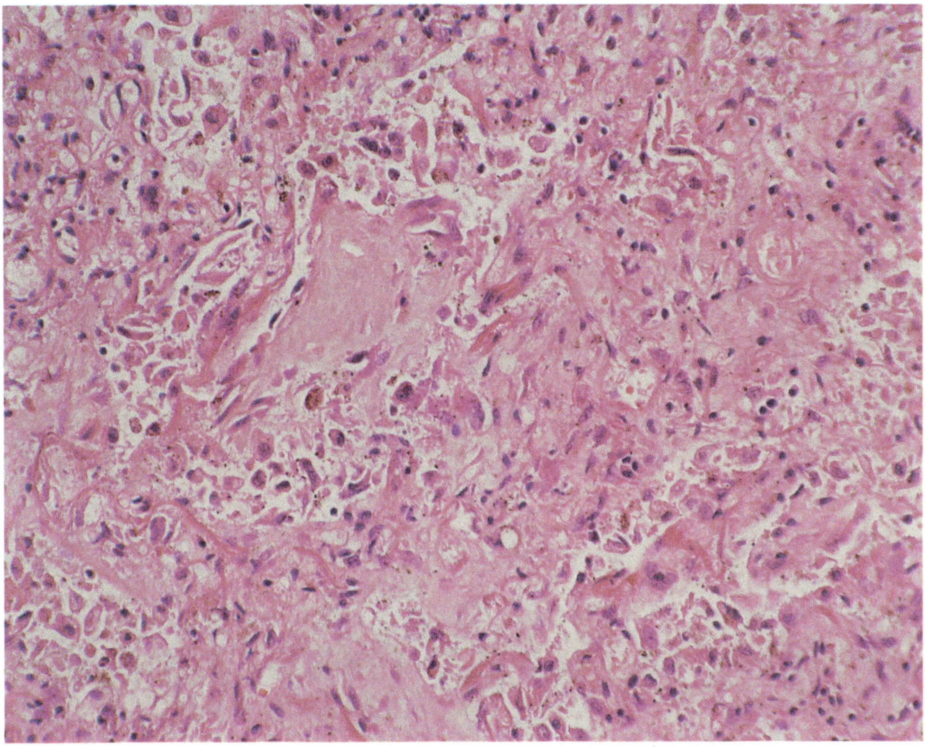

Fig. 5. Acute lung injury that has gone on to organisation with fibrosis, obliterating the alveoli (H&E).

It is unresolved why some patients with DAD in whom the infecting agent is identified and treated promptly still go on to the repair phase and died of pulmonary fibrosis (Wheeler & Bernard 2007). This is particularly seen in patients presenting as advanced HIV disease with *Pneumocystis* infection, and despite co-trimoxazole plus steroid cover become progressively hypoxic; at autopsy the lungs show combined intra-alveolar and interstitial fibrosis.

10.3.1 Ventilator-associated pneumonia (VAP)

VAP is an important entity in ICU, as the development of lung infection during respiratory support demands a change in therapy. There have been several studies of the diagnostic criteria for VAP in vivo (microbiology and cytopathology) and at autopsy (histopathology), and the results are unsettling (Corley et al. 1997) (4177):

- There are no agreed criteria for diagnosing pneumonia in man by histology
- Pathologists do not agree amongst themselves whether there is pneumonia or not
- Quantitative pre-mortem bacteriology does not correlate with clinical symptoms or autopsy histopathology
- Bronchiolar lavage fluid with few neutrophils does correlate with absence of histological pneumonia

Evidently pathology is not yet serving clinical science optimally in this area.

10.3.2 Neutropaenic sepsis

This is a common terminal condition in patients with treated cancer. Bacteria proliferate in many organs and blood vessels, and in the lung they are visible in the alveoli with fibrin and mononuclear cells (Fig 6).

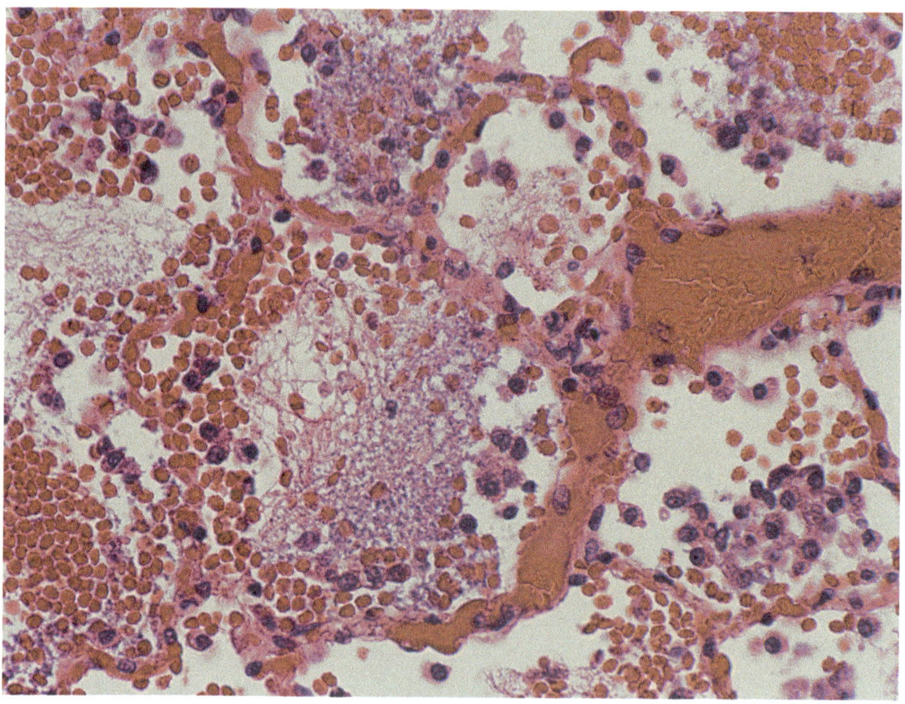

Fig. 6. Lung alveoli in neutropaenic sepsis. There are abundant bacteria in the lumens, some haemorrhage, but only scanty inflammation (H&E)

10.4 Liver

The liver in septic shock has no specific features (Table 6). Clinically, there is cholestatic jaundice. If the source of the sepsis is the biliary tract (cholangitis) there may be abscesses centred on portal tracts. Otherwise, the liver is usually heavier than normal, bile stained, and soft. Histologically, autolysis with cell plate separation is often more advanced than expected from the time since death (perhaps due to high levels of TNFα). There is often fatty change, but usually little parenchymal inflammation, although the sinusoid Kupffer cells and endothelial cells are prominent, and there may haemophagocytosis. Centriacinar necrosis is often prominent.

Several patterns of bile duct histopathology are described, although none are specific to sepsis (Scheuer & Lefkowitch 2006):

- Intracanalicular cholestasis in the perivenular areas
- Ductular cholestasis, proliferating ductules, and surrounding portal neutrophilic inflammation, in addition to canalicular cholestasis
- Non-bacterial cholangitis, with proliferating bile ductules; this is seen in the toxic shock syndrome (Fig 7).

	Liver abscess	Bacterial cholangitis	Bile duct obstruction	Severe sepsis patterns		
				Canalicular cholestasis	Ductular cholestasis & inflammation	Non-bacterial cholestasis
Perivenular cholestasis	+/-	-	+	+	+	-
Canal of Hering & ductular cholestasis	-	-	-	-	+	-
Ductular proliferation	-	+	+	-	+	+
Ductular acute inflammation	+/-	+	+/-	-	+	+
Parenchymal necrosis	+	+	+/-	-	-	-

Table 6. Liver histopathology in sepsis

10.5 Kidney

Acute renal failure occurs in one fifth of patients becoming septic, rising to 50% in septic shock (Munford 2005) (Racusen & Kashgarian 2007). It is the commonest organ dysfunction, manifesting as oliguria and azotaemia. The pathogenesis of the damage in sepsis includes systemic hypotension, renal vasoconstriction, toxic drugs (eg antibiotic aminoglycosides), and inflammatory cytokines.

The pathological lesion is acute tubular injury (ATI), which replaces the older term 'acute tubular necrosis' (Racusen & Kashgarian 2007). Grossly the kidneys are enlarged (oedematous cortex) and typically pale, with blurred cortico-medullary junctions. Focal pyaemic lesions, ascending acute pyelonephritis lines, and (where arterial thrombi are formed) regional cortical infarctive necrosis may also be seen in some cases.

ATI can only be reliably evaluated microscopically. The glomeruli may be collapsed but otherwise show no damage. The tubular damage is conceptually divided into 'ischaemic' and 'toxic' (Racusen & Kashgarian 2007), with more extensive proximal tubule lesions, and more evident cell death, in the latter. In septic shock, with the aetio-pathogenesis often multi-factorial, the distinction becomes blurred. Moreover, autopsy kidneys are notoriously autolysed unless analysed rapidly after death. The main features of ATI are (Fig 8):

- Interstitial oedema with separation of tubules
- Tubular cell swelling
- Loss of nuclei of tubular cells or apoptosis
- Shedding of tubule cells into the lumen

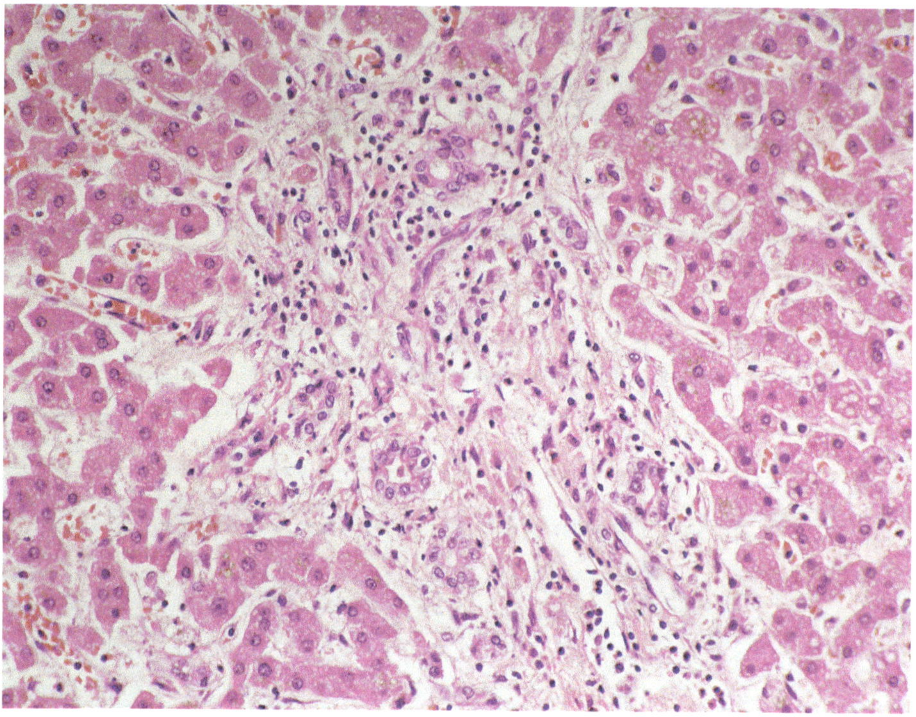

Fig. 7. The portal ductular prolferative reaction in systemic sepsis, with inflammation (H&E)

- Attenuation of the tubular epithelium thickness
- Regeneration of tubular cells: hyperchromatic enlarged nuclei, often adjacent; mitoses
- Insignificant interstitial inflammation
- Accumulation of nucleated cells in the vasa recta in the outer medulla; lymphocytes, myeloid precursors, and nucleated red cell precursors

All too often, the time delay to autopsy precludes confirmation of these features through autolysis. Microvesicular vacuolation of proximal tubules is not ATI, but the result of medical drugs and dextrose-containing plasma expanders.

10.6 Adrenal glands

The adrenals may show the following features

- Lipid depletion and hyperplasia
- Atrophy (if prolonged steroid therapy has been given)
- Parenchymal haemorrhages, small or large
- Thromboses in small arterioles

11. Haemophagocytic syndromes

There is a group of conditions termed 'haemophagocytic syndromes' (HPS) where the driving process is excessive phagocytosis of formed blood cells by macrophages in the marrow, spleen and lymph nodes (Fig 9). The clinical outcomes include:

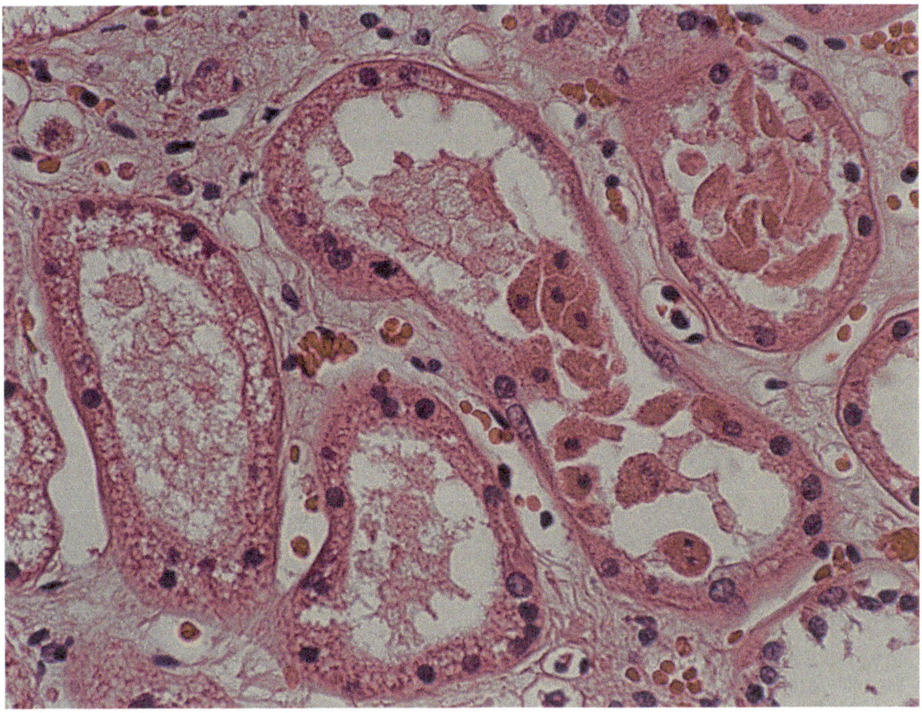

Fig. 8. Kidney in acute tubular necrosis (acute tubular injury). The necrosing epithelium is sloughing into the lumen (H&E)

- High fever
- Pancytopaenia
- Liver dysfunction
- Clotting abnormalities including raised fibrin degradation products and hypofibrinogenaemia
- Hepatosplenomegaly
- Hyperferritinaemia

Thus HPS overlaps clinically with septic shock by case definition (Fisman 2000). The mortality is high, up to 70% (Takahashi et al. 2001) (Ningsanond 2000) From personal experience, many cases that turn out to be HPS have been patients presenting acutely with SIRS, infection screens are negative, and the patients die within a week, of multi-organ failure, despite antibiotics, steroids and standard ICU support procedures.

The pathogenesis of HPS is considered to be an aberrant immunological over-reaction, the hyperstimulation of macrophages by cytokines (particularly TNFα, IL-6, IL-1 and IFNγ) as result of T-cell activation. In addition to a rare familial HPS, the aetiologies include infections, autoimmune disease (particularly SLE) and lymphoma (particularly T-cell lymphoma, but also B-cell). The potential causative infections are legion (Takahashi, Chubachi, Kume, & et al 2001) (Ningsanond 2000) (Fisman 2000):

- Viral - eg EBV, HHV8, HIV (multi-centric Castleman disease), CMV, B19, rubella, viral hepatitis

- Bacteria - eg pneumococcal, typhoid
- Mycobacteria - tuberculosis
- Fungi - eg histoplasmosis
- Protozoa - eg leishmaniasis

Bone marrow haemophagocytosis is found in one third of ICU non-survivors, associated positively with sepsis and blood transfusion, and negatively with cardiovascular disease (Stauss et al. 2004). Thus the distinction between a non-specific reactive process and a syndrome is currently blurred.

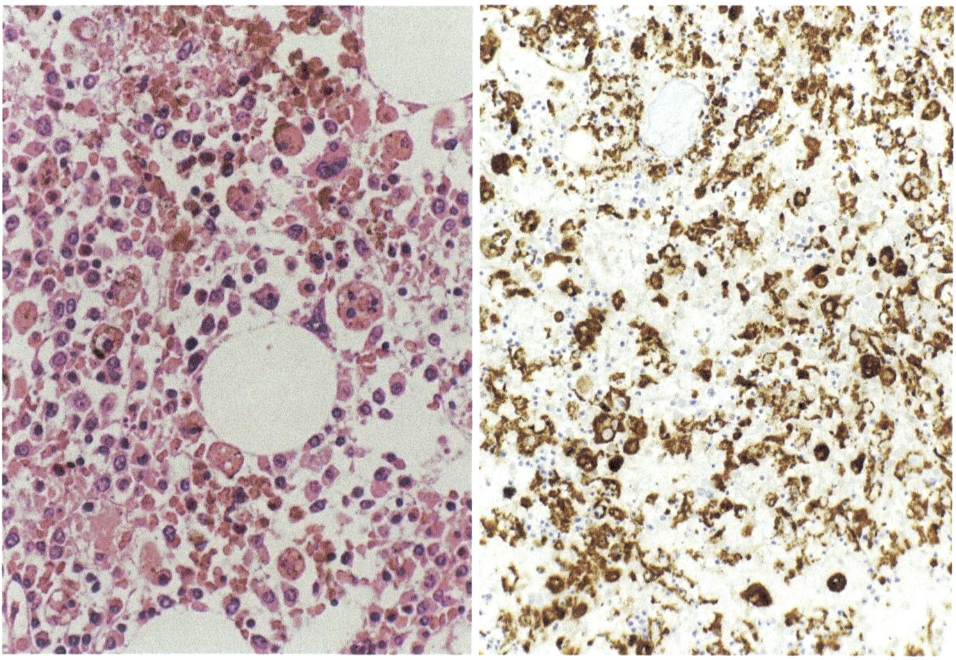

Fig. 9. Bone marrow with haemophagocytosis. Left: numerous large macrophages with engulphed red cells and nuclei (H&E). Right: CD68 immunostaining to highlight the excess number of large macrophages.

12. Thrombotic microangiopathy syndromes

Thombi are frequently encountered in small vessels in sepsis and other conditions. The thrombi are composed of fibrin and platelets in varying proportions. There are two groups of conditions to consider: disseminated intravascular coagulation (DIC) and thrombotic microangiopathy (TTP variant).

12.1 Disseminated intravascular coagulation (Toh & Dennis 2003)

The thrombi are predominantly composed of fibrin and it is accompanied by coagulopathy with depletion of coagulation factors in the blood. DIC (as defined by laboratory criteria) occurs in up to half of patients with severe sepsis (van der Poll.T &

Opal 2008). The pathogenesis is not well understood but may be endothelial injury and the expression of tissue factor on infected monocytes, and initiation of the clotting cascade (Munford 2005). With the exception of meningococcal septicaemia, autopsy studies do not show a correlation of organ dysfunction and deposition of microthrombi in DIC. When thrombi are seen, the kidney glomeruli and lung alveolar capillaries are the commonest location (Fig 10).

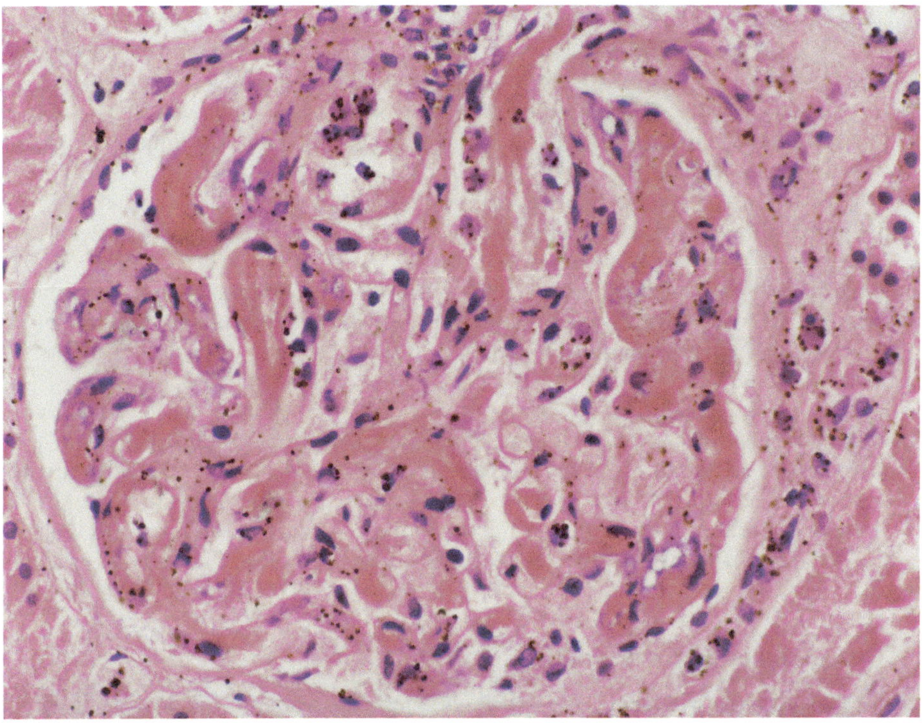

Fig. 10. DIC in pneumococcal sepsis. In this renal glomerulus, all the capillaries are blocked by thrombi (H&E).

Neisseria meningitidis infection causes a fulminant meningococcaemia (and this is often found without a meningitis). Here DIC is the norm, and bacteria may be found within dermal vessels (Fig 3). Meningococci are different from other gram-negative bacilli as they shed membrane blebs that active complement and coagulation directly. Widespread skin and internal organ haemorrhages are seen, associated with small vessel DIC, and the adrenal shows haemorrhages (though rarely a massive destructive haematoma).

A prototype TMA is thrombotic thrombocytopaenic purpura (TTP) and the related haemolytic uraemic syndrome (Hosler, Cusumano, & Hutchins 2003). Unlike DIC, the clotting factors are not affected, and the thrombi are predominantly platelets. Clinically TMA may simulate septic shock. Using immunocytochemistry to quantify fibrin versus platelets (anti-fibrin and anti-CD61 antibodies respectively) and thus distinguish TMA from DIC is not always helpful: the staining intensities can be similar in both conditions.

13. End-stage liver disease (ESDL)

The adverse impact of cirrhosis is well-attested in many medical and surgical conditions. The Child-Pugh liver score (a measure of hepatic and extra-hepatic dysfunction based on combined biochemical markers and clinical signs) predicts non-survival in cirrhotic patients admitted to ICU. Overall, the one-year mortality of such patients is 69-74%, with median survival of one month (Gildea et al. 2004) (Arabi et al. 2004).

Cardiac operations are hazardous in cirrhotic patients, with those on cardio-pulmonary bypass particularly liable to die (Hayashida et al. 2004) and – if they are Child-Pugh class C – approach a 100% mortality. Similarly, abdominal trauma patients have ICU post-operative mortality rates increasing from 15-63% as the severity liver failure increases (Christmas et al. 2005). In these patients a major cause of death is sepsis and septic shock. The abnormal blood circulation to cirrhotic liver tissue renders the Kupffer cell macrophages less able to clear bacteria from the blood.

It is the experience of pathologists examining patients who die in ICU that cirrhosis is significantly under-diagnosed pre-mortem, and that clinicians would like better methods of identifying the patients who have cirrhosis. There are several implications. First, consider liver disease carefully in ICU and sepsis deaths. The eyeball confident diagnosis of cirrhosis - or not - is not always possible. Secondly, in the formulation of cause of death in these cases, 'cirrhosis' should be included as a contributor to mortality in the death certificate.

Thirdly, liver biopsy is the only pre-autopsy definitive marker of liver fibrosis and cirrhosis; but it is invasive and has a mortality rate. Imaging, standard biochemical tests, serum markers of fibrosis, and more specialised tests of liver function only identify a proportion of cirrhotic patients (Rockey & Bissell 2006), and these non-invasive tests have not been validated for 'normal' patients about to undergo cardiac surgery or those already in ICU for other reasons. Further research into better indicators of cirrhosis is urgently needed.

14. Outcomes and co-morbidities

Mortality in patients with septic shock is highly variable, from 35-70% depending on many variables that include (Annane, Bellisant, & Cavaillon 2005)

- age & sex
- co-morbidities and other altered physiological states
  - sickle cell disease and other hyposlenic states (Di Sabatino, Carsetti, & Corrazza 2011)
  - immunosuppression (Morris, Masur, & Huang 2006) (Combes, Mokhtari, Couvelard, & et al 2004)
  - chronic obstructive pulmonary disease
  - ischaemic heart disease
  - end-stage liver disease
  - pregnancy
- the combined total of failing organs, particularly lung and kidney
- whether the infection is nosocomial or polymicrobial
- whether the infection is a fungus
- ethnicity and inherited variables (Villar, Maca-Meyer, Perez-Mendez, & Flores 2004)

14.1 Pregnancy

The subject of susceptibility to infection during pregnancy is under-investigated epidemiologically. The depressed cell-mediated immunity during gestation does predispose to certain infections such as tuberculosis, *Listeria* and some viral infections. But despite the importance of bacterial infections in peri-partum sespsis, particularly *Streptococcus pyogenes*, it is unclear whether the pregnant state per se confers an increased susceptibility to them (Lucas 2011).

15. The treatment of sepsis

ICU treatment of patients in sepsis and shock has four main approaches

- Anti-microbial therapy of known or suspected infective agents
- Failing organ support - eg pulmonary, renal, hepatic, cardiac
- Indirect therapies aimed at the systemic inflammatory response and its consequences: immunomodulatory and anti-inflammatory therapies
- Surgical treatment - excision of septic foci and removal of necrotic tissue (eg infarcted bowel, necrotising fasciitis)

As well as inotropic and renal support, a major function of ICU is ventilatory support. In DAD, the alveoli shut down on expiration and require a higher pressure to re-open. Mechanical ventilation thus exerts its stresses on the delicate lung tissue. Tidal volumes appear to be a critical variable in the causation of lung damage (Wheeler & Bernard 2007). In conjunction with the high oxygen concentration required to keep a reasonable blood PO_2, this can further damage the lung.

15.1 Specific drug treatments in sepsis

Many trials of anti-inflammatory chemotherapy have been held in septic shock, including against (Riederman, Guo, & Ward 2003): immune regulation, endotoxin, TNFα, NO, IL-1, oxidants, neutrophil activity, complement, and coagulation. In practice, only steroid therapy and activated protein C (APC) have been validated as useful in improving survival. The reasons why the other therapeutic avenues have not proven successful include a) non-homogeneity of the study populations, and b) the ill-understood multifactorial complexity of the sepsis syndromes. However, newer approaches to suppressing pro-inflammatory processes are being experimented with, such as anti-HMGB1 antibodies; these could suppress the late-acting pro-inflammatory cytokine High-Mobility Group Box-1 protein. It is know that this increases survival in the caecal puncture model of sepsis (van der Poll.T & Opal 2008).

Steroid therapy has its known complications. APC acts as an anti-coagulant (thus important in DIC) as well as an inhibitor of production of IL-1, IL-6 and TNFα. The side effects are intracerebral (Recombinant human Protein C Worldwide Evaluation in Severe Sepsis (PROWESS) study group. 2001) and pulmonary haemorrhage (personal observations) (Fig 11). Another specific complication in modern chemotherapy is the increased susceptibility to certain pathogens with immunodulatory drugs. An example is the negative impact of adalimumab if the patient has tuberculosis as a co-morbidity (Lever & Mackenzie 2007).

The known increase in apoptosis in the lymphoid population (Hotchkiss, Swanson, Freeman, & et al 1999) has prompted consideration of anti-apoptotic chemotherapy. However, the potential of uncontrolled cell growth has to be evaluated first.

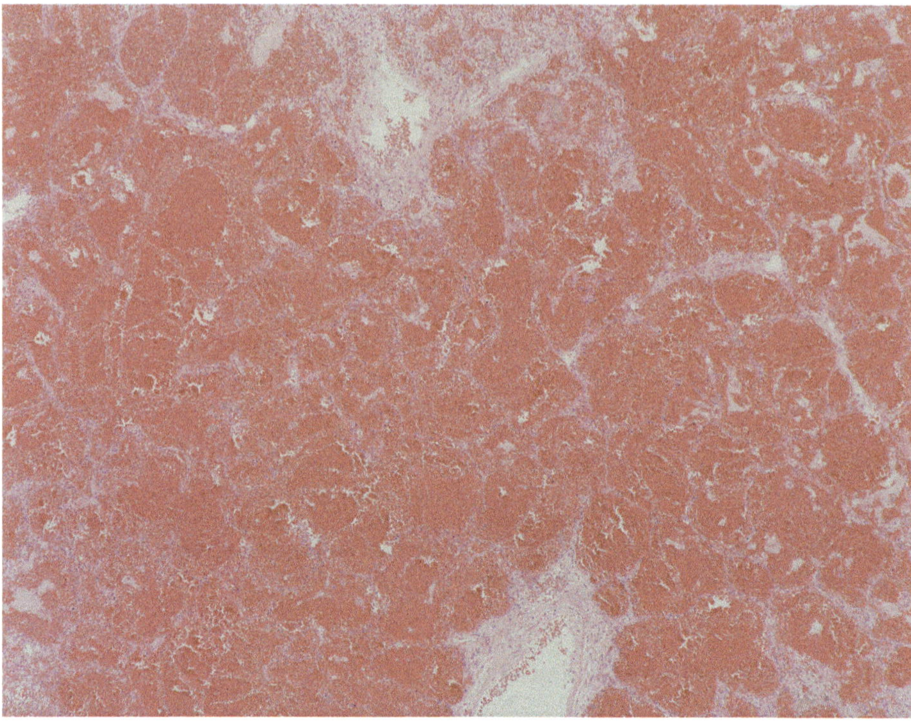

Fig. 11. Lung with massive haemorrhage, associated with administration of activated protein C in a patient with sepsis (H&E)

An epidemiological analysis of outcomes in cardiovascular disease patients demonstrated that statin therapy was associated with reduced rates of sepsis and fatality from sepsis (Hackam et al. 2006). As well as being lipid-lowering agents, statins have many other effects: anti-inflammatory, modulation of cellular immunity, improvement of endothelial cell function, and increasing the bio-availability of NO. Apart from suggesting further strategies in sepsis therapy, this observation reminds pathologists to look at the treatments patients are on when they undergo autopsy.

16. Conclusion

This brief review of septic shock autopsy pathology and its differential diagnosis has focussed on the major conditions. There are less obvious pathologies whose contribution to the disease and outcome are uncertain. For example, apoptosis of neurones and glial cells in the cardiovascular centres of the brain. Patients who died of septic shock showed more such apoptosis in the amygdala and medullary autonomic nuclei than those dying of non-septic shock and sudden extra-cranial trauma. This was strongly associated with endothelial iNOS expression (Sharshar et al. 2003). Does this significantly contribute to outcome over and above direct organ damage?

In conclusion, there is much to be studied still in the morbid anatomy of sepsis syndromes. If pathologists are to be useful in sepsis research, careful documentation of autopsy organ pathology and microbiology, and the correlation of outcome with clinical features and the various therapeutic modalities, is essential. New treatments for severe sepsis are being trialled to raise the poor survival rates in intensive care. The role of the autopsy is thus threefold: to describe carefully the organ lesions and identify microbiological agents directly and through the particular host reactions (Table 5; Fig 12,13); to identify co-morbidities and complications of treatments; and to collaborate with clinicians in audit and improving the outcomes of septic patients.

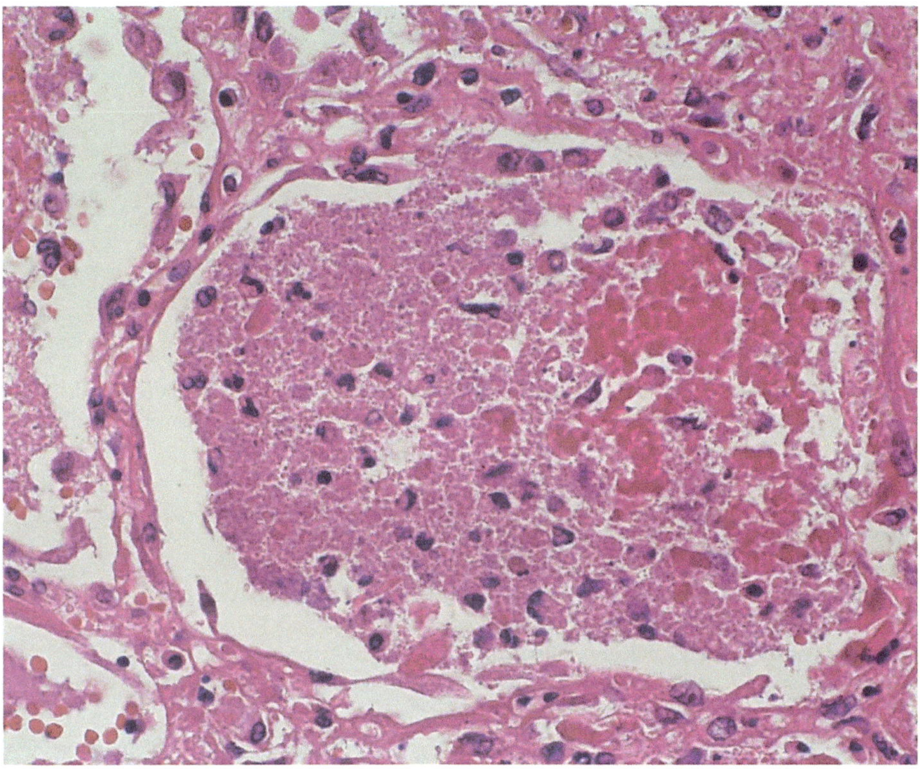

Fig. 12. Autopsy lung of an HIV+ve patient who died with lung and multi-organ failure of uncertain aetiology. The lung alveoli are filled with granular necrotic debris and minimal cellular reaction. This is non-reactive (anergic) tuberculosis infection - see Fig 13 (H&E).

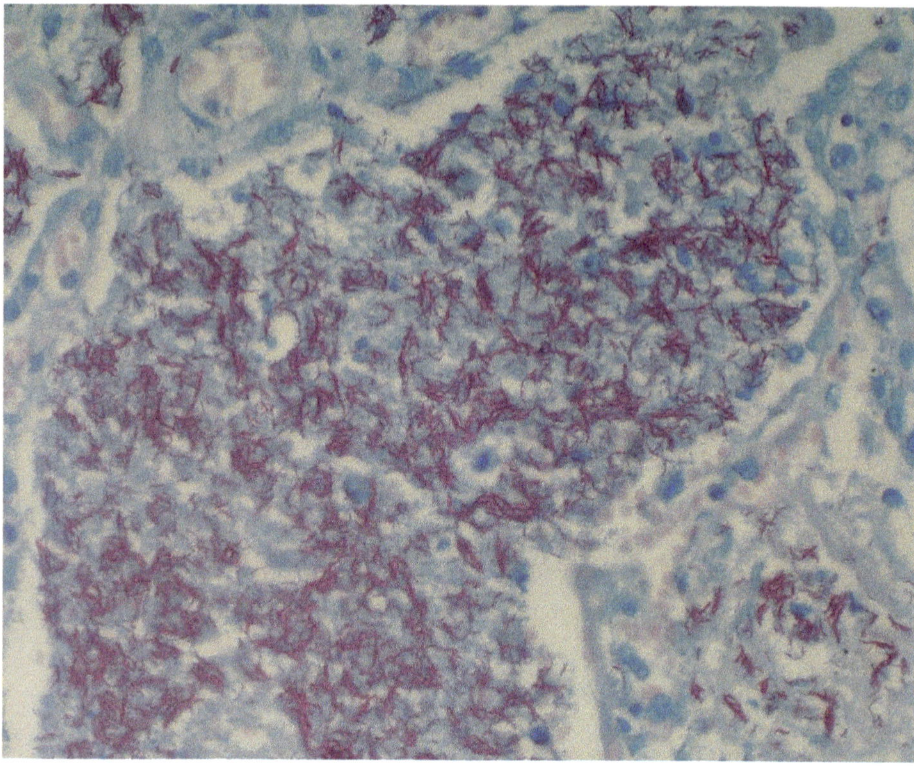

Fig. 13. Same lung as in Fig 12. The Ziehl-Neelsen stain reveals huge numbers of acid-fast bacilli. The 'granular debris' seen in Fig 12 H&E stain is comprised of clumped bacilli.

17. References

Annane, D., Bellisant, E., & Cavaillon, J.-M. 2005, "Septic shock", *Lancet*, vol. 365, pp. 63-78.

Arabi, Y., Ahmed, Q. A., Haddad, S., Aljumah, A., & Al-Shimemeri, A. 2004, "Outcome predictors of cirrhosis patients admitted to the intensive care unit.", *European Journal of Gastroenterology & Hepatology*, vol. 16, pp. 333-339.

Arismendi-Morrillo, G. J., Briceno-Garcia, A. E., Romero-Amaro, Z. R., & et al 2004, "Acute non-specific splenitis as indicator of systemic infection. Assessment of 71 autopsy cases.", *Invest.Clin.*, vol. 45, pp. 131-135.

Baroldi, G. 2006, "Basic pathophysiologic changes," in *Pathology of the Heart and Sudden Death in Forensic Medicine*, V. Fineschi, G. Baroldi, & M. D. Silver, eds., CRC Press, Taylor & Francis Group, Boca Raton, Fl, pp. 31-76.

Bisno, A. K. & Stevens, D. L. 2005, "*Streptococcus pyogenes*," in *Mandell, Douglas, and Bennett's Principles and Practice of Infectious Diseases*, 6 edn, G. L. Mandell, J. E. Bennet, & R. Dolin, eds., Elsevier Churchill Livingstone, Philadelphia, pp. 2362-2379.

Blosser, S. A., Zimmerman, H. E., & Stauffer, J. L. 1998, "Do autopsies of critically ill patients reveal important findings that were clinical undetected?", *Critical Care Medicine*, vol. 26, pp. 1332-1336.

Calandra, T., Cohen, J., & et al 2005, "The International Sepsis Forum Consensus Conference on Definitions of Infection in the Intensive Care Unit.", *Critical Care Medicine*, vol. 33, pp. 1538-1548.

Christmas, A. B., Wilson, A. K., Franklin, G. A., & et al 2005, "Cirrhosis and trauma: a deadly duo.", *American Surgery*, vol. 71, pp. 996-1000.

Combes, A., Mokhtari, M., Couvelard, A., & et al 2004, "Clinical and autopsy diagnoses in the intensive care unit: a prospective study.", *Archives of Internal Medicine*, vol. 164, pp. 389-392.

Corley, D. E., Kirtland, S. H., Winterbauer, R. H., & et al 1997, "Reproducibility of the histologic diagnosis of pneumonia among a panel of four pathologists.", *Chest*, vol. 112, pp. 458-465.

Corrin, B. & Nicholson, A. G. 2011, "Diffuse alveolar damage," in *Pathology of the Lung*, 3 edn, B. Corrin & A. G. Nicholson, eds., Churchill Livingstone, Elsevier, London, pp. 131-149.

Danai, P. & Martin, G. S. 2005, "Epidemiology of sepsis: recent advances.", *Current Infectious Disease Reports*, vol. 7, pp. 329-334.

Dellinger, P., Carlet, J. M., Masur, H., & et al 2004, "Surviving Sepsis Campaign guidelines for management of severe sepsis and septic shock.", *Critical Care Medicine*, vol. 32, pp. 858-878.

Dellinger.R.P., Levy, M. M., Carlet, J. M., & et al 2008, "Surviving sepsis campaign: international guidelines for management of severe sepsis and septic shock: 2008", *Critical Care Medicine*, vol. 36, pp. 296-327.

Di Sabatino, A., Carsetti, R., & Corrazza, G. R. 2011, "Post-splenectomy and hyposplenic states.", *Lancet*, vol. 378, pp. 86-97.

Fisman, D. N. 2000, "Hemophagocytic syndromes and infection.", *Emerging Infectious Diseases*, vol. 6, pp. 601-608.

Fowler, A., Collins, L., de Ruiter, A., & et al 2006, "Multicentric Castleman's disease in a patient with HIV.", *International Journal of STD and AIDS*, vol. 17, pp. 63-64.

Gildea, T. R., Cook, W. C., Nelson, D. R., & et al 2004, "Predictors of long-term mortality in patients with cirrhosis of the liver admitted to a medical ICU.", *Chest*, vol. 126, pp. 1598-1603.

Goldman, L., Sayson, R., Robbins, S., Cohn, L. H., Bettman, M., & Weisberg, M. 1983, "The value of the autopsy in three medical eras.", *New England Journal of Medicine*, vol. 308, pp. 1000-1005.

Ha, T., Grant, D., Xia, Y., & et al 2006, "Glucan phosphate attenuates cardiac dysfunction and inhibits cardiac MIF expression and apoptosis in septic mice.", *American Journal of Physiology Heart Circulatory Physiology*, vol. 291, p. H1910-H1918.

Hackam, D. G., Mamdani, M., Li, P., & Redelmeier, D. A. 2006, "Statins in patients with cardiovascular disease: a population-based cohort analysis.", *Lancet*, vol. 367, pp. 413-418.

Hayashida, M., Shoujima, T., Teshima, H., & et al 2004, "Clinical outcome after cardiac operations in patients with cirrhosis.", *Annals of Thoracic Surgery*, vol. 77, pp. 500-505.

Hirata, K., Miyagi, S., Tome, M., & et al 1988, "Cor pulmonale due to tumour cell microemboli.", *Archives of Internal Medicine*, vol. 148, pp. 2287-2289.

Hosler, G. A., Cusumano, A. M., & Hutchins, G. M. 2003, "Thrombotic thrombocytopenia purpura and hemolytic uremic syndrome are distinct pathologic entities. A review of 56 autopsy cases.", *Archives of Pathology and Laboratory Medicine*, vol. 127, pp. 834-839.

Hotchkiss, R. S., Swanson, P. E., Freeman, B., & et al 1999, "Apoptotic cell death in patients with sepsis, shock, and multiple organ dysfunction.", *Critical Care Medicine*, vol. 27, pp. 1230-1251.

Lever, A. & Mackenzie, I. 2007, "Sepsis: definition, epidemiology, and diagnosis", *Bmj*, vol. 335, pp. 879-883.

Levy, M. M. & et al 1992, "SCCM/ESICM/ACCP/ATS/SIS International Sepsis Definitions Conference.", *Critical Care Medicine*, vol. 31, pp. 1250-1256.

Levy, R. J., Piel, D. A., ACton, P. D., & et al 2005, "Evidence of myocardial hibernation in the septis subject.", *Critical Care Medicine*, vol. 33, pp. 2752-2756.

Lucas, S. B. 2007, "The autopsy pathology of sepsis-related death", *Current Diagnostic Pathology*, vol. 13, pp. 375-388.

Lucas, S. B. 2011, "Saving Mothers' Lives: Sepsis in pregnancy. Annex 7.1. A possible future approach to case definitions.", *British Journal of Obstetrics and Gynaecology*, vol. 118, no. supplement 1, March 2011, pp. 97-101.

Mitchell, R. N. 2005, "Hemodynamic disorders, Thromboembolic disease, and Shock.," in *Robbins and Contran Pathologic Basis of Disease*, 7 edn, V. Kumar, A. K. Abbas, & N. Fausto, eds., Elsevier Saunders, Philadelphia, pp. 119-144.

Moreillon, P., Que, Y.-A., & Glauser, M. P. 2005, "*Staphylococcus aureus* (including staphylococcal toxic shock)," in *Mandell, Douglas, and Bennett's Principles and Practice of Infectious Diseases*, 6 edn, G. L. Mandell, J. E. Bennet, & R. Dolin, eds., Elsevier Churchill Livingstone, Philadelphia, pp. 2321-2351.

Morris, A., Masur, H., & Huang, L. 2006, "Current issues in critical care of the HIV-infected patient.", *Critical Care Medicine*, vol. 34, pp. 42-49.

Morris, J. A., Harrison, L. M., & Partridge, S. M. 2006, "Postmortem bacteriology: a re-evaluation", *Journal of Clinical Pathology*, vol. 59, no. 1, p. 9.

Munford, R. S. 2005, "Sepsis, severe sepsis, and septic shock," in *Mandell, Douglas and Bennett's Principles and Practice of Infectious Diseases*, 6 edn, G. L. Mandell, J. E. Bennet, & R. Dolin, eds., Elsevier Churchill Livingstone, Pennsylvania, pp. 906-925.

National Confidential Enquiry into Patient Outcome and Death 2006, *The Coroner's Autopsy: Do we deserve better?* www.ncepod.org.uk.

Ningsanond, V. 2000, "Infection associated hemophagocytic syndrome: a report of 50 children.", *Journal of the Medical Association of Thailand*, vol. 83, pp. 1141-1149.

Nishida, N., Chiba, T., Ohtani, K., Ikeda, N., Katayama, Y., & Yoshioka, N. 2006, "Relationship between cardiopulmonary resuscitation and injuries of the cardiac conduction system: pathological features and pathogenesis of such injuries.", *Critical Care Medicine*, vol. 34, pp. 363-367.

Perkins, G. D., McAuley, D. F., Davies, S., & Gao, F. 2003, "Discrepancies between clinical and postmortem diagnoses in critically ill patients: an observationsl study.", *Critical Care*, vol. 7, p. R129-R132.

Racusen, L. & Kashgarian, M. 2007, "Ischemic and toxic acute tubular damage and other ischemic renal injury.," in *Heptinstall's Pathology of the Kidney*, 6 edn, J. C. Jennette et al., eds., Lippincott, Williams & Wilkins, Philadelphia, pp. 1139-1186.

Recombinant human Protein C Worldwide Evaluation in Severe Sepsis (PROWESS) study group. 2001, "Efficacy and safety of recombinant human activated protein C for severe sepsis.", *New England Journal of Medicine*, vol. 344, pp. 699-709.

Riederman, N. C., Guo, R.-F., & Ward, P. A. 2003, "The enigma of sepsis.", *Journal of Clinical Investigation*, vol. 112, pp. 460-467.

Rockey, D. C. & Bissell, M. 2006, "Non-invasive measures of liver fibrosis.", *Hepatology*, vol. 43, p. S113-S120.

Roosen, J., Frans, E., Wilmer, A., Knockaert, D. C., & Bobbaers, H. 2000, "Comparison of premortem clinical diagnoses in critically ill patients and subsequent autopsy findings.", *Mayo Clin Proc*, vol. 75, pp. 562-567.

Royal College of Pathologists 2005, *Sudden death with likely cardiac pathology* www.rcpath.org.

Scheuer, P. & Lefkowitch, J. H. 2006, "The liver in systemic disease and pregnancy," in *Liver Biopsy Interpretation*, 7 edn, Elsevier Saunders, pp. 331-332.

Schnadig, V. J., Molina, C. P., & Aronson, J. F. 2007, "Cytodiagnosis in the autopsy suite: a tool for improving autopsy quality and resident education.", *Arch Pathol Lab Med*, vol. 131, pp. 1056-1062.

Sharshar, T., Gray, F., de la Grandmaison, G. L., & et al 2003, "Apoptosis of neurons in cardiovascular autonomic centres triggered by inducible nitric oxide after death from septic shock.", *Lancet*, vol. 362, pp. 1799-1805.

Singer, M., De Santis, V., Vitale, D., & Jeffcoate, W. 2004, "Multiorgan failure is an adaptive, endocrine-mediated, metabolic response to overwhelming systemic inflammation.", *Lancet*, vol. 364, pp. 545-548.

Stauss, R., Neureiter, D., Westenburger, B., & et al 2004, "Multifactorial risk analysis of bone marrow histiocytic hyperplasia with hemophagocytosis in critically ill medical patients - a postmortem clinicopathologic analysis.", *Critical Care Medicine*, vol. 32, pp. 1316-1321.

Stebbing, J., Adams, C., Mletzko, S., & et al 2011, "Plasma HHV8 DNA predicts relapse in individuals with HIV-associated multicentric Castleman disease.", *Blood*, vol. 118, pp. 271-275.

Takahashi, N., Chubachi, A., Kume, M., & et al 2001, "A clinical analysis of 52 adult patients with hemophagocytic syndrome: the prognostic significance of the underlying diseases.", *International Journal of Haematology*, vol. 74, pp. 209-213.

Tissari, P., Zumla, A., Tarkka, E., & et al 2010, "Accurate and rapid identificatino of bacterial species from positive blood cultures with a DNA-based microarray platform: an observational study.", *Lancet*, vol. 375, pp. 224-230.

Toh, C. H. & Dennis, M. 2003, "Disseminated intravascular coagulation: old disease, new hope", *British Medical Journal*, vol. 327, pp. 974-977.

Tsokos, M. 2003, "Immunohistochemical detection of sepsis-induced lung injury in human autopsy material.", *Legal Medicine*, vol. 5, pp. 73-86.

van der Poll.T & Opal, S. M. 2008, "Host-pathogen interactions in sepsis.", *Lancet Infectious Diseases*, vol. 8, pp. 32-43.

Villar, J., Maca-Meyer, N., Perez-Mendez, L., & Flores, C. 2004, "Bench-to-bedside review: understanding genetic predisposition to sepsis.", *Critical Care*, vol. 8, pp. 180-189.

Vincent, J. L. & Singer, M. 2010, "Critical care: advances and future prospects", *Lancet*, vol. 376, pp. 1354-1361.

Wheeler, A. P. & Bernard, G. R. 2007, "Acute lung injury and teh acute respiratory distress syndrome: a clinical review", *Lancet*, vol. 369, pp. 1553-1565.

Whitwell, H. 2005, "Techniques.," in *Forensic Neuropathology*, H. Whitwell, ed., Hodder Arnold, London, pp. 20-35.

Zhu, B. L., Ishikawa, T., Michiue, T., Quan, L., & Maeda, H. 2005, "Postmortem serum endotoxin level in reiation to the causes of death.", *Legal Medicine*, vol. 7, pp. 103-109.

Part 4

Pathophysiology

5

Biomarkers and Physiological Agents in Severe Sepsis and Septic Shock

D. Paramythiotis, E. Digkas and G. Dryllis
1st Propedeutic Surgical Department
Aristotle University of Thessaloniki
A.H.E.P.A. University Hospital
Thessaloniki
Greece

1. Introduction

The term sepsis implies the presence of infection with signs of systemic body response (tachycardia, tachypnea, fever, etc.) and conditions of severe sepsis and septic shock, further disturbance in organ perfusion (impaired consciousness, hypoxia, oliguria) required fluid administration and inotropic and / or vasopressor drugs, respectively (Levy et al. 2003, Bone et al.1992).

Sepsis is an enormously complex clinical syndrome that arises from the activation of an innate host response to danger. Sepsis is associated with infections of bacteria, viruses, fungi and endotoxins, whether or not being evidenced by culture. The above systematic inflammatory response in humans occurs not only in sepsis but also in other non-infectious conditions such as pancreatitis, ischemia, severe trauma, etc. The host responds in the same way in infectious as in non-infectious events, which is described by the term systemic inflammatory response syndrome (SIRS). Insights into the biology of innate immunity suggest that in terms of impact on outcomes, the specific insult evoking the response is less important than the nature of the response itself. The terms sepsis and septicemia were- until relatively recently- used indiscriminately. However, researchers tend to use those two terms with different and distinct meanings according to several conditions under which each of this condition happens (Pezilli et al, 2010, Dhar et al, 2008, Hoover et al, 2006, Matzinger et al, 2002, Bone et al, 1992). Sepsis is a very complex chain of events including inflammatory and anti-inflammatory processes, circulatory abnormalities and humoral and cellular reactions. Its complexity, in addition to high variability of its non-specific signs and symptoms, make early diagnosis and determination of its severity very important, as sepsis can be lethal for patients. Early diagnosis increases the possibility of starting a specific therapy in time (Lever et al, 2007, Hotchkiss and Karl, 2003, Zambon et al., 2008).

As mentioned above, sepsis may be initialized by local inflammation in order to inactivate invading factors. At first the host recruits and activates leukocytes at infectious foci. During that phase, innate immune cells recognize invading factors through pattern recognition receptors (PRRs) on the cells. Toll-like receptors (TLRs), which belong to PRRs, activate immune cells. This activation is caused by the production of pro-inflammatory cytokines and chemokines. Bacterial products and viral proteins are linked to various and distinct TLRs and are the main cause of cytokine and chemokine production. Following the complement is activated which activates leukocytes. Cells activated through all this process produce and secrete many agents such as leukotriene, nitric oxide and inducible nitric oxide synthase (iNOS) and free radicals. All this process is initiated by many proinflammatory mediators (cytokines, adhesion molecules, vasodilating mediators and reactive oxygen species). If the above body reaction fails to achieve its goals, then some of the invading factors may invade into the bloodstream and trigger a systemic inflammatory reaction. This happens mainly through overproduction of inflammatory cytokines (eg TNF, IFNs and IL-1,6). In all the inflammatory process many agents are overproduced and are of high importance for patients health. Apoptosis has a key role in sepsis and it is influenced by many factors such as caspases, pro-inflammatory cytokines release –such as TNF-a, IFN-γ, IL-1β - and anti-inflammatory cytokines e.g. TGFβ, IL-10 and IL-13, many different pathogenic toxins, such as LPS, CLP and CASP, while it happens in many organs such as heart, glomeruli, liver, bone marrow, thymus, spleen, lungs and gut. The TNFR- CD40-TRADD- FADD pathway –activated by TNF-a- leads to inhibition of cas-8, which is an initiator factor of apoptosis, and therefore that pathway inhibits apoptosis. Additionally, neutrophile and monocyte activation leads to inhibition of Bfl-1, which belongs to Bcl-2 family and inhibits apoptosis. On the contrary, activation of Cardinal and Fas death receptor by Bim (of the Bcl-2 family), which leads to activation of lymphocyte apoptosis, causes a decline of inflammatory response. Apoptosis inhibition leads to SIRS, while its activation leads to immunoparalysis and MODS. However, apoptosis inhibition may have a beneficial role for septic patient. Immunodeficiency is another characteristic of sepsis, which happens due to increased apoptosis of CD4 T cells, dendritic cells and B cells and leads to immunoparalysis. The coagulation system is activated by cytokines and oxidants through tissue factor induction. Antithrombin III plays a dominant role among antithrombotic and fibrinolytic agents. Protein C or autoprothrombin IIA, protect cells from sepsis and it has strong anticoagulative effects through inactivating Va and VIIIa factors of the coagulation system (Remick, 2007, Okazaki and Matsukawa, 2009, Hotchkiss et al, 2003, McDonald, et al 2000, Sohn et al 2003, Hildeman et al 2002, O'Neill et al 2000). (**Figure 1**)

Physiological agents participating in sepsis pathophysiology cascades are used as biomarkers in sepsis diagnosis. Biomarker is "a characteristic that is objectively measured and evaluated as an indicator of normal biological processes, pathogenic process or pharmacologic responses to a therapeutic intervention (BDWG, 2001). The exact role of biomarkers in septic patient's management is not yet defined. Nevertheless, biomarkers can play an important role in early diagnosis and severity determination of sepsis. Moreover they can differentiate bacterial from viral and fungal infection and systemic from local infection. Differentiation of Gram-positive from Gram-negative microorganisms as cause of sepsis is a potential use of biomarkers. Biomarkers may also be used in guiding antibiotic therapy, guiding therapy, and evaluating the response to therapy. Other possible biomarker applications are prediction of sepsis complications and development of organ dysfunction (BDWG, 2001, Marshall and Reinhart, 2009, Dellinger et al, 2008). It has been shown that various biomarkers are very useful in clinical practice in sepsis diagnosis and some of them are thought superior to clinical signs as far as diagnosis.

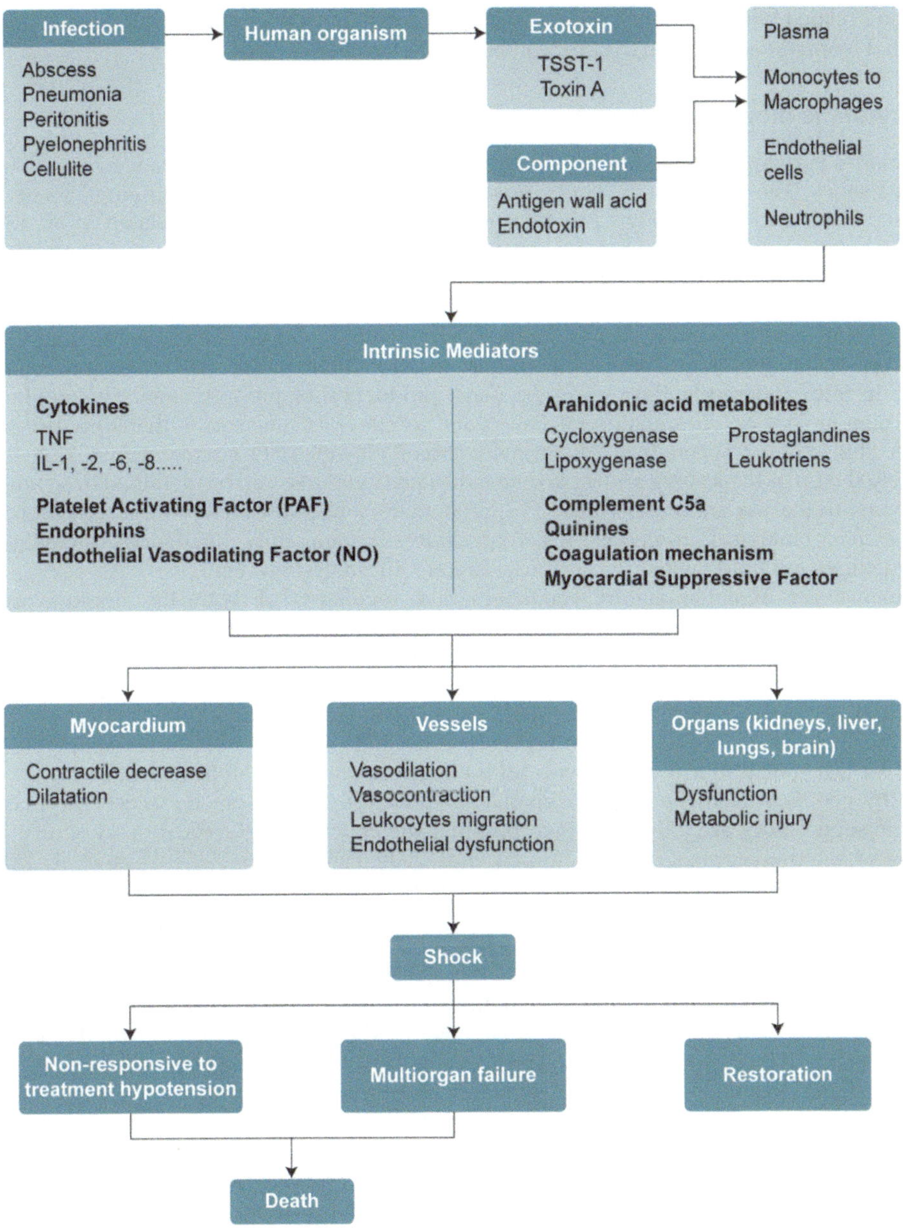

Fig. 1. Pathogenetic mechanism of sepsis (improved figure by Parillo et al, 1993)

Biomarkers of sepsis can be divided in nine categories, which are: 1. Cytokine biomarkers, 2. Coagulation biomarkers, 3. Acute phase protein biomarkers, 4. Receptor biomarkers, 5. Cell marker related biomarkers, 6. Vascular and endothelial damage biomarkers, 7. Vasolidation related biomarkers, 8. Organ dysfunction biomarkers, 9. Genetic biomarkers.

2. Cytokine biomarkers

Cytokines participate in the pro-inflammatory as in the inflammatory cascade of sepsis and septic shock. The release of pro-inflammatory mediators characterizes the initial phase of sepsis. Persistence of the latter provokes acquired immunodepression, related to an anti-inflammatory profile, and hence to a delayed decrease in hypersensitivity, an incapacity to cope with the infection and the onset of inflammation. The first human defence mechanism which is activated is the intrinsic immune system (innate immune system). It is the first line of defence and it is motivated by both exogenous (e.g. Gram-, Gram + bacteria) and endogenous factors (e.g. Heat shock protein, direct cellular injury, ischemia-reperfusion). Both in SIRS and sepsis, there is an excessive production of pro-inflammatory cytokines, adhesion molecules, vasodilating mediators and reactive oxygen species, therefore they are detectable in blood, where they are normally absent. However, the circulating cytokines are merely the tip of the iceberg and leukocyte-associated cytokines can be identified even when amounts in plasma are undetectable. Pro-inflammatory responses lead to the activation of successive biological reactions which include: Inflammatory mediators (cytokines, chemokines and lipid mediators) and coagulation / fibrinolysis system.

Cytokines act as inflammatory mediators and regulators of both the immune and inflammatory reactions. Pro-inflammatory cytokines are released in a cascade, with TNF-a and IL-1β being the initial cytokines. These cytokines stimulate the production of other cytokines such as IL-6, IL-8, IL-10 and MIP-1a (macrophage inflammatory protein-1a). TNFa, IL-1b, IL-6, IL-8 and IL-10 are linked to morbidity and mortality in septic patients. IL-6 levels in plasma rise according to sepsis severity, but that does not always happen. The median levels of IL-6 in patients with SIRS are approximately 10-fold higher than that of healthy people, in sepsis are approximately 20-fold higher, in severe sepsis 60-fold higher and in septic shock are 100-fold higher. But, in some patients IL-6 levels are very similar to those of healthy people (3pg/ml). (Socha et al, 2006, Halter et al, 2005, Akira et al, 2003, Mokart et al, 2002, Paterson et al, 2000, Hack et al, 1997, Casey et al, 1993, Pinsky et al, 1993).

IL-6 is induced by TNF-a and has a longer half-life, reliably measured in blood after insult to the host. IL-6, as a marker of infection, is relatively nonspecific as it is elevated in a variety of inflammatory states. IL-6 is one of the initial cytokines released in inflammation, as mentioned above, and may be an early predictor of more downstream effects, such as organ dysfunction. IL-6 may perform well as a diagnostic and prognostic tool of sepsis. IL-6 levels of more than 1000 ng/mL are highly predictive of sepsis related death. The diagnostic and prognostic accuracy of IL-6 may depend on time and frequency of measurement and underlying illness severity, perhaps suggesting the importance of trending cytokine levels with clinical course and therapy As IL-6, IL-8 is not so a good indicator of systemic infection, although elevated IL-8 levels are indicative of multiple organ failure and an increased likelihood of death. Measurement of IL-6 and IL-8 is not optimal for discriminating patients with infectious from those with noninfectious conditions (Chiesa et al, 2003, Iglesias et al, 2003, Harbarth, 2001, Muller et al, 2000, Panacek, 1999, Martin, 1997, De werra, 1997).

Tumor Necrosis Factor-a (TNF-a), which is mainly produced by macrophages, lymphocytes and fibroblasts, causes fever and elevated liver enzymes among others and activates three main cell signaling pathways, which lead to inflammation and cell death, by binding to its receptor. Plasma levels of TNF-a are increased rapidly after infection and that's how TNF-a activates the inflammation cascade. Additionally, TNF-a levels in plasma are increased due to the elevated production of Haemoxygenase-1 (HO-1), which is implicated by lung injury and organ perfusion (Socha et al, 2006, Kalil et al, 2004, Kan et al, 1999). There are two types of TNFa receptors: TNF-R type 1 (CD120a) - which binds only to TNFα- and TNF-R type 2 (CD120b) - which binds both to TNFα and TNFβ. The three cell signaling pathways, leading to inflammation, activated by TNF-a are the following:

1. TRADD- RIP- TRAF2 pathway stimulates NF-κb pathway and production of antiapoptotic factors, such as Bcl-2.
2. TRADD- RIP-TRAF2-ASK1-MAPK pathway leads mainly to AP-1 production and downstream to the production of pro-apoptotic factors and cell proliferation and cell maturation.

TNFR- CD40 TRADD- FADD pathway leads to cell apoptosis by triggering caspase family cascade (Jaffer et al, 2010) (**Figure 2**).

Cytokines also participate in anti-inflammatory cascade. When the inflammatory response is triggered, anti-inflammatory mechanisms are simultaneously activated. Elevated production of pro-inflammatory cytokines causes the simultaneous production of specific cytokines such as IL-4, IL-10, IL-13, soluble TNF receptor and reduction of lymphocyte cells production. Th1 lymphocytes secrete TNF-a, IL-2 and IFN-γ, while T17 lymphocytes secrete IL-17 leading neutrophils to the infection field, unlike Th2 lymphocytes secrete IL-4, IL-6 and IL-10, while regulatory T-cells (Treg) mediate cytokine secretion amplifying the anti-inflammatory response. Especially IL-10 -produced also by monocytes- is suspensory to Th1-cytokines secretion (and mainly to TNF-a) and inhibits the NF-kB JAK-STAT pathway. IL-13 is secreted by Th-cells and leads to elevated production of IgE, matrix-metalloproteinases (MMPs) and neutrophils while it regulates TNF-a and leucocyte response to SIRS. TNF-a and IL-10 levels are found increased in patients with bad prognosis and the increase is higher in patients with positive blood culture. IL-10 levels can be used to discriminate sepsis from sever sepsis (Jaffer et al 2010, Giamarellos- Bourboulis 2010, Freitas et al 2009, Sobieski et al 2008, Van der Poll et al 2008, Munford et al 2001, Rodriguez-Gaspar et al 2001, Socha et al 2006, Whitlock et al 2006).

3. Coagulation biomarkers

Macrophage Migration Inhibitory Factor (MIF) has a critical role in activating the immune system and accelerating the pro-inflammatory response in sepsis (that is why it is thought that in the near future MIF will be a significant target in the treatment of sepsis). Tissue factor activates coagulation cascade (**figure 3**) and fibrinolysis system. Antithrombin III plays a dominant role among antithrombotic and fibrinolytic agents. Antithrombin III is involved in the formation of a complex constituted by activated FVIIa, FIXa, Fxa and FXIa factors and kallikrein. When antithrombin III is inhibited e.g by prostacyclin, Disseminated Intravascular Coagulation (DIC) is caused -which is considered as an important factor in Multi Organ Dysfunction (MODS) development because its normal function is to lower platelet adhesion and activate monocytes. Finally, we must refer to protein C or autoprothrombin IIA, which protects cells from sepsis and it has strong anticoagulative effects through inactivating Va and VIIIa factors of the coagulation system (Mosnier et al, 2007, Hotchkiss et al, 2003, Nicolaes et al, 2003, Mather et al, 1996).

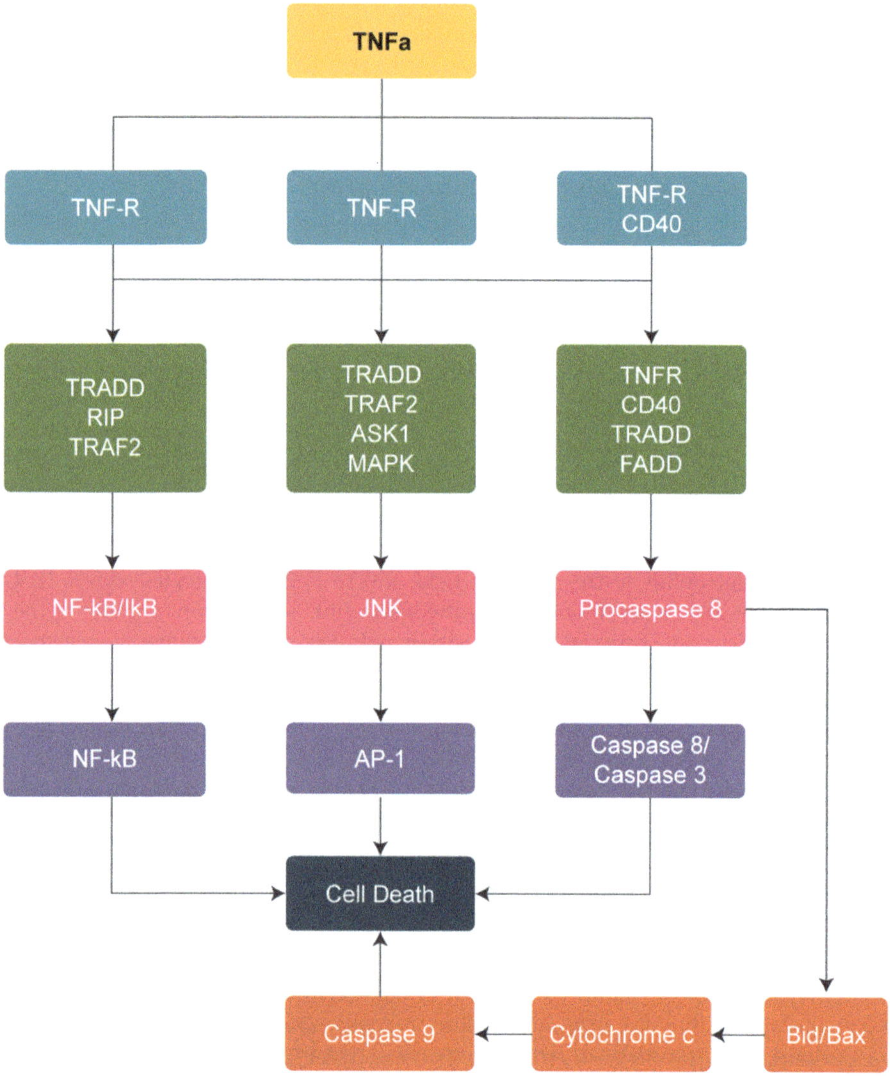

Fig. 2. TNFa activated cellular pathways

The more interesting coagulation factors for sepsis, whose levels have been proposed to be in accordance to sepsis severity and have some prognostic use for septic patient, are easily counted in clinical practice. Activated partial thromboplastin time (aPTT) measurement waveform has been correlated to sepsis. An atypical biphasic transmittance waveform due to decreased light transmission has been observed and it is more common in patients with sepsis. This phenomenon may be due to the formation and precipitation of a calcium dependent complex among C-reactive protein (CRP) and very low density lipoprotein

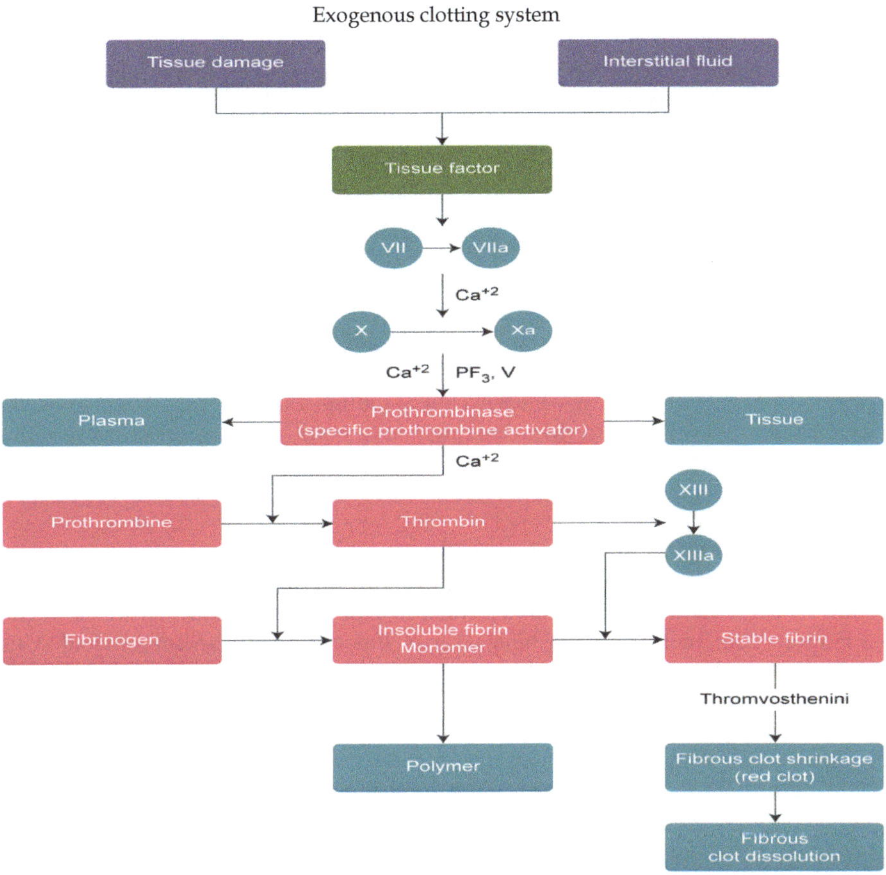

Fig. 3. The exogenous clotting system

(VLDL) in serum of septic patients. That waveform is correlated with negative prediction, sepsis induced disseminated intravascular coagulation and multiorgan failure. Plasminogen activator inhibitor-1 high levels have predictive value for the development of multiorgan failure in septic patients and they are strong correlated with bad prognosis of septic patients with sepsis induced disseminated intravascular coagulation especially when plasminogen activator inhibitor levels are higher than 90 ng/ml. Antithrombin III concentration has been proposed as a prognostic factor, as its levels are lower in septic patients who are not possible to survive. Low protein C levels in septic patient's blood are indicative of increased risk of morbidity and mortality (Zakariah et al, 2008, Madoiwa et al, 2006, Petilla et al, 2002, Fisher et al, 2000).

4. Acute phase protein biomarkers

Acute phase protein biomarkers have been more extensively correlated with prognosis of sepsis, compared to other biomarkers. The two main acute phase protein biomarkers which are related to sepsis are procalsitonin (PCT) and C-reactive protein (CRP). PCT has a bigger sensitivity and specificity in prognosis of sepsis compared to CRP, but CRP is more available and most widely used in clinical practice. Also, PCT is generally elevated in various conditions correlated with inflammatory response, whether CRP has a better prognostic value in the response of therapy in septic patients. However, there are contradictory views for the utility of both biomarkers in prognosis of sepsis and further clinical studies must be demonstrated in this direction. Serum CRP may be used as a biomarker as its concentrations increase in response to inflammation, its half-life is short but its kinetics are not as good as those of PCT. CRP levels are increased in sepsis, but its use as a diagnostic biomarker is not yet established. CRP is proposed to be used as a discriminating factor between septic from non septic shock while it is less accurate than PCT in SIRS from sepsis differentiation. CRP is a poor predictive biomarker of sepsis outcome. Many experimental and clinical trials suggest that PCT is a specific marker for severe bacterial infection and it may be used to distinguish patients who have sepsis from patients who have SIRS in clinical routine. PCT has been shown to be a better biomarker than IL-6 and CRP in characterizing noinfectious from infectious acute respiratory distress syndrome. PCT remains among the most promising biomarkers in sepsis (Jensen, 2006, Castelli, 2004, Clec'h, 2004, Povoa, 2004, Luzzani, 2003, Claeys, 2002, Harbarth, 2001, Muller, 2000, Assicot, 1993).

Other acute phase protein biomarkers which are widely used in clinical practice, are ceruloplasmin - which is correlated with great liver dysfunction in septic patients- and hepcidin which is shown significantly elevated in septic patients and patients with chronic renal failure. Also, another critical biomarker of this category is serum amyloid A (SAA) which is associated with the elevated levels of CRP in septic patients. Finally, there must be a reference on lipopolysacharide binding protein (LBP), which is generally elevated in septic patients compared to the healthy population, but –on the other hand- cannot be used as a prognostic marker in the development of sepsis. (Li et al 2009, Cicarreli et al 2008, Schmit et al 2008, Couto et al 2007, Seller-Perez et al 2005, Oude Nijhuis et al 2003, Becker et al 2008).

5. Receptor biomarkers

Many cell receptors have been proposed to have prognostic value for septic patients. Their reliability for clinical routine use is under investigation and only some experimental findings are indicative of receptor biomarkers quality for usage in septic patient diagnosis. Receptor biomarkers that will be further discussed are IL-2 receptor, Toll-like receptor (TLR2 and TLR 4), TNF receptor and TREM-1 receptor. However, many other receptors have been investigated and proposed as possible biomarkers of sepsis, such as CSL2, Fas Receptor and group II phospholipase A2 receptor. Increased serum levels of soluble IL-2 receptor in patients with gram-negative sepsis may behave as predictive indices of shock. Soluble IL-2 receptor is released in biological fluids mostly from T and B lymphocytes that seem to participate in pathogenesis of sepsis. Soluble IL-2 receptor measurement can be easily performed by the use of diagnostic kits and it is suggested to be routinely measured in sera from patients with gram-negative sepsis in order to identify those, who have the strongest risk to develop septic shock. Microorganisms consist of conserved sequences called Pathogen-Associated Molecular Patterns (PAMPs) such as endotoxin/ lipopolysaccharide (LPS) which are located in Gram- negative bacteria cell wall. These PAMPs bind to specific Pattern Recognition Receptors (PRRs) (there are 15 known subtypes), named Toll-like receptors (TLRs) and especially TLR2 and TLR4. TLRs have an intracellular domain, homologous with IL-1 and the IL-18 receptors. Adaptor proteins facilitate binding to IL-1 receptor-associated kinase, which in turn induces TNF receptor-associated factor-6, leading to nuclear translocation of nuclear factor-kB (NF-kB) and ultimately to activation of cytokine gene promoters, resulting in advanced proinflammatory cytokine production (Rittisch et al, 2008, Brunn et al, 2006, Cornell et al, 2005, Delogu et al, 1995, Willatts et al, 1994). Initially in inflammatory response, LPS is bound by a lipopolysaccharide binding protein which is located to CD14 and TLR4. TLR4 and CD14 are receptors of macrophages and circulating monocytes and they are activated by LPS binding. Their activation causes signal transduction through Toll Inerleukin-1 Receptor (TIR) domain which is referred as myeloid differentiation protein 88. Afterwards, the IL-1 receptor-associated kinase (IRAK) is activated and in turn activates the TNFa-receptor associated factor (TRAF) and the TRAF-associated kinase (TAK). That is the role of TLRs in sepsis. But what is their diagnostic use as biomarkers, if there is any? TLR-2 and TLR-4 expressions are relatively increased in septic critically ill patients, as it was found in experiments using mice. Moreover, the increased levels of those two TLRs were related to advanced possibility to death.

In septic patients, soluble TNFRs plasma levels have been found increased. In the same study it was suggested that the increased levels of the receptor correlate in the same way with multiple organ failure, as with mortality. Elevated soluble TNFR levels may be used as a biomarker for severity of sepsis, in a predicting manner. But more information and clinical trials are needed in order TNFR to be used in clinical routine. Soluble TREM-1 is a reliable marker of bacterial infection, while it participates in the septic process. A decrease in soluble TREM-1 concentration may be indicative of treatment effectiveness. On the contrary, when sTREM-1 levels are persistenly increased the therapy administered to patient is not effective or patients are not in a good condition. Moreover, sTREM-1 concentration is indicative of the prognosis of the patients and they can be used in predicting septic patient outcome. The receptors levels on the 28th day from diagnosis are significantly different in patients with good prognosis from those with not such a good prognosis, which may lead them to death (Rittisch et al, 2008, Annane et al, 2005, Gibot, 2005, Williams et al, 2003, McCuskey et al, 1996 Ertel, 1994).

6. Cell marker related biomarkers

Cells that bear on their membrane surface special proteins have been used in experiments in sepsis trials, in order to find some special patterns of expression of those proteins during sepsis and try to combine these findings with sepsis diagnosis and prognosis. So, CD10, CD11, CD14, CD18, CD25, CD28, CD40, CD48, CD54, CD60, CD80 and CD163 are the cell marker proteins which levels have been correlated to sepsis and septic shock prognosis. From those CD10 and CD11c are found in decreased levels in septic patients. Neutrophil CD11b and CD64 appear to be promising markers for diagnosis of early and late onset infections. CD11b is normally expressed in low concentration on the surface of neutrophils and its expression is increased 2-4 times more in infants and adults with positive blood culture for sepsis. CD11b seems to be very useful in early diagnosis of neonatal sepsis. CD14, CD25, CD28, CD40 and CD163 are significant different between septic patients with good prognosis and those with very bad prognosis in the 28th day from sepsis diagnosis. CD69 and CD48 are increased in septic patients (Giamarelos et al, 2010,Nolan et al, 2008, Kaneko et al, 2003, Mishra, 2006).

7. Vascular and endothelial damage dysfunction biomarkers

Activated macrophages in sepsis produce early response cytokines TNF-a and IL-1 which stimulate vascular endothelial cells to express Intercellular Adhesion Molecules-1 (ICAM-1), E-selectin and tissue factor. In addition, the adhesion of neutrophils to endothelium involves interaction between endothelial ICAM-1 and beta2 integrin of neutrophils. Adhesion molecules expression is increased in the most severely ill septic patients and it reaches its peak in patients with Multi Organ Failure (MOF). According to these findings, vascular cell adhesion molecule (VCAM-1), E-selectin, P-selectin and endocan are fine prognostic biomarkers in the development of multi-organ dysfunction (MODS) and septic shock in septic patients. Also, L-laminin shows a significant increase in septic patients and ADAMTS-13 is increased in septic patients without disseminated intravascular coagulopathy (DIC) compared to septic patients with DIC. Additionally, there is an existing increase in other biomarkers of this category like cellular and soluble endothelial leukocyte adhesion molecule (ELAM)-1 and vascular endothelial growth factor (VEGF) in septic patients with very poor prognosis, but further clinical studies must be demonstrated. (Drake et al 1993, Mimuro et al 2008, Seidelin et al 2002, Lopez et al 1999, Whalen et al 2000, Cowley et al, 1994, Moss et al, 1996).

8. Vasolidation related biomarkers

There are several biomarkers of sepsis related to vasodilation which have been already identified in patients. Firstly, C-type natriuretic peptide (CNP), anandamide, angiotesin converting enzyme (ACE), 2- arachidonoglykerol and neuropeptide Y are shown to be significantly increased in septic patients comparing to the healthy population, although further clinical studies must be done to ensure this finding. Also, 47 kD high molecular weight kininogen (HK) shows a critical correlation with more severe sepsis. Furthermore, proadrenomedulin and andrenomedulin are correlated with development of sepsis. But, the most critical vasodilatory factor which is correlated with development of sepsis is nitric oxide and its derivatives. In the metabolic pathway of inducible (or induced) NO synthase (Inducible Nitric Oxide Synthetase: iNOS), the inducible NO synthetase overproduces nitric oxide by reacting with L-Arginine, which results to relaxation of smooth muscle cells. Its concentration increases as a result of gene activation, which in turn produces high levels of nitric oxide (NO). NO activates guanylyl cyclase enzyme. Guanylyl cyclase increases the production of cyclic guanosine monophosphate (cGMP). However, if NO production is inhibited by blockading the NOS enzyme, then it is associated with poor prognosis in septic patients. Also, nitric oxide is being hugely produced after the activation of iNOS gene by Hypoxia Inducible Factor-1 (HIF-1). Finally, there are tetrahydrobiopterin which is shown increased in critically ill septic patients and vasoactive intestinal peptide (VIP) which is shown quite increased in tissues of patients with severe peritonitis. Elastin is shown decreased in septic patients compared to healthy population (Jacob et al 2007, Levy, et al 2005, Faury et al, 2005, Jang et al, 2004, Hama et al 1994, Beer et al 2002, Amalich et al 1995, Deitz et al, 1987).

9. Organ dysfunction biomarkers

Specific organ dysfunction biomarkers which are shown significantly increased in septic patients compared to healthy population are myocardial angiotensin II, pancreatitis-associated protein-I, pre B cell colony-enhancing factor (PBEF), glial fibrillary acidic protein

(GFAP) and Gc-globulin. Even most, Gc-globulin - which acts as an actin scavenger- has a good prognostic value in the development of multi-organ dysfunction, as it is found in low concentrations in patients developing sepsis and respiratory failure (Hsu et al 2008, Ji et al 1996, Tribl et al 2004, Ye et al 2005).

In sepsis it is highly possible that the balance between inflammatory and anti-inflammatory mechanisms becomes unbalanced so organ dysfunction and cardiovascular dysfunction, metabolic disturbances, renal dysfunction and haematological dysfunction are possible to happen. All the above clinical conditions combined are leading to multiple organ dysfunction. So, after an insult, the balance between inflammatory response and immunoparalysis determine the prognosis of the septic patient, which makes the above biomarkers of vital importance for them (Paterson et al, 2000, Poderoso et al, 1996, Neumann et al, 1997, Baudo et al, 1998, Karima et al, 1999, Grover et al, 1999,) **(figure 4)**.

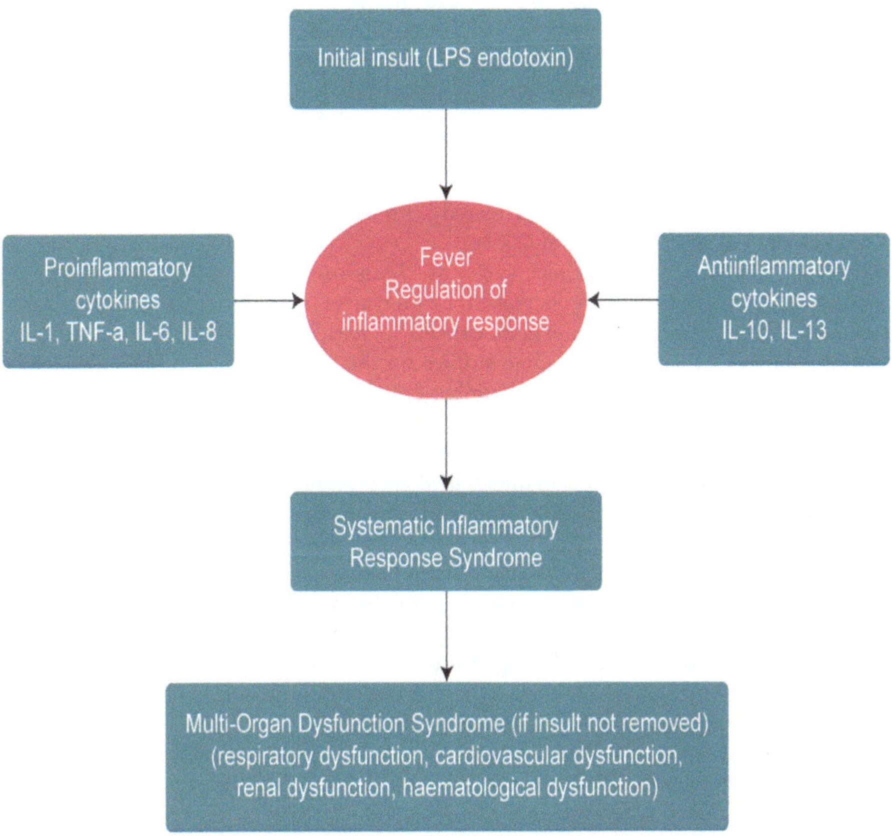

Fig. 4. The process of sepsis

10. Genetic biomarkers-single nucleotide polymorphisms

As in almost every other disease, genetic predisposition seems to play an important role in susceptibility in sepsis. Despite modern treatment of sepsis (eg, hydrocortisone) important genetic factors may be responsible even for death by sepsis. Also, along with genetic predisposition, comorbidity and age seem to play a significant role (Alberti et al 2002, Yende et al 2008, Pachot et al 2006, Wong et al 2007, Calvano et al 2005, Annane et al.1998, Bollaert et al.1998, Briegel et al.1999).

In recent years, there have been many clinical studies using modern methods and techniques of molecular genetics, such as genotyping to correlate gene expression with inflammatory response. Specific polymorphisms in some genes express proteins involved in the cascade of systematic inflammatory response and they have an important role in sepsis. These polymorphisms participating in sepsis are Single nucleotide polymorphisms (SNPs). SNPs of a gene is a DNA sequence variation which occurs whenever there is a difference in a single nucleotide position in genome and this one differs between members of a species. The simplest change of this kind is the substitution of one nucleotide by another which is not similar to the previous one. Single nucleotide polymorphisms have a minor allele frequency of >1% (or 0.5% etc.) A large number of SNPs in several genes involved in inflammatory response have been found to vary in their clinical outcomes during infection (Arcaroli et al 2005, Waterer et al 2003, Holmes et al 2003, Stuber et al 1996, Barber et al 2006). The major genetic agents that have been studied are the following:

Toll-like receptors: Polymorphisms found in TLR5 and TLR2 are correlated with bacterial infections, and those in TLR4 are correlated with susceptibility in sepsis (Sutherland et al. 2005, Skinner et al 2005, Hawn et al. 2003).

Collectins: There are collectins, such as Mannose binding lectine (MBL) whose polymorphisms associate with increased incidence of systemic inflammatory syndrome caused by infectious and noninfectious causes, increased severity of sepsis, and increased mortality although the results of some studies on this topic are contradictory (Garred et al. 2003, Roy et al. 2002, Gong et al 2007, Kronborg et al. 2002).

Tumor Necrosis Factor-a (TNF-a): TNF-a gene is polymorphic and there are various polymorphisms in its products. TNF-308 polymorphism with A-allele substitution is of high importance (the most common is G-allele) as it is correlated with increasing risk of death in septic patients. On the other hand, some studies state that there is no correlation between TNF polymorphism and sepsis (O'Keefe et al. 2002, Nakada et al. 2005, Azim et al. 2007, Schueller et al. 2006, Waterer et al. 2001).

Interleukin-1 (IL-1) Family: Polymorphisms in IL1β may correlate with sepsis according to its cause, as in some cases they are associated with sepsis development and in some cases they are not. Also, there are conflicting studies of variants of IL-1 receptor antagonist gene (IL-1RN) and its correlation with mortality in patients with septic shock (Arnalich et al. 2002, Ma et al. 2002, Fang et al. 1999, Turner et al. 1997).

Interleukin-10 (IL-10): IL-10-1082 G polymorphic allele presence is correlated to sensitivity to pneumonia and susceptibility to septic shock as well as with multiorgan dysfunction (Stanilolva et al. 2006, Gallagher et al. 2003, Schaaf et al. 2003).

Furthermore, SNPs have also been found in genes expressing proteins participating into the inflammatory response. These genes, which SNPs may show correlation with septic shock are: *Lymphotoxin Alpha (LTA) gene, Immunoglobin Receptors genes, Heat shock protein gene, Protein C gene* and *Plasminogen activation inhibitor (PAI) -1 gene, Lippopollysaccharide binding protein (LBP) gene*, *CD14 gene* and *Myeloid differentiation protein-2 (MD-2) gene* (Gu et al. 2007, Temple et al. 2004, Yuan et al. 2003, Ye et al. 1995, Binder et al. 2007, Geishofer et al. 2005, Haralambous et al. 2003, Hermans et al. 1999, Van der Poll et al. 2001, Hubacek et al. 2001, Waterer et al. 2001).

As discussed in this chapter there are many biomarkers of sepsis. All of them are very promising in sepsis diagnosis and prognosis, but more evidence is needed so as to be valuable for in every day clinical routine. Sepsis severity and its high incidence to patient's death make extremely difficult every decision in using one and only one clue as the absolute biomarker for sepsis diagnosis and prognosis. Sepsis is such a complex syndrome that every oversimplified approach may become lethal for patients. Multi-biomarker control is the best approach till now. As research continues newer and more advanced biomarkers may be found helping in sepsis diagnosis and therapeutics.

11. References

Akira S, Sato S (2003). Toll-like receptors and their signalling mechanisms. *Scand J Infect Dis*; 35:555-562.

Alberti C, Brun-Buisson C, Burchardi H, Martin C, Goodman S, Artigas A, Sicignano A, Palazzo M, Moreno R, Boulmé R, Lepage E, Le Gall R (2002). Epidemiology of sepsis and infection in ICU patients from an international multicentre cohort study. *Intensive Care Med*; 28:108-121.

Annane D, Bellissant E, Cavaillon J-M (2005). Septic shock. *Lancet*; 365:63-78.

Annane D, Bellissant E, Sebille V, Lesieur O, Mathieu B, Raphael JC, Gajdos P (1998). Impaired pressor sensitivity to noradrenaline in septic shock patients with and without impaired adrenal function reserve. *Br J Clin Pharmacol*; 46:589-597.

Arcaroli J, Fessler MB, Abraham E (2005). Genetic polymorphisms and sepsis. *Shock*; 24(4):300-312.

Arnalich F, Sanchez JF, Martinez M, Jimenez M, Lopez J, Vazquez JJ, Hernanz A (1995). Changes in plasma concentrations of vasoactive neuropeptides in patients with sepsis and septic shock. *Life Sci*, 56:75-81.

Arnalich F, Lopez-Maderuelo D, Codoceo R, Lopez J, Solis-Garrido LM, Capiscol C, Fernandez-Capitan C, Madero R, Montiel C (2002). Interleukin-1 receptor antagonist gene polymorphism and mortality in patients with severe sepsis. *Clin Exp Immunol*; 127:331-336.

Assicot M, Gendrel D (1993). High serum procalcitonin concentrations in patients with sepsis and infection. *Lancet*; 341:515-518.

Azim K, McManus R, Brophy K, Ryan A, Kelleher D, Reynolds JV (2007). Genetic polymorphisms and the risk of infection following esophagectomy. Positive association with TNF-alpha gene -308 genotype. *Ann Surg*; 246:122-128.

Barber RC, Chang LY, Arnoldo BD, Purdue GF, Hunt JL, Horton JW, Aragaki CC (2006). Innate immunity SNPs are associated with risk for severe sepsis after burn injury. *Clin Med Res*; 4(4):250-255.

Baudo F, Caimi TM, deCataldo F (1998). Antithrombin III (ATIII) replacement therapy in patients with sepsis and/or postsurgical complications: a controlled double-blind, randomized, multicenter study. *Intensive Care Med*; 24:336-342.

Becker KL, Snider R, Nylen ES (2008). Procalcitonin assay in systemic inflammation, infection, and sepsis: clinical utility and limitations. *Crit Care Med*; 36:941-952.

Beer S, Weighardt H, Emmanuilidis K, Harzenetter MD, Matevossian E, Heidecke CD, Bartels H, Siewert JR, Holzmann B (2002). Systemic neuropeptide levels as predictive indicators for lethal outcome in patients with postoperative sepsis. *Crit Care Med*; 30:1794-1798.

Binder A, Endler G, Muller M, Mannhalter C, Zenz W (2007). 4G4G genotype of the plasminogen activator inhibitor-1 promoter polymorphism associates with disseminated intravascular coagulation in children with systemic meningococcemia. *J Thromb Haemost*; 5:2049-54.

Biomarkers Definitions Working Group (2001): Biomarkers and surrogate endpoints: Preferred definitions and conceptual framework. *Clin Pharmacol Ther*; 69:89-95.

Bollaert PE, Charpentier C, Debouverie M, Audibert G, Larcan A (1998). Reversal of late septic shock with supraphysiologic doses of hydrocortisone. *Crit Care Med*; 26:645-650.

Bone RC, Balk RA, Cerra FB , Cerra FB, Dellinger RP, Fein AM, Knaus WA, Schein RM, Sibbald WJ; ACCP/SCCM Consensus Conference Committee (1992). ACCP/SCCM Consensus Conference. Definitions for sepsis and organ failure and guidelines for the use of innovative therapies in sepsis. *Chest*; 101:1644-1655.

Briegel J, Forst H, Haller M, Schelling G, Kilger E, Kuprat G, Hemmer B, Hummel T, Lenhart A, Heyduck M, Stoll C, Peter K (1999). Stress doses of hydrocortisone reverse hyperdynamic septic shock: A prospective, randomized, double-blind, single-center study. *Crit Care Med*; 27:723-732.

Brunkhorst FM, Heinz U, Forycki ZF (1998). Kinetics of procalcitonin in iatrogenic sepsis. *Intensive Care Med*; 24:888-889.

Brunn GJ, Platt JL (2006). The aetiology of sepsis: turned inside out. *Trends Mol Med*; 12:10-16.

Calvano SE, Xiao W, Richards DR, Felciano RM, Baker HV, Cho RJ, Chen RO, Brownstein BH, Cobb JP, Tschoeke SK, Miller-Graziano C, Moldawer LL, Mindrinos MN, Davis RW, Tompkins RG, Lowry SF; Inflamm and Host Response to Injury Large Scale Collab. Res. Program (2005). A network-based analysis of systemic inflammation in humans. *Nature*; 437:1032–1037.

Casey LC, Balk RA, Bone RC (1993). Plasma cytokines and endotoxin levels correlate with survival in patients with the sepsis syndrome. *Ann Intern Med*; 119:771-778.

Castelli GP, Pognani C, Meisner M, Stuani A, Bellomi D, Sgarbi L (2004). Procalcitonin and C-reactive protein during systemic inflammatory response syndrome, sepsis and organ dysfunction. *Crit Care*; 8:R234-242.

Chiesa C, Pellegrini G, Panero A, Osborn JF, Signore F, Assumma M, Pacifico L (2003). C-reactive protein, interleukin-6, and procalcitonin in the immediate postnatal period: influence of illness severity, risk status, antenatal and perinatal complications, and infection. *Clin Chem*; 49:60-68.

Cicarelli DD, Vieira JE, Bensenor FE (2008). Comparison of C-reactive protein and serum amyloid a protein in septic shock patients. *Mediators Inflamm*; 2008:631414.

Claeys R, Vinken S, Spapen H, ver Elst K, Decochez K, Huyghens L, Gorus FK (2002). Plasma procalcitonin and C-reactive protein in acute septic shock: clinical and biological correlates. *Crit Care Med*; 30:757-762.

Clec'h C, Ferriere F, Karoubi P (2004). Diagnostic and prognostic value of procalcitonin in patients with sepsis and septic shock. *Crit Care Med*; 32:1166-1169.

Cornell Timothy T, Wynn James, Shanley Thomas P, Wheeler Derek S, Wong Hector R (2010). Mechanisms and Regulation of the Gene-Expression Response to Sepsis. *Pediatrics*; 125:1248.

Couto RC, Barbosa JA, Pedrosa TM, Biscione FM (2007). C-reactive protein-guided approach may shorten length of antimicrobial treatment of cultureproven late-onset sepsis: an intervention study. *Braz J Infect Dis*; 11:240-245.

Cowley HC, Heney D, Gearing AJ, Hemingway I, Webster NR (1994). Increased circulating adhesion molecules concentration in patients with the systemic inflammatory response syndrome: a prospective cohort study. *Crit Care Med*; 22: 651-657.

De Werra I, Jaccard C, Corradin SB, Chioléro R, Yersin B, Gallati H, Assicot M, Bohuon C, Baumgartner JD, Glauser MP, Heumann D (1997). Cytokines, nitrite/nitrate, soluble tumor necrosis factor receptors, and procalcitonin concentrations: comparisons in patients with septic shock, cardiogenic shock, and bacterial pneumonia. *Crit Care Med;* 25:607-613.

Deitz DM, Swartz KR, Wright M, Murphy E, Connell RS, Harrison MW (1987). Effects of E. coli endotoxin on rat plasma angiotensin converting enzyme activity in vitro and in vivo. *Circ Shock*; 21:23-29.

Dellinger RP, Levy MM, Carlet JM, Bion J, Parker MM, Jaeschke R, Reinhart K, Angus DC, Brun-Buisson C, Beale R, Calandra T, Dhainaut JF, Gerlach H, Harvey M, Marini JJ, Marshall J, Ranieri M, Ramsay G, Sevransky J, Thompson BT, Townsend S, Vender JS, Zimmerman JL, Vincent JL (2008). Surviving Sepsis Campaign: international guidelines for management of severe sepsis and septic shock: 2008. *Crit Care Med*; 36:296-327.

Delogu G, Casula MA, Mancini P, Tellan G, Signore L (1995). Serum neopterin and soluble interleukin-2 receptor for prediction of a shock state in gramnegative sepsis. *J Crit Care*; 10:64-71.

Dhar R, Diringer MN (2008). The burden of the systemic inflammatory response predicts vasospasm and outcome after subarachnoid hemorrhage. *Neurocrit Care*; 8(3):404-412.

Drake TA, Cheng J, Chang A, Taylor FB Jr (1993). Expression of tissue factor, thrombomodulin, and E-selectin in baboons with lethal Escherichia coli sepsis. *Am J Pathol*; 142:1458-1470.

Ertel W, Scholl FA, Gallati H, Bonaccio M, Schildberg FW, Trentz O (1994). Increased release of soluble tumor necrosis factor receptors into blood during clinical sepsis. *Arch Surg*; 129:1330-1336.

Fang XM, Schroder S, Hoeft A, Stuber F (1999). Comparison of two polymorphisms of the interleukin-1 gene family: interleukin-1 receptor antagonist polymorphism contributes to susceptibility to severe sepsis. *Crit Care Med;* 27:1330-1334.

Faury G, Wynnychenko TM, Cand F, Leone M, Jacob MP, Verdetti J, Boyle WA (2005). Decreased circulating elastin peptide levels in humans with sepsis. *Pathol Biol (Paris)*; 53:443-447.

Fisher CJ Jr, Yan SB (2000). Protein C levels as a prognostic indicator of outcome in sepsis and related diseases. *Crit Care Med*; 28:S49-S56.

Freitas A, Alves-Filho JC, Victoni T, Secher T, Lemos HP, Sônego F, Cunha FQ, Ryffel B (2009). IL- -17 receptor signaling is required to control polymicrobial sepsis. *J Immunol*; 182(12):7846-7854.

Gallagher PM, Lowe G, Fitzgerald T, Bella A, Greene CM, McElvaney NG, O'Neill SJ (2003). Association of IL-10 polymorphism with severity of illness in community acquired pneumonia. *Thorax;* 58:154-156.

Garred P, Strom J, Quist L, Taaning E, Madsen H (2003). Association of mannose-binding lectin polymorphisms with sepsis and fatal outcome, in patients with systemic inflammatory response syndrome. *J Infect Dis;* 188:1394-1403.

Geishofer G, Binder A, Muller M, Zohrer B, Resch B, Muller W, Faber J, Finn A, Endler G, Mannhalter C, Zenz W, C. E. M. G. S. Group (2005). 4G/5G promoter polymorphism in the plasminogen-activator-inhibitor-1 gene in children with systemic meningococcaemia. *Eur J Pediatr;* 164:486-490.

Giamarellos-Bourboulis EJ (2010). What is the pathophysiology of the septic host upon admission? *Int J Antimicrob Agents;* S2:S2-S5.

Gibot S, Cravoisy A, Kolopp-Sarda MN, Bene MC, Faure G, Bollaert PE, Levy B (2005). Time-course of sTREM (soluble triggering receptor expressed on myeloid cells)-1, procalcitonin, and C-reactive protein plasma concentrations during sepsis. *Crit Care Med;* 33:792-796.

Gong MN, Zhou W, Williams PL, Thompson BT, Pothier L, Christiani DC (2007). Polymorphisms in the mannose binding lectin-2 gene and acute respiratory distress syndrome. *Crit Care Med* 35:48-56.

Grover R, Lopez A, Lorente J (1999). Multi-center, randomized, placebo-controlled, double blind study of the nitric oxide synthase inhibitor 546C88: effect on survival in patients with septic shock. *Crit Care Med;* 27: A33.

Gu W, Shan Y, Zhou J, Jiang D, Zhang L, Du D, Wang Z, Jiang J (2007). Functional significance of gene polymorphisms in the promoter of myeloid differentiation-2. *Ann Surg;* 246:151-158.

Hack CE, Aarden LA, Thijs LG (1997). Role of cytokines in sepsis. *Adv Immunol;* 66: 101-195.

Halter J, Steinberg J, Fink G, Lutz C, Picone A, Maybury R, Fedors N, DiRocco J, Lee HM, Nieman G (2005). Evidence of systemic cytokine release in patients undergoing cardiopulmonary bypass. *J Extra Corpor Technol;* 37: 272-277.

Hama N, Itoh H, Shirakami G, Suga S, Komatsu Y, Yoshimasa T, Tanaka I, Mori K, Nakao K (1994). Detection of C-type natriuretic peptide in human circulation and marked increase of plasma CNP level in septic shock patients. *Biochem Biophys Res Commun;* 198(3):1177-1182.

Haralambous E, Hibberd ML, Hermans PW, Ninis N, Nadel S, Levin M (2003). Role of functional plasminogen-activator-inhibitor-1 4G/5G promoter polymorphism in susceptibility, severity, and outcome of meningococcal disease in Caucasian children. *Crit Care Med;* 31:2788-2793.

Harbarth S, Holeckova K, Froidevaux C, Pittet D, Ricou B, Grau GE, Vadas L, Pugin J; Geneva Sepsis Network (2001). Diagnostic value of procalcitonin, interleukin-6, and interleukin- 8 in critically ill patients admitted with suspected sepsis. *Am J Respir Crit Care Med;* 164:396-402.

Hawn TR, Verbon A, Lettinga KD, Zhao LP, Li SS, Laws RJ, Skerrett SJ, Beutler B, Schroeder L, Nachman A, Ozinsky A, Smith KD, Aderem A (2003). A common dominant TLR5 stop codon polymorphism abolishes flagellin signaling and is associated with susceptibility to legionnaires' disease. *J Exp Med;* 198:1563-1572.

Hermans PW, Hibberd ML, Booy R, Daramola O, Hazelzet JA, de Groot R, Levin M (1999). 4G/5G promoter polymorphism in the plasminogen-activator-inhibitor-1 gene and outcome of meningococcal disease. Meningococcal Research Group. *Lancet;* 354 (9178):556-560.

Hildeman DA, Zhu Y, Mitchell TC, Kappler J, Marrack P (2002). Molecular mechanisms of activated T cell death in vivo. *Curr Opin Immunol;* 14:354-359.

Holmes CL, Russell JA, Walley KR (2003). Genetic polymorphisms in sepsis and septic shock: role in prognosis and potential for therapy. *Chest;* 124(3):1103-111.

Hoover L, Bochicchio GV, Napolitano LM, Joshi M, Bochicchio K, Meyer W, Scalea TM (2006). Systemic inflammatory response syndrome and nosocomial infection in trauma. *J Trauma;* 61(2):310-316.

Hotchkiss RS, Tinsley KW, Karl IE (2003). Role of apoptotic cell death in sepsis. *Scand J Infect Dis;* 35:585-592.

Hotchkiss RS, Coopersmith CM, Karl IE (2005). Prevention of lymphocyte apoptosis--a potential treatment of sepsis? *Clin Infect Dis;* 41 Suppl 7:S465-469.

Hotchkiss RS, Karl IE (2003). The pathophysiology and treatment of sepsis. *N Engl J Med;* 348:138-150.

Hsu AA, Fenton K, Weinstein S, Carpenter J, Dalton H, Bell MJ (2008). Neurological injury markers in children with septic shock. *Pediatr Crit Care Med;* 9:245-251.

Hubacek JA, Stuber F, Frohlich D, Book M, Wetegrove S, Ritter M, Rothe G, Schmitz G (2001). Gene variants of the bactericidal/permeability increasing protein and lipopolysaccharide binding protein in sepsis patients: gender-specific genetic predisposition to sepsis. *Crit Care Med;* 29:557-561.

Iglesias J, Marik PE, Levine JS (2003). Elevated serum levels of the type I and type II receptors for tumor necrosis factor-alpha as predictive factors for ARF in patients with septic shock. *Am J Kidney Dis;* 41:62-65.

Jacob P, Mueller MH, Hahn J, Wolk I, Mayer P, Nagele U, Hennenlotter J, Stenzl A, Konigsrainer A, Glatzle J (2007). Alterations of neuropeptides in the human gut during peritonitis. *Langenbecks Arch Surg;* 392:267-271.

Jaffer U, Wade RG, Gourlay T (2010). Cytokines in the systemic inflammatory response syndrome: a review. Hammersmith Hospital, London, UK; University of East Anglia, Norwich, Norfolk, UK; University of Strathclyde, Glasgow, Scotland. *HSR Proceedings in Intensive Care and Cardiovascular Anesthesia;* 2:161-175.

Jensen JU, Heslet L, Jensen TH, Espersen K, Steffensen P, Tvede M (2006). Procalcitonin increase in early identification of critically ill patients at high risk of mortality. *Crit Care Med;* 34:2596-2602.

Ji Y, Ren X, Zhao Y, Dong L, Wu L, Su J (1996). Role of intracardiac angiotensin II in cardiac dysfunction of rat during septic shock. *Chin Med J (Engl);* 109:864-867.

Jiang W, Jiang HF, Cai DY, Pan CS, Qi YF, Pang YZ, Tang CS (2004). Relationship between contents of adrenomedullin and distributions of neutral endopeptidase in blood and tissues of rats in septic shock. *Regul Pept;* 118:199-208.

Joshi VD, Kalvakolanu DV, Cross AS (2003). Simultaneous activation of apoptosis and inflammation in pathogenesis of septic shock: a hypothesis. *FEBS Letters;* 555:180-184.

Kalil AC, Coyle SM, Um JY, LaRosa SP, Turlo MA, Calvano SE, Sundin DP, Nelson DR, Lowry SF (2004). Effects of drotrecogin alfa (activated) in human endotoxemia. *Shock*; 21:222-229.

Kan H, Xie Z, Finkel MS (1999). TNF-alpha enhances cardiac myocyte NO production through MAP kinasemediated NF-kappaB activation. *Am J Physiol*; 277:1641-1646.

Kaneko T, Stearns-Kurosawa DJ, Taylor F Jr, Twigg M, Osaki K, Kinasewitz GT, Peer G, Kurosawa S (2003). Reduced neutrophil CD10 expression in nonhuman primates and humans after in vivo challenge with E. coli or lipopolysaccharide. *Shock*; 20:130-137.

Karima R, Matsumoto S, Hidemitsu H, Matsushima K (1999). The molecular pathogenesis of endotoxic shock and organ failure. *Mol Med Today*; 98: 123-133.

Kronborg G, Weis N, Madsen H, Pedersen S, Wejse C, Nielsen H, Skinhøj P, Garred P (2002). Variant mannose- binding lectin alleles are not associated with susceptibility to or outcome of invasive pneumococcal infection in randomly included patients. *J Infect Dis*; 185:1517-1520.

Lever A, Mackenzie I (2007). Sepsis: definition, epidemiology, and diagnosis. *BMJ*; 335:879-883.

Levy MM, Fink MP, Marshall JC, Abraham E, Angus D, Cook D, Cohen J, Opal SM, Vincent JL, Ramsay G, SCCM/ESICM/ACCP/ATS/SIS (2003). "2001 SCCM/ESICM/ACCP/ATS/SIS International Sepsis Definitions Conference". *Crit. Care Med.* 31 (4): 1250-1256.

Levy RM, Prince JM, Billiar TR (2005). Nitric oxide: a clinical primer. *Crit Care Med*; 33:S492-S495.

Li H, Rose MJ, Tran L, Zhang J, Miranda LP, James CA, Sasu BJ (2009). Development of a method for the sensitive and quantitative determination of hepcidin in human serum using LC-MS/MS. *J Pharmacol Toxicol Methods*; 59(3):171-180.

Lopez S, Prats N, Marco AJ (1999). Expression of E-selectin, P-selectin, and intercellular adhesion molecule-1 during experimental murine listeriosis. *Am J Pathol*; 155:1391-1397.

Luzzani A, Polati E, Dorizzi R, Rungatscher A, Pavan R, Merlini A (2003). Comparison of procalcitonin and C-reactive protein as markers of sepsis. *Crit Care Med*; 31:1737-1741.

Ma P, Chen D, Pan J, Du B (2002). Genomic polymorphism within interleukin-1 family cytokines influences the outcome of septic patients. *Zhonghua Yi Xue Za Zhi*; 82:1237-1241.

Madoiwa S, Nunomiya S, Ono T, Shintani Y, Ohmori T, Mimuro J, Sakata Y (2006). Plasminogen activator inhibitor 1 promotes a poor prognosis in sepsisinduced disseminated intravascular coagulation. *Int J Hematol*; 84:398-405.

Marshall JC, Reinhart K (2009). Biomarkers of sepsis. *Crit Care Med*; 37:2290-2298.

Martin C, Boisson C, Haccoun M, Thomachot L, Mege JL (1997). Patterns of cytokine evolution (tumor necrosis factor-alpha and interleukin-6) after septic shock, hemorrhagic shock, and severe trauma. *Crit Care Med*; 25:1813-1819.

Mather T, Oganessyan V, Hof P, Huber R, Foundling S, Esmon C, Bode W -December (1996). "The 2.8 Å crystal structure of Gla-domainless activated protein C". *EMBO J.* 15 (24): 6822-6831.

Matzinger P (2002).The danger model: A renewed sense of self. *Science*; 96:301-305.

McCuskey RS, Urbaschek R, Urbaschek B (1996). The microcirculation during endotoxemia. *Cardiol Res*; 32:752-763.
McDonald TE, Grinman MN, Carthy CM, Walley KR (2000). Endotoxin infusion in rats induces apoptotic and survival pathways in hearts. *Am J Physiol Heart Circ Physiol*; 79:H2053- H2061.
Mimuro J, Niimura M, Kashiwakura Y, Ishiwata A, Ono T, Ohmori T, Madoiwa S, Okada K, Matsuo O, Sakata Y (2008). Unbalanced expression of ADAMTS13 and von Willebrand factor in mouse endotoxinemia. *Thromb Res*; 122:91-97.
Mishra UK, Jacobs SE, Doyle LW, Garland SM (2006). Newer approaches to the diagnosis of early onset neonatal sepsis. *Arch Dis Child Fetal Neonatal*; 91(3):F208-212.
Mokart D, Capo C, Blache JL, Delpero JR, Houvenaeghel G, Martin C, Mege JL (2002). Early postoperative compensatory anti-inflammatory response syndrome is associated with septic complications after major surgical trauma in patients with cancer. *Br J Surg*; 89: 1450-1456.
Mori K, Nakao K (1994). Detection of C-type natriuretic peptide in human circulation and marked increase of plasma CNP level in septic shock patients. *Biochem Biophys Res Commun*; 198:1177-1182.
Mosnier LO, Zlokovic BV, Griffin JH (2007). The cytoprotective protein C pathway". *Blood*; 109 (8): 3161-3172.
Moss M, Gillespie MK, Ackerson L, Moore FA, Moore EE, Parsons PE (1996). Endothelial cell activity varies in patients at risk for the adult respiratory distress syndrome. *Crit Care Med*; 24: 1782-1786.
Muller B, Becker KL, Schachinger H, Rickenbacher PR, Huber PR, Zimmerli W, Ritz R (2000). Calcitonin precursors are reliable markers of sepsis in a medical intensive care unit. *Crit Care Med*; 28:977-983.
Munford RS, Pugin J (2001). Normal responses to injury prevent systemic inflammation and can be immunosuppressive. *Am J Respir Crit Care Med*; 163:316-21.
Nakada TA, Hirasawa H, Oda S, Shiga H, Matsuda KI, Nakamura M, Watanabe E, Abe R, Hatano M, Tokuhisa T (2005). Influence of toll-like receptor 4, CD14, tumor necrosis factor, and interleukine-10 gene polymorphisms on clinical outcome in Japanese critically ill patients. *J Surg Res*; 129:322-328.
Neumann F, Ott I, Marx N, Marx N, Luther T, Kenngott S, Gawaz M, Kotzsch M, Schömig A (1997). Effect of human recombinant interleukin-6 and interleukin-8 on monocyte procoagulant activity. *Arterioscler Thromb Vasc Biol*;17:3399-3405
Nicolaes GA, Dahlbäck B (2003). Congenital and acquired activated protein C resistance. *Semin Vasc Med*; 3 (1): 33-46.
Nolan A, Weiden M, Kelly A, Hoshino Y, Hoshino S, Mehta N, Gold JA (2008). CD40 and CD80/86 act synergistically to regulate inflammation and mortality in polymicrobial sepsis. *Am J Respir Crit Care Med*; 177:301-308.
O'Keefe GE, Hybki DL, Munford RS (2002). The G→A single nucleotide polymorphismat the -308 position in the tumor necrosis factor-alpha promoter increases the risk for severe sepsis after trauma. *J Trauma*; 52:817-825. discussion 825-826.
O'Neill S, O'Neill AJ, Conroy E, Brady HR, Fitzpatrick JM, Watson RW (2000). Altered caspase expression results in delayed neutrophil apoptosis in acute pancreatitis. *J Leukoc Biol*; 68:15-20.

Okazaki Y, Matsukawa A (2009). Pathophysiology of sepsis and recent patents on the diagnosis, treatment and prophylaxis for sepsis. *Recent Pat Inflamm Allergy Drug Discov;* 3(1):26-32.

Oude Nijhuis CS, Vellenga E, Daenen SM, Graaf van der WT, Gietema JA, Groen HJ, Kamps WA, De Bont ES (2003). Lipopolysaccharide-binding protein: apossible diagnostic marker for Gram-negative bacteremia in neutropenic cancer patients. *Intensive Care Med;* 29:2157-2161.

Pachot A, Lepape A, Vey S, Bienvenu J, Mougin B, Monneret G (2006). Systemic transcriptional analysis in survivor and nonsurvivor septic shock patients: A preliminary study. *Immunol Lett;* 106:63-71.

Panacek EA, Kaul M (1999). IL-6 as a marker of excessive TNF-a activity in sepsis. *Sepsis;* 3:65-73.

Parrillo J (1993). Pathogenetic Mechanisms of Septic *Shock. N Engl J Med 1993;* 328:1471-1477.

Paterson RL, Webster NR (2000). Sepsis and the systemic inflammatory response syndrome. *J R Coll Surg Edinb;* 45(3):178-182.

Pettila V, Pentti J, Pettila M, Takkunen O, Jousela I (2002). Predictive value of antithrombin III and serum C-reactive protein concentration in critically ill patients with suspected sepsis. *Crit Care Med;* 30:271-275.

Pezzilli R, Zerbi A, Di Carlo V, Bassi C, Delle Fave GF (2010). Working Group of the Italian Association for the Study of the Pancreas on Acute Pancreatitis. Practical guidelines for acute pancreatitis. *Pancreatology;* 10(5):523-535.

Pierrakos C, Vincent JL (2010).Sepsis biomarkers: a review. *Crit Care;* 14(1):R15.

Pinsky MR, Vincent JL, Deviere J, Alegre M, Kahn RJ, Dupont E (1993). Serum cytokine levels in human septic shock. Relation to multiple-system organ failure and mortality. *Chest;* 103:565-575.

Poderoso JJ, Carreras MC, Lisdero C (1996). Nitric oxide inhibits electron transfer and increases superoxide radical production in rat mitochondria and submitochondrial particles. *Arch Biochem Biophys;* 328: 85-92.

Povoa P, Coelho L, Almeida E, Fernandes A, Mealha R, Moreira P, Sabino H (2004). C-reactive protein as a marker of infection in critically ill patients. *Clin Microbiol Infect;* 11:101-108.

Remick DG (2007). Pathophysiology of sepsis. *Am J Pathol;*170(5):1435-44

Rittisch D, Flierl MA, Ward PA (2008). Harmful molecular mechanisms in sepsis. *Nat Immunol;* 8:776-786.

Rodriguez-Gaspar M, Santolaria F, Jarque-Lopez A, González-Reimers E, Milena A, de la Vega MJ, Rodríguez-Rodríguez E, Gómez-Sirvent JL (2001). Prognostic value of cytokines in SIRS general medical patients. *Cytokine;* 15:232-236.

Roy S, Knox K, Segal S, Griffiths D, Moore C, Welsh K, González-Reimers E, Milena A, de la Vega MJ, Rodríguez-Rodríguez E, Gómez-Sirvent JL (2002). MBL genotype and risk of invasive pneumococcal disease: a case–control study. *Lancet;* 359(9317):1569-1573.

Schaaf BM, Boehmke F, Esnaashari H, Seitzer U, Kothe H, Maass M, Zabel P, Dalhoff K (2003). Pneumococcal septic shock is associated with the interleukin-10-1082 gene promoter polymorphism. *Am J Respir Crit Care Med;* 168:476-480.

Schmit X, Vincent JL (2008). The time course of blood C-reactive protein concentrations in relation to the response to initial antimicrobial therapy in patients with sepsis. *Infection*; 36:213-219.

Schueller AC, Heep A, Kattner E, Kroll M, Wisbauer M, Sander J, Bartmann P, Stuber F (2006). Prevalence of two tumor necrosis factor gene polymorphisms in premature infants with early onset sepsis. *Biol Neonate*; 90:229-232.

Seidelin JB, Nielsen OH, Strom J (2002). Soluble L-selectin levels predict survival in sepsis. *Intensive Care Med*; 28:1613-1618.

Seller-Perez G, Herrera-Gutierrez ME, Lebron-Gallardo M, Toro-Peinado I, Martin-Hita L, Porras-Ballesteros JA (2005): [Serum C-reactive protein as a marker of outcome and infection in critical care patients]. *Med Clin (Barc)*; 125:761-765.

Skinner NA, MacIsaac CM, Hamilton JA, Visvanathan K (2005). Regulation of toll-like receptor (TLR)2 and TLR4 on CD14dimCD16+ monocytes in response to sepsis-related antigens. *Clin Exp Immunol*; 141:270-278.

Sobieski MA, Graham JD, Pappas PS, Tatooles AJ, Slaughter MS (2008). Reducing the effects of the systemic inflammatory response to cardiopulmonary bypass: can single dose steroids blunt systemic inflammatory response syndrome? *ASAIO J*; 54:203-206.

Socha LA, Gowardman J, Silva D, Correcha M, Petrosky N (2006). Elevation in interleukin 13 levels in patients diagnosed with systemic inflammatory response syndrome. *Intensive Care Med*; 32:244-250.

Sohn SJ, Rajpal A, Winoto A (2003). Apoptosis during lymphoid development. *Curr Opin Immunol*;15:209-216.Spriggs DR, Sherman ML, Frei E 3rd, Kufe DW. (1987). Clinical studies with tumour necrosis factor. *Ciba Found Symp*; 131:206-227.

Stanilova SA, Miteva LD, Karakolev ZT, Stefanov CS (2006). Interleukin-10-1082 promoter polymorphism in association with cytokine production and sepsis susceptibility. *Intensive Care Med*; 32:260-266.

Stuber F, Petersen M, Bokelmann F, Schade U (1996). A genomic polymorphism within the tumor necrosis factor locus influences plasma tumor necrosis factor-alpha concentrations and outcome of patients with severe sepsis. *Crit Care Med*; 24:381-384.

Sutherland AM, Russell JA (2005). Issues with polymorphism analysis in sepsis. *Clin Infect Dis*; 41(7 Suppl):S396-S402.

Temple SE, Cheong KY, Ardlie KG, Sayer D, Waterer GW (2004). The septic shock associated HSPA1B1267 polymorphism influences production of HSPA1A and HSPA1B. *Intensive Care Med*; 30:1761-1767.

Tribl B, Filipp D, Bodeker H, Yu P, Hammerrmuller I, McKerlie C, Keim V, Sibbald WJ (2004). Pseudomonas pneumonia-mediated sepsis induces expression of pancreatitis-associated protein-I in rat pancreas. *Pancreas*; 29:33-40.

Turner DM, Williams DM, Sankaran D, Lazarus M, Sinnott PJ, Hutchinson IV (1997). An investigation of polymorphism in the interleukin-10 gene promoter. *Eur J Immunogenet*; 24:1-8.

Van der Pol WL, Huizinga TW, Vidarsson G, Van der Linden MW, Jansen MD, Keijsers V, de Straat FG, Westerdaal NA, de Winkel JG, Westendorp RG (2001). Relevance of Fcgamma receptor and interleukin-10 polymorphisms for meningococcal disease. *J Infect Dis*; 184:1548-1555.

Van der Poll T, Opal SM (2008). Host-pathogen interactions in sepsis. *Lancet Infect Dis*; 8:32-43.

Waterer GW, ElBahlawan L, Quasney MW, Zhang Q, Kessler LA, Wunderink RG (2003). Heat shock protein 70–2+1267 AA homozygotes have an increased risk of septic shock in adults with community-acquired pneumonia. *Crit Care Med;* 31:1367-1372.

Waterer GW, Quasney MW, Cantor RM, Wunderink RG (2001). Septic shock and respiratory failure in community-acquired pneumonia have different TNF polymorphism associations. *Am J Respir Crit Care Med;* 163:1599-1604.

Whalen MJ, Doughty LA, Carlos TM, Wisniewski SR, Kochanek PM, Carcillo JA (2000). Intercellular adhesion molecule-1 and vascular cell adhesion molecule-1 are increased in the plasma of children with sepsis-induced multiple organ failure. *Crit Care Med*; 28:2600-2607.

Whitlock RP, Young E, Noora J, Farrokhyar F, Blackall M, Teoh KH (2006). Pulse low dose steroids attenuate post-cardiopulmonary bypass SIRS; *SIRS I J Surg Res*; 132:188-194.

Willatts SM, Speller DC, Winter RJ (1994). Incidence of gram-negative bacteraemia in sepsis syndrome. *Implications for immunotherapy. Anaesthesia*; 49:751-754.

Williams DL, Ha T, Li C, Kalbfleisch JH, Schweitzer J, Vogt W, Browder IW (2003). Modulation of tissue Toll-like receptor 2 and 4 during the early phases of polymicrobial sepsis correlates with mortality. *Crit Care Med;* 31:1808-1818.

Wong HR, Shanley TP, Sakthivel B, Lin R, Allen GL, Thomas NJ, Doctor A, Kalyanaraman M, Tofil NM, Penfil S, Monaco M, Tagavilla MA, Odoms K, Dunsmore K, Barnes M, Aronow BJ; Genomics of Pediatric SIRS/Septic Shock Investigators (2007). Genome-level expression profiles in pediatric septic shock indicate a role for altered zinc homeostasis in poor outcome. *Physiol Genomics*; 30:146-155.

Ye S, Green FR, Scarabin PY, Nicaud V, Bara L, Dawson SJ, Humphries SE, Evans A, Luc G, Cambou JP, et al (1995). The 4G/5G genetic polymorphism in the promoter of the plasminogen activator inhibitor-1 (PAI-1) gene is associated with differences in plasma PAI-1 activity but not with risk of myocardial infarction in the ECTIM study. Etude CasTemoins de I'nfarctus du Mycocarde. *Thromb Haemost;* 74:837-841.

Ye SQ, Simon BA, Maloney JP, Zambelli-Weiner A, Gao L, Grant A, Easley RB, McVerry BJ, Tuder RM, Standiford T, Brower RG, Barnes KC, Garcia JG (2005). Pre-Bcell colony-enhancing factor as a potential novel biomarker in acute lung injury. *Am J Respir Crit Care Med*; 171:361-370.

Yende S, D'Angelo G, Kellum JA, Weissfeld L, Fine J, Welch RD, Kong L, Carter M, Angus DC, GenIMS Investigators (2008). Inflammatory markers at hospital discharge predict subsequent mortality after pneumonia and sepsis. *Am J Respir Crit Care Med*; 177:1242-1247.

Yuan FF, Wong M, Pererva N, Keating J, Davis AR, Bryant JA, and Sullivan JS (2003). FcgammaRIIA polymorphisms in Streptococcus pneumoniae infection. *Immunol Cell Biol* 81:192-195.

Zakariah AN, Cozzi SM, Van Nuffelen M, Clausi CM, Pradier O, Vincent JL (2008). Combination of biphasic transmittance waveform with blood procalcitonin levels for diagnosis of sepsis in acutely ill patients. *Crit Care Med*; 36:1507-1512.

Zambon M, Ceola M, Almeida-de-Castro R, Gullo A, Vincent JL (2008). Implementation of the Surviving Sepsis Campaign guidelines for severesepsis and septic shock: we could go faster. J *Crit Care;* 23:455-460.

6

Immune Cell Dysfunction as a Consequence of Severe Sepsis

William F. Carson IV and Steven L. Kunkel
Department of Pathology, University of Michigan Medical School
U.S.A.

1. Introduction

The pathophysiology of severe sepsis is unique among immunological conditions in that the immune system is ultimately the root cause of the disease, and yet in certain aspects it is the immune system that suffers the most severe after effects following resolution of disease. During the acute phase of the disease, unchecked activation of the immune system results in severe physiological stress, which can lead to multi-organ dysfunction (MODS) and death (G. P. Patel et al., 2003). However, both during the acute phase and following recovery from severe sepsis, the immune system can suffer from significant deficiencies in activation and effector function that can render the patient susceptible to secondary, nosocomial and opportunistic infections (Reddy et al., 2001). This immune suppression is most readily apparent in regards to cellular responses, as both innate and adaptive immune cells exhibit deficiencies in effector responses following the onset of severe sepsis, both *in vitro* and *in vivo*. In certain cases, these deficiencies appear tied to the overstimulation of immune responses during the acute phase of the disease; for example, as macrophages become unresponsive to further stimulation with lipopolysaccharide (LPS) despite Gram-negative organisms being the (one of many possible) root cause(s) of the onset of sepsis (Fujihara et al., 2003). These phenomena may be considered an instance of immune tolerance as a consequence of overstimulation (e.g. "LPS tolerance" in macrophages both *in vivo* and *in vitro*). In addition, many instances of cellular dysfunction persist in survivors of severe sepsis long after the resolution of the acute phase of the disease; these cellular deficiencies are correlated in experimental models of sepsis, and play a key role in the development of post-septic immunosuppression.

Cellular dysfunction following severe sepsis proceeds from the intense inflammatory response triggered by exposure to large quantities of microbes, microbial products, and/or dead and dying cells and tissues. Suppression of activation and effector function of immune cells can be mediated through negative regulation of signalling pathways involved in the sensing of microbes and dead tissues, via direct suppression of immune responses through the signalling activity of anti-inflammatory cytokines, and in the long term, via modifications to the regulation of gene expression necessary for proper activation and effector function of immune cells. The end result of these phenomena is an immune system that lacks the ability to properly mount directed inflammatory responses in the context of secondary infections and other pathologies (such as cancer). The observed cellular dysfunction following the initial onset of sepsis can be loosely grouped into two distinct categories: acute deficiencies in the context of the systemic inflammatory response syndrome (SIRS), and chronic deficiencies in the context of the compensatory anti-inflammatory response syndrome (CARS) and beyond (N. S. Ward et al., 2008).

1.1 Pathophysiology of SIRS and CARS

The initial onset of severe sepsis can be due to numerous factors, many of which are derived from infectious agents but are not necessarily of infectious origin. For example, LPS derived from Gram-negative bacterial cell walls is a potent initiator of the septic response through its ability to stimulate large amounts of proinflammatory cytokines through Toll-like receptor (TLR)-4 signalling pathways (Zhang & Ghosh, 2000). Additionally, Gram-positive cell wall components (e.g. lipoteichoic acid) can signal through TLR2, initiating many of the same proinflammatory responses as LPS stimulation (Henneke et al., 2008). Shared components of both Gram-negative and -positive bacteria are the presence of unmethylated CpG motifs within the bacterial genome; these CpG motifs can be sensed by TLR9 (Wagner, 2002). Several types of RNA species, especially double-stranded RNA (dsRNA) from viruses, and intracellular RNA released from necrotic host cells (Cavassani et al., 2008), can activate TLR3 (Sen & Sarkar, 2005) as well as intracellular dsRNA sensors such as RIG-I and MDA-5 (Takeuchi & Akira, 2008). Additionally, bacterial superantigens (SAgs) can activate peripheral T cells in a non-specific, polyclonal manner, leading to the undirected production of proinflammatory cytokines and the development of sepsis (Ferry et al., 2005; Fraser & Proft, 2008). Despite the disparity in the instigating agent(s), the pathophysiology of the disease follows a biphasic progression, based on the generalized immune responses to the original stimuli and the subsequent "cytokine storm," respectively.

The systemic inflammatory response syndrome (SIRS) is defined clinically as the presence of two of the following four symptoms: hyper/hypothermia, tachycardia, tachypnea and leukocytosis/leukopenia with exaggerated neutrophils (>10% of peripheral white blood cells) (Conference:, 1992). From an immunological perspective, SIRS is a result of the exaggerated production of proinflammatory chemokines and cytokines by large numbers of activated immune cells. For example, early inflammatory mediators such as Tumor Necrosis Factor-alpha (TNFα), Interleukin-1 beta (IL-1β), IL-6 and IL-8 (CXCL8) are responsible for the variation in body temperature, breathing rate and peripheral white blood cell count, and the overproduction of these mediators can result in further exacerbation of inflammatory responses as well as immune cell apoptosis (Unsinger, McDonough, et al., 2009). Overproduction of proinflammatory chemokines and cytokines by the innate immune system (e.g. macrophages, granulocytes and dendritic cells) can feed back on the adaptive immune system, resulting in amplification of SIRS through production of type I (Kelly-Scumpia et al., 2010) and type II interferons (IFN) (Romero et al., 2010; Silva & Cohen, 1992) and T-cell derived cytokines such as IL-17(Flierl et al., 2008). The "cytokine storm" of SIRS is multifaceted, and reflects the multiple possible instigating agents and the multiple immune cell types participating in the response.

The cytokine storm of SIRS results in morbidity and mortality through the stresses caused by the unchecked inflammation on the host's physiology. For example, SIRS results in a massive apoptotic/necrotic cell death event observable in primary and secondary lymphoid tissues, as well as in the peripheral blood (Wesche-Soldato et al., 2005). This widespread cell death has two major outcomes. First, by significantly reducing the number of available leukocytes, this cytokine-storm induced cell death leaves the patient susceptible to secondary infections (C. Oberholzer et al., 2001). Secondly, cell components released by dying cells (especially nucleic acids and mitochondrial proteins) can further amplify the cytokine storm through stimulation of TLRs on remaining immune cells - this is especially true in the case of necrosis (Cavassani et al., 2008). Extreme variations in body temperature, heart rate and breathing rate are also mediated by the unchecked production of proinflammatory chemokines and cytokines (Sriskandan & Altmann, 2008). Ultimately, these physiological stresses, combined with adverse coagulation events and damage to the vasculature, can result in SIRS-induced mortality.

The initiation of SIRS is ultimately a result of immune cell activation; as a result, the immune system will often attempt to overcompensate for the overproduction of proinflammatory chemokines and cytokines by upregulating anti-inflammatory mediators. These anti-inflammatory mediators can be immunosuppressive cytokines, such as IL-10 or transforming growth factor-beta (TGFβ), or immune-deviating cytokines, such as T-helper type 2 cytokines (such as IL-4 and IL-13) which attempt to counteract the largely T-helper type 1 response initiated by SIRS cytokines (such as IL-12 and IFNγ) (Adib-Conquy & Cavaillon, 2009). Unfortunately, these compensatory mechanisms often fail to restrict the damaging effects of the cytokine storm of SIRS; instead, they often render those leukocytes that survive the initial apoptotic/necrotic event unable to respond to further infectious stimuli. This is especially dangerous at timepoints proximal to the onset of severe sepsis, as it renders hospitalized patients (undergoing treatment for SIRS) at risk for developing nonsocomial infections. Recent epidemiological studies also suggest that the CARS response may persist in some form for days, months and years following the resolution of severe sepsis and discharge from hospital care, as the both the survival rates and quality of life of survivors of severe sepsis are significantly reduced when compared to the healthy age-matched population (Perl et al., 1995; Quartin et al., 1997).

Cellular immune dysfunction as a result of severe sepsis can therefore be further conceptualized as three distinct phases, all following the initial onset of SIRS due to overstimulation of the immune system. In the first phase, anti-microbial responses are blunted due to "exhaustion" of the inflammatory responses of cells responding to the septic insult. In the second phase, the upregulation of anti-inflammatory responses by the immune system, in an attempt to regulate SIRS, renders the immune system unable to deal with secondary infections; this can be thought of as early-phase CARS, or compensatory immunosuppression. In the third phase, immune cells that have survived severe sepsis retain deficiencies in activation and effector function even after the resolution of disease; this can be thought of as late-phase CARS or post-septic immunosuppression. These last two phases occur as a direct response to cytokine storm of CARS, and are defined loosely based on their proximity to the initiation of severe sepsis. In all three cases, the phenotypic responses of the human patient or animal model (susceptibility to secondary, nosocomial and opportunistic infections) follows in part from the inability of the cells of the immune system to properly respond to challenges following sepsis. The specific mechanisms underlying the immunoparalysis observed in survivors of severe sepsis are specific to both the cell type and the phase of disease progression, but all ultimately deal with deficiencies in the activation, differentiation and effector function of post-septic immune cells.

1.2 Immune dysfunction in sepsis – clinical and experimental outcomes

Epidemiologically, immune suppression following sepsis manifests as a significant decrease in the long-term survival of patients recovered from severe sepsis; this decrease is seen years after the resolution of the inflammatory episode, as compared to the healthy age-matched population. Additionally, patients who do survive severe sepsis report lower quality of life scores as compared to healthy control populations (Winters et al., 2010). Of the patients that succumb to increased morbidity and mortality following sepsis, there are numerous infectious and non-infectious comorbidities that are correlated with decreased life expectancy. For example, opportunistic infections are commonly associated with patients recovering from septic shock (Benjamim et al., 2004). The long-term decrease in life expectancy observed in patients post-sepsis is described in epidemiological studies, and the underlying etiology of this post-septic mortality is less clear; however, the increase in mortality observed in post-septic patients appears unreleated to associated comorbidities, and is a direct result of the severity of the initial septic episode (Quartin et al., 1997).

Experimentally, post-septic immunosuppression can be studied by utilizing "two-hit" models of disease, whereby experimental animals are subjected to severe sepsis and then challenged with a secondary infection or immunity-stimulating event (such as solid tumor challenge). These models have been critical for both the identification of long term immunosuppression in survivors of severe sepsis, as well as for discerning the underlying mechanisms of cellular immune dysfunction following sepsis. Classical "two-hit" models often utilize a sepsis-triggering effect (such as high dose LPS injection or surgical induction of sepsis, also known as cecal ligation and puncture, CLP) in combination with airway challenges with opportunistic micro-organisms. The use of the lung microenvironment to study secondary infections and post-septic immunosuppression is of particular importance. By utilizing secondary infections that originate in the lung, researchers can study the immune environment in the lung during sepsis, where immune responses can both initiate septic shock and exacerbate deleterious outcomes (such as in the case of acute respiratory distress syndrome) (Hudson et al., 1995).

Experimental models of "two-hit" post-septic immunosuppression often utilize opportunistic pathogens for the second challenge, as healthy animals (untreated, or subjected to sham surgery as a control) would be expected to clear the microorganism without difficulty. One classic example of such an opportunistic pathogen is the fungi *Aspergillus fumigatus,* whose infectious conidia are ubiquitous in the environment and are normally controlled by a fully functioning immune system (Walsh et al., 2005). In immunocompromised individuals, these condidia can germinate in the lung and result in invasive infection. In mice, *A. fumigatus* airway challenge results in little discernible pathology, with the conidia unable to germinate prior to clearance by innate immune cells with phagocytotic activity (such as macrophages and neutrophils). In contrast, mice that have recovered from severe sepsis are unable to generate protective immune responses to *A fumigatus* conidia; these animals ultimately succumb to invasive aspergillosis, characterized by tissue damage mediated by hyphal outgrowth in the lungs (Benjamim et al., 2003). Deficiencies in cellular immune responses in post-septic animals are directly responsible for the susceptibility of post-septic animals to *A. fumigatus*-induced mortality. In addition to fungal challenge, other microorganisms are utilized to study post-septic immunosuppression in murine models. Secondary bacterial challenges are especially useful for modelling nosocomial infections in human patients; susceptibility to secondary infections has been identified in mouse models using *Pseudomonas aeruginosa* or *Listeria monocytogenes,* among others (Delano et al., 2011). Post-septic animals are also more susceptible to the implantation of solid tumors, as tumor size is increased in post-septic animals as compared to controls(Cavassani et al., 2010).

Impaired immune cell function plays a key role in mediating post-septic immunosuppression in all the experimental models discussed previously. In addition, these same deficiencies in immune cell function underlie the susceptibility of human patients to secondary, nosocomial and opportunistic infections following the onset of severe sepsis. Cell populations within the innate and adaptive immune system exhibit distinct phenotypes that mediate the different phases of post-septic immunosuppression, and the interplay between these various celluar deficiencies results in the susceptibility to infection observed in both human patients and animal models.

2. Immune cell dysfunction during SIRS

Despite immune activation being the root cause of severe sepsis, the cytokine storm associated with acute inflammation also feeds back on peripheral immune cells to mediate immunosuppression. This immunosuppression is mediated through two general mechanisms. First, widespread apoptosis of peripheral leukocytes limits the population of immune cells (and immune cell progenitors) available to respond to secondary infections. Second, overstimulation of surviving leukocytes - due to exposure to large amounts of microbial products, apoptotic/necrotic cell products and/or chemokines & cytokines - results in a refractory response to secondary stimulation, as is the case with a concurrent nosocomial infection during severe sepsis. The combination of these two factors results in susceptibility to secondary infections proximal to the onset of sepsis. In human patients, this response manifests as nosocomial infections that present soon after the admittance of the patient to emergency/intensive care; in animal models, this early immunosuppression is modelled with secondary infections early after the onset of sepsis (24-72 hours following induction).

The physiological stress caused by the cytokine storm of sepsis results in a widespread apoptotic event, coupled with (and amplified by) the necrosis of damaged tissues and subsequent release of intracellular components (e.g. proteins and nucleic acids). This apoptotic event is mediated both cell-contact dependent (such as Fas-Fas ligand interactions) and cell contact-independent mechanisms (Mahidhara & Billiar, 2000). In regards to cell contact-independent mechanisms, instead of a single causative event, the combined stress of the multiple chemokines and cytokines upregulated by severe sepsis combine to induce apoptosis in multiple immune cell types. In addition, adverse coagulation events caused by unchecked activation of the complement cascade can also induce immune cell death, especially in the vasculature and susceptible immune organs (such as the bone marrow and spleen) (P. A. Ward, 2008). Within a relatively short time following the onset of sepsis - hours to days - primary and secondary lymphoid organs are significantly depleted of cells as a result of this apoptosis. For example, cell density is significantly reduced in the bone marrow, thymus and spleen during acute sepsis; this is especially striking in the thymus, where the organ shrinks in size dramatically during the early inflammatory response of severe sepsis (Riedemann et al., 2002; Wang et al., 1994). In addition, peripheral tissue-resident immune cells, such as dendritic cells (DCs), decrease in number during the acute phase of sepsis, in part due to cytokine storm-induced cell death(Tinsley et al., 2003).

The widespread immune cell apoptosis significantly limits the number of cells available to combat a secondary infection. Complicating this response is the limited activation potential of immune cells that survive the initial apoptotic event. As mentioned previously, severe sepsis is induced through widespread activation of pattern recognition receptors (such as TLRs) and/or indiscriminate activation of nominally antigen-specific pathways (such as the case with polyclonal activation of T cells with superantigen). As a result of this excessive stimulation, the surviving immune cells become refractory to further stimulation through these specific pathways - this results in blunted responses to microbes and microbial products, leading to impaired immunity to secondary infections. This phenomenon is particularly evident in phagocytic cells of the innate immune system, manifested as a reduction in proinflammatory responses to secondary exposure to microbial products.

In macrophages, for example, prolonged exposure to high doses of LPS, as can be seen during severe sepsis, can result in refractory responses to further TLR signalling (Biswas & Lopez-Collazo, 2009). This suppressed TLR-mediated response is evidenced by a reduction in proinflammatory chemokine and cytokine production (Fujihara et al., 2003), as well as modulations in costimulatory ligand expression (Newton et al., 2004). This response is particularly prevalent in sepsis cases with a predominantly Gram-negative etiology, and high-dose LPS exposure in experimental models either *in vivo* or *in vitro* is often used to mimic this suppressed response (Medvedev et al., 2006). The phenomenon of "LPS tolerance" is intimately linked with the level of LPS exposure, as relatively low amounts (approximately 1 ng/ml in *in vitro* experiments) of LPS pre-treatment can enhance rather than suppress subsequent proinflammatory responses (West & Koons, 2008). However, high doses of LPS can result in suppressed extracellular signal-regulated kinase activity during subsequent secondary LPS exposures, including mitogen-activated protein kinases (MAPKs) and c-Jun NH_2-terminal kinase (JNK), with subsequent decreases in NF-κB and AP-1 transcription factor activity (Adib-Conquy et al., 2000; Fan & Cook, 2004; West et al., 2007). This decrease in TLR4-mediated signal transduction can lead to decreased production of proinflammatory genes such as Tumor Necrosis Factor-alpha (TNFα), interleukin(IL)-1β and IL-12, among others (Munoz et al., 1991; Spolarics et al., 2003).

Prolonged exposure to microbial products (and LPS in particular) also has a deleterious effect on the proinflammatory responses of neutrophils, although this response is distinct from the phenotype of "LPS tolerized" macrophages. Neutrophils play a critical role in initiating the septic response, as the early activation of neutrophils can lead to organ and tissue damage through the overproduction of reactive oxygen species (ROS) and highly active proteases such as neutrophil elastase (Fujimi et al., 2002; Sabroe et al., 2005). Additionally, accumulation of neutrophils in the vasculature and peripheral organs can result in non-specific cell and tissue damage, further complicating sepsis-induced organ dysfunction (Brown et al., 2006). Paradoxically, however, decreased neutrophil function during acute phase sepsis (characterized by decreased chemotactic responses and impaired surface receptor expression) is correlated with decreased survival in human patients, suggesting that the suppression of the antimicrobial functions of neutrophils is not enough to protect against sepsis-induced mortality (Chishti et al., 2004; Muller Kobold et al., 2000). Importantly, neutrophils are critical for the clearance of many nosocomial infections, as well as central to the innate immune responses against many experimental models of "two-hit" post-septic immunosuppression. Exhaustion of neutrophil functions during the acute phase of sepsis can therefore lead to susceptibility to secondary infections. For example, neutrophils that survive the early apoptotic event exhibit decreased chemotactic responses to neutrophil chemoattractants, most notably via CXCR1, which mediates neutrophil responses to CXCL8/IL-8 (Duffy et al., 2000). This reduced sensitivity to CXCL8 is similar to reduced TLR4 signalling in septic macrophages, as surface levels of CXCR1 are not reduced on septic neutrophils; rather, the ability of CXCR1 to signal through G-protein coupled receptor (GPCR) signalling pathways appears impaired (Arraes et al., 2006; Reddy et al., 2008). Therefore, in a similar fashion to "LPS tolerized" macrophages, septic neutrophils are impaired in their ability to respond to secondary microbial stimuli, leaving the septic patient susceptible to secondary infections.

In addition, a form of passive immune suppression can be seen during early phase sepsis in the increase in immature neutrophils - also known as "band cells" or "banded neutrophils" - in peripheral blood and immune organs of patients and animal models. Banded neutrophils are immature neutrophils that have differentiated from granulocyte/monocyte precursors in the bone marrow, but have yet to fully differentiate into mature neutrophils (Klut et al., 1998). Increases in peripheral banded neutrophils have long been used as a simple diagnostic tool for inflammatory responses; while their use as a predictive tool for sepsis severity (and subsequent mortality) is under question, their presence as a result of severe inflammatory responses is well characterized (Cavallazzi et al., 2010; Cornbleet, 2002; M. J. Ward et al., 2010). The increase in peripheral banded neutrophils appears to be a response of the bone marrow to the widespread apoptosis of mature neutrophils in response to the cytokine storm of sepsis - however, while the newly released neutrophils are rapidly produced, they lack many of the functional aspects of fully differentiated neutrophils (Pillay et al., 2010). The increased number of banded neutrophils therefore may arise at the loss of fully differentiated and functional neutrophils. Just as the loss of leukocytes due to apoptosis renders septic patients and animal models susceptible to secondary infections, the increase of banded neutrophils can contribute to post-septic immunosuppression, as these cells are not able to control secondary infections in the same manner as mature, functional neutrophils.

It may appear paradoxical to identify cellular immune suppression in the context of uncontrolled inflammation, particularly in the population of peripheral innate immune cells (such as macrophages and neutrophils) that are largely responsible for the cytokine storm of severe sepsis. It is therefore important to consider that the peripheral innate immune compartment during the acute phase of sepsis is a heterogeneous mixture of pro-inflammatory cells, "exhausted" cells (as mentioned previously) and in addition, cells which have converted to a regulatory or suppressive phenotype in an attempt to counteract the uncontrolled inflammatory response. In the hours and days proximal to the onset of severe sepsis, this combination of immune cell phenotypes results in the multifaceted disease phenotype of sepsis, whereby uncontrolled inflammation both results in tissue damage and mortality, and renders bystander immune cells unable to respond to secondary infections.

3. Immune cell dysfunction during CARS and beyond

Despite the immunosuppressive phenomena discussed previously (LPS tolerance, chemokine desensitization, etc), the acute phase of sepsis is primarily defined by the over activation of proinflammatory mechanisms, in particular cytokine and chemokine production by activated immune cells. The widespread immune cell apoptosis and anergy (unresponsiveness to immunogenic stimuli) often fails to completely control the cytokine storm of sepsis; as a compensatory mechanism, the immune system attempts to switch to active mechanisms of immune suppression, in an attempt to resolve the SIRS response. These active mechanisms, including the production of anti-inflammatory cytokines and the generation, activation and differentiation of suppressor cells, are considered hallmarks of the compensatory anti-inflammatory response syndrome (CARS) (A. Oberholzer et al., 2001). Classically, the CARS response was considered to be the generalized switch from pro- to anti-infl ammatory cytokines during the acute phase of sepsis; this is evidenced by increased production of suppressive cytokines (such as IL-10) and cytokines which counteract the primarily T_H1-type inflammation of severe sepsis (such as T_H2 type cytokines IL-4, -5 and -13) (Miller et al., 2007). Recent epidemiological studies in human patients, along with studies of experimental animal models of sepsis, have identified the CARS response as being maintained in immune cells for extended timepoints, long after the resolution of sepsis. These responses still retain components of early-phase CARS, such as the T_H2 cytokine shift, but are also characterized by cell-intrinsic defects in activation, differentiation and effector function that blunt the effectiveness of post-septic immune cells to protect the host from opportunistic infections. In this conception, CARS can be defined as a multifaceted immunosuppression following the onset of severe sepsis that leaves the patient susceptible to increased morbidity and mortality as compared to healthy individuals. In a generalized categorization, early-phase CARS can be described in terms of directed immune cell suppression via cytokine and the directed activity of suppressor cells, while late-phase CARS can be described as cell-intrinsic defects in activation, differentiation and effector function.

3.1 Early phase CARS: Suppressor cells and immunosuppressive cytokines

The switch from SIRS to CARS represents a directed effort by the immune system to regulate the production of proinflammatory chemokines and cytokines that are mediating physiological stress and tissue damage. When considering the cellular mediators of SIRS, such as innate immune cells (e.g. macrophages and neutrophils), cell-extrinsic suppression of their effector function can proceed through cell contact-dependent and –independent mechanisms. In terms of cell contact-dependent mechanisms, the development and expansion of myeloid and lymphoid suppressor cells is one of the hallmarks of CARS, and the persistent presence of these cells can restrict cellular immune responses to secondary infections. In terms of cell contact-independent mechanisms, the production of suppressive cytokines (e.g. IL-10), cytokine-sequestering factors (e.g. soluble TNF receptor type II) and immune-deviating cytokines (e.g. IL-4 and IL-13) all serve to restrict immune responses to secondary infections as well. One important hallmark of these early phase responses is their direct correlation with the uncontrolled cytokine storm of SIRS; these early phase CARS responses are directly triggered by the proinflammatory cascade of acute sepsis, and may represent a final effort by the immune system to restrict the cytokine- and chemokine-driven inflammation of SIRS.

The development and expansion of suppressor cells during CARS is multifaceted, and encompasses both myeloid-derived and lymphoid-derived suppressor cells. In certain cases, the expansion of suppressor cells is due to the directed development of cells with suppressive phenotypes from bone marrow progenitor cells; this is postulated to be the case with the heterogeneous population of myeloid-derived suppressor cells (MDSCs) seen in the periphery of survivors of severe sepsis (Cuenca et al., 2011). In other cases, the relative expansion of cells with suppressive phenotypes is thought to be due to the deletion of effector cells during SIRS due to cytokine driven apoptosis; this is often described with the increase in peripheral regulatory T cells (T_{regs}) following sepsis (Venet et al., 2004). In either case, the resulting suppressor cells are defined by their ability to directly regulate the activation of immune cells, including suppression of antigen presentation by accessory myeloid cells such as DCs, and restriction of the antigen-specific proliferation and effector function of T lymphocytes. The development of suppressor cells is a compensatory mechanism by the host to restrict the widespread inflammation of SIRS, both through biasing the peripheral immune cell pool towards cells with suppressive phenotypes, as well as utilizing those suppressive cells to directly regulate those proinflammatory cells that have failed to restrict their own activation through previously discussed mechansims (e.g. tolerance induction, apoptosis, etc).

Much of what is understood about MDSCs in humans comes from studies in cancer patients, where studies of peripheral blood leukocytes have identified a heterogeneous population of cells with stem cell markers on their surface (i.e. CD34) (Marigo et al., 2008). These cells are heterogeneous, both in terms of surface marker expression and in morphology, consisting of both monocyte and granulocyte subtypes. As a heterogeneous population, MDSCs have the ability to suppress the immune responses of other leukocytes, most notably T cells; co-cultures of MDSCs with CD4+ T cells result in decreased cell surface marker expression and cytokine production in response to antigen stimulation (Lechner et al., 2010). Their presence in the context of cancer is thought to arise through the modulatory activity of the malignancy, in an attempt to shield the growing tumor from immune surveillance (in a similar fashion as the development of tumor-associated macrophages) (Mantovani et al., 2009). In animal models of sepsis, MDSCs appear in peripheral immune organs in the days following experimental onset of the disease; these cells mimic the human MDSCs in their heterogenicity, their mixed monocyte and granulocyte morphology, and their ability to suppress antigen-specific lymphocyte responses *in vitro* (Delano et al., 2007).

While there remains a paucity of data concerning direct observation of MDSCs in human patients during severe sepsis and following recovery, techniques have been developed to generate MDSCs from peripheral blood mononuclear cells, utilizing a cocktail of cytokines that are also key players in the cytokine storm of severe sepsis (such as IL-6, IL-1β and TNF-α) (Lechner et al., 2010). The majority of experimental data concerning MDSCs in sepsis comes from experimental models, especially in the mouse - peripheral MDSCs can be induced by high dose LPS treatment, and these cells exhibit multifaceted immunosuppressive capabilities, including suppression of antigen-specific responses (Bronte, 2009; De Wilde et al., 2009). The source of peripheral MDSCs appears to be from progenitor cells in the bone marrow, although their presence as a terminally differentiated cell population vs. a mobilized population of immature leukocytes in response to inflammation and subsequent peripheral cell apoptosis (often referred to as "emergency myelopoiesis") remains in question. In addition, their role as mediators of post-septic immunosuppression is unclear, both due to the paucity of MDSC data from human septic patients, and in the difficulty inherent in eliminating MDSCs from the periphery of experimental animals. This difficulty arises from the lack of a definitive marker for MDSCs, in particular one that is not shared by other immune cells (e.g. macrophages and neutrophils). For example, many published studies in animal models utilize anti-Gr1 antibodies to deplete peripheral MDSCs to study their impact on disease (Nausch et al., 2008; Ribechini et al., 2009); however, this antibody also depletes mature neutrophils, and anti-Gr1 treatment on its own can render mice susceptible to opportunistic infections due to the depletion of these neutrophils (Mehrad et al., 1999). However, the correlative data from human patients, in context with the studies in animal models of sepsis, suggest that severe sepsis can result in an increase in peripheral MDSCs. When coupled with their ability to suppress antigen-specific activation and effector function of lymphocytes, MDSCs become a strong candidate for mediating post-septic immunosuppression.

In addition to myeloid-based suppressive cells, restriction of immune cell function post-sepsis is mediated by suppressive lymphoid cells as well. Arguably the best understood of these suppressive lymphocytes is the CD4+ regulatory T cell (T_{reg}). T_{regs} are themselves relatively heterogeneous, based on cell surface marker phenotype, tissue of residence, and/or the disease (or disease model) where the cells are studied. While T_{regs} are nominally defined by their suppressive activity (both *in vivo* and *in vitro*), they are identified by the expression of the transcription factor Foxp3 (Campbell & Ziegler, 2007), and are correlated with the expression of specific cell surface markers (most notably CD25, but also CTLA-4 and GITR, among others) (Wilczynski et al., 2008). T_{regs} have the capacity to suppress antigen-specific responses by effector T cells, as well as inflammatory responses by innate immune cells (Suzuki et al., 2010). T_{regs} are critical for the maintenance of peripheral immune tolerance, and deletion of T_{regs} in animal models results in the development of autoimmunity (Suri-Payer & Fritzsching, 2006). In humans, genetic mutations in the *Foxp3* gene results in the development of autoimmune disease (i.e. IPEX syndrome), due to a breakdown of T_{reg}-mediated suppression of self-antigen responses in the periphery (van der Vliet & Nieuwenhuis, 2007). Additionally, accumulations of T_{regs} in peripheral organs can help suppress immune responses and promote tolerance induction; examples of this phenomenon include inflammatory bowel disorders (Uhlig et al., 2006), allergic asthma (W. F. Carson et al., 2008) and transplant tolerance (Ge et al., 2010). In a negative context, peripheral T_{regs} can also suppress tumor surveillance by the adaptive immune system, indicating that in certain disease contexts, T_{regs} can promote rather than reduce pathology (Nishikawa & Sakaguchi, 2010).

Phenotypic analysis of peripheral blood from patients suffering from severe sepsis indicates an increase in CD4+ T_{regs} (Venet et al., 2009). This increase is seen rapidly following the onset of disease, and can persist throughout recovery (defined as the resolution of the cytokine storm), especially in animal models of sepsis. The origin of the increased T_{regs} is controversial, as certain studies describe the increase as being a directed expansion of T_{regs} and others as a result of the depletion of effector T cells due to sepsis-induced apoptosis (Venet et al., 2004; Wisnoski et al., 2007). Interestingly, *in vivo* studies utilizing PBMCs indicate that bacterial SAgs have the capacity to induce Foxp3 expression, suggesting that certain types of polyclonal stimuli associated with severe sepsis can directly modulate T_{reg} numbers (Taylor & Llewelyn, 2010). Regardless of the nature of this increase, however, it is clear that peripheral T_{regs} are enhanced in number in post-septic patients. At present, experimental modulation in T_{regs} has focused on their role in mediating the severity of acute sepsis; however, recent studies have begun to shed light on the role of T_{regs} in mediating post-septic immunosuppression. For example, increases in peripheral T_{reg} numbers in humans correlates with the development of suppressive phenotypes in peripheral lymphocytes from the same patients (Monneret et al., 2003). In animal models of sepsis, *ex vivo* blockade of Foxp3 via treatment with silencing RNAs (siRNA) can restore the proliferative responses of splenocytes, suggesting that Foxp3-dependent mechanisms are mediating lymphocyte anergy in post-septic animals (Venet et al., 2009). The direct effect of peripheral T_{regs} in mediating post-septic immunosuppression remains unclear; however, similar experimental models of secondary infections following trauma suggest an important role for T_{regs} in mediating immunosuppression following uncontrolled inflammation. For example, in animal models of severe burn injury, secondary infection with *Pseudomonas aeruginosa* results in increased mortality as compared to healthy control mice. Importantly, experimental neutralization of T_{reg} *in vivo* in these animals reverses this susceptibility (Liu et al., 2011).

Of particular interest to the study of post-septic immunosuppression is the nature of T_{reg} generation. Functional T_{regs} can be generated in two distinct pathways; either in the thymus ("natural" T_{regs}) or in the periphery in response to antigen stimulation in the context of tolerance-promoting signals, such as immunosuppressive cytokines ("adaptive" or "induced" T_{regs}) (Bluestone & Abbas, 2003). As mentioned previously, one possible explanation for the observed increase in peripheral T_{regs} following sepsis is the concurrent apoptosis of effector T cells; this would suggest that it is natural T_{regs} that are the primary regulatory T cell type following sepsis. However, studies of peripheral CD4+ T cells in animal models of sepsis suggest that following the onset of inflammation, peripheral effector T cells may have an increased propensity to become T_{regs} in response to secondary stimulus, due to modulations in their gene regulation patterns (Cavassani et al., 2010). This suggests that severe sepsis may condition the peripheral T cell pool to respond in a more regulatory fashion to secondary antigen challenges, which would ultimately result in an increase in immune suppression at the cost of protective pro-inflammatory responses. These modulated gene regulatory events will be discussed in the following sections dealing with late-phase CARS, as similar gene regulatory events underlie cell-intrinsic defects in the activation and effector function of other leukocytes during long-term sepsis-induced immunosuppression.

In concert with the increase in suppressive immune cells, imbalances in cytokine production by the immune system during the switch from SIRS to CARS can also contribute to post-septic immunosuppression. Characterization of the upregulation of these soluble mediators comes from studies at the physiological level, i.e. analysis of peripheral blood samples from human patients or peripheral tissues from animal models. The relative increase in these soluble anti-inflammatory mediators is observed in survivors of severe sepsis, and the presence of these mediators has a profound effect on the ability of leukocytes to respond to secondary infections. Soluble mediators of post-septic immunosuppression can be grouped into three general categories based on their mechanism of action: anti-inflammatory cytokines, soluble cytokine-sequestering receptors and immune-deviating cytokines. While the ultimate function of each grouping is different (i.e. direct suppression vs. immune-deviating), all three types of soluble factors contribute to post-septic immunosuppression.

The most well understood of the many immunosuppressive cytokines produced during CARS is arguably IL-10 (Bazzoni et al., 2010). Signalling via IL-10 proceeds through a heterodimeric receptor (IL-10R1/IL-10R2 complex), and the intracellular signalling pathways associated with IL-10 receptor activation (including involvement of tyrosine kinases and the transcription factor STAT3) have the ability to directly regulate cytokine gene expression induced by LPS; this makes IL-10 an intriguing candidate for mediating post-septic immunosuppression, especially in regards to LPS-dependent secondary responses (Crepaldi et al., 2001). Supporting this concept is the kinetics of IL-10 expression in human patients and animal models, where increased levels of IL-10 can be observed following the onset of sepsis (van der Poll et al., 1997). Blockade of IL-10 has been shown to have a protective effect in many experimental models of severe sepsis (Latifi et al., 2002; Oberholzer et al., 2002). Interestingly, however, increased IL-10 production in human patients is often correlated with poor outcomes, suggesting that IL-10 may be a potent regulator of the CARS response (Abe et al., 2008). IL-10 has potent suppressive effects on a wide range of leukocytes, including suppression of proliferation, surface receptor expression and cytokine/chemokine production (Akdis & Blaser, 2001; Williams et al., 2004). Of particular interest is IL-10's potent effect on monocytes and macrophages, primarily mediated by the antagonistic effect of IL-10 signalling on LPS-dependent gene induction (Cavaillon & Adib-Conquy, 2006). IL-10 has dramatic suppressive effects on the pro-inflammatory responses of macrophages, including inhibition of cytokine production (Brandtzaeg et al., 1996; Gerard et al., 1993). IL-10 can also negatively impact neutrophil activation in the context of LPS stimulation (as seen with Gram-negative sepsis), as neutrophils only expresses the IL-10R following LPS stimulation; in this fashion, IL-10 serves as a negative regulator of activated neutrophils (Cassatella et al., 2005; Tamassia et al., 2008). In a normal physiological context, limited by either the kinetics of stimulation or the restricted microenvironment of a given inflammatory insult, the IL-10-dependent negative feedback look allows the immune system to properly regulate the potentially damaging anti-inflammatory effects of macrophages and neutrophils following the clearance of infectious micro-organisms. However, the high levels of IL-10 produced during CARS can drastically shift the balance away from pro-inflammatory responses, leaving peripheral macrophages and neutrophils unable to respond to secondary bacterial challenges unrelated to the causative agent of septic shock.

In addition to IL-10, the shift from SIRS to CARS is also associated with an increase in transforming growth factor-beta (TGFβ). TGFβ is a potent cytokine that is normally involved with wound healing and the development of fibrosis in damaged tissues (Leask & Abraham, 2004). TGFβ also has the ability to direct the activation and differentiation of many cell types, including but not limited to immune cells. In the context of immune responses, TGFβ is a potent immunosuppressive cytokine, with the ability to suppress the antigen-specific activation and effector function of leukocytes (Prud'homme & Piccirillo, 2000). Additionally, TGFβ signalling in the context of T-cell receptor signalling can direct the development of CD4+ T_{regs} from effector T cell precursors (Li & Flavell, 2008). In the context of severe sepsis, TGFβ is significantly increased in the systemic circulation (Marie et al., 1996); this increase is both due to the directed production of TGFβ by immune cells, but also as a byproduct of sepsis-induced apoptosis, as TGFβ is produced by apoptotic cells (T cells in particular) during programmed cell death (Chen et al., 2001). TGFβ isoforms (of which there are 3 primary forms) signal through cell surface receptors through SMAD transcription factors, which regulate numerous genes, including those responsible for mediating apoptosis (for example, through downregulation of anti-apoptotic genes such as Bcl-xl) (Kanamaru et al., 2002; Spender et al., 2009). TGFβ signalling can also limit chemokine and cytokine production by immune cells, in particular T lymphocytes and activated macrophages (Letterio, 2005; Yang et al., 2010). In particular, TGFβ is a potent suppressor of the anti-microbial activity of macrophages; this is manifest via TGFβ-mediated suppression of cytotoxic activity, superoxide production and nitric oxide synthase (iNOS) activity (Mitra & Khar, 2004). This increase in TGFβ during sepsis can therefore suppress secondary anti-microbial responses by macrophages, limiting the ability of these cells to respond to secondary infections. In addition, as TGFβ signalling is important for the differentiation of effector CD4+ T cells into T_{regs}, there appears to be a role for increased TGFβ production post-sepsis in mediating the increase in peripheral T_{regs} observed in human patients and animal models. Therefore, in addition to TGFβ's direct immunosuppressive properties (as with IL-10), TGFβ can also mediate immunosuppression through the development of cells with intrinsic immunosuppressive properties.

The immunosuppression observed during early phase CARS proceeds both through the production of anti-inflammatory cytokines, but also through the production of soluble factors that can limit the ability of pro-inflammatory cytokines to signal cells and mediate inflammation. Of particular importance to the switch from SIRS to CARS is the production of soluble receptors and antagonists that interfere with the signalling of the proinflammatory cytokines IL-1β, IL-6 and TNFα. All three cytokines are central mediators of SIRS through their ability to drive the acute phase response, fever, cytotoxic activity of immune cells (e.g. phagocytosis) and ultimately septic shock (Jean-Baptiste, 2007). As a result, during the switch from SIRS to CARS, the immune system upregulates the production of cytokine antagonists which attempt to block the activity of these inflammatory mediators. For example, in septic patients, plasma levels of soluble IL-1ra receptor antagonist (IL-1ra), soluble TNFα receptors I and II (sTNFRI/sTNFRII), and soluble IL-6 receptor (sIL-6R) are all increased as compared to healthy patients (Gogos et al., 2000; Marie et al., 1997). IL-1ra binds the IL-1 receptor in competition with IL-1β, resulting in functional inhibition of IL-1β signalling (Bresnihan & Cunnane, 1998). In a similar fashion, the sTNFRs and sIL-6R achieve functional inhibition of their respective cytokines by binding and sequestering the soluble proteins from interacting with cell surface receptors on circulating leukocytes (Jones & Rose-John, 2002). As with the upregulation of anti-inflammatory cytokines, the production of receptor antagonists and soluble receptors is an attempt by the immune system to restrict the cytokine storm of SIRS. However, blockade of the functional activity of these cytokines can result in vulnerability to secondary infections, especially when placed in context with the upregulation of anti-inflammatory cytokines such as IL-10 and TGFβ.

For cellular immune responses to be protective, they must be conditioned to produce the proper inflammatory response for the specific infectious agent. The cytokine storm of SIRS can be loosely categorized as a T helper type-1 response (T_H1), geared towards cytotoxic activity and anti-microbial responses. Many cytokines central to sepsis responses, such as TNFα, IL-6, IL-12 and IFNγ, are normally considered to be T_H1-type cytokines, as they promote the cytotoxic activity of macrophages, neutrophils and CD8+ cytotoxic T cells. T-helper type-2 responses (T_H2) are associated with immunity to parasites, as well as allergic responses, and are characterized by antibody production (primarily immunoglobulin type E) and eosinophilopoiesis (at the expense of neutrophils). T_H2 cytokines have the ability to directly regulate T_H1 responses through their ability to suppress T_H1 gene expression in CD4+ T cells, as well as by modulating the granulocyte output of the bone marrow in response to inflammation (i.e. eosinophils vs. neutrophils) Summaries of the T-helper cytokine response and its role in inflammation are available in the literature (Cameron et al., 2001; DiPiro, 1997; Miller et al., 2007). As a third cytokine-dependent mechanism, the cytokine milleu of CARS is also characterized by an upregulation of T_H2 cytokine responses (Mack et al., 1996). This upregulation of T_H2 cytokines serves to blunt the T_H1-dominant SIRS response through the modulation of leukocyte gene expression. In human patients, immune responses post-sepsis are observed to have a generalized shift towards T_H2 responses, especially in regards to adaptive immune cell activation (O'Sullivan et al., 1995). IL-4 in particular has potent effects on macrophages, with the ability to suppress cytotoxic activity as well as promote the production of IL-1ra and sTNFRs, resulting in an autocrine feedback loop that further restricts macrophage activity (Nicod et al., 1994). In addition, T_H2 cytokines like IL-4 and IL-13 are key factors in the development of alternatively activated macrophages (aaMΦ, or M2-type macrophages), which promote wound healing and fibrosis at the expense of anti-microbial activity (Gordon & Martinez, 2010). Animal models of sepsis have identified that bone-marrow derived macrophages from survivors of sepsis exhibit a M2 phenotype as compared to control animals, suggesting that the T_H2 cytokine-dependent development of M2 macrophages can be maintained for timepoints distal from the acute inflammatory event (Takahashi et al., 2004).

Because a majority of the studies dealing with soluble mediators of the CARS phenotype are done on the physiological level (i.e. with analysis of peripheral blood samples), it is often difficult to directly identify the source of the immunomodulatory cytokines mediating CARS. In the case of soluble receptors and receptor antagonists, the root source is often considered to be macrophages and other phagocytotic innate immune cells, especially in response to circulating IL-10 levels. As mentioned previously, increases in TGFβ production are often the result of lymphocyte apoptosis during sepsis; however, many T cells, especially T_{regs}, can produce both TGFβ and IL-10 when mediating immunosuppression. Many of the T_H2 cytokines observed during CARS are normally produced by CD4+ T cells, and it is hypothesized that these cells are at the root of the T_H12 shift observed in survivors of severe sepsis. Conceptually, the shift from SIRS to CARS may result from a negative feedback loop whereby the proinflammatory cytokine storm results in the apoptosis of cells, resulting in increased TGFβ production that then leads to the development of T_{regs} that produce IL-10, which then go on to stimulate anti-inflammatory responses (i.e. IL-1ra, sTNFR & sIL-6R) from macrophages, and so on. This type of model may explain the mechanisms underlying the switch from SIRS to CARS; however, they do not fully explain the maintenance of post-septic immunosuppression in patients for the months and years following recovery. Investigations into the long-term maintenance of the CARS phenotype have identified many cell-intrinsic defects in activation and effector function that maintain the immunsuppressive phenotype once the relative levels of anti-inflammatory cytokines and antagonistic factors have returned to baseline levels in the periphery. It is hypothesized that these cell-intrinsic factors may be programmed by the cytokine milleu of either SIRS or CARS; additionally, they may utilize modulation in gene regulation as an underlying mechanism for the maintenance of these defects.

3.2 Late phase CARS: Cellular dysfunction and epigenetic reprogramming

Sepsis-induced immunosuppression during SIRS and the early switch to CARS relies on active mechanisms, such as cytokine-induced apoptosis, anergy induction, suppression of signal transduction and modulation of bone marrow hematopoiesis. Ultimately, however, these mechanisms of suppression resolve as the patient recovers from the septic episode. For example, despite the widespread apoptosis & necrosis of immune cells observed during the acute phase of sepsis, immune cells are ultimately re-seeded into immune tissues and peripheral blood & lymph following recovery. Interestingly, the re-seeding of T lymphocytes to peripheral organs does not appear to favor specific T cell-receptor subtypes (Unsinger, Kazama, et al., 2009). This phenomenon suggests that the repopulation of lymphocytes is not due simply to the expansion of cells primed during the acute phase of septic shock. However, despite the return of the immune system to a state comparable to conditions pre-sepsis, both human patients and experimental animals continue to exhibit signs of immunosuppression. As mentioned previously, the long term survival curves of survivors of severe sepsis are significantly reduced as compared to the healthy age-matched population, and this increased morbidity and mortality is observable even in the presence of co-morbidities. Additionally, self-reported quality of life measurements are significantly reduced in survivors of severe sepsis, indicating negative physiological outcomes even in the absence of secondary infection. Taken in context, these results suggest that the cellular immune response in post-septic individuals remains dysregulated even once the major mediators of CARS have subsided.

Experimental studies aimed at identifying cell-intrinsic defects in activation and effector function of immune cells following severe sepsis have described numerous immunosuppressive phenomena that are maintained even after the resolution of SIRS and CARS. These deficiencies in activation and effector function are considered to be cell-intrinsic as they manifest both *in vivo* and *in vitro*, are often preserved in adoptive transfer models, and are in many cases resistant to treatment with optimized culture conditions (e.g. polyclonal stimulus and exogenous recombinant cytokines). In "two-hit" models of post-septic immunosuppression, these cell-intrinsic defects contribute directly to the susceptibility of survivors of severe sepsis to opportunistic infections, as adoptive transfer of immune cells from control animals can confer protect in these immunosuppressed animals. The current working hypothesis for this phenomenon deals with gene regulation in post-septic cells, in particular with the expression of proinflammatory cytokines that are necessary for protection against secondary infection. In this model, immune cells that have survived septic shock are no longer able to effectively respond to secondary infectious stimuli due to the repression of gene expression following activation. While many disparate yet interrelated molecular mechanisms may be involved in this dysregulation of gene expression, recent studies have implicated epigenetic reprogramming of immune cells (and possibly hematopoietic progenitor cells) as a major player in long-term immunosuppression post-sepsis (W. F. Carson et al., 2011).

Perhaps the most well-characterized immune cell deficiency following sepsis is concerning the activation of DCs. As mentioned previously, DCs are rapidly depleted from peripheral tissues following the onset of sepsis, and as DCs are critical for the antigen-specific activation of T cells, this loss of peripheral DCs severely restricts the activation potential of the adaptive immune system (Tinsley et al., 2003). Interestingly, peripheral DCs that do return following the resolution of SIRS and early-phase CARS continue to exhibit an immunosuppressive phenotype following sepsis, highlighted by a significant reduction in their ability to produce IL-12 in response to TLR stimulation (Wen et al., 2006). IL-12 is a potent pro-inflammatory cytokine that is critical for the development of T_H1 responses and T_H1-type CD4+ T cells (Watford et al., 2003). This inability to produce IL-12 results in susceptibility to pathogens that are normally cleared by a T_H1 immune response. Experimentally, this response can be studied using airway challenges with *Aspergillus fumigatus* in post-septic mice - the reduction in DC-dependent IL-12 production in these animals restricts the development of T_H1 responses, resulting in uncontrolled fungal growth and *Aspergillus*-induced mortality (Benjamim et al., 2003). When bone-marrow derived DCs from control animals are transferred into post-septic animals prior to airway challenge, resistance to fungal infection can be restored (Benjamim et al., 2005). Interestingly, this suppression of IL-12 production does not appear to be due to increased IL-10 production; while *ex vivo* stimulated post-septic DCs exhibit increased IL-10 production (an expected CARS-type cytokine response), neutralization of IL-10 *in vitro* with blocking antibodies fails to restore IL-12 production (Wen, Dou, et al., 2008). Importantly, this suppression of IL-12 production is maintained long past the resolution of severe sepsis, with lung DCs exhibiting deficiencies in IL-12 production up to six weeks following the experimental onset of sepsis (Wen, Dou, et al., 2008). From a therapeutic standpoint, this long-term suppression of IL-12 production is problematic, as it does not follow from the upregulation of anti-inflammatory cytokines that can themselves be blocked (as with *in vitro* inhibition of IL-10).

DCs are critical accessory cells for the activation of T cells, through the presentation of antigen to T-cell receptors in the context of MHC. In addition, DCs instruct T cells to differentiate into one of several effector/regulatory cell lineages (characterized by distinct families of effector cytokines and downstream immunomodulatory functions); this instruction occurs both through cell-contact dependent mechanisms and the production of instructional cytokines (such as IL-12). As mentioned previously, post-septic immune responses are characterized by a generalized shift away from T_H1 cytokines towards T_H2 cytokines. This phenomenon may be due at least in part to the immunomodulatory properties of post-septic DCs, as these cells promote T_H2 cytokines such as IL-4, IL-5 and IL-13 at the expense of T_H1 cytokines such as IFNγ (Wen et al., 2006). This skewing to T_H2 occurs in an antigen-specific fashion, and is not a result of pre-conditioning of the responder T cells during severe sepsis, as the responder cells used in these *in vitro* experiments were naïve and specific for an antigen that is unrelated to polymicrobial sepsis (ovalbumin). This reduction in T_H1 polarizing capabilities may also negatively regulate innate immune system functions, as T_H1 CD4+ T cell-derived IFNγ is critical for the activation of phagocytotic activity by macrophages (Kasten et al., 2010).

In addition to DC-mediated suppression, CD4+ T cell exhibit deficiencies in activation, differentiation and effector function following sepsis, even in the context of polyclonal stimulus or nominally functioning DCs. One of the hallmarks of CD4+ T cells from septic patients is the development of anergy, or unresponsives to antigen stimulation (Heidecke et al., 1999). CD4+ T cells from septic animals also exhibit this anergic phenotype, and the proliferative capacity of these cells is not recovered by the addition of exogenous cytokines, such as the potent T cell proliferative factor IL-2 (W. F. Carson et al., 2010). In addition, their gene expression is drastically altered as compared to CD4+ T cells from healthy animals. For example, mRNA for IFNγ, IL-4 and the T_H17 cytokine IL-17 can be upregulated in naïve CD4+ T cells from post-septic mice following polyclonal stimulus, as compared to levels in cells from control animals. Concurrently, these cells downregulate mRNA for cell surface receptors critical for T cell activation, including CD4 and CD28. As these differences in gene expression are observed following optimized polyclonal stimulus in the absence of accessory cells such as DCs, it appears that the changes in gene expression are due to cell-intrinsic factors (W. F. Carson et al., 2010).

This modulated cytokine response by post-septic CD4+ T cells becomes even more apparent once these cells are tasked with committing to specific T-helper lineages. When studied *in vitro*, post-septic CD4+ T cells exhibit deficiencies in their ability to properly commit to either the T_H1 or T_H2 lineage, as evidenced by cytokine production. For example, when expanded in an optimized T_H1-promoting environment (including exogenous IL-12 and blocking antibodies to IL-4), post-septic CD4+ T cells produce significantly less IFNγ in recall responses, as compared to CD4+ T cells from control animals. If these same cells are expanded in a T_H2 culture (exogenous IL-4 and blocking antibodies to IL-12 and IFNγ), post-septic CD4+ T cells produce both T_H1 and T_H2 cytokines upon recall, whereas CD4+ T cells from control animals only make T_H2 cytokines (W. F. Carson et al., 2010). This modulation in T-helper subtype cytokine responses represents an inability of post-septic CD4+ T cells to properly commit to either the T_H1 or T_H2 effector lineage.

This modulated cytokine production is also apparent *in vivo*, when post-septic CD4+ T cells are transferred into lymphopenic animals (i.e. Rag2$^{-/-}$ mice, which lack mature peripheral lymphocytes). As mentioned previously, post-septic myeloid cells exhibit numerous deficiencies in activation and cytokine production throughout SIRS, early and late phase CARS; as these cells are critical for the activation of CD4+ T cells, any deficiencies observed in lymphocyte activation *in vivo* in post-septic animals may be due to myeloid deficiencies, and not necessarily due to CD4+ cell-intrinsic factors. Adoptive transfer experiments allow post-septic CD4+ T cells to be studied in the context of a functional myeloid immune cell response, as both macrophages and DCs develop and function normally in (genetically engineered) lymphopenic mice. When post-septic CD4+ T cells are challenged with *in vivo* models of T_H1 or T_H2 lung inflammation, a similar pattern of cytokine expression emerges. Histological examination of lung granuloma formation in response to embolized antigen-coupled beads indicates that post-septic CD4+ T cells mediate smaller T_H1 and T_H2 type lesions, as expected based on the generalized shift to T_H2 responses following sepsis (W. F. Carson et al., 2011). Interestingly, when lymph nodes from mice that received post-septic CD4+ T cells were restimulated with cognate antigen, they produced increased amounts of a wide range of T-helper cytokines, including IL-4 in a T_H1 context, and IFNγ in T_H2 context. Additionally, in both T_H1 and T_H2 disease models, lymph nodes from mice that received post-septic CD4+ T cells produced increased IL-17 as compared to those that received CD4+ T cells from control mice. In both cases, this inability to properly commit to a T-helper lineage results in measurable differences in both *in vivo* inflammatory processes and *ex vivo* cytokine production (W. F. Carson et al., 2011). While it may be counter-intuitive to suggest that increased pro-inflammatory cytokine production is indicative of immunosuppression, it is important to place this increase in the context of productive inflammation. Adaptive immunity requires directed cytokine production to initiate proper immune responses directed against the specific infectious agent (i.e. T_H1 responses for intracellular bacterial and viral infections vs. T_H2 responses for helminth infections). Increases in T-helper cytokines can be counterproductive when they promote incorrect inflammatory responses (as seen with the T_H1 granuloma studies) or exacerbate inflammation past the level of protection (as seen with the T_H2 granulomas). When coupled with the shift towards T_H2 responses observed with DCs post-sepsis, this dysregulation of cytokine expression can ultimately result in decreased immunity to secondary infections, which normally require T_H1 responses for clearance.

During late phase CARS, both myeloid cells (specifically DCs) and lymphoid cells (specifically CD4+ T cells) exhibit deficiencies in cytokine production in response to stimulation with microbes, microbial products and antigens. As mentioned previously, following the apoptotic response during SIRS, both DCs and CD4+ T cells are re-seeded to the periphery, in many cases to levels similar to those found in control animals or healthy individuals. These results suggest that the mechanisms governing cytokine responses in post-septic cells are both cell-intrinsic and not reliant on exogenous factors, such as soluble mediators of early phase CARS (e.g. IL-10, IL-1ra, etc). Recent studies in animal models have identified one possible molecular pathway governing this dysregulation of gene expression and cytokine production, epigenetics. The study of epigenetics involves any and all molecular mechanisms that can modulate gene expression without changing the underlying genetic information present in a cell or organism. Epigenetic mechanisms include chemical modifications to DNA and DNA-associated histone proteins that can either activate or suppress gene transcription, as well as expression of small RNA species (called microRNAs/miRNAs) that can post-transcriptionally regulate gene expression through the targeted degradation of mRNA (Delcuve et al., 2009). Epigenetics plays a critical role during embryogenesis and development, particularly when multipotent stem cells commit to defined lineages during the development of tissues and organs (Roloff & Nuber, 2005; Shafa et al., 2010). The differentiation process requires tight regulation of gene expression, as the differentiation of stem cells into cells with defined phenotypes requires not only the activation of essential genes, but also the suppression of genes unrelated to the function of the new daughter cell. In a similar fashion, the immune system relies on epigenetic mechanisms to guide the development of peripheral blood leukocytes from hematopoietic cell precursors (Bergman & Cedar, 2010; Fernandez-Morera et al., 2010). In addition, the activation, differentiation and effector function of peripheral immune cells also relies on epigenetic mechanisms. For example, modifications in the tails of histones associated with the promoter regions of essential gene families correlates with the decision of macrophages to become either classically activated (i.e. anti-microbial) or alternatively activated (i.e. fibrotic/wound healing) (Ishii et al., 2009). In addition, CD4+ T cells utilize similar histone modification processes to govern the expression of T-helper cytokines during the differentiation to T_H1 or T_H2 (Ansel et al., 2003). When these processes are disrupted in immune cells, disease can often result; for example, modulations in DNA methylation patterns (DNA methylation results in the suppression of gene expression) are often correlated with the development of systemic lupus erythematosus (D. R. Patel & Richardson, 2010). Regulation of gene expression is essential for the proper function of the immune system, and changes in the epigenetic landscape of an immune cell can have a profound effect on immune responses and subsequent disease.

Recent studies in animal models have identified a number of epigenetic modifications in immune cells following severe sepsis. These modifications are often found associated with genes essential for immune cell effector function, such as cytokine genes or transcription factors, and they correlate with deficiencies in activation, differentiation and effector function in these cells. Additionally, these modifications are found in both myeloid and lymphoid cells, suggesting a common molecular mechanism for the modification of epigenetic marks in leukocytes following sepsis. At present, the best described epigenetic mechanism governing post-septic immunosuppression is via histone modification events, in particular changes in histone acetylation and methylation. Post-translational modifications of the protein tails of histone core proteins can have a direct effect on gene expression, depending on the type of modification and its location on the histone tail (Cosgrove & Wolberger, 2005). For example, acetylation of histone tails is often associated with transcriptional activation, regardless of the location of the modification on the histone tail. In contrast, the functional result of the methylation of histone tails is site specific; transcriptional activation or repression can occur depending on the location of the methylation event on the histone tail. Studies of both myeloid and lymphoid cells post-sepsis have identified modulations in both histone acetylation and methylation following sepsis, in particular in the promoter regions of genes essential for mediating protective immune responses against secondary infections.

In DCs, for example, modulations in histone methylation events in the promoter regions of IL-12 are observable following sepsis (Wen, Schaller, et al., 2008). When tissue-resident DCs from post-septic animals are compared to those from healthy controls, the pattern of histone methylation is skewed towards gene repression. This includes decreases in methylation of lysine 4 on the tail of histone 3 (H3K4me), which is considered an activating epigenetic mark, as well as increases in methylation of lysine 27 on the tail of histone 3 (H3K27me), which is considered a repressive epigenetic mark. These marks are maintained for a significant amount of time following the resolution of severe sepsis, as tissue-resident DCs from post-septic animals retain these modulated methylation marks six weeks after the experimental onset of severe sepsis. In addition, the chromatin modifying enzymes responsible for the addition of these histone methylation marks is significantly altered in post-septic DCs, with the H3K4me machinery decreased and the H3K27me machinery increased in the promoter regions of both IL-12a and IL-12b . This increase in repressive histone methylation marks correlates with decreased IL-12 production both *in vitro* and *in vivo*, and provides one explanation for the observed reduction in proinflammatory cytokine production that is unrelated to the presence of anti-inflammatory cytokines (i.e. IL-10) (Wen, Dou, et al., 2008).

While the data concerning epigenetic reprogramming in macrophages is less robust in regards to long-term immunosuppression, modulations in histone modifications can be observed in macrophages following the onset of severe sepsis, and these modulations affect proinflammatory responses by these cells. For example, macrophages recovered from experimental models of severe sepsis exhibit increased levels of methylation at lysine 9 of histone 3 (H3K9, repressive) at the promoter region of both IL-1β and TNFα, resulting in decreased production of both inflammatory mediators (Lyn-Kew et al., 2010). This increase in repressive histone methylation appears to be a mechanism whereby the immune system is attempting to limit proinflammatory cytokine production; however, as both of these cytokines are critical for immunity against bacteria, their decreased production by macrophages can leave the immune system less able to properly respond to secondary infections. In addition, decreases in H3K4me and increases in acetylation of the tail of histone 4 (AcH4) are observed both in the TNFα and iNOS promoter; reductions in iNOS expression severely limit the ability of the macrophage to produce nitric oxide, a critical component of the cytotoxic response. To date, few studies have been performed to determine if these aberrant histone modification events remain present in macrophages long after the resolution of SIRS. However, recent studies identifying an epigenetic role for the development of the alternatively activated macrophage (decreases in H3K27 methylation mediated by the histone demethylase KDM6B) may provide a mechanism for the increased propensity of post-septic macrophages to become alternatively activated, as the increase in KDM6B expression and activation is driven by T_H2 cytokines that are upregulated during CARS, most notably IL-4 (Ishii et al., 2009).

Epigenetic reprogramming of CD4+ T cells following sepsis is also apparent, both in regards to cytokine production and T-helper lineage commitment. As mentioned previously, CD4+ T cells from post-septic animals exhibit deficiencies in their ability to properly commit to either the T_H1 or T_H2 lineage, as evidenced by modulations in cytokine production during recall/re-challenge both *in vivo* and *in vitro*. These deficiencies in lineage commitment correlate with modulations in histone modifications, specifically increases in H3K27me levels in promoter regions of T-helper subtype genes. For example, post-septic CD4+ T cells exhibit increased levels of H3K27me in the promoter region of *Ifng*, correlating with the decreased production of IFNγ during skewing and restimulation experiments *in vitro*. In addition, these same cells exhibit increased levels of H3K27me in the promoter region of *Gata3*, a transcription factor critical for the development of T_H2 T cells. This increase in repressive histone methylation correlates with the reduced capacity of post-septic T cells to fully commit to the T_H2 lineage, as evidenced by the continued production of IFNγ in T_H2

inflammatory contexts both *in vitro* and *in vivo (W. F. Carson et al., 2010; W. F. Carson et al., 2011)*. In addition to modulations in histone methylation, histone acetylation is also modulated in post-septic CD4+ T cells, in particular the CD4+ CD25- T cell subset that is thought to consist primarily of effector cells. CD4+ CD25- T cells from post-septic animals exhibit increases in H3K9 acetylation (H3K9ac) in the promoter region of *Foxp3* (Cavassani et al., 2010); Foxp3 is a transcription factor considered to be a master regulator of T_{reg} function, and expression of Foxp3 is essential for the suppressive activity of T_{regs}. In addition, CD4+ CD25- T cells from post-septic mice exhibit increased expression of Kat2a mRNA; Kat2a is the chromatin modifying enzyme responsible for the addition of the H3K9ac mark. The concurrent increase in both H3K9ac and Kat2a in post-septic CD4+ T cells correlates with the increase in both T_{reg} numbers and functional activity in post-septic mice; in terms of post-septic immunosuppression, this increase in T_{reg} results in increased susceptibility to solid tumor challenge. Taken together, these studies indicate that following severe sepsis, CD4+ T cells exhibit modulations in the epigenetic regulation of gene expression, via changes in histone modifications, and that these changes can have significant effects on the activation, differentiation and effector function of these cells at timepoints post-sepsis.

Clearly, post-septic immunosuppression is a chronic condition, and can manifest itself in survivors of severe sepsis long after the resolution of SIRS and CARS-associated cytokine, chemokine and soluble mediator production. Of particular importance is the ability of post-septic immunosuppression to manifest itself even after the resolution of active suppressive mechanisms, such as with the increase in peripheral IL-10 and TGFβ observed during CARS. Studies of leukocyte function in experimental models of severe sepsis have identified numerous activation deficiencies in post-septic cells, centred on dysregulated cytokine and transcription factor expression. One possible explanation of the maintenance of this immunosuppressive phenotype is via changes in gene expression due to modulations in the epigenetic signatures of post-septic leukocytes. However, these studies have up to now been limited in scope, even within the field of epigenetics, as there remains many other epigenetic mechanisms (such as histone phosphorylation, DNA methylation, miRNA expression, etc) that may also be playing a role in mediating post-septic immunosuppression. In addition, much work remains to be done in correlating the gene regulatory events observed during late-phase CARS in animals with the phenotypes of peripheral blood leukocytes in patients who have recovered from severe sepsis. However, studies in animal models provide experimental data to bolster the findings from epidemiological studies in humans - namely, that post-septic immunosuppression can last far beyond the resolution of CARS, and the long-term survival of severe sepsis patients can be adversely effected by the improper function of the post-septic immune system.

4. Conclusion

Following the onset of severe sepsis, the cellular immune system is tasked with responding to both the septic insult, and any subsequent secondary infections or challenges, while also balancing the need to restrict the same pro-inflammatory responses that are mediating sepsis-induced mortality. The initial molecular mechanisms intended to resolve sepsis-induced mortality - namely, the increase in anti-inflammatory and immune-deviating cytokines observed during CARS - can render the cellular immune system unable to respond to secondary infections. In addition, apoptosis of immune cells during SIRS may remove those cells from participating in the cytokine storm of severe sepsis, but it reduces the number of functional immune cells able to respond to opportunistic and nosocomial infections. Following recovery from sepsis, the cellular immune system retains many deficiencies in activation and effector function, resulting in persistent immunosuppression that can adversely affect the long-term survival of patients who have recovered from severe sepsis. Ultimately, the cellular immune system is faced with a seemingly unsolvable paradox, in that limiting cellular activation can protect the organism from sepsis-induced mortality, only to leave the door open for mortality based on secondary infections during recovery.

Despite what is known about the nature of cellular immunosuppression following severe sepsis, many questions still remain to be answered. Of particular importance is the apparent link between the severity of the septic response (i.e. the cytokine storm) and the development of post-septic immunosuppression. It appears that the severity of the septic response, presumably as measured by the qualitative severity of the cytokine storm, is directly related to the development of post-septic immunosuppression. However, it is not clearly understood whether the development of immunosuppression is due to the increased level of a specific cytokine, or due to the combined presence of multiple proinflammatory cytokines acting in concert. Clearly, neutralization of individual cytokines during SIRS (for example, by utilizing mice that are genetically deficient) can have a dramatic effect on the sepsis-induced mortality; however, it remains to be seen whether the resulting effects on post-septic immunosuppression are due to the neutralization of the specific proinflammatory cytokine or a generalized effect of reducing the severity of the septic shock. In addition, much work remains to be done on the role of the cytokine storm of SIRS in modulating long-term immunosuppression, in particular the setting of epigenetic marks in post-septic leukocytes. It remains to be seen if the setting of specific epigenetic marks - along with the up- or down-regulation of chromatin modifying enzymes - is mechanistically driven by the cytokine milleu during SIRS.

From a clinical perspective, the persistence of post-septic immunosuppression presents a challenge for both diagnosis and treatment. Treatments aimed at reducing the severity of the acute phase of severe sepsis may help reduce sepsis-induced mortality at the expense of exacerbating CARS-associated mortality. Modulation of epigenetic mechanisms may prove useful for restoring immune function post-sepsis, but the available pharmacological approaches against histone modifications are limited. In addition, the diagnostic tools available to diagnose post-septic immunosuppression remain few, as not all survivors of severe sepsis go on to develop immunosuppressive phenotypes. To date, there are few described markers useful for the diagnosis of post-septic immunosuppression, aside from either functional analysis of peripheral blood leukocytes or, unfortunately, the development of secondary, opportunistic or nosocomial infections in the patient. Ultimately, these challenges associated with the proper diagnosis and treatment of post-septic immunosuppression makes this phenomenon a significant human health concern.

In summary, immune cell dysfunction is an important sequela of severe sepsis. This dysfunction manifests in three distinct phases following the onset of disease: during SIRS as a result of cell apoptosis and exhaustion, during the switch from SIRS to CARS as a result of directed immunosuppression by cells and soluble factors, and for the long term (CARS and beyond) due to cell-intrinsic defects in activation, differentiation and effector function. As a result, survivors of severe sepsis remain susceptible to secondary infections long after recovery from the acute phase of the inflammatory response. Despite the current understanding of the mechanisms governing post-septic immunosuppression, much remains to be understood concerning the development of this phenomenon and the proper treatments and therapies to recover the proper function of the immune system in post-septic patients.

5. Acknowledgment

This work was funded by National Institutes of Health (NIH) grants HL031237, HL089216, HL31963 and HL007517.

6. References

Abe, R., Hirasawa, H., Oda, S., Sadahiro, T., Nakamura, M., Watanabe, E., Nakada, T. A., Hatano, M., & Tokuhisa, T. (2008). Up-regulation of interleukin-10 mRNA expression in peripheral leukocytes predicts poor outcome and diminished human leukocyte antigen-DR expression on monocytes in septic patients. *J Surg Res, 147*(1), 1-8.

Adib-Conquy, M., Adrie, C., Moine, P., Asehnoune, K., Fitting, C., Pinsky, M. R., Dhainaut, J. F., & Cavaillon, J. M. (2000). NF-kappaB expression in mononuclear cells of patients with sepsis resembles that observed in lipopolysaccharide tolerance. *Am J Respir Crit Care Med, 162*(5), 1877-1883.

Adib-Conquy, M., & Cavaillon, J. M. (2009). Compensatory anti-inflammatory response syndrome. *Thromb Haemost, 101*(1), 36-47.

Akdis, C. A., & Blaser, K. (2001). Mechanisms of interleukin-10-mediated immune suppression. *Immunology, 103*(2), 131-136.

Ansel, K. M., Lee, D. U., & Rao, A. (2003). An epigenetic view of helper T cell differentiation. *Nat Immunol, 4*(7), 616-623.

Arraes, S. M., Freitas, M. S., da Silva, S. V., de Paula Neto, H. A., Alves-Filho, J. C., Auxiliadora Martins, M., Basile-Filho, A., Tavares-Murta, B. M., Barja-Fidalgo, C., & Cunha, F. Q. (2006). Impaired neutrophil chemotaxis in sepsis associates with GRK expression and inhibition of actin assembly and tyrosine phosphorylation. *Blood, 108*(9), 2906-2913.

Bazzoni, F., Tamassia, N., Rossato, M., & Cassatella, M. A. (2010). Understanding the molecular mechanisms of the multifaceted IL-10-mediated anti-inflammatory response: lessons from neutrophils. *Eur J Immunol, 40*(9), 2360-2368.

Benjamim, C. F., Hogaboam, C. M., & Kunkel, S. L. (2004). The chronic consequences of severe sepsis. *J Leukoc Biol, 75*(3), 408-412.

Benjamim, C. F., Hogaboam, C. M., Lukacs, N. W., & Kunkel, S. L. (2003). Septic mice are susceptible to pulmonary aspergillosis. *Am J Pathol, 163*(6), 2605-2617.

Benjamim, C. F., Lundy, S. K., Lukacs, N. W., Hogaboam, C. M., & Kunkel, S. L. (2005). Reversal of long-term sepsis-induced immunosuppression by dendritic cells. *Blood, 105*(9), 3588-3595.

Bergman, Y., & Cedar, H. (2010). Epigenetic control of recombination in the immune system. *Semin Immunol, 22*(6), 323-329.

Biswas, S. K., & Lopez-Collazo, E. (2009). Endotoxin tolerance: new mechanisms, molecules and clinical significance. *Trends Immunol, 30*(10), 475-487.

Bluestone, J. A., & Abbas, A. K. (2003). Natural versus adaptive regulatory T cells. *Nat Rev Immunol, 3*(3), 253-257.

Brandtzaeg, P., Osnes, L., Ovstebo, R., Joo, G. B., Westvik, A. B., & Kierulf, P. (1996). Net inflammatory capacity of human septic shock plasma evaluated by a monocyte-based target cell assay: identification of interleukin-10 as a major functional deactivator of human monocytes. *J Exp Med, 184*(1), 51-60.

Bresnihan, B., & Cunnane, G. (1998). Interleukin-1 receptor antagonist. *Rheum Dis Clin North Am, 24*(3), 615-628.

Bronte, V. (2009). Myeloid-derived suppressor cells in inflammation: uncovering cell subsets with enhanced immunosuppressive functions. *Eur J Immunol, 39*(10), 2670-2672.

Brown, K. A., Brain, S. D., Pearson, J. D., Edgeworth, J. D., Lewis, S. M., & Treacher, D. F. (2006). Neutrophils in development of multiple organ failure in sepsis. *Lancet, 368*(9530), 157-169.

Cameron, S. B., Nawijn, M. C., Kum, W. W., Savelkoul, H. F., & Chow, A. W. (2001). Regulation of helper T cell responses to staphylococcal superantigens. *Eur Cytokine Netw, 12*(2), 210-222.

Campbell, D. J., & Ziegler, S. F. (2007). FOXP3 modifies the phenotypic and functional properties of regulatory T cells. *Nat Rev Immunol, 7*(4), 305-310.

Carson, W. F., Cavassani, K. A., Dou, Y., & Kunkel, S. L. (2011). Epigenetic regulation of immune cell functions during post-septic immunosuppression. *Epigenetics, 6*(3), 273-283.

Carson, W. F., Cavassani, K. A., Ito, T., Schaller, M., Ishii, M., Dou, Y., & Kunkel, S. L. (2010). Impaired CD4+ T-cell proliferation and effector function correlates with repressive histone methylation events in a mouse model of severe sepsis. *Eur J Immunol, 40*(4), 998-1010.

Carson, W. F., Guernsey, L. A., Singh, A., Vella, A. T., Schramm, C. M., & Thrall, R. S. (2008). Accumulation of regulatory T cells in local draining lymph nodes of the lung correlates with spontaneous resolution of chronic asthma in a murine model. *Int Arch Allergy Immunol, 145*(3), 231-243.

Carson, W. F., Ito, T., Schaller, M., Cavassani, K. A., Chensue, S. W., & Kunkel, S. L. (2011). Dysregulated Cytokine Expression by CD4+ T cells from Post-Septic Mice Modulates both Th1 and Th2-Mediated Granulomatous Lung Inflammation. *PLoS One, 6*(5), e20385.

Cassatella, M. A., Tamassia, N., Crepaldi, L., McDonald, P. P., Ear, T., Calzetti, F., Gasperini, S., Zanderigo, F., & Bazzoni, F. (2005). Lipopolysaccharide primes neutrophils for a rapid response to IL-10. *Eur J Immunol, 35*(6), 1877-1885.

Cavaillon, J. M., & Adib-Conquy, M. (2006). Bench-to-bedside review: endotoxin tolerance as a model of leukocyte reprogramming in sepsis. *Crit Care, 10*(5), 233.

Cavallazzi, R., Bennin, C. L., Hirani, A., Gilbert, C., & Marik, P. E. (2010). Is the band count useful in the diagnosis of infection? An accuracy study in critically ill patients. *J Intensive Care Med, 25*(6), 353-357.

Cavassani, K. A., Carson, W. F. t., Moreira, A. P., Wen, H., Schaller, M. A., Ishii, M., Lindell, D. M., Dou, Y., Lukacs, N. W., Keshamouni, V. G., Hogaboam, C. M., & Kunkel, S. L. (2010). The post sepsis-induced expansion and enhanced function of regulatory T cells create an environment to potentiate tumor growth. *Blood, 115*(22), 4403-4411.

Cavassani, K. A., Ishii, M., Wen, H., Schaller, M. A., Lincoln, P. M., Lukacs, N. W., Hogaboam, C. M., & Kunkel, S. L. (2008). TLR3 is an endogenous sensor of tissue necrosis during acute inflammatory events. *J Exp Med, 205*(11), 2609-2621.

Chen, W., Frank, M. E., Jin, W., & Wahl, S. M. (2001). TGF-beta released by apoptotic T cells contributes to an immunosuppressive milieu. *Immunity, 14*(6), 715-725.

Chishti, A. D., Shenton, B. K., Kirby, J. A., & Baudouin, S. V. (2004). Neutrophil chemotaxis and receptor expression in clinical septic shock. *Intensive Care Med, 30*(4), 605-611.

Conference:, A. C. o. C. P. S. o. C. C. M. C. (1992). American College of Chest Physicians/Society of Critical Care Medicine Consensus Conference: definitions for sepsis and organ failure and guidelines for the use of innovative therapies in sepsis. *Crit Care Med, 20*(6), 864-874.

Cornbleet, P. J. (2002). Clinical utility of the band count. *Clin Lab Med, 22*(1), 101-136.

Cosgrove, M. S., & Wolberger, C. (2005). How does the histone code work? *Biochem Cell Biol, 83*(4), 468-476.

Crepaldi, L., Gasperini, S., Lapinet, J. A., Calzetti, F., Pinardi, C., Liu, Y., Zurawski, S., de Waal Malefyt, R., Moore, K. W., & Cassatella, M. A. (2001). Up-regulation of IL-10R1 expression is required to render human neutrophils fully responsive to IL-10. *J Immunol, 167*(4), 2312-2322.

Cuenca, A. G., Delano, M. J., Kelly-Scumpia, K. M., Moreno, C., Scumpia, P. O., Laface, D. M., Heyworth, P. G., Efron, P. A., & Moldawer, L. L. (2011). A paradoxical role for myeloid-derived suppressor cells in sepsis and trauma. *Mol Med, 17*(3-4), 281-292.

De Wilde, V., Van Rompaey, N., Hill, M., Lebrun, J. F., Lemaitre, P., Lhomme, F., Kubjak, C., Vokaer, B., Oldenhove, G., Charbonnier, L. M., Cuturi, M. C., Goldman, M., & Le Moine, A. (2009). Endotoxin-induced myeloid-derived suppressor cells inhibit alloimmune responses via heme oxygenase-1. *Am J Transplant, 9*(9), 2034-2047.

Delano, M. J., Scumpia, P. O., Weinstein, J. S., Coco, D., Nagaraj, S., Kelly-Scumpia, K. M., O'Malley, K. A., Wynn, J. L., Antonenko, S., Al-Quran, S. Z., Swan, R., Chung, C. S., Atkinson, M. A., Ramphal, R., Gabrilovich, D. I., Reeves, W. H., Ayala, A., Phillips, J., Laface, D., Heyworth, P. G., Clare-Salzler, M., & Moldawer, L. L. (2007). MyD88-dependent expansion of an immature GR-1(+)CD11b(+) population induces T cell suppression and Th2 polarization in sepsis. *J Exp Med, 204*(6), 1463-1474.

Delano, M. J., Thayer, T., Gabrilovich, S., Kelly-Scumpia, K. M., Winfield, R. D., Scumpia, P. O., Cuenca, A. G., Warner, E., Wallet, S. M., Wallet, M. A., O'Malley, K. A., Ramphal, R., Clare-Salzer, M., Efron, P. A., Mathews, C. E., & Moldawer, L. L. (2011). Sepsis induces early alterations in innate immunity that impact mortality to secondary infection. *J Immunol, 186*(1), 195-202.

Delcuve, G. P., Rastegar, M., & Davie, J. R. (2009). Epigenetic control. *J Cell Physiol, 219*(2), 243-250.

DiPiro, J. T. (1997). Cytokine networks with infection: mycobacterial infections, leishmaniasis, human immunodeficiency virus infection, and sepsis. *Pharmacotherapy, 17*(2), 205-223.

Duffy, A. J., Nolan, B., Sheth, K., Collette, H., De, M., & Bankey, P. E. (2000). Inhibition of alveolar neutrophil immigration in endotoxemia is macrophage inflammatory protein 2 independent. *J Surg Res, 90*(1), 51-57.

Fan, H., & Cook, J. A. (2004). Molecular mechanisms of endotoxin tolerance. *J Endotoxin Res, 10*(2), 71-84.

Fernandez-Morera, J. L., Calvanese, V., Rodriguez-Rodero, S., Menendez-Torre, E., & Fraga, M. F. (2010). Epigenetic regulation of the immune system in health and disease. *Tissue Antigens, 76*(6), 431-439.

Ferry, T., Thomas, D., Genestier, A. L., Bes, M., Lina, G., Vandenesch, F., & Etienne, J. (2005). Comparative prevalence of superantigen genes in Staphylococcus aureus isolates causing sepsis with and without septic shock. *Clin Infect Dis, 41*(6), 771-777.

Flierl, M. A., Rittirsch, D., Gao, H., Hoesel, L. M., Nadeau, B. A., Day, D. E., Zetoune, F. S., Sarma, J. V., Huber-Lang, M. S., Ferrara, J. L., & Ward, P. A. (2008). Adverse functions of IL-17A in experimental sepsis. *FASEB J, 22*(7), 2198-2205.

Fraser, J. D., & Proft, T. (2008). The bacterial superantigen and superantigen-like proteins. *Immunol Rev, 225*, 226-243.

Fujihara, M., Muroi, M., Tanamoto, K., Suzuki, T., Azuma, H., & Ikeda, H. (2003). Molecular mechanisms of macrophage activation and deactivation by lipopolysaccharide: roles of the receptor complex. *Pharmacol Ther, 100*(2), 171-194.

Fujimi, S., Ogura, H., Tanaka, H., Koh, T., Hosotsubo, H., Nakamori, Y., Kuwagata, Y., Shimazu, T., & Sugimoto, H. (2002). Activated polymorphonuclear leukocytes enhance production of leukocyte microparticles with increased adhesion molecules in patients with sepsis. *J Trauma, 52*(3), 443-448.

Ge, W., Jiang, J., Liu, W., Lian, D., Saito, A., Garcia, B., Li, X. C., & Wang, H. (2010). Regulatory T cells are critical to tolerance induction in presensitized mouse transplant recipients through targeting memory T cells. *Am J Transplant, 10*(8), 1760-1773.

Gerard, C., Bruyns, C., Marchant, A., Abramowicz, D., Vandenabeele, P., Delvaux, A., Fiers, W., Goldman, M., & Velu, T. (1993). Interleukin 10 reduces the release of tumor necrosis factor and prevents lethality in experimental endotoxemia. *J Exp Med, 177*(2), 547-550.

Gogos, C. A., Drosou, E., Bassaris, H. P., & Skoutelis, A. (2000). Pro- versus anti-inflammatory cytokine profile in patients with severe sepsis: a marker for prognosis and future therapeutic options. *J Infect Dis, 181*(1), 176-180.

Gordon, S., & Martinez, F. O. (2010). Alternative activation of macrophages: mechanism and functions. *Immunity, 32*(5), 593-604.

Heidecke, C. D., Hensler, T., Weighardt, H., Zantl, N., Wagner, H., Siewert, J. R., & Holzmann, B. (1999). Selective defects of T lymphocyte function in patients with lethal intraabdominal infection. *Am J Surg, 178*(4), 288-292.

Henneke, P., Dramsi, S., Mancuso, G., Chraibi, K., Pellegrini, E., Theilacker, C., Hubner, J., Santos-Sierra, S., Teti, G., Golenbock, D. T., Poyart, C., & Trieu-Cuot, P. (2008). Lipoproteins are critical TLR2 activating toxins in group B streptococcal sepsis. *J Immunol, 180*(9), 6149-6158.

Hudson, L. D., Milberg, J. A., Anardi, D., & Maunder, R. J. (1995). Clinical risks for development of the acute respiratory distress syndrome. *Am J Respir Crit Care Med, 151*(2 Pt 1), 293-301.

Ishii, M., Wen, H., Corsa, C. A., Liu, T., Coelho, A. L., Allen, R. M., Carson, W. F. t., Cavassani, K. A., Li, X., Lukacs, N. W., Hogaboam, C. M., Dou, Y., & Kunkel, S. L. (2009). Epigenetic regulation of the alternatively activated macrophage phenotype. *Blood, 114*(15), 3244-3254.

Jean-Baptiste, E. (2007). Cellular mechanisms in sepsis. *J Intensive Care Med, 22*(2), 63-72.

Jones, S. A., & Rose-John, S. (2002). The role of soluble receptors in cytokine biology: the agonistic properties of the sIL-6R/IL-6 complex. *Biochim Biophys Acta, 1592*(3), 251-263.

Kanamaru, C., Yasuda, H., & Fujita, T. (2002). Involvement of Smad proteins in TGF-beta and activin A-induced apoptosis and growth inhibition of liver cells. *Hepatol Res, 23*(3), 211-219.

Kasten, K. R., Tschop, J., Adediran, S. G., Hildeman, D. A., & Caldwell, C. C. (2010). T cells are potent early mediators of the host response to sepsis. *Shock, 34*(4), 327-336.

Kelly-Scumpia, K. M., Scumpia, P. O., Delano, M. J., Weinstein, J. S., Cuenca, A. G., Wynn, J. L., & Moldawer, L. L. (2010). Type I interferon signaling in hematopoietic cells is required for survival in mouse polymicrobial sepsis by regulating CXCL10. *J Exp Med, 207*(2), 319-326.

Klut, M. E., van Eeden, S. F., & Hogg, J. C. (1998). Neutrophil structural changes associated with chronic endotoxemia and lung injury. *J Inflamm, 48*(1), 1-12.

Latifi, S. Q., O'Riordan, M. A., & Levine, A. D. (2002). Interleukin-10 controls the onset of irreversible septic shock. *Infect Immun, 70*(8), 4441-4446.

Leask, A., & Abraham, D. J. (2004). TGF-beta signaling and the fibrotic response. *FASEB J, 18*(7), 816-827.

Lechner, M. G., Liebertz, D. J., & Epstein, A. L. (2010). Characterization of cytokine-induced myeloid-derived suppressor cells from normal human peripheral blood mononuclear cells. *J Immunol, 185*(4), 2273-2284.

Letterio, J. J. (2005). TGF-beta signaling in T cells: roles in lymphoid and epithelial neoplasia. *Oncogene, 24*(37), 5701-5712.

Li, M. O., & Flavell, R. A. (2008). TGF-beta: a master of all T cell trades. *Cell, 134*(3), 392-404.

Liu, Q. Y., Yao, Y. M., Yu, Y., Dong, N., & Sheng, Z. Y. (2011). Astragalus Polysaccharides Attenuate Postburn Sepsis via Inhibiting Negative Immunoregulation of CD4CD25 T Cells. *PLoS One, 6*(6), e19811.

Lyn-Kew, K., Rich, E., Zeng, X., Wen, H., Kunkel, S. L., Newstead, M. W., Bhan, U., & Standiford, T. J. (2010). IRAK-M regulates chromatin remodeling in lung macrophages during experimental sepsis. *PLoS One, 5*(6), e11145.

Mack, V. E., McCarter, M. D., Naama, H. A., Calvano, S. E., & Daly, J. M. (1996). Dominance of T-helper 2-type cytokines after severe injury. *Arch Surg, 131*(12), 1303-1308; discussion 1308-1309.

Mahidhara, R., & Billiar, T. R. (2000). Apoptosis in sepsis. *Crit Care Med, 28*(4 Suppl), N105-113.

Mantovani, A., Sica, A., Allavena, P., Garlanda, C., & Locati, M. (2009). Tumor-associated macrophages and the related myeloid-derived suppressor cells as a paradigm of the diversity of macrophage activation. *Hum Immunol, 70*(5), 325-330.

Marie, C., Cavaillon, J. M., & Losser, M. R. (1996). Elevated levels of circulating transforming growth factor-beta 1 in patients with the sepsis syndrome. *Ann Intern Med, 125*(6), 520-521.

Marie, C., Losser, M. R., Fitting, C., Kermarrec, N., Payen, D., & Cavaillon, J. M. (1997). Cytokines and soluble cytokine receptors in pleural effusions from septic and nonseptic patients. *Am J Respir Crit Care Med, 156*(5), 1515-1522.

Marigo, I., Dolcetti, L., Serafini, P., Zanovello, P., & Bronte, V. (2008). Tumor-induced tolerance and immune suppression by myeloid derived suppressor cells. *Immunol Rev, 222*, 162-179.

Medvedev, A. E., Sabroe, I., Hasday, J. D., & Vogel, S. N. (2006). Tolerance to microbial TLR ligands: molecular mechanisms and relevance to disease. *J Endotoxin Res, 12*(3), 133-150.

Mehrad, B., Strieter, R. M., Moore, T. A., Tsai, W. C., Lira, S. A., & Standiford, T. J. (1999). CXC chemokine receptor-2 ligands are necessary components of neutrophil-mediated host defense in invasive pulmonary aspergillosis. *J Immunol, 163*(11), 6086-6094.

Miller, A. C., Rashid, R. M., & Elamin, E. M. (2007). The "T" in trauma: the helper T-cell response and the role of immunomodulation in trauma and burn patients. *J Trauma, 63*(6), 1407-1417.

Mitra, R., & Khar, A. (2004). Suppression of macrophage function in AK-5 tumor transplanted animals: role of TGF-beta1. *Immunol Lett, 91*(2-3), 189-195.

Monneret, G., Debard, A. L., Venet, F., Bohe, J., Hequet, O., Bienvenu, J., & Lepape, A. (2003). Marked elevation of human circulating CD4+CD25+ regulatory T cells in sepsis-induced immunoparalysis. *Crit Care Med, 31*(7), 2068-2071.

Muller Kobold, A. C., Tulleken, J. E., Zijlstra, J. G., Sluiter, W., Hermans, J., Kallenberg, C. G., & Tervaert, J. W. (2000). Leukocyte activation in sepsis; correlations with disease state and mortality. *Intensive Care Med, 26*(7), 883-892.

Munoz, C., Carlet, J., Fitting, C., Misset, B., Bleriot, J. P., & Cavaillon, J. M. (1991). Dysregulation of in vitro cytokine production by monocytes during sepsis. *J Clin Invest, 88*(5), 1747-1754.

Nausch, N., Galani, I. E., Schlecker, E., & Cerwenka, A. (2008). Mononuclear myeloid-derived "suppressor" cells express RAE-1 and activate natural killer cells. *Blood, 112*(10), 4080-4089.

Newton, S., Ding, Y., Chung, C. S., Chen, Y., Lomas-Neira, J. L., & Ayala, A. (2004). Sepsis-induced changes in macrophage co-stimulatory molecule expression: CD86 as a regulator of anti-inflammatory IL-10 response. *Surg Infect (Larchmt), 5*(4), 375-383.

Nicod, L. P., Galve-De-Rochemonteix, B., & Dayer, J. M. (1994). Modulation of IL-1 receptor antagonist and TNF-soluble receptors produced by alveolar macrophages and blood monocytes. *Ann N Y Acad Sci, 725*, 323-330.

Nishikawa, H., & Sakaguchi, S. (2010). Regulatory T cells in tumor immunity. *Int J Cancer, 127*(4), 759-767.

O'Sullivan, S. T., Lederer, J. A., Horgan, A. F., Chin, D. H., Mannick, J. A., & Rodrick, M. L. (1995). Major injury leads to predominance of the T helper-2 lymphocyte phenotype and diminished interleukin-12 production associated with decreased resistance to infection. *Ann Surg, 222*(4), 482-490; discussion 490-482.

Oberholzer, A., Oberholzer, C., & Moldawer, L. L. (2001). Sepsis syndromes: understanding the role of innate and acquired immunity. *Shock, 16*(2), 83-96.

Oberholzer, A., Oberholzer, C., & Moldawer, L. L. (2002). Interleukin-10: a complex role in the pathogenesis of sepsis syndromes and its potential as an anti-inflammatory drug. *Crit Care Med, 30*(1 Suppl), S58-63.

Oberholzer, C., Oberholzer, A., Clare-Salzler, M., & Moldawer, L. L. (2001). Apoptosis in sepsis: a new target for therapeutic exploration. *FASEB J, 15*(6), 879-892.

Patel, D. R., & Richardson, B. C. (2010). Epigenetic mechanisms in lupus. *Curr Opin Rheumatol, 22*(5), 478-482.

Patel, G. P., Gurka, D. P., & Balk, R. A. (2003). New treatment strategies for severe sepsis and septic shock. *Curr Opin Crit Care, 9*(5), 390-396.

Perl, T. M., Dvorak, L., Hwang, T., & Wenzel, R. P. (1995). Long-term survival and function after suspected gram-negative sepsis. *JAMA, 274*(4), 338-345.

Pillay, J., Ramakers, B. P., Kamp, V. M., Loi, A. L., Lam, S. W., Hietbrink, F., Leenen, L. P., Tool, A. T., Pickkers, P., & Koenderman, L. (2010). Functional heterogeneity and differential priming of circulating neutrophils in human experimental endotoxemia. *J Leukoc Biol, 88*(1), 211-220.

Prud'homme, G. J., & Piccirillo, C. A. (2000). The inhibitory effects of transforming growth factor-beta-1 (TGF-beta1) in autoimmune diseases. *J Autoimmun, 14*(1), 23-42.

Quartin, A. A., Schein, R. M., Kett, D. H., & Peduzzi, P. N. (1997). Magnitude and duration of the effect of sepsis on survival. Department of Veterans Affairs Systemic Sepsis Cooperative Studies Group. *JAMA, 277*(13), 1058-1063.

Reddy, R. C., Chen, G. H., Tekchandani, P. K., & Standiford, T. J. (2001). Sepsis-induced immunosuppression: from bad to worse. *Immunol Res, 24*(3), 273-287.

Reddy, R. C., Narala, V. R., Keshamouni, V. G., Milam, J. E., Newstead, M. W., & Standiford, T. J. (2008). Sepsis-induced inhibition of neutrophil chemotaxis is mediated by activation of peroxisome proliferator-activated receptor-{gamma}. *Blood, 112*(10), 4250-4258.

Ribechini, E., Leenen, P. J., & Lutz, M. B. (2009). Gr-1 antibody induces STAT signaling, macrophage marker expression and abrogation of myeloid-derived suppressor cell activity in BM cells. *Eur J Immunol, 39*(12), 3538-3551.

Riedemann, N. C., Guo, R. F., Laudes, I. J., Keller, K., Sarma, V. J., Padgaonkar, V., Zetoune, F. S., & Ward, P. A. (2002). C5a receptor and thymocyte apoptosis in sepsis. *FASEB J, 16*(8), 887-888.

Roloff, T. C., & Nuber, U. A. (2005). Chromatin, epigenetics and stem cells. *Eur J Cell Biol, 84*(2-3), 123-135.

Romero, C. R., Herzig, D. S., Etogo, A., Nunez, J., Mahmoudizad, R., Fang, G., Murphey, E. D., Toliver-Kinsky, T., & Sherwood, E. R. (2010). The role of interferon-gamma in the pathogenesis of acute intra-abdominal sepsis. *J Leukoc Biol, 88*(4), 725-735.

Sabroe, I., Dower, S. K., & Whyte, M. K. (2005). The role of Toll-like receptors in the regulation of neutrophil migration, activation, and apoptosis. *Clin Infect Dis, 41 Suppl 7*, S421-426.

Sen, G. C., & Sarkar, S. N. (2005). Transcriptional signaling by double-stranded RNA: role of TLR3. *Cytokine Growth Factor Rev, 16*(1), 1-14.

Shafa, M., Krawetz, R., & Rancourt, D. E. (2010). Returning to the stem state: epigenetics of recapitulating pre-differentiation chromatin structure. *Bioessays, 32*(9), 791-799.

Silva, A. T., & Cohen, J. (1992). Role of interferon-gamma in experimental gram-negative sepsis. *J Infect Dis, 166*(2), 331-335.

Spender, L. C., O'Brien, D. I., Simpson, D., Dutt, D., Gregory, C. D., Allday, M. J., Clark, L. J., & Inman, G. J. (2009). TGF-beta induces apoptosis in human B cells by transcriptional regulation of BIK and BCL-XL. *Cell Death Differ, 16*(4), 593-602.

Spolarics, Z., Siddiqi, M., Siegel, J. H., Garcia, Z. C., Stein, D. S., Denny, T., & Deitch, E. A. (2003). Depressed interleukin-12-producing activity by monocytes correlates with adverse clinical course and a shift toward Th2-type lymphocyte pattern in severely injured male trauma patients. *Crit Care Med, 31*(6), 1722-1729.

Sriskandan, S., & Altmann, D. M. (2008). The immunology of sepsis. *J Pathol, 214*(2), 211-223.

Suri-Payer, E., & Fritzsching, B. (2006). Regulatory T cells in experimental autoimmune disease. *Springer Semin Immunopathol, 28*(1), 3-16.

Suzuki, J., Ricordi, C., & Chen, Z. (2010). Immune tolerance induction by integrating innate and adaptive immune regulators. *Cell Transplant, 19*(3), 253-268.

Takahashi, H., Tsuda, Y., Takeuchi, D., Kobayashi, M., Herndon, D. N., & Suzuki, F. (2004). Influence of systemic inflammatory response syndrome on host resistance against bacterial infections. *Crit Care Med, 32*(9), 1879-1885.

Takeuchi, O., & Akira, S. (2008). MDA5/RIG-I and virus recognition. *Curr Opin Immunol, 20*(1), 17-22.

Tamassia, N., Calzetti, F., Menestrina, N., Rossato, M., Bazzoni, F., Gottin, L., & Cassatella, M. A. (2008). Circulating neutrophils of septic patients constitutively express IL-10R1 and are promptly responsive to IL-10. *Int Immunol, 20*(4), 535-541.

Taylor, A. L., & Llewelyn, M. J. (2010). Superantigen-induced proliferation of human CD4+CD25- T cells is followed by a switch to a functional regulatory phenotype. *J Immunol, 185*(11), 6591-6598.

Tinsley, K. W., Grayson, M. H., Swanson, P. E., Drewry, A. M., Chang, K. C., Karl, I. E., & Hotchkiss, R. S. (2003). Sepsis induces apoptosis and profound depletion of splenic interdigitating and follicular dendritic cells. *J Immunol, 171*(2), 909-914.

Uhlig, H. H., Coombes, J., Mottet, C., Izcue, A., Thompson, C., Fanger, A., Tannapfel, A., Fontenot, J. D., Ramsdell, F., & Powrie, F. (2006). Characterization of Foxp3+CD4+CD25+ and IL-10-secreting CD4+CD25+ T cells during cure of colitis. *J Immunol, 177*(9), 5852-5860.

Unsinger, J., Kazama, H., McDonough, J. S., Hotchkiss, R. S., & Ferguson, T. A. (2009). Differential lymphopenia-induced homeostatic proliferation for CD4+ and CD8+ T cells following septic injury. *J Leukoc Biol, 85*(3), 382-390.

Unsinger, J., McDonough, J. S., Shultz, L. D., Ferguson, T. A., & Hotchkiss, R. S. (2009). Sepsis-induced human lymphocyte apoptosis and cytokine production in "humanized" mice. *J Leukoc Biol, 86*(2), 219-227.

van der Poll, T., de Waal Malefyt, R., Coyle, S. M., & Lowry, S. F. (1997). Antiinflammatory cytokine responses during clinical sepsis and experimental endotoxemia: sequential measurements of plasma soluble interleukin (IL)-1 receptor type II, IL-10, and IL-13. *J Infect Dis, 175*(1), 118-122.

van der Vliet, H. J., & Nieuwenhuis, E. E. (2007). IPEX as a result of mutations in FOXP3. *Clin Dev Immunol, 2007*, 89017.

Venet, F., Chung, C. S., Kherouf, H., Geeraert, A., Malcus, C., Poitevin, F., Bohe, J., Lepape, A., Ayala, A., & Monneret, G. (2009). Increased circulating regulatory T cells (CD4(+)CD25 (+)CD127 (-)) contribute to lymphocyte anergy in septic shock patients. *Intensive Care Med, 35*(4), 678-686.

Venet, F., Pachot, A., Debard, A. L., Bohe, J., Bienvenu, J., Lepape, A., & Monneret, G. (2004). Increased percentage of CD4+CD25+ regulatory T cells during septic shock is due to the decrease of CD4+CD25- lymphocytes. *Crit Care Med, 32*(11), 2329-2331.

Wagner, H. (2002). Interactions between bacterial CpG-DNA and TLR9 bridge innate and adaptive immunity. *Curr Opin Microbiol, 5*(1), 62-69.

Walsh, T. J., Roilides, E., Cortez, K., Kottilil, S., Bailey, J., & Lyman, C. A. (2005). Control, immunoregulation, and expression of innate pulmonary host defenses against Aspergillus fumigatus. *Med Mycol, 43 Suppl 1*, S165-172.

Wang, S. D., Huang, K. J., Lin, Y. S., & Lei, H. Y. (1994). Sepsis-induced apoptosis of the thymocytes in mice. *J Immunol, 152*(10), 5014-5021.

Ward, M. J., Fertel, B. S., Bonomo, J. B., Smith, C. L., Hart, K. W., Lindsell, C. J., & Wright, S. W. (2010). The degree of bandemia in septic ED patients does not predict inpatient mortality. *Am J Emerg Med.*

Ward, N. S., Casserly, B., & Ayala, A. (2008). The compensatory anti-inflammatory response syndrome (CARS) in critically ill patients. *Clin Chest Med, 29*(4), 617-625, viii.

Ward, P. A. (2008). Sepsis, apoptosis and complement. *Biochem Pharmacol, 76*(11), 1383-1388.

Watford, W. T., Moriguchi, M., Morinobu, A., & O'Shea, J. J. (2003). The biology of IL-12: coordinating innate and adaptive immune responses. *Cytokine Growth Factor Rev, 14*(5), 361-368.

Wen, H., Dou, Y., Hogaboam, C. M., & Kunkel, S. L. (2008). Epigenetic regulation of dendritic cell-derived interleukin-12 facilitates immunosuppression after a severe innate immune response. *Blood, 111*(4), 1797-1804.

Wen, H., Hogaboam, C. M., Gauldie, J., & Kunkel, S. L. (2006). Severe sepsis exacerbates cell-mediated immunity in the lung due to an altered dendritic cell cytokine profile. *Am J Pathol, 168*(6), 1940-1950.

Wen, H., Schaller, M. A., Dou, Y., Hogaboam, C. M., & Kunkel, S. L. (2008). Dendritic cells at the interface of innate and acquired immunity: the role for epigenetic changes. *J Leukoc Biol, 83*(3), 439-446.

Wesche-Soldato, D. E., Lomas-Neira, J. L., Perl, M., Jones, L., Chung, C. S., & Ayala, A. (2005). The role and regulation of apoptosis in sepsis. *J Endotoxin Res, 11*(6), 375-382.

West, M. A., & Koons, A. (2008). Endotoxin tolerance in sepsis: concentration-dependent augmentation or inhibition of LPS-stimulated macrophage TNF secretion by LPS pretreatment. *J Trauma, 65*(4), 893-898; discussion 898-900.

West, M. A., Koons, A., Crandall, M., Skinner, R., Worley, M., & Shapiro, M. B. (2007). Whole blood leukocyte mitogen activated protein kinases activation differentiates intensive care unit patients with systemic inflammatory response syndrome and sepsis. *J Trauma, 62*(4), 805-811.

Wilczynski, J. R., Radwan, M., & Kalinka, J. (2008). The characterization and role of regulatory T cells in immune reactions. *Front Biosci, 13*, 2266-2274.

Williams, L. M., Ricchetti, G., Sarma, U., Smallie, T., & Foxwell, B. M. (2004). Interleukin-10 suppression of myeloid cell activation--a continuing puzzle. *Immunology, 113*(3), 281-292.

Winters, B. D., Eberlein, M., Leung, J., Needham, D. M., Pronovost, P. J., & Sevransky, J. E. (2010). Long-term mortality and quality of life in sepsis: a systematic review. *Crit Care Med, 38*(5), 1276-1283.

Wisnoski, N., Chung, C. S., Chen, Y., Huang, X., & Ayala, A. (2007). The contribution of CD4+ CD25+ T-regulatory-cells to immune suppression in sepsis. *Shock, 27*(3), 251-257.

Yang, L., Pang, Y., & Moses, H. L. (2010). TGF-beta and immune cells: an important regulatory axis in the tumor microenvironment and progression. *Trends Immunol, 31*(6), 220-227.

Zhang, G., & Ghosh, S. (2000). Molecular mechanisms of NF-kappaB activation induced by bacterial lipopolysaccharide through Toll-like receptors. *J Endotoxin Res, 6*(6), 453-457.

7

Microparticles and Exosomes: Are They Part of Important Pathways in Sepsis Pathophysiology?

Luciano C. P. Azevedo
Research and Education Institute, Hospital Sírio-Libanês and University of São Paulo School of Medicine
Brazil

1. Introduction

Microparticles are a heterogeneous population of small membrane-coated vesicles released by several cell lines upon activation or apoptosis. Microparticles generation seems to be a well regulated process, although these vesicles are highly variable in size, composition and function. Despite being previously considered inert debris without specific function, recent data demonstrated important pathophysiological mechanisms orchestrated by microparticles in vascular diseases associated with endothelial dysfunction. These vesicles have been implicated, among others, in the pathogenesis of thrombosis, inflammation, atherosclerosis and vascular cell proliferation. In addition to microparticles, activation of the endocytic-lisosomal cellular system of circulating cells induce the release of smaller vesicles denominated exosomes that can also participate in vascular derangement. This role of microparticles and exosomes in mediating vascular dysfunction suggests that they may represent novel pathways in short or long-distance paracrine transcellular signaling in vascular environment. The mechanisms involved in the origin of microparticles and exosomes, their composition and participation in the pathogenesis of sepsis will be discussed in this review.

2. Origin of microparticles

Circulating cells in vascular environment as well as endothelial cells after activation or apoptosis are capable of releasing membranous fragments (vesicles), of size varying from 100 nm to 1000 nm (Fig. (**1**)). These vesicles present, on their surfaces, at least some of the antigenic markers of the parent cell (Azevedo et al., 2007). The first description of these vesicles was made in 1967, with the reports of a "platelet dust" (platelet membrane fragments) in human plasma (Wolf et al., 1967). After a more precise characterization on their origin, composition and function, these vesicles were called microparticles (or microvesicles) and there is now increasing evidence for their role in transcellular communication in microvascular environment. However, the precise functions of these fragments and their interaction with cells in vasculature remain incomplete.
The release of microparticles has been described in several circumstances in normal physiology as well as in disease states. In health, it has been reported that 80% of

circulating microparticles express membrane antigens that suggest a platelet origin. These vesicles have also been implicated to play a role in inflammation, coagulation and diseases associated with impairment of vascular function, e.g. atherosclerosis, diabetes and hypertension (Tushuizen et al., 2011). Usually, microparticles release is the result of cell activation or apoptosis, although it is not known whether these events lead to the formation of similar microparticles, in terms of size, lipid and protein composition and pathophysiological effects. Microparticles release is an integral part of the membrane-remodeling process in which the asymmetric distribution of constitutive phospholipids between the two leaflets of the cell membrane is lost, with released microparticles exposing phosphatidylserine in the outer membrane, which acts as a template for the prothrombinase complex assembly and for their role in coagulation activation (Zwaal & Schroit, 1997).

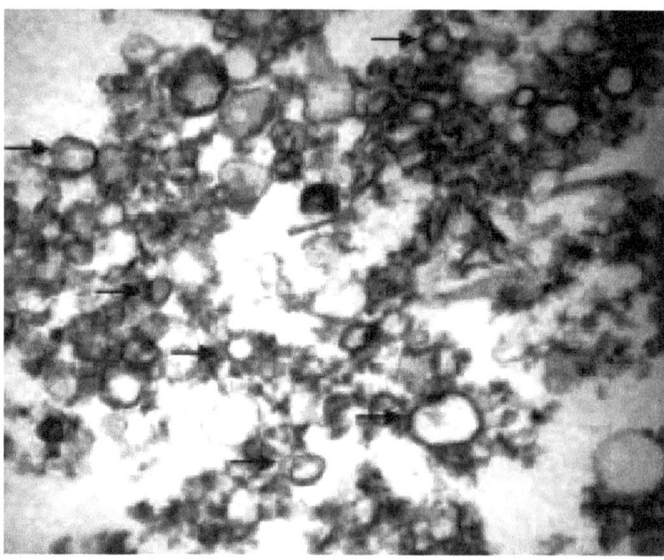

Fig. 1. Microparticles (arrows) isolated from plasma of a patient 24 hours after percutaneous coronary angioplasty. Electron micrography depicts a heterogeneous population of vesicles ranging in size from 80 to 200 nm (original magnification X39000). Adapted from Azevedo et al., 2007 with permission.

It is important to note, in first place, that circulating microparticles are a population of vesicles from different cell types and from different cellular compartment origins. As already discussed, the most common mechanism of microparticle release is cell activation or apoptosis, which induces plasma membrane budding, leading to the formation of membrane blebs. However, apoptosis can also induce the formation of apoptotic bodies, which are sometimes considered as members of microparticles' family. Apoptotic bodies are cell fragments many times larger in diameter and volume than microparticles that are consequence of cell fragmentation in the final stages of apoptosis, in contrast with microparticles, that are released in the early moments of programmed cell death. These apoptotic bodies also expose phosphatidylserine in the outer membrane, but unlike microparticles, have poor prothrombotic properties. Probably, the role of phosphatidylserine in these corpuscles is to recruit phagocytic cells to the site of apoptotic death (Janiszewski et al, 2004).

Other type of vesicle released after cell activation that can sometimes overlap microparticle function is the exosome. Dissimilar to microparticles that are fragments of cell membranes, exosomes are vesicles produced in the endocytic-lysosomal system of several cell lines. Exosomes are smaller than microparticles (usually less than 0.1 μm), have different surface antigens and poor clotting capacity (Azevedo et al, 2007). The role of exosomes in sepsis will be discussed in more details below.

Virtually all cell types subjected to activation can release microparticles after blebbing of plasma membrane. The most common cell types associated with microparticle release are platelets, endothelial cells, neutrophils, smooth muscle cells, monocytes and T lymphocytes. (Azevedo et al, 2007). Their ubiquity has suggested a more general role for microparticles in cellular regulation, possibly with functions reminiscent of their original cell.

3. Composition of microparticles

The membrane of microparticles, which is derived from the parental cell plasma membrane, consists primarily of lipids and proteins, in variable amounts. The precise content of lipids and proteins is dependent on the cell they originate from and the type of stimulus involved in their formation.

Microparticles are surrounded by a phospholipid bilayer. During the budding process, the normal phospholipid asymmetry of the membrane is lost, with microparticles exposing negatively charged phospholipids such as phosphatidylserine (PS) and phosphatidylethanolamine (PE) in their outer membrane leaflet. Exposure of PS plays a role in the in vivo effects of microparticles, since PS is an efficient site for coagulation factor activation. Analysis of components of microparticles from blood of healthy donors indicates that phosphatidylcholine represents more than 60% of their lipid content (Weerheim et al, 2002). Other lipids present in minor concentrations are sphingomyelin, PS and PE. Although these microparticles are in the vast majority derived from platelets (~75%), their phospholipid composition is different from parental cell.

Protein composition in the surface of microparticles is dependent of parental cell type. These surface antigens are specific for the cell they originate from and can help to identify the origin of microparticle. However, microparticle can differ in the expression of cell surface molecules from their parental cells. This is particularly important when microparticles express molecules upregulated or translocated by cell activation or apoptosis. For example, IL-1 alpha-activated cultured endothelial cells can release microparticles displaying E-selectin and endothelial cell adhesion molecule 1 in significantly higher concentrations than resting cultivated endothelial cells (Abid Hussein et al, 2003). There are also data depicting different protein composition of microparticles in response to different agonists and with the same parental cell stimulated with the same agonist (Hughes et al, 2000). Taken together, these differences indicate that shedding seems to be a well-regulated process that originates unique microparticle characteristics depending on the cell source, stimulus, scenario and pathophysiological conditions.

More recent data demonstrate that, besides proteins and lipid composition on the surface of microparticles, the inner portion of these vesicles also contain several enzymes and genetic material capable of interacting and producing effects on the target cell (Meziani et al, 2010). Subunits of enzymes with superoxide producing activity like NADPH oxidase have been identified on microparticles originated from platelets (Janiszewski et al, 2004). In addition, microparticles and exosomes from cultured cells and normal individuals have been demonstrated to contain mRNA and microRNA, which suggests that these vesicles may play a role on the cell to cell transfer of genetic contents (Hunter et al, 2008 and Valadi et al, 2007).

4. Mechanisms of microparticle release

Platelets release microparticles after activation by thrombin, ADP plus collagen, calcium ionophore A23187 and high shear stress. Endothelial cells, monocytes and vascular smooth cells can release microparticles after activation by bacterial lipopolysaccharide, inflammatory cytokines, complement complex C5b-9 or reactive oxygen species (Boulanger et al, 2006).

The mechanisms governing plasma membrane shedding and consequent microparticle release are only partially understood. Usually, the shedding starts within minutes after addition of an agonist, by a calcium-dependent process that can be blocked by calcium chelators. One of the possible molecules governing this process is calpain μ, which is a calcium-dependent cytosolic-protease that cleaves talin and α-actin. Inhibition of calpain by calpeptin or calcium chelators prevents the release of microparticles (Azevedo et al, 2007). However, molecules other than calpain may be involved in calcium-dependent microparticles release, since blockade by calpeptin did not induce an inhibition of microparticle release to the same extent as EGTA, suggesting a role for other calcium dependent processes. Cytosolic calcium increase may also activate kinases and inhibit phosphatases, which together with calpain activation, are responsible for cytoskeleton disruption. Membrane skeleton disruption is the result of several mechanisms, such as myosin light-chain phosphorylation mediated by myosin light-chain kinase (MLCK) upon activation or Rho-associated kinase I (ROCK-I), in apoptosis. Phosphorilation of myosin light chains (MLC) stimulates the contractile activity of myosin, with myosin ATPase activation creating movement between actin and myosin filaments (Azevedo et al, 2007). This movement may tensionate plasma membrane and cause detachment of the cytoskeleton from the membrane, with the formation of blebs and the subsequent release of microparticles. However, the precise interaction between cell membrane and cytoskeleton, which permits microparticle formation, is still unknown. Recent data has implicated ROCK-II (an isoform of ROCK-I) in thrombin-induced microparticle release from endothelial cells. These new data recently incorporated indicates that the knowledge on mechanisms inducing cytoskeleton rearrangement during bleb formation is still scarce.

Another important feature in microparticle formation is the loss of phospholipid asymmetry of membranes after cell activation. Usually, PS and PE are specifically segregated in the inner leaflet, whereas phosphatidylcholine and sphingomyelin are enriched in the external one. This distribution is controlled by three enzymes: an inward-directed pump, a flippase (aminophospholipid translocase), specific for PS and PE; an outward-directed pump referred to as "floppase"; and a lipid scramblase, promoting unspecific bidirectional redistribution across the bilayer. The increase in calcium content after cell activation may lead to collapse of the membrane asymmetry by stimulating scramblase and floppase activities and concomitantly inhibiting the flippase. The increase in PS exposure in the outer leaflet that follows microparticle formation enhances coagulative properties and facilitates removal of apoptotic bodies by phagocytic cells. PS also binds annexin-5, which has been used in several studies for microparticle quantification (Azevedo et al, 2007).

Whether microparticles release is the result of cell membrane shedding, the release of exosomes from the parental cell is mainly orchestrated by the endocytic-lisossomal system. Endocytosis is a range of processes performed by the cell in order to internalize specific regions of the plasma membrane as well as small amounts of extracellular fluid. In this process, intracellular compartments of endocytic pathway called multivesicular bodies (MVB) composed of numerous vesicles are able to fuse with the plasma membrane, releasing these vesicles abroad. After incorporation into the cell, the absorbed material is accumulated in endosomes, which are major sites of entry for the captured molecules. The endosomes then become MVB, which are characterized by being more spherical, had lower intra-luminal pH and a different protein distribution. It is unclear the mechanism by which endosomes become MVB. In MVB, the presence of vesicular bodies inside is better characterized and once formed, these structures are destined for several processes: they can serve as storage sites; They can direct proteins to be degraded through their fusion with lysosomes (organelles that constitute, together with the MVB, the major site of protein and lipid degradation in the cell); Or they can fuse with the plasma membrane, thereby releasing their vesicles (exosomes) into the extracellular medium (Azevedo et al, 2007).

5. Microparticles in inflammatory conditions and sepsis

There is now emerging evidence that microparticles and exosomes participate actively in regulation of vascular function in several healthy and disease states. Microparticles, regardless their cell origin, can transfer biological information between cells, therefore acting as vectors of signaling molecules. Most of the exchange of information from microparticles takes place at the level of endothelium and contributes to their (patho)physiological role. Microvesicles (microparticles and exosomes) have been reported to be part of the disease mechanisms in several conditions, such as inflammation, thrombosis and vascular dysfunction, all elements that are reported to be extremely involved in the pathogenesis of sepsis.

It is now demonstrated from in vitro and in vivo studies that microparticles may play a role in inflammatory conditions, since they display a variety of proinflammatory activities. Microparticles from endothelial cells, platelets and leukocytes can promote adhesion and rolling of leukocytes, contain proinflammatory cytokines and trigger the release of microparticles from several cell types in vitro (Huber at el, 2002, Forlow et al, 2000). In addition, oxidized phospholipids from endothelial microparticles released by oxidative stress may cause monocyte adherence to endothelial cells and neutrophil activation (Huber et al, 2002). A recent study demonstrated also that microparticles isolated from septic shock patients injected into rats induce the expression of inducible nitric oxide synthase, nuclear factor kappa B and cyclooxygenase-2 in the lungs and hearts of these animals (Mastronardi et al, 2011).

Besides endothelial microparticles, other vesicles released from different cell sources may have a role in mediating cellular interactions in vascular milieu. Platelet-derived microparticles, for instance, can enhance the binding of neutrophils to other neutrophils under flow conditions. This effect seems to be mediated by an interaction between P-selectin on microparticles and P-selectin-glycoprotein ligand 1 on neutrophils, since the blockade of these surface molecules can reduce this binding (Forlow et al, 2000). Microparticles derived from platelets can also stimulate monocyte-endothelial interactions, by delivering arachidonic acid to endothelial cells, which induces the upregulation of expression of cellular adhesion molecules (ICAM-1) on endothelium and CD11a/CD18 and CD11b/CD18 on monocytes (Barry et al, 1998).

Platelet-derived microparticles, as well as vesicles from other cell lines, can contribute to inflammation by stimulating the production of several cytokines. Microparticles derived from leukocytes can increase the production of IL-6, monocyte chemotactic protein 1 (MCP-1) and Tissue Factor (TF) in endothelial cells (Mesri & Altieri, 1999). Platelet-derived microparticles have been associated with increased production of IL-8, IL-1beta and TNF-alpha by a monocytic cell line (THP-1) and endothelial cells in high shear stress conditions (Nomura et al, 2004). In leukocytes, endotoxin stimulation induced the shedding of microvesicles containing platelet-activating factor (PAF), a known inducer of inflammatory response (Watanabe et al, 2003).

Evidence that microparticles participate in the genesis of inflammatory diseases is supported by studies that depicted increased number of microparticles in inflammatory conditions in vivo. Meningococcal sepsis, for instance, is associated with increased levels of microparticles released mainly from granulocytes and platelets (Nieuwland et al, 2000). These vesicles are highly procoagulant, which demonstrates the correlation among inflammation and coagulation in the pathogenesis of several vascular diseases. In patients with sepsis and multiple organ dysfunction syndrome, Joop et al found increased number of microparticles released from granulocytes, and diminished levels of microparticles derived from platelets and erythrocytes were also found. Trauma patients have also increased levels of leukocyte microparticles with enhanced expression of adhesion molecules on days 2 to 5 after injury (Fujimi et al, 2003). In addition, in sepsis, circulating levels of endothelial and platelet microparticles were negatively correlated with unfavorable outcomes during multiple organ dysfunction syndrome (Soriano et al, 2005).

Sepsis has also been associated with significant endothelial dysfunction. Many studies have isolated microparticles from blood of patients with disease states marked by vascular dysfunction, and these vesicles were associated with this impairment in isolated arteries (Martin et al, 2004, Tesse et al 2005). Microparticles released from T-lymphocytes are capable of impairing endothelial function after 12 or 24 hours of incubation, also decreasing eNOS expression and increasing caveolin-1 expression of endothelial cells in culture (Martin et al, 2004). Another investigation reported impairment of vascular function with microparticles released from an apoptotic T cell line in a mechanism associated with transcription factor NF-κB production and proinflammatory protein upregulation (Tesse et al, 2005). Microparticles originated from endothelial cells in culture induce superoxide production by aortic rings associated with impairment of acethylcoline-induced vasorelaxation. These microvesicles also inhibit NO production by aortic rings and display p22(phox), a subunit of superoxide-producing enzyme NADPH oxidase, thus demonstrating an important role for oxidative stress in vascular dysfunction (Brodsky et al, 2004). However, there is still a lot to be discovered on the mechanisms of microparticles induced endothelial dysfunction.

Another hallmark of sepsis is activation of coagulation. The most known property of microparticles is their ability to induce coagulation activation with subsequent thrombosis of vascular beds. There is substantial in vitro evidence of the involvement of microparticles in activation of coagulation system (Muller et al, 2003). In vivo studies depicting increased concentrations of microparticles in diseases associated with coagulation activation corroborate the in vitro data (Nieuwland et al, 2000).

Circulating microparticles provide an additional procoagulant phospholipid surface for the assembly of the clotting enzymes complexes that promote thrombin generation. The assembly of vitamin-K dependent tenase and prothrombinase complexes in microparticles is known as platelet factor 3 activity. Platelet microparticles also display activated factor V in their surface, which may contribute to activation of clotting. Endothelial microparticles, in turn, released after stimulation of endothelial cells in culture with plasminogen activator inhibitor-1 (PAI-1) become procoagulant with an accelerated thrombin production (Brodsky et al, 2002). This activation of coagulation that occurs after microparticle release culminates with the generation of thrombin, which consequently induces hemostasis or a prothrombotic state. The stimulation of clotting that follows microparticle release requires a tight control exerted by natural anticoagulant systems. Indeed, binding of protein S to microparticle surface has already been described, with subsequent binding of protein C and activated protein C.

A more direct mechanism relating microparticles and initiation of coagulation was described when TF was reported to be present in the surface of platelet-derived microvesicles (Muller et al, 2003). TF has also been described in microparticles derived from monocytes and smooth muscle cells after apoptosis (Azevedo et al, 2007). Moreover, microparticles are capable of inducing TF expression on monocytes (Sturk-Maquelin et al, 2003). Since TF mRNA has not been demonstrated in megakaryocytes, platelet-derived and microparticles-derived TF is likely to originate from other cell lines, incorporated in platelets by transcelular exchange (Scholz et al, 2002). Tissue factor production in microparticles has also been associated with inflammatory conditions such as meningococcal disease (Nieuwland et al, 2000), thus demonstrating the continuous interplay between inflammation and coagulation activation.

The evidence for microparticle contribution to coagulation in vivo is circumstantial. There are reports of increase in microparticle numbers in several diseases associated with hypercoagulation such as heparin induced thrombocytopenia and acute coronary syndromes. Moreover, several diseases related with hypercoagulation are associated with production of microparticles exposing TF, such as disseminated intravascular coagulation ((Nieuwland et al, 2000). This demonstrates a probable role of microparticles as contributors of vascular dysfunction in cardiovascular diseases and sepsis.

6. Exosomes are a special type of microparticles

Exosomes are frequently referred as a specialized category of microparticles with specific functions in immune response and protein sorting. They are released mainly from antigen presenting cells, although exosomes have been identified after platelet (Heijnen et al, 1999) and mast cell (Denzer et al, 2000) activation and in body fluids, such as urine (Zhou et al, 2006) or bronchoalveolar lavage (Admyre et al, 2003). Dissimilar to microparticles, exosomes are more homogeneous in size (diameters ranging from 60 to 100 nm) and composition, and are enriched in tetraspaning proteins (Azevedo et al, 2007). They are also derived from endocytic-lisosomal cellular system, whereas microparticles are fragments of plasmatic membrane. Platelet-derived exosomes display PS in a much less extent than microparticles, thus they are poor coagulation activators (Heijnen et al, 1999). However, they exhibit major histocompatibility complex (MHC) class I or II molecules in their surface, which demonstrate their role in antigen presentation (Théry et al, 2002). Common filtration and centrifugation processes used to separate microparticles frequently cannot eliminate these small particles. Thus, some of the biologic effects of microparticles observed in the literature may be due to the presence of exosomes in the preparation. The major differences between microparticles and exosomes regarding origin and composition are described in table 1.

Property	Microparticles	Exosomes
Origin	Plasma Membrane	Endocytic-lisosomal system
Type of Generation	Regulated	Constitutive
Mechanism of Release	Shedding from plasma membrane	Exocytosis of MVB
Intracellular Storage	No	Yes
Protein Composition	Annexin 2, caspases	CD9, CD63, cytokines, Integrins
Lipid Composition	Cholesterol	Cheramides, cholesterol

Table 1. Main differences between microparticles and exosomes

The role of exosomes in sepsis remains deeply unexplored. One previous study from our laboratory identified in septic patients' plasma exosomes derived predominantly from platelets. These vesicles have been associated with vascular dysfunction of sepsis, due to their effects in inducing apoptosis of endothelial cells and vascular smooth muscle cells in culture, in a mechanism mediated by oxidative stress (Janiszewski et al, 2004; Gambim et al, 2007). They display components of NADPH oxidase in their membrane and are capable of production of reactive oxygen species *per se* (Janiszewski et al, 2004; Gambim et al, 2007). In addition, these vesicles may induce contractile dysfunction in isolated hearts as well as in isolated papillary muscle preparations. This dysfunction is enhanced by previous treatment of the animals with LPS and the mechanism associated is probably NO-mediated (Azevedo et al, 2007). Thus, in a condition associated with severe vascular dysfunction such as sepsis, exosomes may play a role in regulating cardiovascular function.

7. Conclusions

In this review we have assessed the current knowledge on microparticles formation, composition and function, as well as their role in sepsis. Accumulating data suggest that these microvesicles play a role in inflammation, thrombosis and vascular dysfunction, three pathways clearly involved in the pathogenesis of sepsis. Additional studies that clarify the composition of these vesicles as well as the underlying mechanisms involved in their effects will probably help in the development of additional interventional strategies for prevention and treatment of sepsis.

8. References

Abid-Hussein, M.N.; Meesters, E.W.; Osmanovic, N.; Romijn, F.P.; Nieuwland, R.; Sturk, A. (2003). Antigenic characterization of endothelial cell-derived microparticles and their detection ex vivo. *Journal of Thrombosis and Haemosthasis.* Vol. 1, No. 11, (November), pp. 2434–2443

Admyre, C.; Grunewald, J.; Thyberg, J.; Gripenbäck, S.; Tornling, G.; Eklund, A.; Scheynius, A.; Gabrielsson, S. (2003). Exosomes with major histocompatibility complex class II and co-stimulatory molecules are present in human BAL fluid. *European Respiratory Journal.* Vol. 22, No. 4, (April), pp. 578-583

Azevedo, L.C.; Pedro, M.A.; Laurindo, F.R. (2007). Circulating microparticles as therapeutic targets in cardiovascular diseases. *Recent Patents Cardiovascular Drug Discovery* Vol.2, No.1, (January), pp. 41-51

Azevedo, L.C.; Janiszewski, M.; Pontieri, V.; Pedro, M. de A.; Bassi, E.; Tucci, P.J.; Laurindo, F.R. (2007). Platelet-derived exosomes from septic shock patients induce myocardial dysfunction. *Critical Care,* Vol. 11, No. 6, pp. R120

Barry, O.P.; Pratico, D.; Savani, R.C.; Fitzgerald, G.A. (1998). Modulation of monocyte-endothelial cell interactions by platelet microparticles. *Journal of Clinical Investigation.* Vol. 102, No. 1, (july), pp. 136-144

Boulanger, C.M.; Amabile, N.; Tedgui, A. (2006). Circulating microparticles - A potential prognostic marker for atherosclerotic vascular disease. *Hypertension.* Vol. 48, No. 2 (august), PP. 180-186

Brodsky, S.V.; Malinowski, K.; Golightly, M.; Jesty, J.; Goligorsky, M.S. (2002). Plasminogen activator inhibitor-1 promotes formation of endothelial microparticles with procoagulant potential. *Circulation.* Vol. 106, No. 18, (October), pp. 2372-2378

Brodsky, S.V.; Zhang, F.; Nasjletti, A.; Goligorsky, M.S. (2004). Endothelium derived microparticles impair endothelial function in vitro. *American Journal of Physiology Heart and Circulatory Physiology.* Vol. 286, No. 5, (May), pp. H1910-1915

Denzer, K.; Kleijmeer, M.J.; Heijnen, H.F.; Stoorvogel, W.; Geuze, H.J. (2000). Exosome: from internal vesicle of the multivesicular body to intercellular signaling device. *Journal of Cell Science.* Vol. 113, No. 19, (October), pp. 3365-3374

Forlow, S.B.; McEver, R.P.; Nollert, M.U. (2000) Leukocyte–leukocyte interactions mediated by platelet microparticles under flow. *Blood.* Vol. 95, No. 4, (February), pp. 1317–1323

Fujimi, S.; Ogura, H.; Tanaka, H.; Koh, T.; Hosotsubo, H.; Nakamori, Y.; Kuwagata, Y.; Shimazu, T.; Sugimoto, H. (2003). Increased production of leukocyte microparticles with enhanced expression of adhesion molecules from activated polymorphonuclear leukocytes in severely injured patients. *Journal of Trauma.* Vol. 54, No. 1, (January), pp. 114-119

Gambim, M.H.; do Carmo, A. de O.; Marti, L.; Veríssimo-Filho, S.; Lopes, L.R.; Janiszewski, M. (2007). Platelet-derived exosomes induce endothelial cell apoptosis through peroxynitrite generation: experimental evidence for a novel mechanism of septic vascular dysfunction. *Critical Care.* Vol. 11, No. 6, pp. R107

Heijnen, H.F.; Schiel, A.E.; Fijnheer, R.; Geuze, H.J.; Sixma, J.J. (1999). Activated platelets release two types of membrane vesicles: microvesicles by surface shedding and exosomes derived from exocytosis of multivesicular bodies and alpha-granules. *Blood.* 1999; Vol. 94, No. 11, (December), pp. 3791-3799

Huber, J.; Vales, A.; Mitulovic, G.; Blumer, M.; Schmid, R.; Witztum, J.L.; Binder, B.R.; Leitinger, N. (2002). Oxidized membrane vesicles and blebs from apoptotic cells contain biologically active oxidized phospholipids that induce monocyte-endothelial interactions. *Arteriosclerosis Thrombosis and Vascular Biology* . Vol. 22, No. 1, (January), pp. 101-107

Hughes, M.; Hayward, C.P.M.; Warkentin, T.E.; Horsewood, P.; Chorneyko, K.A.; Kelton, J.G. (2000). Morphological analysis of microparticle generation in heparin-induced thrombocytopenia. *Blood,* Vol. 96, No. 1, (July), pp. :188-194

Hunter, M.P.; Ismail, N.; Zhang, X.; Aguda, B.D.; Lee, E.J.; Yu, L.; Xiao, T.; Schafer, J.; Lee, M.L.; Schmittgen, T.D.; Nana-Sinkam, S.P.; Jarjoura, D.; Marsh, C.B. (2008). Detection of microRNA expression in human peripheral blood microvesicles. *PLoS One.* Vol. 3, No. 11, pp. e3694

Janiszewski, M.; Do Carmo, A.O.; Pedro, M.A.; Silva, E.; Knobel, E.; Laurindo, F.R. (2004) Platelet-derived exosomes of septic individuals possess proapoptotic NAD(P)H oxidase activity: A novel vascular redox pathway. *Critical Care Medicine* . Vol.32, No. 3, (march), pp. 818-825

Martin, S.; Tesse, A.; Hugel, B.; Martínez, M.C.; Morel, O.; Freyssinet, J.M.; Andriantsitohaina, R (2004). Shed membrane particles from T lymphocytes impair endothelial function and regulate endothelial protein expression. *Circulation.* Vol. 109, No. 13, (April), pp. 1653–1659

Mastronardi M.L.; Mostefai, H.A.; Meziani, F.; Martínez, M.C. ; Asfar, P.; Andriantsitohaina, R. (2011). Circulating microparticles from septic shock patients exert differential tissue expression of enzymes related to inflammation and oxidative stress. *Critical Care Medicine.* Vol. 39, No. 7, (july), pp. 1739-1748.

Mesri, M.; Altieri, D.C. (1999). Leukocyte microparticles stimulate endothelial cell cytokine release and tissue factor induction in a JNK1 signaling pathway. *Journal of Biological Chemistry.* Vol. 274, No. 33, (august), pp. 23111-23118

Meziani, F.; Xavier Delabranche, X. ; Asfar, P. ; Toti, F. (2010). Bench-to-bedside review: Circulating microparticles - a new player in sepsis? *Critical Care.* Vol. 14, No. 5, pp. 236

Muller, I.; Klocke, A.; Alex, M.; Kotzsch, M.; Luther, T.; Morgenstern, E.; Zieseniss, S.; Zahler, S.; Preissner, K.; Engelmann B. (2003). Intravascular tissue factor initiates coagulation via circulating microparticles and platelets. *FASEB Journal.* Vol. 17, No. 3, (March), pp. 476-478

Nieuwland, R.; Berckmans, R.J.; McGregor, S.; Böing, A.N.; Romijn, F.P.; Westendorp, R.G.; Hack, C.E.; Sturk A. (2000) Cellular origin and procoagulant properties of microparticles in meningococcal sepsis. *Blood.*Vol. 95, No. 3, (February), pp. 930-935

Nomura, S.; Shouzu, A.; Omoto, S.; Nishikawa, M.; Iwasaka, T.; Fukuhara, S. (2004). Activated platelet and oxidized LDL induce endothelial membrane vesiculation: clinical significance of endothelial cell-derived microparticles in patients with type 2 diabetes. *Clinical Applications in Thrombosis and Hemosthasis* . Vol.10, No. 3, (july), pp. 205-215.

Scholz, T.; Temmler, U.; Krause, S.; Heptinstall, S.; Losche, W. (2002). Transfer of tissue factor from platelets to monocytes: role of platelet-derived microvesicles and CD62P. *Thrombosis and Haemosthasis.* Vol. 88, No. 6, (December), pp. 1033-1038

Soriano, A.O. ; Jy, W. ; Chirinos, J.A.; Valdivia, M. A.; Velasquez, H.S.; Jimenez, J.J.; Horstman, L.L. ; BS; Kett, D.H.; Schein, R. M.; Ahn, Y. S. (2005). Levels of endothelial and platelet microparticles and their interactions with leukocytes negatively correlate with organ dysfunction and predict mortality in severe sepsis. *Critical Care Medicine.* Vol. 33, No. 11, (November), pp. 2540-2546.

Sturk-Maquelin, K.N.; Nieuwland, R.; Romijn, F.P.; Eijsman, L.; Hack, C.E.; Sturk, A. (2003) Pro- and non-coagulant forms of non-cell-bound tissue factor in vivo. *Journal of Thrombosis and Haemosthasis* Vol. 1, No. 9, (September), pp. 1920-1926

Tesse, A.; Carmen Martinez, M.; Hugel, B.; Chalupsky, K.; Muller, C.D.; Meziani, F.; Mitolo-Chieppa, D.; Freyssinet, J.M.; Andriantsitohaina, R. (2005) Upregulation of proinflammatory proteins through NF-kappaB pathway by shed membrane microparticles results in vascular hyporeactivity *Arteriosclerosis Thrombosis and Vascular Biology.* Vol. 25, No. 12, (December), pp. 2522-2527

Thery, C.; Zitvogel, L.; Amigorena, S. (2002) Exosomes: composition, biogenesis and function. *Nature Reviews Immunology* Vol. 2,. No. 8, (August), pp. 569-579

Tushuizen, M.E.; Diamant, M.; Sturk, A.; Nieuwland, R. (2011). Cell-derived microparticles in the pathogenesis of cardiovascular disease: friend or foe? *Arteriosclerosis Thrombosis and Vascular Biology.* Vol. 31, No. 1, (January), pp.4-9

Valadi, H.; Ekström, K.; Bossios, A.; Sjöstrand, M.; Lee, J.J.; Lötvall, J.O. (2007). Exosome-mediated transfer of mRNAs and microRNAs is a novel mechanism of genetic exchange between cells. *Nature Cell Biology.* Vol. 9, No. 6, (June), pp.654-659

Watanabe, J.; Marathe, G.K.; Neilsen, P.O.; Weyrich, A.S.; Harrison, K.A.; Murphy, R.C.; Wolf, P. (1967). The nature and significance of platelet products in human plasma. *British Journal of Haematology* . Vol. 13, No. 3, (may), pp. 269-288

Weerheim, A.M.; Kolb, A.M.; Sturk, A.; Nieuwland, R. (2002) Phospholipid composition of cell-derived microparticles determined by one-dimensional high-performance thin-layer chromatography. *Anal Biochemistry.*Vol. 302, No. 2, (march), pp. 191-198

Zhou, H.; Yuen, P.S.; Pisitkun, T.; Gonzales, P.A.; Yasuda, H.; Dear, J.W.; Gross, P.; Knepper, M.A.; Star, R.A. (2006). Collection, storage, preservation, and normalization of human urinary exosomes for biomarker discovery. *Kidney International.* Vol. 69, No. 8, (April), pp. 1471-1476

Zimmerman, G.A.; McIntyre, T.M.(2003). Endotoxins stimulate neutrophil adhesion followed by synthesis and release of platelet-activating factor in microparticles. *Journal of Biological Chemistry. Vol.* 278, No. 35, (august), pp:33161-33168.

Zwaal, R.F.; Schroit, A.J. (1997). Pathophysiologic implications of membrane phospholipids asymmetry. *Blood* 1997; Vol. 89, No. 4, (February), pp. 1121-1132

8

Cellular Mechanisms of MOF During Severe Sepsis and Septic Shock

Barbara Assenzio and Erica L. Martin-Conte
University of Turin
Italy

1. Introduction

Severe sepsis and septic shock continue to plague intensive care units, leading to significant morbidity and mortality (Vincent et al., 2007). During the pathogenesis of sepsis, patients often develop multiple organ failure (MOF), which is believed to be the main cause of death (Vincent et al., 2007), indicating that either treatment or prevention of MOF could have profound therapeutic implications. However, despite extensive research in this field, the mechanisms and cellular pathophysiology involved in the transition of sepsis to MOF remain unclear, likely due to their immense complexity and cross-talk between signalling pathways.

This chapter aims to highlight the current knowledge regarding the pathophysiology of sepsis-induced organ dysfunction and failure, specifically outlining the current state of knowledge regarding septic-induced dysfunction of the lung, liver, kidney, cardiovascular system and brain For each of these organ systems, we will identify the major cell types prone to damage and briefly describe the key molecular pathways thought to contribute to this phenomenon, thereby ascertaining possible novel therapeutic targets.

2. LPS-TLR4 signalling pathway

Septic shock is initiated by a complex set of pathophysiological responses to the invasion of foreign microbial pathogens in the body. The most common organisms isolated during septic shock are gram-negative bacteria, which contain large quantities of lipopolysaccharide (LPS) in their cellular membranes (Legrand et al., 2010). LPS and its interaction with the Toll-like receptor 4 (TLR-4), is believed to be the major trigger of the septic signalling cascade (Salomao et al., 2008). To briefly describe this important cellular interaction; LPS, in association with LPS-binding protein and the receptor CD14, forms a complex with TLR-4 (Salomao et al., 2008). This complex then recruits the Toll-IL-1 resistance (TIR)-domain-containing adaptor molecules to the cytosolic surface of TLR-4. The four known adaptor proteins include 1) myeloid differentiation factor 88 (MyD88), 2) MyD88 adaptor-like protein, 3) TIR-domain-containing adaptor molecule 1 (TRIF) and 4) TRIF-related adaptor molecule. Depending on which of these adaptor molecules are involved, LPS-TLR4 signalling can be categorized as either early MyD88-dependent responses or delayed MyD88-independent responses. Of these, the more commonly characterized MyD88-dependent pathway initiates the phosphorylation of various signalling kinases, induces the nuclear translocation of the transcription factor NF-κB and ultimately the up-regulation of inflammatory cytokines and mediators (Salomao et al., 2008; Baumgarten et al., 2006). In general, these cytokines (including tumor necrosis factor (TNF), interlukin-1 (IL-1), IL-6, IL-8) and inflammatory mediators (coagulation factors, complement, nitric oxide, ROS) can induce cellular dysfunction and apoptosis resulting in tissue injury and organ failure (Baumgarten et al., 2006; Rittirsch et al., 2008; Cunningham et al., 2004). Other micro-organisms, such as gram-positive bacteria, viruses and fungi, can also induce a strong inflammatory reaction; however, this is often induced through modified signalling mechanisms, such as the TLR-2 pathway (Salomao et al., 2008; Legrand et al., 2010).

This chapter will attempt to review the mechanisms and pathophysiology involved in the cellular injury and tissue dysfunction of the main organ systems affected during severe sepsis and septic shock. Moreover, this manuscript will highlight target molecules that are unique or of particular importance to the development of organ injury, to outline current evidence regarding the development and application of novel therapeutic targets in the clinical treatment of septic shock.

3. Lung

3.1 Pathophysiology

The lung is often the first organ to undergo dysfunction during sepsis, due to its early involvement in the inflammatory process, leading to the culmination of acute lung injury (ALI) or acute respiratory distress syndrome (ARDS) (Bellingan, 2002). The development of ARDS significantly worsens patient outcome, with associated mortality rate rising to between 30-60% (Ware & Matthay, 2000). This process is believed to be initiated by activation of resident alveolar macrophages, which produce inflammatory mediators causing the activated leukocytes of the circulation to be recruited towards the lung (Abraham & Singer, 2007). This army of phagocytes invades the pulmonary interstitium causing the breakdown of endothelial and epithelial barriers thereby leading to significant tissue edema (Bhatia & Moochhala, 2004). This plague of leukocytes both responds and contributes to inflammation by producing various cytokines, reactive oxygen species (ROS), protein kinases, and transcription factors which perpetuate the influx of more leukocytes, causes direct injury to lung tissue and provokes cellular apoptosis (Bhatia & Moochhala, 2004; Abraham & Singer, 2007; Marshall, 2001). The consequence of these cellular alterations is the formation of hyaline membranes, fibrin deposition, surfactant alterations and impaired gas exchange, leading to the therapeutic requirement of mechanical ventilation support (Abraham & Singer, 2007). As if this damage was not enough, mechanical ventilation itself, while being a necessary life-saving intervention, can act as a "secondary hit", causing additional injury known as ventilator-induced lung injury (VILI), which occurs due to excessive stretch of pulmonary alveoli (Vlahakis & Hubmayr, 2005).

3.2 Major cell types involved

The major cell types involved include alveolar macrophages that initiate the pulmonary inflammatory response, leukocytes, including neutrophils and monocytes that are recruited to the lung, pulmonary endothelial and epithelial cells (both type I and type II) that regulate the barriers of the lung, and fibroblasts that are involved in injury-repair processes.

3.3 Key molecular pathways and possible therapeutic targets

3.3.1 TLR-4 and inflammation

As described above, TLR-4 signalling plays role in the septic response of most organs, but has been intensely studied in the specific context of ALI and ARDS (Bhatia & Moochhala, 2004). TLR-4 signalling is known to activate either directly or indirectly through MyD88 the nuclear translocation of NFκB, which in turn stimulates the production of a vast array of inflammatory proteases and cytokines (Salomao et al., 2008). The central role of TLR in the septic response is further supported by genetic studies that demonstrate that polymorphic variations in TLR-4 can predispose patients to gram-negative bacteremia and septic shock (Agnese et al., 2002; Lorenz et al., 2002). The importance of downstream NFκB signalling has also been emphasized by the clinical observation that in neutrophils from patients with septic-induced ARDS the amount of NFκB activity is associated with fewer ventilator-free days (Yang et al., 2003) and decreased survival (Bohrer et al., 1997). Of the cytokines stimulated by TLR-4, TNFα and IL-1β are believed to be the major mediators of septic shock (Bhatia & Moochhala, 2004). Both of these mediators are release in the very early stages of the inflammatory response, appearing within 30-90 minutes, and in turn activate a second level of the inflammatory cascade including other cytokines, lipid mediators and reactive oxygen species (Bhatia & Moochhala, 2004). The specific role TNFα is highlighted by several studies which report that the ratio of TNFα to its receptor TNFR is significantly correlated with increased organ dysfunction and patient mortality (Pellegrini et al., 1996), and genetic polymorphisms in TNF both increase the amount of circulating TNF and worsen patient outcome (Stuber et al., 1996). Furthermore, there is currently a prospective, randomized, double-blind, multi-center, phase II clinical trial underway testing the efficacy of an anti-TNF antibody (ALT-836) versus placebo in the prevention of septic-induced ALI/ARDS, with the primary outcomes being patient safety and ventilator-free days (clinicaltrials.gov NCT00879606). In addition to TNFα and IL-1β, other cytokines and inflammatory mediators thought to play an important role in the pathogenesis of ARDS during septic shock include, but is not limited to, IL-6, IL-8, IL-10, IL-4, granulocyte colony-stimulating factor (G-CSF), inter-cellular adhesion molecule-1 (ICAM-1), complement component 5a (C5a) and various pro-coagulation molecules (Bhatia & Moochhala, 2004; Bozza et al., 2007).

3.3.2 The RAGE axis

The receptor for advanced glycation end-products, or RAGE, is an inflammation perpetuating receptor with a diverse range of ligands, for which there is compelling evidence for its role in the development of systemic inflammation and ALI (Creagh-Brown et al., 2010). While RAGE is expressed at low levels in all cells, it has a uniquely high constitutive expression in the lung (Buckley & Ehrhardt, 2010), which is further up-regulated upon activation by its various ligands (Schmidt et al., 2000), including S100 proteins, high mobility group proteins and advanced glycation end-products. RAGE signalling has been described to involve NFκB, mitogen-activated protein kinases (MAPK), and phosphoinositide 3-kinases (PI3K) which in turn lead to increased production of inflammatory cytokines, proteases and oxidative stress (Creagh-Brown et al., 2010). Interestingly, genetic ablation or inhibition of RAGE has consistently shown to increase survival in several different animal models of severe sepsis and septic shock (Creagh-Brown et al., 2010), and has additionally been reported to decrease septic-induced lung injury even when blocked therapeutically up to 24hrs following the initiation of sepsis (Lutterloh et al.,

2007). In accordance, similar results are found regarding the RAGE ligand HMGB1, which is known to be a late mediator of sepsis released from injured and stressed cells (Creagh-Brown et al., 2010). Similar to RAGE, inhibition of HMGB1 during sepsis has also been shown to decrease lung injury and improve survival (Sawa et al., 2006; Yang et al., 2008). In clinical studies, patients with ALI have been observed to have increased soluble RAGE (sRAGE) in bronchioalveolar lavage fluid (BAL), and sRAGE levels correlated in severity of illness, ALI and mortality (Calfee et al., 2008; Uchida et al., 2006). Furthermore, ALI patients also display increased levels of various RAGE ligands (Creagh-Brown et al., 2010). While the benefits of RAGE inhibition have not been tested in the context of septic shock or ARDS, it is currently being assessed in the treatment of Alzheimer's dementia (clinicaltrials.gov NCT00566397), which will provide valuable information regarding patient safety, which could assist in establishing future trails in the treatment of septic shock.

3.3.3 Phosphoinositide 3-kinase gamma (PI3Kγ)

Various phosphorylation molecules have been shown to significantly contribute to lung injury during the pathogenesis of severe sepsis and septic shock. In 2001, Yum et al. first showed that specific loss of PI3Kγ induced protection against acute lung injury in an experimental model of LPS-induced sepsis (Yum et al., 2001). While this paper was later challenged by a contradictory study using a model of *E.coli* (Ong et al., 2005), these original findings have since been confirmed in an extensive study by Martin et al. (Martin et al., 2010). In this most recent study, both the genetic and pharmacological blockade of the kinase activity of PI3Kγ activity was shown to decrease lung inflammation, edema, and neutrophil invasion, and improve survival, even when pharmacological inhibition occurred up to 9 hours following the initiation of sepsis (Martin et al., 2010). Furthermore, this study demonstrated that these effects are likely due to decreased GRK2 phosphorylation and consequent maintenance of the receptor CXCR2 expression on neutrophils (Martin et al., 2010). This, in turn, improves neutrophil recruitment to the origin of infection during severe sepsis, allowing for improved bacterial control and decreased decompartmentalization of the infection into the systemic circulation (Martin et al., 2010). Moreover, PI3Kγ is known to lie upstream to other phosphorylation molecules including Akt (or PKB), MAP kinases and NFκB, which have each been identified as contributors to lung injury during severe sepsis and septic shock (Martin & Ranieri, 2011).

3.3.4 Fas

Apoptosis, or programmed-cell death, occurs frequently in tissues under stress or injury as an attempt to limit necrosis; however in several disease pathologies including severe sepsis and septic shock, high levels of apoptosis can in itself be destructive (Wheeler, 2009). Apoptosis occurs through two distinct pathways; the intrinsic pathway involving mitochondrial signalling and the extrinsic pathway involving activation of cell surface death receptors (Wheeler, 2009). Fas is a type of death receptor for which there is compelling evidence for its fundamental role in pulmonary epithelial cells in the pathogenesis of septic-induced ALI and ARDS (Chopra et al., 2009). In patients with ALI or ARDS, high levels of soluble Fas and its ligand (FasL) in BAL fluid correlate with increased mortality (Albertine et al., 2002; Matute-Bello et al., 1999). This role is supported by the fact that mice deficient in either Fas or FasL are protected from lung injury (Neff et al., 2005). More recent studies have shown that silencing the expression of Fas or the related Fas-associated death domain

(FADD) decreases lung apoptosis, injury and inflammation during sepsis (Perl et al., 2007; Matsuda et al., 2009). In addition this apoptotic pathway appears to be particularly dominant in this context, since silencing Fas, but not caspase-8 of the intrinsic pathway, in lung epithelial cells ameliorated pulmonary apoptosis, inflammation and neutrophil influx in a model of hemorrhage shock and sepsis (Perl et al., 2005). Moreover, in pulmonary epithelium, Fas can directly induce the production and release of inflammatory mediators, which further perpetuates the cycle of destruction (Perl et al., 2007). Together these data make Fas a potential therapeutic target that should be further explored in future studies.

3.3.5 Activated protein C (APC)

Activated protein C (APC) is a plasma serum protease that plays a central role in endogenous anti-coagulation. The PROWESS study, published in 2001, demonstrated the clinical significance of this molecule in the pathogenesis of sepsis, since administration of human recombinant APC (rhAPC) was found to significantly reduce mortality in patients with severe sepsis (Bernard et al., 2001). The specific role of APC in septic-induced ALI or ARDS has also been explored since protein C levels are documented to be decreased in ALI patients of both septic or non-septic origin, and that these reduced levels correlated with poor clinical outcome (Shorr et al., 2006; Matthay & Ware, 2004). These clinical finding are supported by studies in sheep, demonstrating that treatment with rhAPC in endotoxin or peritoneal-induced sepsis can reduce lung edema and injury (Waerhaug et al., 2008; Wang et al., 2007). Although APC is known for its anti-coagulative effects, these alone can not account for the improved clinical outcome in septic patients, since targeting of either activated factor X, anti-thrombin or tissue factor inhibitors has failed to produce a comparative protection (Sarangi et al., 2010). As such, APC has also been described to induce several cytoprotective effects which likely contribute to its success in the treatment of sepsis. These mechanisms include: 1) decreasing apoptosis (Mosnier et al., 2007), 2) the ability to bind to nuclear ribonucleoproteins, thereby facilitating the clearance of nuclear material from injured and necrotic tissue (Jean-Baptiste, 2007), 3) mediating the protection of the endothelial barrier, which prevents the destructive massive infiltration of neutrophils (Rittirsch et al., 2008), 4) a number anti-inflammatory effects including the decrease of tissue factor and thrombin, which in turn can induce inflammation, and the blockade of NFκB, which subsequently decreases the direct up-regulation of cytokines (Sarangi et al., 2010). Future studies, including the current multi-centered, phase III clinical trial PROWESS SHOCK (clinicaltrials.gov NCT00604214), are likely to further investigate and clarify the various mechanisms involved in APC-induced ALI protection during sepsis.

4. Liver

4.1 Pathophysiology

The liver is the largest solid organ in the body, comprising 2-5% of the body weight of a normal adult. Its function is believed to play a major role in the development of multiple organ dysfunction syndrome due to its central control of metabolism and host defence mechanisms (Van Amersfoort et al., 2003); however it remains one of the most poorly characterized and understood organs involved in MOF. During septic shock the evolution of liver dysfunction can be divided in two phases. The early phase involves hepatocyte dysfunction induced by gut-derived norepinephrine, which activates α_2-adrenoceptors, which stimulate Kupffer cells to enhance TNF-α release and depresses hepatocellular function in the absence of hepatic blood flow alterations (Yang et al., 2001). In contrast, the late phase results mainly from a decreased hepatic perfusion, which mechanistically has been linked with increased coagulation, inflammation and derangement of endothelial nitric oxide synthase (eNOS) signalling (Dhainaut et al., 2001; Mookerjee, 2011). In addition, Kupffer cells can play either a protective or destructive role in the septic response of the liver, in that they are important in the removal and detoxification of LPS, while they can also initiate an exaggerated inflammatory response which can cause further liver damage (Van Amersfoort et al., 2003). Specifically, excessive inflammatory mediators can induce endothelial damage causing barrier breakdown and permeability, and are thought to be the driving force behind increased intra-hepatic resistance (Dhainaut et al., 2001; Mookerjee, 2011). Furthermore, the development of hyperlipidemia in response to sepsis is believed to result from pathomorphological changes in sinusoidal endothelial cells (Cheluvappa et al., 2010). Moreover, recent animal studies have shown that liver injury and dysfunction during sepsis is associated with G1 cell cycle arrest of hepatocytes and that hepatic function recovery was furthermore accompanied by cell cycle progression (Yang et al., 2011). Overall, these cellular defects result in loss of metabolic function, hypoglycaemia, lactic acidosis and coagulopathy.

4.2 Major cell types involved

In the pathogenesis of septic-induced liver dysfunction several hepatic cell types have been shown to be involved. This includes the parenchymal cells or hepatocytes, which are the main structural cell type of the liver comprising about 60% of the liver. These cells are highly metabolically active regulating lipids, bile and glucose. In addition, endothelial cells, which line the many sinusoids, and Kupffer cells, which are the resident macrophages of the liver, are also known to be significantly involved in the progression of sepsis to MOF. Moreover, circulating neutrophils which are recruited to the liver due to the high production of inflammatory cytokines have also been shown to contribute to this pathology.

4.3 Key molecular pathways and possible therapeutic targets

4.3.1 Tumor necrosis factor

While several inflammatory cytokines including IL-6 and IL-1β have been implicated in the pathogenesis of liver dysfunction during sepsis, there is overwhelming evidence for a predominant role of TNF-α in this process. TNF-α is produced in large quantities primarily by Kupffer cells during the very early phase of hepatocyte dysfunction, following α_2-adrenergic stimulation (Yang et al., 2001; Fong et al., 1990). These high levels of TNF-α are shown to induce a variety of effects including the production of acute phase proteins (APPs), which serve several physiological function of the immune response (Dhainaut et al., 2001). However, the high up-regulation of APPs has also been associated with the development of liver failure (Ananian et al., 2005). Both TNF-α and their induced APPs also enhance pro-coagulant activity of vascular endothelial cells (Bevilacqua et al., 1986), which in turn can decrease hepatic perfusion, leading to further injury, as well as further ignite the inflammatory cascade (Dhainaut et al., 2001). TNF-α also up-regulates the expression adhesion molecules facilitating an excessive recruitment of activated neutrophils, which through the production of destructive proteases and reactive oxygen species, amplifies the damage to hepatocytes and endothelial cells (Zhang et al., 1994; Malmros et al., 1994; Holman, Jr. & Saba, 1988).

4.3.2 Thrombin/ anti-thrombin

Coagulation, resulting from an imbalance between pro- and anti-thrombin in the liver, occurs within the early phases of sepsis and significantly contributes to patient mortality (Stearns-Kurosawa et al., 2011). *In vivo* animal studies have described that microthrombi develop in the hepatic microcirculation with five minutes of an endotoxin challenge (Asaka et al., 1996). Furthermore, if the endotoxin dose is sublethal, clot lysis occurs with a few hours and hepatic architecture is conserved, while if endotoxin exposure continues, there develops clot accumulation, hypoperfusion, coagulation necrosis and irreversible tissue injury (Asaka et al., 1996). In addition, many studies have demonstrated that coagulation can further activate the inflammatory cascade, and visa versa, leading to a positive-feedback interaction (Stearns-Kurosawa et al., 2011; Jagneaux et al., 2004; Dhainaut et al., 2001). Novel treatments targeting thrombin activity during sepsis has been shown to decrease serum bilirubin concentrations and prevent liver dysfunction (Nitescu et al., 2007; Inthorn et al., 1997); however its overall role in reducing septic mortality is still unclear (Wiedermann et al., 2006).

4.3.3 Activated protein C (APC)

Protein C is a zymogenic protein that is produced by the liver and later converted to the active serine proteinase, which degrades Factors Va and VIIIa of the coagulation cascade, thereby preventing excessive thrombin formation (Stearns-Kurosawa et al., 2011). During septic shock the synthesis of protein C is significantly decreased due to hepatocyte dysfunction, which correlates with disease severity and poor patient prognosis (Stearns-Kurosawa et al., 2011). Apart from coagulation, APC has also been described to possess several cytoprotective effects including the ability to degrade damaging histones, anti-inflammatory and anti-apoptotic activities and stabilization of endothelial barriers (Mosnier et al., 2007; Xu et al., 2009), which can each limit hepatic injury. In addition, treatment of septic patients with rhAPC can decrease liver dysfunction (Rinaldi et al., 2008), which in animal experiments has been shown to result from an ability of APC to attenuate leukocyte trafficking into the liver (Huynh et al., 2010).

4.3.4 Complement system

The complement system is a family of proteins produced mainly by the liver that at normal physiological levels assist phagocytic cell to clear invading pathogens (Ward & Gao, 2009). However, during the pathogenesis of sepsis, the liver is stimulated to produce exceedingly high concentrations of complement factors, such as C5a, which in large quantities produce an array of detrimental effects (Ward & Gao, 2009). These include the up-regulation of tissue factor leading to intensified coagulation, the induction of neutrophil paralysis that causes uncontrolled bacterial expansion, as well as increased inflammation and apoptosis, which all contribute to the development of MOF (Ward & Gao, 2009). Furthermore, several organs, including the liver, increase the expression of the C5a receptor during sepsis, which if blocked by an antagonist has been shown to improve organ function and survival in various animal models (Guo & Ward, 2006; Riedemann et al., 2002).

5. Kidney

5.1 Pathophysiology

Acute kidney injury (AKI), a complex disorder with clinical manifestations ranging from a minimal elevation in serum creatinine to anuric renal failure, and is a frequent and serious complication of sepsis in intensive care unit (ICU) patients (Lafrance & Miller, 2010). Moreover, there is strong evidence that septic AKI, accounting for 50% or more of cases of AKI in ICUs, is associated with a very high mortality (Uchino et al., 2005). Despite extensive research and progress in several other fields, the incidence, as well as mortality of septic AKI, remains at unacceptable levels (Silvester et al., 2001). A possible explanation of failure in the treatment of septic AKI is the relative lack of histopathologic information and reliance on creatinine measurements for assessment of kidney function, both leading to an incomplete understanding of the pathogenesis of this condition (Wan et al., 2008). AKI has been traditionally thought to be induced by ischemia secondary to decreased cardiac output and hypotension, which in turn leads to renal vasoconstriction and exacerbate the ischemia. Most of our understanding regarding renal blood flow (RBF) during sepsis relies on animal models. Across these studies, the heterogeneous nature of animals used, methods of inducing sepsis, and observed changes in RBF that vary from unchanged, decreased, and markedly increased all translate to uncertainty regarding their applicability to humans (Langenberg et al., 2007; Bagshaw et al., 2007). The characteristic pattern of RBF in human sepsis is for the most part largely unknown because RBF cannot be measured continuously in humans, and even its intermittent measurement requires a high level of invasiveness (Langenberg et al., 2007; Licari et al., 2007). Only a small study with limited patients has measured RBF in patients with sepsis, and reported that RBF was either preserved or increased in these patients (Bradley et al., 1976) However, recent findings suggest that, although hemodynamic factors may play a role in the loss of glomerular filtration, they do not necessary involve renal ischemia. In addition, other mechanisms including immunologic, toxic and inflammatory factors seem to affect the microvasculature and the tubular cell function. Apoptosis induced by LPS or cytokines, for instance, has emerged as a possible cause of loss of function of both endothelial and epithelial tubular cells (Humphrey et al., 1991).

5.2 Major cell types involved

The major cell types involved in the development of septic AKI includes all the cells forming the functional unit of the nephron. Tubular epithelium, podocytes, endothelium, and mesangial cells have been found to be directly affected by exposure to LPS , as well as susceptible to the inflammatory state induced by sustained bacterial infection.

5.3 Key molecular pathways and possible therapeutic targets

5.3.1 Apoptosis pathway

LPS can directly cause apoptosis of tubular cells through the Fas-mediated and caspase-mediated pathways and increased plasma levels of soluble Fas has been described in septic patients (Jo et al., 2002). Additionally, experimental models of sepsis have shown that increased caspase activation is associated with the presence of AKI (Guo et al., 2004). In recent studies it has been demonstrated that plasma of septic patients can induce apoptosis of tubular cells and that the amount of this cell death correlates with the extent of proteinuria, which in turn is related with the severity of the septic process, with the impairment of renal function and with patient outcome (Cantaluppi et al., 2008). The extrinsic pathway is not the sole mechanism responsible for sepsis induced apoptosis in the kidney. As a matter of fact, it has been found that also the intrinsic pathway is activated in endothelial and tubular cells exposed to LPS (Mariano et al., 2008; Cantaluppi et al., 2008). This mechanism involves the oligomerization of the pro-apoptotic members of the Bcl-2 family proteins, such as Bax, which translocates to the mitochondria and forms pores in the outer mitochondrial membrane that allow the release of cytochrome C from the mitochondria. Cytosol cytochrome C binds to the adaptor protein apoptosis protease activating factor (APAF-1) and this complex binds to pro-caspase 9, forming the apoptosome. This in turn results in the auto-activation of caspase-9 (Mariano et al., 2008; Cantaluppi et al., 2008). One of the proposed mechanisms of protection induced by APC treatment in septic patients could also be due to its anti-apoptotic effects. Recent studies demonstrated that recombinant human APC directly modulates patterns of endothelial gene expression clustering into cell survival pathway and modulate several genes, including Bcl-2. Moreover, it normalizes Bax/Bcl-2 ratio and reduces caspase-3 signalling. Also the decrease in sepsis-AKI found in patients treated with the aggressive insulin therapy could be due by his powerful anti-apoptotic effect. Conversely, it has been demonstrated that high glucose concentration induces oxidative-stress-mediated apoptosis in tubular cells (Allen et al., 2003).

5.3.2 Permeability molecules

Proteinuria found in AKI patients is usually in the nephrotic range with a mixed glomerular and tubular pattern (Schiavon et al., 1988), suggesting a simultaneous defect of tubular reabsorption and an increase of glomerular permeability. Megalin is an endocytic receptor that regulates the physiological reabsorption of glomerular-filtered low molecular weight proteins (Christensen & Birn, 2001). It has been shown that plasma derived from septic patients decreases the expression of megalin, suggesting that the impaired expression of this molecule may contribute to proteinuria resulting in a failure of tubular handling of filtered proteins (Mariano et al., 2008; Cantaluppi et al., 2008). Physiological tubular handling of electrolytes is based on the maintenance of cell polarity and on the integrity of tight junction protein expression (Lee et al., 2006). After challenge of tubular cells with septic plasmas, it has been observed a marked decrease of ZO-1 expression with a simultaneous alteration of trans-electrical resistance (TER) (Cantaluppi et al., 2008). These functional changes may alter the ability of tubular cells to maintain compositionally distinct fluid-filled compartments with precise electrolyte concentrations. Moreover, albumin diffusion across podocytes increases in the presence of septic plasma and this phenomenon is associated with decreased expression of nephrin, a slit diaphragm protein known to modulate glomerular permeability (Cantaluppi et al., 2008). Another molecule playing an important role in the correct organization and function of podocytes is nestin, able to stably link the intermediate filaments to other cytoskeleton proteins (Chen et al., 2006). The alterations in nephrin and cytoskeleton distribution may also account for the altered cell polarity and albumin transport across the podocyte monolayer observed after challenge with septic AKI plasma (Mariano et al., 2008; Cantaluppi et al., 2008).

6. Cardiovascular

6.1 Pathophysiology

The worsening of sepsis toward septic shock is characterized by hypotension refractory to fluid resuscitation. An important component of this process is the development of progressive cardiac and hemodynamic dysfunction. Traditionally, these disturbances have been described in a biphasic spectrum: early hyperdynamic shock characterized by increased cardiac output, decreased systemic vascular resistance (SVR) and warm, perfused skin, followed by cold hypodynamic shock, during which SVR increases to compensate for worsened cardiac output, resulting in tissue hypoperfusion, cool skin and eventual organ failure (Hoesel et al., 2007). However, it is now generally accepted that, after adequate volume resuscitation, patients develop a hyperdynamic circulatory state associated with high cardiac output, decreased systemic vascular resistance, and biventricular dilatation (Hunter & Doddi, 2010). Experimental models of sepsis showed clear evidence of myocardial contractile disturbance both *in vivo* and *in vitro*. These disturbances are present even in early hyperdynamic shock, when aggressive volume replacement and adaptive left ventricular dilatation can combine to preserve cardiac output (Grocott-Mason & Shah, 1998). What exactly triggers septic cardiomyopathy is still unknown. Cardiac dysfunction in sepsis is characterized by decreased contractility, impaired ventricular response to fluid therapy, and in some patients ventricular dilatation (Bouhemad et al., 2009). The hemodynamic instability is mainly due to dysfunction of vascular autoregulatory mechanisms in microcirculation and subsequently enhanced perfusion of large arteriovenous shunts (Matsuda & Hattori, 2007).

6.2 Major cell types involved

The pathophysiology of cardiovascular dysfunction during sepsis involves a highly complex, integrated response that includes activation of number of cell types, inflammatory mediators and the hemostatic system. Central to this process is alterations in vascular endothelial, smooth muscle cells and cardiomyocyte function.

6.3 Key molecular pathways and possible therapeutic targets

6.3.1 Nitric oxide (NO)

NO is produced by all types of cardiac and endothelial cells and has a multitude of cardiovascular effects both in healthy and disease states. Effects of NO relevant to sepsis-induced cardiovascular dysfunction include vasodilation, depression of mitochondrial respiration, and further release of pro-inflammatory cytokines (Massion et al., 2003). NO is produced from conversion of L-arginine to L-citrulline by nitric oxide synthase (NOS). In mammals, NOS has three isoforms: neuronal (nNOS/ NOS1), inducible (iNOS/ NOS2) and constitutive (cNOS/ NOS3). Current evidence suggests that early myocardial dysfunction in sepsis may occur through the over-production of NO and resultant cyclic guanosine monophosphate (cGMP) through cNOS activation in cardiac cells. Activation of iNOS and resultant nitric oxide may be more important in late sepsis-induced cardiovascular dysfunction. Peroxynitrite, a by-product of nitric oxide, has also been proposed as an important modulator of prolonged myocardial depression (Pacher et al., 2007). As a reflection of the complexity of the role of NO is in sepsis-induced myocardial depression, myocardial over-expression of cNOS has been shown to attenuate myocardial depression in sepsis models utilizing genetically modified mice (Fraccarollo et al., 2008). Unfortunately, initial attempts to block nitric oxide production as a therapeutic target have failed, likely due to vascular and other actions of NO in sepsis.

6.3.2 Contractility pathway

The concept of circulating myocardial depressant factors was first proposed by Parrillo et al. In this study the authors found myocardial depression in isolated myocytes exposed to serum obtained from septic patients with clinical manifestations of sepsis-induced myocardial dysfunction. Septic shock patients during the acute phase showed a significant lower extent of shortening compared with other patient groups including septic shock patients in the recovery phase (Parrillo et al., 1985). There was also a correlation between *in vitro* depression of contractility and *in vivo* myocardial depression measured by left ventricular ejection fraction. Further studies have identified cytokines such as TNF-α, IL-1-β, and IL-6 as circulating causative factors of myocardial depression in sepsis. Lysozyme c has been shown to have cardiac depressant actions in animal models of sepsis (Mink et al., 2008). Furthermore, competitive inhibition of lysozyme c in these animal models was observed to be protective and prevented sepsis-induced myocardial dysfunction. Early studies suggest a potential role for endothelin-1 (ET-1) in the development of sepsis-induced myocardial depression (Konrad et al., 2004; Schuetz et al., 2007). Moreover calcium is thought to play an important role in the myocardial depression. Current evidence suggests that reductions in cytosolic calcium levels during sepsis lead to reduced contractility (Rudiger & Singer, 2007). Calcium signalling and metabolism are linked to mitochondrial function, which is also altered in sepsis.

7. Brain

7.1 Pathophysiology

Several studies have demonstrated that sepsis survivors present long-term cognitive impairment, including alteration in memory, attention, concentration and/or global loss of cognitive function (Heyland et al., 2000; Hopkins et al., 1999; Hough & Curtis, 2005). Most investigations have tried to understand the pathogenetic mechanisms of sepsis encephalopathy (SE) using animals or cell cultures (Jacob et al., 2011) due to obvious limitations in humans. Although these studies have expanded the understanding of central nervous system (CNS) cellular response to endotoxin or cytokines, the way in which these mechanisms relate to clinical brain injury remains obscure. It is important to note that the reciprocal interaction between the CNS and the immune response is considered one of the main components of the host response during sepsis. The brain mediates via the autonomic nervous system and neurohormones the growth and proliferation of most if not all tissues involved in immunity, and all immune cells have membrane or cytosolic receptors for a number of neuromediators. The systemic inflammatory response to infection results in brain activation, which subsequently generates an appropriate anti-inflammatory response. However, excess in pro-inflammatory mediators entering the brain can cause cerebral damage. In turn, dysfunction of the autonomic nervous and neuroendocrine systems may alter immunity in a vicious circle resulting in metabolic derangements and organ failure (Streck et al., 2008).

7.2 Major cell types involved

The anatomical substrate of the blood brain barrier (BBB) is the cerebral microvascular endothelium, which together with astrocytes, pericytes, neurons and the extracellular matrix, constitute a "neurovascular unit" that is essential for the health and function of the CNS. All the cell types forming the BBB are immunologically active and can be influenced by systemic inflammatory reactions and responses, such as those resulting from sepsis. Inflammatory mediators released by leukocytes in sepsis have profound effects on endothelial cells and astrocytes; damage to these cells results in impaired neuronal function.

7.3 Key molecular pathways and possible therapeutic targets

7.3.1 Oxidative stress

One important factor that can lead to cognitive impairment due to SE is oxidative stress. Studies on oxidative stress showed cerebral damage caused by active species of oxygen in some regions of the brain after sepsis induced by CLP. It has been demonstrated that, differently from other organs involved in septic response, CNS oxidative stress is restricted to earlier times after sepsis induction (Barichello et al., 2006). It has also been demonstrated an increase in superoxide dismutase activity without a proportional increase in catalase activity with a consequent increase in the relation of superoxide dismutase/catalase. Based on this evidence, the same authors also measured oxidative stress parameters in brains of rats after CLP and treated with antioxidants NAC (N-acetylcysteine) and/or DFX (deferoxamine) in the first hours after surgery. Ten and thirty days after CLP, behavior tests involving step down inhibitory avoidance, continuous multiple-trials step-down inhibitory avoidance and habituation to an open-field were conducted. It has been found that antioxidant treatment could significantly attenuate late cognitive deficits in sepsis survivors from CLP. In addition, the combined use of antioxidants attenuated oxidative damage in the hippocampus in early periods after sepsis induction. These results suggested a role of early CNS oxidative damage in the development of long-term cognitive deficits. In addition the authors demonstrated a new role to antioxidant treatment in an animal model of sepsis (Barichello et al., 2007).

7.3.2 Inflammation

Inflammation is being considered an important biological event that might increase the risk of major depressive episodes much like more traditional psychosocial factors. In this context, it is possible that pro-inflammatory cytokines, which are peripherally produced during the septic response, could contribute to the development of long-term cognitive dysfunction and behavioural symptoms related to sickness behaviour. When the activation of the peripheral immune system continues such as during systemic infections, the immune signalling to the brain may lead to an exacerbation of sickness and the development of symptoms of depression (Dantzer et al., 2008). Many studies suggest that these phenomena account for increased prevalence of clinical depression in critically ill people (Dantzer et al., 2008). Some studies also link pro-inflammatory cytokines and neuronal death. However, the mechanisms underlying pro-inflammatory cytokines and neuronal death are still poorly understood (Glass et al., 2010).

7.3.3 Blood Brain Barrier (BBB)

The BBB is established through specialized tight junctions of the endothelial cells, which are induced and maintained through interactions between astrocytes, pericytes and endothelial cells (Abbott et al., 2006). BBB dysfunction is found in patients and rodent models of sepsis and causes increased infiltration of inflammatory cells and increased exposure of the brain to toxins (Nishioku et al., 2009). The BBB impairment may be caused by disruption of the normal interaction between endothelial cells, astrocytes and pericytes leading to increased pineocytosis and disruption of tight junctions. Additionally, neuroinflammation with LPS exposure may also facilitate active directed transport of cytokines across the BBB (Nishioku et al., 2009). In sepsis, leukocytes are activated, adhere to the blood vessel and move into the tissue, a process mediated by adhesion molecules such as intercellular adhesion molecule (ICAM). The expression of ICAM is increased in septic encephalopathy, whereas platelet endothelial cell adhesion molecule (PECAM) remains unaltered (Hofer et al., 2008). One of the key inflammatory mediators is TNF-α, which is also produced intrinsically in the brain where it regulates aquaporin 4 (AQP4) and alters transport of water into the brain resulting in edema (Alexander et al., 2008).

7.3.4 Complement activation

It has been shown that the complement cascade, especially C5a generated by complement activation, is an integral part of the central hub of the inflammatory response in sepsis (Rittirsch et al., 2008). It also induces apoptosis in the adrenomedullary cells, which are responsible for the bulk of endogenous catecholamines (Flierl et al., 2008). The cross talk between the complement cascade and coagulation, which is generally activated during sepsis, could further amplify complement activation in sepsis (Rittirsch et al., 2008). In addition to complement activation, glial activation induces the expression of Toll-like receptor 2 (TLR-2), IL-1β, IL-6 and indoleamine 2, 3 dioxygenase (IDO) that could be prevented by the microglial inhibitor minocycline, modulating sickness (Henry et al., 2008). Both blocking C5a or its receptor, and inhibiting the alternative complement pathway, attenuates neuronal death in experimental traumatic brain injury (Sewell et al., 2004; Leinhase et al., 2007).

8. Conclusion

In summary, since MOF in the late stages of septic shock is the major contributor to patient death, further understanding of the cellular mechanisms involved in the development and progression of MOF is imperative to identify novel treatment strategies.

9. Acknowledgements

The authors would like to thank their colleagues, E. Tonoli, C. Muraca and F. Civiletti for assistance in researching, modifying and discussing various sections of this chapter, and Prof. V.M. Ranieri for his continued support.

10. References

Vincent JL, Taccone F, Schmit X. Classification, incidence, and outcomes of sepsis and multiple organ failure. Contrib Nephrol 2007;156:64-74.

Legrand M, Klijn E, Payen D, Ince C. The response of the host microcirculation to bacterial sepsis: does the pathogen matter? J Mol Med 2010;88:127-133.

Salomao R, Martins PS, Brunialti MK, Fernandes ML, Martos LS, Mendes ME, Gomes NE, Rigato O. TLR signaling pathway in patients with sepsis. Shock 2008;30 Suppl 1:73-77.

Baumgarten G, Knuefermann P, Wrigge H, Putensen C, Stapel H, Fink K, Meyer R, Hoeft A, Grohe C. Role of Toll-like receptor 4 for the pathogenesis of acute lung injury in Gram-negative sepsis. Eur J Anaesthesiol 2006;23:1041-1048.

Rittirsch D, Flierl MA, Ward PA. Harmful molecular mechanisms in sepsis. Nat Rev Immunol 2008;8:776-787.

Cunningham PN, Wang Y, Guo R, He G, Quigg RJ. Role of Toll-like receptor 4 in endotoxin-induced acute renal failure. J Immunol 2004;172:2629-2635.

Bellingan GJ. The pathogenesis of ALI/ARDS. Thorax 2002;57:540-546.

Ware LB, Matthay MA. The acute respiratory distress syndrome. N Engl J Med 2000;342:1334-1349.

Abraham E, Singer M. Mechanisms of sepsis-induced organ dysfunction. Crit Care Med 2007;35:2408-2416.

Bhatia M, Moochhala S. Role of inflammatory mediators in the pathophysiology of acute respiratory distress syndrome. J Pathol 2004;202:145-156.

Marshall JC. Inflammation, coagulopathy, and the pathogenesis of multiple organ dysfunction syndrome. Crit Care Med 2001;29:S99-106.

Vlahakis NE, Hubmayr RD. Cellular stress failure in ventilator-injured lungs. Am J Respir Crit Care Med 2005;171:1328-1342.

Agnese DM, Calvano JE, Hahm SJ, Coyle SM, Corbett SA, Calvano SE, Lowry SF. Human toll-like receptor 4 mutations but not CD14 polymorphisms are associated with an increased risk of gram-negative infections. J Infect Dis 2002;186:1522-1525.

Lorenz E, Mira JP, Frees KL, Schwartz DA. Relevance of mutations in the TLR4 receptor in patients with gram-negative septic shock. Arch Intern Med 2002;162:1028-1032.

Yang KY, Arcaroli JJ, Abraham E. Early alterations in neutrophil activation are associated with outcome in acute lung injury. Am J Respir Crit Care Med 2003;167:1567-1574.

Bohrer H, Qiu F, Zimmermann T, Zhang Y, Jllmer T, Mannel D, Bottiger BW, Stern DM, Waldherr R, Saeger HD, Ziegler R, Bierhaus A, Martin E, Nawroth PP. Role of NFkappaB in the mortality of sepsis. J Clin Invest 1997;100:972-985.

Pellegrini JD, Puyana JC, Lapchak PH, Kodys K, Miller-Graziano CL. A membrane TNF-alpha/TNFR ratio correlates to MODS score and mortality. Shock 1996;6:389-396.

Stuber F, Petersen M, Bokelmann F, Schade U. A genomic polymorphism within the tumor necrosis factor locus influences plasma tumor necrosis factor-alpha concentrations and outcome of patients with severe sepsis. Crit Care Med 1996;24:381-384.

Bozza FA, Salluh JI, Japiassu AM, Soares M, Assis EF, Gomes RN, Bozza MT, Castro-Faria-Neto HC, Bozza PT. Cytokine profiles as markers of disease severity in sepsis: a multiplex analysis. Crit Care 2007;11:R49.

Creagh-Brown BC, Quinlan GJ, Evans TW, Burke-Gaffney A. The RAGE axis in systemic inflammation, acute lung injury and myocardial dysfunction: an important therapeutic target? Intensive Care Med 2010;36:1644-1656.

Buckley ST, Ehrhardt C. The receptor for advanced glycation end products (RAGE) and the lung. J Biomed Biotechnol 2010;2010:917108.

Schmidt AM, Yan SD, Yan SF, Stern DM. The biology of the receptor for advanced glycation end products and its ligands. Biochim Biophys Acta 2000;1498:99-111.

Lutterloh EC, Opal SM, Pittman DD, Keith JC, Jr., Tan XY, Clancy BM, Palmer H, Milarski K, Sun Y, Palardy JE, Parejo NA, Kessimian N. Inhibition of the RAGE products increases survival in experimental models of severe sepsis and systemic infection. Crit Care 2007;11:R122.

Sawa H, Ueda T, Takeyama Y, Yasuda T, Shinzeki M, Nakajima T, Kuroda Y. Blockade of high mobility group box-1 protein attenuates experimental severe acute pancreatitis. World J Gastroenterol 2006;12:7666-7670.

Yang ZY, Ling Y, Yin T, Tao J, Xiong JX, Wu HS, Wang CY. Delayed ethyl pyruvate therapy attenuates experimental severe acute pancreatitis via reduced serum high mobility group box 1 levels in rats. World J Gastroenterol 2008;14:4546-4550.

Calfee CS, Ware LB, Eisner MD, Parsons PE, Thompson BT, Wickersham N, Matthay MA. Plasma receptor for advanced glycation end products and clinical outcomes in acute lung injury. Thorax 2008;63:1083-1089.

Uchida T, Shirasawa M, Ware LB, Kojima K, Hata Y, Makita K, Mednick G, Matthay ZA, Matthay MA. Receptor for advanced glycation end-products is a marker of type I cell injury in acute lung injury. Am J Respir Crit Care Med 2006;173:1008-1015.

Yum HK, Arcaroli J, Kupfner J, Shenkar R, Penninger JM, Sasaki T, Yang KY, Park JS, Abraham E. Involvement of phosphoinositide 3-kinases in neutrophil activation and the development of acute lung injury. J Immunol 2001;167:6601-6608.

Ong E, Gao XP, Predescu D, Broman M, Malik AB. Role of phosphatidylinositol 3-kinase-gamma in mediating lung neutrophil sequestration and vascular injury induced by E. coli sepsis. Am J Physiol Lung Cell Mol Physiol 2005;289:L1094-L1103.

Martin EL, Souza DG, Fagundes CT, Amaral FA, Assenzio B, Puntorieri V, Del Sorbo L, Fanelli V, Bosco M, Delsedime L, Pinho JF, Lemos VS, Souto FO, Alves-Filho JC, Cunha FQ, Slutsky AS, Ruckle T, Hirsch E, Teixeira MM, Ranieri VM. PI3K{gamma} Kinase Activity Contributes to Sepsis and Organ Damage by Altering Neutrophil Recruitment. Am J Respir Crit Care Med 2010.

Martin EL, Ranieri VM. Phosphorylation mechanisms in intensive care medicine. Intensive Care Med 2011;37:7-18.

Wheeler DS. Death to sepsis: targeting apoptosis pathways in sepsis. Crit Care 2009;13: 1010.

Chopra M, Reuben JS, Sharma AC. Acute lung injury:apoptosis and signaling mechanisms. Exp Biol Med (Maywood) 2009;234:361-371.

Albertine KH, Soulier MF, Wang Z, Ishizaka A, Hashimoto S, Zimmerman GA, Matthay MA, Ware LB. Fas and fas ligand are up-regulated in pulmonary edema fluid and lung tissue of patients with acute lung injury and the acute respiratory distress syndrome. Am J Pathol 2002;161:1783-1796.

Matute-Bello G, Liles WC, Steinberg KP, Kiener PA, Mongovin S, Chi EY, Jonas M, Martin TR. Soluble Fas ligand induces epithelial cell apoptosis in humans with acute lung injury (ARDS). J Immunol 1999;163:2217-2225.

Neff TA, Guo RF, Neff SB, Sarma JV, Speyer CL, Gao H, Bernacki KD, Huber-Lang M, McGuire S, Hoesel LM, Riedemann NC, Beck-Schimmer B, Zetoune FS, Ward PA. Relationship of acute lung inflammatory injury to Fas/FasL system. Am J Pathol 2005;166:685-694.

Perl M, Chung CS, Perl U, Lomas-Neira J, de Paepe M, Cioffi WG, Ayala A. Fas-induced pulmonary apoptosis and inflammation during indirect acute lung injury. Am J Respir Crit Care Med 2007;176:591-601.

Matsuda N, Yamamoto S, Takano K, Kageyama S, Kurobe Y, Yoshihara Y, Takano Y, Hattori Y. Silencing of fas-associated death domain protects mice from septic lung inflammation and apoptosis. Am J Respir Crit Care Med 2009;179:806-815.

Perl M, Chung CS, Lomas-Neira J, Rachel TM, Biffl WL, Cioffi WG, Ayala A. Silencing of Fas, but not caspase-8, in lung epithelial cells ameliorates pulmonary apoptosis, inflammation, and neutrophil influx after hemorrhagic shock and sepsis. Am J Pathol 2005;167:1545-1559.

Bernard GR, Vincent JL, Laterre PF, LaRosa SP, Dhainaut JF, Lopez-Rodriguez A, Steingrub JS, Garber GE, Helterbrand JD, Ely EW, Fisher CJ, Jr. Efficacy and safety of recombinant human activated protein C for severe sepsis. N Engl J Med 2001;344:699-709.

Shorr AF, Bernard GR, Dhainaut JF, Russell JR, Macias WL, Nelson DR, Sundin DP. Protein C concentrations in severe sepsis: an early directional change in plasma levels predicts outcome. Crit Care 2006;10:R92.

Matthay MA, Ware LB. Plasma protein C levels in patients with acute lung injury: prognostic significance. Crit Care Med 2004;32:S229-S232.

Waerhaug K, Kuklin VN, Kirov MY, Sovershaev MA, Langbakk B, Ingebretsen OC, Ytrehus K, Bjertnaes LJ. Recombinant human activated protein C attenuates endotoxin-induced lung injury in awake sheep. Crit Care 2008;12:R104.

Wang Z, Su F, Rogiers P, Vincent JL. Beneficial effects of recombinant human activated protein C in a ewe model of septic shock Crit Care Med 2007;35:2594-2600.

Sarangi PP, Lee HW, Kim M. Activated protein C action in inflammation. Br J Haematol 2010;148:817-833.

Mosnier LO, Zlokovic BV, Griffin JH. The cytoprotective protein C pathway. Blood 2007;109:3161-3172.

Jean-Baptiste E. Cellular mechanisms in sepsis. J Intensive Care Med 2007;22:63-72.

Van Amersfoort ES, Van Berkel TJ, Kuiper J. Receptors, mediators, and mechanisms involved in bacterial sepsis and septic shock. Clin Microbiol Rev 2003;16:379-414.

Yang S, Zhou M, Chaudry IH, Wang P. Norepinephrine-induced hepatocellular dysfunction in early sepsis is mediated by activation of alpha2-adrenoceptors. Am J Physiol Gastrointest Liver Physiol 2001;281:G1014-G1021.

Dhainaut JF, Marin N, Mignon A, Vinsonneau C. Hepatic response to sepsis: interaction between coagulation and inflammatory processes. Crit Care Med 2001;29:S42-S47.

Mookerjee RP. Acute-on-chronic liver failure: the liver and portal haemodynamics. Curr Opin Crit Care 2011;17:170-176.

Cheluvappa R, Denning GM, Lau GW, Grimm MC, Hilmer SN, Le Couteur DG. Pathogenesis of the hyperlipidemia of Gram-negative bacterial sepsis may involve pathomorphological changes in liver sinusoidal endothelial cells. Int J Infect Dis 2010;14:e857-e867.

Yang QH, Liu DW, Wang XT, Yang RL, Shi Y, Long Y, Liu HZ, He HW, Zhou X, Tang B. G1 cell cycle arrest signaling in hepatic injury after intraperitoneal sepsis in rats. Inflamm Res 2011.

Fong YM, Marano MA, Moldawer LL, Wei H, Calvano SE, Kenney JS, Allison AC, Cerami A, Shires GT, Lowry SF. The acute splanchnic and peripheral tissue metabolic response to endotoxin in humans. J Clin Invest 1990;85:1896-1904.

Ananian P, Hardwigsen J, Bernard D, Le Treut YP. Serum acute-phase protein level as indicator for liver failure after liver resection. Hepatogastroenterology 2005;52:857-861.

Bevilacqua MP, Pober JS, Majeau GR, Fiers W, Cotran RS, Gimbrone MA, Jr. Recombinant tumor necrosis factor induces procoagulant activity in cultured human vascular endothelium: characterization and comparison with the actions of interleukin 1. Proc Natl Acad Sci U S A 1986;83:4533-4537.

Zhang P, Xie M, Spitzer JA. Hepatic neutrophil sequestration in early sepsis: enhanced expression of adhesion molecules and phagocytic activity. Shock 1994;2:133-140.

Malmros C, Holst E, Hansson L, Martensson L, Thorne J. Dynamic accumulation of neutrophils in lungs and visceral organs during early abdominal sepsis in the pig. World J Surg 1994;18:811-816.

Holman JM, Jr., Saba TM. Hepatocyte injury during post-operative sepsis: activated neutrophils as potential mediators. J Leukoc Biol 1988;43:193-203.

Stearns-Kurosawa DJ, Osuchowski MF, Valentine C, Kurosawa S, Remick DG. The pathogenesis of sepsis. Annu Rev Pathol 2011;6:19-48.

Asaka S, Shibayama Y, Nakata K. Pathogenesis of focal and random hepatocellular necrosis in endotoxemia: microscopic observation in vivo. Liver 1996;16:183-187.

Jagneaux T, Taylor DE, Kantrow SP. Coagulation in sepsis. Am J Med Sci 2004;328:196-204.

Nitescu N, Grimberg E, Ricksten SE, Marcussen N, Nordlinder H, Guron G. Effects of thrombin inhibition with melagatran on renal hemodynamics and function and liver integrity during early endotoxemia. Am J Physiol Regul Integr Comp Physiol 2007;292:R1117-R1124.

Inthorn D, Hoffmann JN, Hartl WH, Muhlbayer D, Jochum M. Antithrombin III supplementation in severe sepsis: beneficial effects on organ dysfunction. Shock 1997;8:328-334.

Wiedermann CJ, Hoffmann JN, Juers M, Ostermann H, Kienast J, Briegel J, Strauss R, Keinecke HO, Warren BL, Opal SM. High-dose antithrombin III in the treatment of severe sepsis in patients with a high risk of death: efficacy and safety. Crit Care Med 2006;34:285-292.

Xu J, Zhang X, Pelayo R, Monestier M, Ammollo CT, Semeraro F, Taylor FB, Esmon NL, Lupu F, Esmon CT. Extracellular histones are major mediators of death in sepsis. Nat Med 2009;15:1318-1321.

Rinaldi L, Marietta M, Mignini MA, Donno L, Busani S, Codeluppi M, Masetti M, Girardis M. Use of activated protein C in liver transplantation patients with septic shock. Liver Transpl 2008;14:1598-1602.

Huynh T, Nguyen N, Keller S, Moore C, Shin MC, McKillop IH. Reducing leukocyte trafficking preserves hepatic function after sepsis. J Trauma 2010;69:360-367.

Ward PA, Gao H. Sepsis, complement and the dysregulated inflammatory response. J Cell Mol Med 2009;13:4154-4160.

Guo RF, Ward PA. C5a, a therapeutic target in sepsis. Recent Pat Antiinfect Drug Discov 2006;1:57-65.

Riedemann NC, Guo RF, Neff TA, Laudes IJ, Keller KA, Sarma VJ, Markiewski MM, Mastellos D, Strey CW, Pierson CL, Lambris JD, Zetoune FS, Ward PA. Increased C5a receptor expression in sepsis. J Clin Invest 2002;110:101-108.

Lafrance JP, Miller DR. Acute kidney injury associates with increased long-term mortality. J Am Soc Nephrol 2010;21:345-352.

Uchino S, Kellum JA, Bellomo R, Doig GS, Morimatsu H, Morgera S, Schetz M, Tan I, Bouman C, Macedo E, Gibney N, Tolwani A, Ronco C. Acute renal failure in critically ill patients: a multinational, multicenter study. JAMA 2005;294:813-818.

Silvester W, Bellomo R, Cole L. Epidemiology, management, and outcome of severe acute renal failure of critical illness in Australia. Crit Care Med 2001;29:1910-1915.

Wan L, Bagshaw SM, Langenberg C, Saotome T, May C, Bellomo R. Pathophysiology of septic acute kidney injury: what do we really know? Crit Care Med 2008;36:S198-S203.

Langenberg C, Wan L, Egi M, May CN, Bellomo R. Renal blood flow and function during recovery from experimental septic acute kidney injury. Intensive Care Med 2007;33:1614-1618.

Bagshaw SM, Langenberg C, Wan L, May CN, Bellomo R. A systematic review of urinary findings in experimental septic acute renal failure. Crit Care Med 2007;35:1592-1598.

Licari E, Calzavacca P, Ronco C, Bellomo R. Fluid resuscitation and the septic kidney: the evidence. Contrib Nephrol 2007;156:167-177.

Bradley VE, Shier MR, Lucas CE, Rosenberg IK. Renal hemodynamic response to furosemide in septic and injured patients. Surgery 1976;79:549-554.

Humphrey TJ, Baskerville A, Chart H, Rowe B, Whitehead A. Salmonella enteritidis PT4 infection in specific pathogen free hens: influence of infecting dose. Vet Rec 1991;129:482-485.

Jo SK, Cha DR, Cho WY, Kim HK, Chang KH, Yun SY, Won NH. Inflammatory cytokines and lipopolysaccharide induce Fas-mediated apoptosis in renal tubular cells. Nephron 2002;91:406-415.

Guo R, Wang Y, Minto AW, Quigg RJ, Cunningham PN. Acute renal failure in endotoxemia is dependent on caspase activation. J Am Soc Nephrol 2004;15:3093-3102.

Cantaluppi V, Assenzio B, Pasero D, Romanazzi GM, Pacitti A, Lanfranco G, Puntorieri V, Martin EL, Mascia L, Monti G, Casella G, Segoloni GP, Camussi G, Ranieri VM. Polymyxin-B hemoperfusion inactivates circulating proapoptotic factors. Intensive Care Med 2008;34:1638-1645.

Mariano F, Cantaluppi V, Stella M, Romanazzi GM, Assenzio B, Cairo M, Biancone L, Triolo G, Ranieri VM, Camussi G. Circulating plasma factors induce tubular and glomerular alterations in septic burns patients. Crit Care 2008;12:R42.

Allen DA, Harwood S, Varagunam M, Raftery MJ, Yaqoob MM. High glucose-induced oxidative stress causes apoptosis in proximal tubular epithelial cells and is mediated by multiple caspases. FASEB J 2003;17:908-910.

Schiavon M, Di Landro D, Baldo M, De Silvestro G, Chiarelli A. A study of renal damage in seriously burned patients. Burns Incl Therm Inj 1988;14:107-112.

Christensen EI, Birn H. Megalin and cubilin: synergistic endocytic receptors in renal proximal tubule. Am J Physiol Renal Physiol 2001;280:F562-F573.

Lee DB, Huang E, Ward HJ. Tight junction biology and kidney dysfunction. Am J Physiol Renal Physiol 2006;290:F20-F34.

Chen J, Boyle S, Zhao M, Su W, Takahashi K, Davis L, Decaestecker M, Takahashi T, Breyer MD, Hao CM. Differential expression of the intermediate filament protein nestin during renal development and its localization in adult podocytes. J Am Soc Nephrol 2006;17:1283-1291.

Hoesel LM, Niederbichler AD, Ward PA. Complement-related molecular events in sepsis leading to heart failure. Mol Immunol 2007;44:95-102.

Hunter JD, Doddi M. Sepsis and the heart. Br J Anaesth 2010;104:3-11.

Grocott-Mason RM, Shah AM. Cardiac dysfunction in sepsis: new theories and clinical implications. Intensive Care Med 1998;24:286-295.

Bouhemad B, Nicolas-Robin A, Arbelot C, Arthaud M, Feger F, Rouby JJ. Acute left ventricular dilatation and shock-induced myocardial dysfunction. Crit Care Med 2009;37:441-447.

Matsuda N, Hattori Y. Vascular biology in sepsis: pathophysiological and therapeutic significance of vascular dysfunction. J Smooth Muscle Res 2007;43:117-137.

Massion PB, Feron O, Dessy C, Balligand JL. Nitric oxide and cardiac function: ten years after, and continuing. Circ Res 2003;93:388-398.

Pacher P, Beckman JS, Liaudet L. Nitric oxide and peroxynitrite in health and disease. Physiol Rev 2007;87:315-424.

Fraccarollo D, Widder JD, Galuppo P, Thum T, Tsikas D, Hoffmann M, Ruetten H, Ertl G, Bauersachs J. Improvement in left ventricular remodeling by the endothelial nitric oxide synthase enhancer AVE9488 after experimental myocardial infarction. Circulation 2008;118:818-827.

Parrillo JE, Burch C, Shelhamer JH, Parker MM, Natanson C, Schuette W. A circulating myocardial depressant substance in humans with septic shock. Septic shock patients with a reduced ejection fraction have a circulating factor that depresses in vitro myocardial cell performance. J Clin Invest 1985;76:1539-1553.

Mink SN, Kasian K, Jacobs H, Cheng ZQ, Light RB. N,N'-diacetylchitobiose, an inhibitor of lysozyme, reverses myocardial depression and lessens norepinephrine requirements in Escherichia coli sepsis in dogs. Shock 2008;29:681-687.

Konrad D, Oldner A, Rossi P, Wanecek M, Rudehill A, Weitzberg E. Differentiated and dose-related cardiovascular effects of a dual endothelin receptor antagonist in endotoxin shock. Crit Care Med 2004;32:1192-1199.

Schuetz P, Christ-Crain M, Morgenthaler NG, Struck J, Bergmann A, Muller B. Circulating precursor levels of endothelin-1 and adrenomedullin, two endothelium-derived, counteracting substances, in sepsis. Endothelium 2007;14:345-351.

Rudiger A, Singer M. Mechanisms of sepsis-induced cardiac dysfunction. Crit Care Med 2007;35:1599-1608.

Heyland DK, Hopman W, Coo H, Tranmer J, McColl MA. Long-term health-related quality of life in survivors of sepsis. Short Form 36: a valid and reliable measure of health-related quality of life. Crit Care Med 2000;28:3599-3605.

Hopkins RO, Weaver LK, Pope D, Orme JF, Bigler ED, Larson-LOHR V. Neuropsychological sequelae and impaired health status in survivors of severe acute respiratory distress syndrome. Am J Respir Crit Care Med 1999;160:50-56.

Hough CL, Curtis JR. Long-term sequelae of critical illness: memories and health-related quality of life. Crit Care 2005;9:145-146.

Jacob A, Brorson JR, Alexander JJ. Septic encephalopathy: inflammation in man and mouse. Neurochem Int 2011;58:472-476.

Streck EL, Comim CM, Barichello T, Quevedo J. The septic brain. Neurochem Res 2008;33:2171-2177.

Barichello T, Fortunato JJ, Vitali AM, Feier G, Reinke A, Moreira JC, Quevedo J, Dal Pizzol F. Oxidative variables in the rat brain after sepsis induced by cecal ligation and perforation. Crit Care Med 2006;34:886-889.

Barichello T, Machado RA, Constantino L, Valvassori SS, Reus GZ, Martins MR, Petronilho F, Ritter C, Quevedo J, Dal Pizzol F. Antioxidant treatment prevented late memory impairment in an animal model of sepsis. Crit Care Med 2007;35:2186-2190.

Dantzer R, O'Connor JC, Freund GG, Johnson RW, Kelley KW. From inflammation to sickness and depression: when the immune system subjugates the brain. Nat Rev Neurosci 2008;9:46-56.

Glass CK, Saijo K, Winner B, Marchetto MC, Gage FH. Mechanisms underlying inflammation in neurodegeneration. Cell 2010;140:918-934.

Abbott NJ, Ronnback L, Hansson E. Astrocyte-endothelial interactions at the blood-brain barrier. Nat Rev Neurosci 2006;7:41-53.

Nishioku T, Dohgu S, Takata F, Eto T, Ishikawa N, Kodama KB, Nakagawa S, Yamauchi A, Kataoka Y. Detachment of brain pericytes from the basal lamina is involved in disruption of the blood-brain barrier caused by lipopolysaccharide-induced sepsis in mice. Cell Mol Neurobiol 2009;29:309-316.

Hofer S, Bopp C, Hoerner C, Plaschke K, Faden RM, Martin E, Bardenheuer HJ, Weigand MA. Injury of the blood brain barrier and up-regulation of icam-1 in polymicrobial sepsis. J Surg Res 2008;146:276-281.

Alexander JJ, Jacob A, Cunningham P, Hensley L, Quigg RJ. TNF is a key mediator of septic encephalopathy acting through its receptor, TNF receptor-1. Neurochem Int 2008;52:447-456.

Flierl MA, Rittirsch D, Chen AJ, Nadeau BA, Day DE, Sarma JV, Huber-Lang MS, Ward PA. The complement anaphylatoxin C5a induces apoptosis in adrenomedullary cells during experimental sepsis. PLoS One 2008;3:e2560.

Henry CJ, Huang Y, Wynne A, Hanke M, Himler J, Bailey MT, Sheridan JF, Godbout JP. Minocycline attenuates lipopolysaccharide (LPS)-induced neuroinflammation, sickness behavior, and anhedonia. J Neuroinflammation 2008;5:15.

Sewell DL, Nacewicz B, Liu F, Macvilay S, Erdei A, Lambris JD, Sandor M, Fabry Z. Complement C3 and C5 play critical roles in traumatic brain cryoinjury: blocking effects on neutrophil extravasation by C5a receptor antagonist. J Neuroimmunol 2004;155:55-63.

Leinhase I, Rozanski M, Harhausen D, Thurman JM, Schmidt OI, Hossini AM, Taha ME, Rittirsch D, Ward PA, Holers VM, Ertel W, Stahel PF. Inhibition of the alternative complement activation pathway in traumatic brain injury by a monoclonal anti-factor B antibody: a randomized placebo-controlled study in mice. J Neuroinflammation 2007;4:13.

9

Impact of Severe Sepsis or Septic Shock on Drug Response

Marta Vázquez, Pietro Fagiolino,
Cecilia Maldonado, Manuel Ibarra and Anna Boronat
Pharmaceutical Sciences Department, Faculty of Chemistry
Therapeutic Drug Monitoring Service, University Hospital, Montevideo
Uruguay

1. Introduction

Several studies conducted in critically ill patients have demonstrated that inappropriate antibiotic treatment was associated with increased mortality (Niederman, 2006; Pea & Viale, 2009; Zilberberg et al., 2008). This fact was always related to the use of the wrong antimicrobial agent. However, the failure of a treatment might be due to inadequate doses that lead to sub-therapeutic concentrations at the infection site.

This last issue is relevant in patients with severe sepsis or septic shock as many factors can influence pharmacokinetic variability and consequently human drug response. Among these factors we can mention the pathology itself. Only the knowledge of the pathogenesis of sepsis can enable us to understand the variability of drug concentrations with the aim of a successful therapeutic outcome avoiding therapeutic failure or toxicity.

The sudden changes observed in severe sepsis or septic shock (increase in capillary permeability, edema formation, vasodilation and hypotension) and the therapeutic action taken to revert the situation (volume resuscitation, vasopressor agents) makes antibiotics or other drug concentrations difficult to interpret.

Due to the lack of stable disease conditions, and consequently marked variations in pharmacokinetics parameters, dose dosage in these patients is a great challenge.

The dynamic status of sepsis in critically ill patients results in alterations in pharmacokinetic parameters so it is of importance drug concentration assessment in this population, different from healthy volunteers or less severe ill patients.

The use of nomograms to provide estimates for dosages is not advisable as they assume normal pharmacokinetic parameters and due to instability of the system, pharmacokinetic parameters are subject to rapid changes.

As the measurement of total drug concentration (free drug plus protein-bound drug) is much easier and cheaper than free drug determination, therapeutic drug monitoring is usually based on total plasma concentrations. However, only the free drug is capable of diffusing into the biophase, only the free drug is responsible for the therapeutic effect. This fact has to be taken into account to see if the changes provoked by sepsis itself impact on both total drug and free drug in the same way. If this is not the case, defining dose regimens only by plasma total drug concentrations could be erroneous.

Measurement of the free drug in plasma is desirable but it is difficult to achieve in practice. Corrective algorithms (Bahn et al., 2002) have been proposed in order to predict unbound drug but with limitations if displacing drugs are present in the treatment. Salivary therapeutic drug monitoring in different populations has extensively been studied by our group (Maldonado et al., 2008, 2011). So, in view of this, this fluid may serve as an alternative to plasma free concentration in this population.
A theoretical multi-compartmental model designed by our group (Fagiolino et al., 2011), was used to understand the rapid changes that occur during sepsis causing highly variable drug concentrations.
The experimental results obtained with two different drugs: vancomycin and phenytoin used in the intensive care setting will be presented in order to study the impact of sepsis on their concentrations in accordance to this model.

2. Pathophysiological characteristics in critically ill patients with severe sepsis or septic shock and the influence on pharmacokinetics

Sepsis itself is characterized by an early response which implies the release of inflammatory mediators (tumor necrosis factor-α, interleukin 6 and chemokines) resulting in a detriment to the host. This constitutes the systemic inflammatory response syndrome (SIRS) (Dinarello, 2000). This release is counterbalanced by the opponent antiinflammatory molecules (interleukin 10, 4, etc) (Figure 1). This later response is referred to as the compensatory antiinflammatory response syndrome (CARS) (Bone, 1996). The magnitude of septic injury is determined by the balance of pro and antiinflammatory mediators.

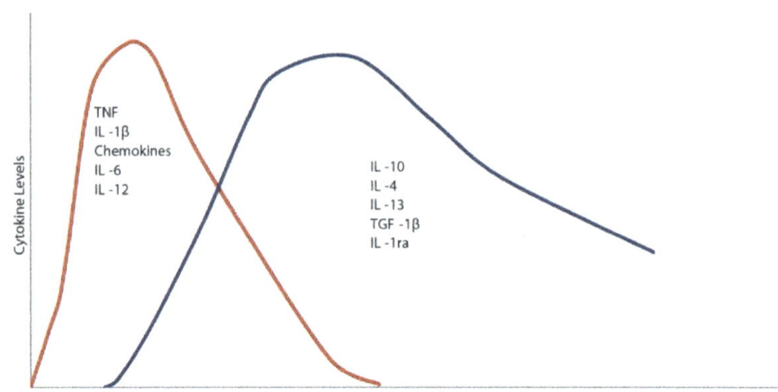

Fig. 1. Cytokines during sepsis. Figure adapted from Reddy et al., 2001. The red curve represents the mediators released during the systemic inflammatory response syndrome (SIRS). The blue curve represents the mediators released during the compensatory anti-inflammatory response syndrome (CARS).

At an initial stage, patients show enhanced inflammation responsible for tissue damage. The subsequent anti-inflammatory response makes the host more vulnerable for a secondary infection (Reddy et al., 2001). This first stage is the one that is going to be referred to in this chapter.

The initial mediators cause an increase in heart rate, an increased cardiac output, a decrease in systemic vascular resistance, an anomalous distribution of blood flow, reduced blood volume and tissue perfusion.

2.1 Alterations in tissue permeability

Endothelial damage provoked by SIRS, may result in an increase in capillary permeability and interstitial edema formation. This generalized increase in capillary permeability may lead to presence of urinary albumin (Fuster-Lluch et al., 2008).

2.2 Glomerular hyperfiltration

The study of the renal function in critically ill patients has always been focused on renal impairment. Nevertheless, glomerular filtration rate may be elevated in certain conditions such as sepsis (Fuster-Lluch et al., 2008). This could be due to the presence of a hyperdynamic circulatory situation by the increased cardiac output, indicating glomerular hyperfiltration and leading to an increase renal clearance of substances.

2.3 Alterations in protein binding

Changes in the plasma protein binding of drugs during sepsis may be caused by many factors such as competition of endogenous substances for binding sites, changes in the binding characteristics that could be the consequence of changes in pH , etc. A reduction in the level of serum albumin in critically ill patients is often seen due to scarce protein intake, increased capillary permeability, reduced hepatic synthesis, renal loss (De Paepe et al., 2002).

The alterations observed in sepsis are of great impact on drug pharmacokinetics. The volume of distribution (Vd) and mainly the clearance (CL) of antimicrobials as well as of many others drugs suffer great variations during the disease. These disturbances can result in an increase in CL for hydrophilic and moderately lipophilic drugs if renal function is not compromised.

On the other hand, advanced status of sepsis is characterized by multiple organ dysfunction, with the kidneys and the liver involved at this stage. Kidney damage is very common and this will affect concentrations of renally-excreted hydrophilic drugs, resulting in higher concentration, total and free plasma concentrations. The effect of liver impairment on drugs eliminated by hepatic metabolism is not well defined and occurred mainly at a final stage as the liver has functional reserve.

3. Drug concentrations in sepsis due to the pathology itself or the medication used to resolve the situation

An appropriate infection control is the priority to manage sepsis and requires an early adequate dose of antibiotics to achieve therapeutic concentrations at the site of infection.

Antiobiotic therapy in critically ill septic patients usually consists of a broad-spectrum beta-lactam combined with a glycopeptide and /or an aminoglycoside.

Their greater efficacy occurs when antimicrobials concentrations are maintained above the minimum inhibitory concentration (MIC) of the pathogens responsible for the infection for extended periods.

Insufficient concentrations of antibiotics in the early phase of severe sepsis or septic shock are commonly observed in patients with normal renal function. Many authors have

confirmed sub therapeutic plasma concentrations of aminoglycosides (Beckhouse et al., 1988; Marik, 1993). So much is written in the literature about an increase in Vd in sepsis, which reduces in turn plasma antibiotic levels (Taccone et al., 2010a). For example for amikacin, the Vd is between 0.2 and 0.3 L/kg in healthy volunteers and in mild infections but in septic patients an increase of 60 % was found compared with normal ranges (Taccone et al., 2010b). But what is interesting from their studies was the fact that trough concentrations at steady state at the initial septic stage remain the same or were lower. Some authors reported lower areas under the plasma concentration -time curve (AUC) of these antibiotics during sepsis (Joukhadar et al., 2001). The latter observations confirm that the main cause of low concentrations of drugs during sepsis is mainly an increase in CL.
Equation 1 refers to the mean steady state concentration, average steady state concentration (C_{avss}) after multiple doses.

$$C_{avss}=\frac{AUC_0^{\tau}}{\tau}=\frac{FD/\tau}{CL} \tag{1}$$

Being CL the total clearance, F the bioavailability factor, D the dose, τ the administration interval, $AUC_{0-\tau}$ (the AUC from zero to the last point of the administration interval).
Since drug administration in critically ill patients is mainly by intravenous route, F=1. So, any change in C_{avss} depends on CL only.
Due to hypoalbuminemia, highly and moderate protein-bound drugs reduce their total plasma concentration but their free plasma levels may also be reduced in sepsis.
If renal or intestinal excretion clearance predominates, a significant decrease in free plasma levels is expected because of the increased generalized permeability at capillaries and increased blood flow fraction derived to these zones.
So, an important fall in concentrations, even free concentrations in plasma, suggests an important increase in CL. This fact could be due to the following reasons:

1. Increase in capillary renal permeability
2. Increase in renal blood fraction
3. Increase in renal cardiac output affecting mainly highly renally extracted drugs.

This is the case of beta-lactams (penicillins, cephalosporins, carbapenems, monobactams), glycopeptides, aminoglycosides which are hydrophilic or moderate lipophilic drugs and can be extrapolated to any drug with the same characteristics.
If hepatic metabolic clearance or hepatic excretion clearance is the main route of elimination, then a discrete free drug level reduction would be expected. This is because hepatic blood flow fraction does not change in sepsis (De Paepe et al., 2002) and the increased capillary permeation in the liver does not change the normal unrestricted diffusion through sinusoid wall.This is the case for some lipophilic antibiotics and could be the case for any other drug with the same behavior.
New sepsis treatment strategies, mainly immune stimulatory therapy, have improved outcomes significantly (Lolis & Bucala, 2003). Nevertheless, antimicrobial therapy is still probably the most influential factor. So, prompt initiation of the correct antibiotic therapy is the cornerstone of therapy in sepsis.
Not only the sudden changes observed in severe sepsis or septic shock (increase in capillary permeability, edema formation, vasodilation and hypotension) make antibiotics or other drug concentrations difficult to analyze, but also the therapeutic action taken to resolve the situation (volume resuscitation, vasopressor agents) plays an important role.

Patients with severe sepsis or septic shock need replacement of the fluid to keep the arterial blood pressure for adequate organ perfusion (Choi et al., 1999). Changes in the water volume caused by the administration of large volumes of fluids, will affect antibiotics that distribute to the extracellular space fluid.

Administration of fluids for volume resuscitation such as crystalloids or colloids, causes an increase in aqueous volume leading to an increase in Vd of hydrophilic drugs. This dilution in drug concentrations is compensated by a slower elimination of drug. Consequently, no changes in CL could be observed.

Vasopressors are usually used (Holmes et al., 2001). This may affect drug concentrations as well. Of note, glomerular hyperfiltration may be a consequence of inotropic agents when hypotension does not revert with fluid therapy.

It is worth noting that the extent of renal and non renal excretion clearance of a drug is the fundamental issue to keep in mind and not how hydrophilic a drug is. Interestingly, it was recently shown (Pea & Viale, 2009; Thallinger et al. 2008) that a lipophilic antibiotic, linezolid, does not reduce significantly its free or tissue level in patients with sepsis and septic shock in relation with healthy volunteers. The explanation was that the intracellular depot of the agent restores its cleared amount. However, in our opinion, no statistical differences were found mainly because of the high inter-individual variability observed among individuals.

Pharmacokinetic data reported in the literature (Slatter et al, 2001; Wagenlehner et al., 2003) reveal an important contribution of renal excretion in linezolid clearance (40% approximately). Therefore, the increased renal clearance in septic patients mentioned above should necessarily diminish free linezolid levels in relation with healthy volunteers. Comparing free plasma C_{avss} of healthy volunteers with septic patients results (Thallinger et al. 2008), a reduction in free plasma levels in sever sepsis could be observed (13.3±5.03 mg/L and 8.37±3.89 mg/L respectively). This could be clinically relevant and may be significant in the same individual. So, standard doses of this antibiotic may be inadequate to reach therapeutic free plasma concentrations

4. Antibiotic administration strategies

It should not be overlooked that bacteria can grow again when antimicrobials concentrations fall below the MIC no matter the antibiotics used (time-dependent or concentration-dependent).

So it may be reasonable to suggest that maintenance of plasma trough concentrations above the MIC ought to be the goal of therapy in daily clinical practice for critically ill patient.

Many studies with different administration strategies for antibiotics were carried out (Petrosillo et al., 2010). One strategy was the case of extended infusion (over 3 to 4 hours) (Lomaestro & Drusano, 2005).

Continuous infusion may be the best approach to improve clinical outcomes in patients with severe infections (James et al., 1996; Lorente et al., 2009). The problem is the stability at room temperature of the drugs. Meropenem and imipenem are not good candidates. On the other hand, some other antibiotics are stable such as piperacillin/tazobactam; ceftazidime and vancomycin (Viaene et al., 2002).

So, not only the appropriate dose, usually larger doses than standard regimen are necessary, but also the right mode of administration could help to resolve this clinical situation.

It is evident that higher doses are required for optimal treatment as free plasma levels responsible for the pharmacological effect, decrease significantly.

Antimicrobials concentrations in septic patients were determined in different studies (Table 1) and thus pharmacokinetic data could be inferred.
Several authors found that antibacterial concentrations of these antibiotics are easily achievable with continuous infusion, thus representing and effective alternative dosing regimen to infusion bolus.
In a recent study (Roberts et al., 2009), continuous versus intermittent infusion of meropenem in critically ill patients with sepsis and without renal dysfunction was compared. In this study, continuous infusion was more successful in achieving the target concentrations despite meropenem instability.

Antibiotics	Suggested doses	Analytical techniques
Piperacillin-tazobactam (Petrosillo et al., 2010; Taccone et al., 2010a)	A loading dose of 2g, then 8g by continuous infusion over 24 h	High performance liquid chromatography with diode array detection
Meropenem (Taccone et al., 2010a)	2g every 8 hours	High performance liquid chromatography with diode array detection
Ceftazidime (Benko et al., 1996; Taccone et al., 2010a)	2 g loading dose followed by a 3-g continuous infusion over 24 h	High performance liquid chromatography with diode array detection
Cefepime (Lipman et al., 1999; Taccone et al., 2010a)	1g every 4 hours	High performance liquid chromatography with diode array detection
Amikacin (Taccone et al., 2010b)	A loading dose ≥25 mg/kg	Fluorescence polarization immunoassay (TDx, Abbott Laboratories, IL, USA)
Gentamicin (Petrosillo et al., 2010)	7 mg /kg once daily	Fluorescence polarization immunoassay (TDx, Abbott Laboratories, IL, USA)
Vancomycin (Vázquez et al., 2008)	1 g loading dose followed by a 3-g continuous infusion over 24 hours	Fluorescence polarization immunoassay (TDx, Abbott Laboratories, IL, USA)
Teicoplanin (Brink et al., 2008)	Loading doses of 6 mg/kg every 12 hours for 48 h	Fluorescence polarization immunoassay (TDx, Abbott Laboratories, IL, USA)

Table 1. Antibiotics used in critically ill patients, dose recommendations and analytical techniques used to measure their levels

5. Background information of vancomycin and phenytoin

Vancomycin is a glycopeptide antibiotic used to treat Gram-positive infections and in particular, methicillin-resistant Staphylococcal species. Therapeutic drug monitoring of vancomycin is commonly based on trough and peak determinations. However, a continuous infusion of vancomycin was reported in the literature (James et al., 1996) and it was the mode of administration in our patients with good outcomes and with the advantage of adjusting the dose easily, proving to be even safer and more effective than intermittent administration.

In critical care units, intravenous phenytoin is the first - line drug in prophylaxis or suppression of seizures. For lipophylic drugs and non significant ionized at biological pH range, the total concentration of drug in saliva is equal to free drug concentration in plasma (Al Zaabi et al., 2003) after loading doses and therefore more reflective of drug concentration in the biophase. So saliva could be a better surrogate for free drug levels, becoming a more advantageous monitoring fluid.

Both drugs are bound to albumin: 50% and 90% for vancomycin and phenytoin respectively. Vancomycin is mainly excreted by the kidneys (80%), whereas hepatic metabolism is predominant for phenytoin with less than 5% excreted as unchanged drug in the urine (Letteri et al., 1971). CYP2C9 and CYP2C19 are the main enzymes responsible for phenytoin elimination (Levy, 1995) and their low distribution in the gut suggests an hepatic metabolism for this drug (Läpple et al., 2003). Phenytoin is also a multidrug resistance protein (MRP2) substrate (Potschka et al., 2003) and is capable of inducing these transporters after multiple doses (Lombardo et al., 2008).

6. Pharmacokinetic modelling

The multi-compartmental model, shown in Figure 2, reflects the pharmacokinetic factors associated with the use of vancomycin and phenytoin in critically ill patients with sepsis.

As it can be observed, different processes of transference of mass could take place after intravenous drug administration, depending on the drug considered. For instance, phenytoin has lower intestinal and negligible renal elimination pathways, while vancomycin has major renal and minor splanchnic excretion processes with practically null intestinal and renal reabsorption of drug. Firstly, the drug enters the body directly into the blood stream which is located within the Central Blood-Plasma compartment. From here the drug is distributed to different extravascular spaces according to the fraction of total blood flow destined to each organ (red arrows). Hence, the higher the blood flow fraction delivered to an organ is, the higher the fraction of total molecules of drug delivered to the corresponding tissue is. This last issue is very important to understand the impact that vasodilatation could have on regional drug distribution. If kidneys receive an increased fraction of the cardiac output, all elimination processes taking place in these organs increase. The same could be the case for the intestinal uptake of drug from blood compartment. At the liver region, the uptake by hepatocytes suffers only a little change. Since hepatic blood flow fraction is regulated by both portal and arterial supply, acting in a compensated way, then drug transference could remain unchanged.

The most important change in sepsis is the increase in capillary permeability. This happens in all the vessels, and consequently there will be a generalized escape to the extravascular space, including the eliminating organs. For this reason, drug clearance is the main

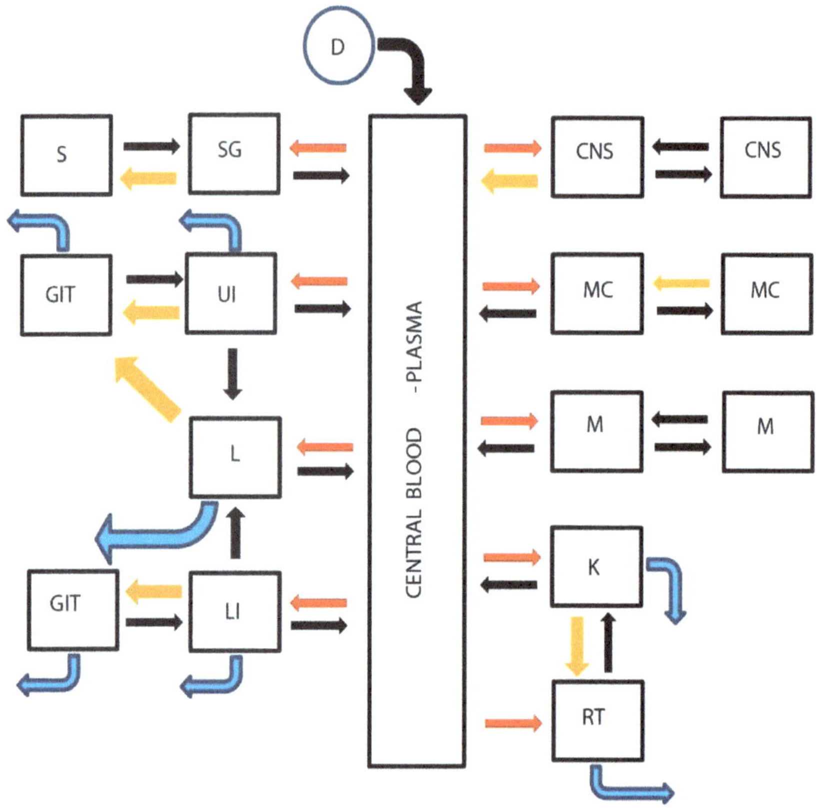

Fig. 2. Multi-compartmental model to explain drug variations during sepsis.Yellow arrows indicate efflux pumps. Red arrows represent blood flow and blood flow fraction to the different zones and blue arrows drug elimination. Some organs/tissues can be represented: (UI) upper intestine; (LI) lower intestine; (L) liver; (K) kidney; (RT) renal tubule; (GIT) gastrointestinal tract; (SG) salivary gland, (S) saliva; (M) muscle; (MC) myocardium; (CNS) central nervous system. (D) is the dose.

pharmacokinetic process affected by this change. Distribution into the intracellular spaces is not affected because both solute and solvent diffuse outside the vessels, so drug concentrations in plasma and in the interstitium remain unchanged. Secretions of fluid containing the drug increase through all secretory organs (gastrointestinal tract, kidneys) and consequently drug excretion increases. Fluid resuscitation does not reverse this phenomenon, because it just re-establishes blood pressure, but the increased clearance of drug persists. In the model, arrows getting mass of drug out of the blood compartment would increase, and those returning it back would decrease.

Loss of plasma proteins from the body, due to the increased permeability and increased clearance of proteins, produces a decrease in plasma protein concentrations. So, a decreased capacity to retain drug in the vasculature contributes to diminish even more drug levels in plasma and all over the body.

To sum up, free drug concentration in plasma decreases during sepsis because of an increased clearance. Total plasma drug concentration could decrease to a greater extent depending on the capacity of plasma protein to bind the drug. If there is a low binding capacity, the decrease in total drug concentration could be significantly higher than its respective free level decrease.

Since phenytoin is mainly eliminated by metabolism, and the hepatic clearance is its major route of elimination, a small decrease in free drug levels could be expected because of an increased blood flow fraction destined to both the intestine and the kidneys. However, saturation in plasma protein binding could be attained in hypoalbuminemic septic patients and then total plasma drug level may be decreased to a greater extent, even though non-significant clinical consequences should be expected. As the figure shows, certain arrows are painted in yellow, denoting a process mediated by efflux carriers. Since phenytoin is a MRP2 substrate, and it could induce its expression after chronic administration, different consequences either in clearance (Fagiolino et al. 2011), or in brain distribution, or in saliva excretion, could be envisaged. Readers should be aware of these increases in yellow arrows to deduce the pharmacokinetic and the therapeutic impact, and the corresponding drug monitoring using free plasma or saliva concentrations.

7. Experimental results

During sepsis the release of inflammatory mediators during the initial stage often results in detrimental effects to the host. The endothelial damage provoked by leucocytes, prostaglandins, leukotrienes or cascade activated complement leads to a generalized increase in capillary permeability and interstitial edema. Abnormalities in the microcirculation result in vasodilation and hypotension.

7.1 Vancomycin

The increase in permeability provokes an increase in renal clearance, thus there is a drop in both total and free plasma concentrations. Due to the hydrophilic characteristics of the drug, the tubular reabsorption is scarce and renal excretion is the augmented elimination pathway.

Vasodilation taking place mainly in the splanchnic and renal region would also produce an increase in drug clearance. In the case of critically ill patients in resting position, the blood flow to this area is already increased, so supplementary reduction in drug concentration is negligible.

Edema and hypovolemia have no further effect on the already low total drug concentrations.

Our data revealed no changes in protein binding for vancomycin . The comparison of the free fraction between 36 patients with sepsis and 24 patients without sepsis (all of them with normal renal function) showed no significant differences The values obtained (mean ± SD) were 34.6 ± 6.3% and 34.5 ± 5.9% respectively (Boronat, 2006). In the septic group a fall in free plasma concentration was observed even though daily doses were higher.

So the fall in vancomycin concentrations, even free concentrations, is mainly due to increased capillary permeability. Only with the eradication of the infection this situation can be reverted. Meanwhile, a higher dose should be administered (Vázquez et al, 2008).

Volume resuscitation did not have impact on free drug concentration but catecholamine administration reverted the slight impact that vasodilation could have on the already low free plasma concentrations.

Importantly, with deterioration in the clinical condition of the patient, lower plasma levels of vancomycin were observed. Conversely, an improvement in the clinical outcome was associated with increases in vancomycin plasma levels.
In this context, daily monitoring of plasma levels of this drug is mandatory to manage the infection.

7.2 Phenytoin

Due to its predominant hepatic elimination, changes in free plasma concentrations caused by capillary permeability modifications are not expected.
Vasodilation in intestine and renal regions with increasing blood flow derived to these areas would not impact significantly on free plasma phenytoin concentration either.
Changes in protein binding were observed in our hypoalbuminemic critically ill patients (Ibarra et al, 2010). For phenytoin, low total blood levels correspond mainly to an increased free drug fraction. Mean free phenytoin fraction in these patients was significantly higher (0.169 ± 0.080) in comparison to the one reported for patients with normal albumin (0.10). Thus, an increase in dose is not necessary and monitoring of the unbound concentration may be desirable.
Limited data are available about the enzymatic functionality during sepsis. De Paepe et al. (2002) reported the findings that long periods under hypoxic conditions decrease cytochrome P450 enzymes activity, but this could not be the case in septic patients because of the prompt hemodynamic and ventilatory measurements taken in order to maintain adequate organ perfusion. Then, conclusions about this issue are not so easily reached.
As the free drug determination is difficult and expensive to achieve in practice, salivary phenytoin monitoring may serve as an alternative to plasma free concentration monitoring in this population due to its good correlation with the effect.
Our results showed significant correlations between saliva (S) and free plasma (P) drug concentrations in critically ill patients when doses were administered for short periods of time. In some of them, when the treatment was maintained and high doses were given, a slight increase in S/P ratio was observed. Despite the strong correlation found between salivary and free plasma concentrations, the induction of efflux transporters in different organs (including salivary glands) by this antiepileptic in chronic treatments could explain the higher S/P ratio obtained.

8. Conclusions

There was consistency of the pharmacokinetic model presented and the clinical data. It could be stated that for hydrophilic drugs both renal and non renal excretion significantly increase in sepsis. Physiopathology of sepsis has little influence on free drug metabolic clearance, which is mainly affected by cardiac output distribution changes. Changes in protein binding should not be taken as a major constraint for achieving the therapeutic goal because these changes themselves, do not affect free drug levels in plasma or in the biophase. So, total blood level shoul not be taken into account to guide therapeutic management of critically ill patients.
In patients without renal impairment, and receiving hydrophilic antibiotics higher doses and continuous or extended infusions are the best approaches to improve clinical outcomes. In the case of vancomycin and according to our studies the recommended daily dose should be 3 g with later adjustments considering clinical evolution.

According to our experience, in neurologic critically ill patients receiving phenytoin, the increase in the loading dose, as a consequence of the diminished total plasma levels, more than a benefit, enhanced drug-related toxicities. In these cases, free plasma or saliva drug monitoring is advisable.

9. References

Al Zaabi, M., Deleu, D. & Batchelor, C. (2003). Salivary free concentration of antiepileptic drugs: an evaluation in a routine clinical setting. *Acta Neurol Belg,* Vol.103, No.1, pp. 19-23, ISSN 0300-9009

Bahn, HL., Burton, ME. & Sperling, MR.(2002). Interpatient and intrapatient variability in phenytoin protein binding. *Ther Drug Monit,* Vol.24, No.3, (June 2002), pp.379-385, ISSN 0163-4356

Beckhouse, MJ., Whyte, IM., Byth, PL., Napier, JC.& Smith AJ. (1988). Altered aminoglycoside pharmacokinetics in the critically ill. *Anaesth Intensive Care,* Vol.16, No.4, (November 1988), pp.418-422, ISSN 0310-057X

Benko, AS; Cappelletty, DM., Kruse, JA. & RyBak, MJ. Continuous infusion versus intermittent administration of ceftazidime in critically ill patients with suspected gram-negative infections. (1996). *Antimicrob Agents Chemother,* Vol. 40, No.3, (March 1996), pp. 691-695, ISSN 0066-4804

Bone, RC. (1996). Sir Isaac Newton, sepsis, SIRS, and CARS. *Crit Care Med,* Vol.24, No.7, (July 1996), pp.1125-1128, ISSN 0090-3493

Boronat, A. (2006). Pharmacokinetic follow-up of antimicrobials therapies in different hospital populations. *Doctoral thesis.* (In Spanish). Faculty of Chemistry, University of the Republic, Uruguay.

Brink, AJ., Richards, GA., Cummins, RR., Lambson, J. & G auteng Undersatnding Teicoplanin Serum levels (GUTS) study group. (2008). Recommendations to achieve rapid therapeutic teicoplanin plasma concentration in adult hospitalized patients treated for sepsis. *Int J Antimicrob Agents,* Vol. 32, No. 5, (November 2008), pp.455-458, ISSN 0924-8579

Choi, PT., Yip, G., Quinonez, LG. & Cook, DJ. (1999). Crystalloids vs colloids in fluid resuscitation: a systematic review. *Crit Care Med,* Vol. 27, No.1, (January 1999), pp. 200-210, ISSN 0090-3493

De Paepe, P., Belpaire, FM. & Buylaert WA. (2002). Pharmacokinetic and pharmacodynamic considerations when treating patients with sepsis and septic shock. *Clin Pharmacokinetic,* Vol. 41, No.14, (January 2002), pp.1135-1151, ISSN 0312-5963

Dinarello, CA. (2000). Proinflammatory cytokines. *Chest,* Vol.118, No.2, (August 2000), pp.503-508, ISSN 0012-3692

Fagiolino, P., Vázquez, M., Eiraldi, R., Maldonado, C. & Scaramelli, A. (2011). Influence of efflux transporters on drug metabolism. Theoretical approach for bioavalilability and clearance prediction. *Clin Pharmacokinet,* Vol. 50, No. 2, (February 2011), pp. 75-80, ISSN 0312-5963

Fuster-Lluch, O., Gerónimo-Pardo, M., Peyró-García, R. & Lizán-García, M. (2008). Glomerular hyperfiltration and albuminuria in critically ill patients. *Anaesth Intensive Care,* Vol. 36, No.5, (September 2008), pp. 674-680, ISSN 0310-057X

Holmes, CL., Patel, BM., Russell, JA. & Wallay, KR. (2001) Physiology of vasopressin relevant to management of septic shock. *Chest,* Vol. 120, No. 3, (September 2001), pp. 989-1002 ISSN 0012-3692

Ibarra, M., Vázquez, M., Fagiolino, P., Mutilva, F.& Canale, A. (2010). Total, unbound plasma and salivary phenytoin levels in critically ill patients. *J Epilepsy Clin Neurophysiol,* Vol.16, No. 2, (April 2010), pp.69-73, ISSN 1676-2649

James, JK., Palmer, SM., Levine, DP. & Rybak, MJ. (1996). Comparison of conventional dosing versus continuous-infusion vancomycin therapy for patients with suspected or documented gram-positive infections. *Agents Chemother,* Vol. 40, No.3, (March 1996), pp. 696-700, ISSN 0006-4971

Joukhadar, C., Frossard, M., Mayer, BX., Brunner, M., Klein, N., Siostrzonek, P., Eichler, HG. & Muller, M. (2001). Impaired target site penetration of beta-lactams may account for therapeutic failure in patients with septic shock. *Crit Care Med,* Vol. 29, No.2, (February 2001), pp. 385-391, ISSN 0090-3493

Läpple, F., von Richter, O., Fromm, MF., Richter, T., Thon, K., Wisser H., Griese EU., Eichelbaum, M. & Kivistö KT. (2003). Differential expression and function of CYP2C isoforms in human intestine and liver. *Pharmacogenetics,* Vol. 13, No.9, (September 2003), pp. 565-575, ISSN 0960-314X

Letteri, JM., Mellk, H., Louis, S., Kutt, H., Durante, P. & Glasko, A. (1971). Diphenylhydantoin metabolism in uremia. *N Engl J Med,* Vol. 285, (September 1971), pp. 648-652, ISSN 0028-4793

Levy, RH. (1995). Cytochrome P450 isoenzymes and antiepileptic drug interactions. *Epilepsia,* Vol. 36, Suppl.5, (May 1995), pp.:S8-S13, ISSN 0013-9580

Lipman, J., Wallis, SC. & Rickard, C.(1999). Low plasma cefepime levels in critically ill septic patients : pharmacokinetic modeling indicates improved troughs with revised dosing. *Antimicrob Agents Chemother,* Vol.43. No. 10, (October 1999), pp. 2559-2561, ISSN 0066-4804

Lolis, E. & Bucala, R. Therapeutic approaches to innate immunity: severe sepsis and septic shock. (2003).*Nature Reviews Drug Discovery,* Vol. 2, (August 2003), pp. 635-645, ISSN 1474-1776

Lomaestro, BM.& Drusano, GL. (2005). Pharmacodynamic evaluation of extending the administration time of meropenem using Monte Carlo simulation. *Antimicrob Agents Chemother,* Vol. 49, No.1, (January 2005), pp. 461-463, ISSN 0066-4804

Lombardo, L., Pellitteri, R., Balazy, M. & Cardile, V. (2008). Induction of nuclear receptors and drug resistance in the brain microvascular endothelial cells treated with antiepileptic drugs. *Curr Neurovasc Res,*Vol. 5, No. 2, (May 2008), pp. 82-92. ISSN 1567-2026.

Lorente, L., Jimenez, A., Martin, MM., Iribarren, JL., Jimenez, JJ. & Mora, MM. (2009). Clinical cure of ventilator-associated pneumonia treated with piperacillin/tazobactam administered by continuous or intermittent infusion. *Int J Antimicrob Agents,* Vol. 33, No.5, (May 2009), pp. 464-468, ISSN 0924-8579

Maldonado, C., Fagiolino, P., Vázquez, M., Rey, A., Olano, I., Eiraldi, E. & Scavone, C. (2008). Therapeutic carbamazepine (CBZ) and valproic acid (VPA) monitoring in children using saliva as a biologic fluid. *J Epilepsy Clin Neurophysiol,* Vol. 14, No.2, (March 2002), pp. 55-58, ISSN 1676-2649

Maldonado, C., Fagiolino, P., Vázquez, M., Eiraldi, R., Alvariza, S., Bentancour, C. & Alvarez, P. (2011). Time-dependent and concentration-dependent upregulation of carbamazepine efflux transporter. A preliminary assessment from salivary drug monitoring. (2011). *Lat Am J Pharm,* Vol.30, No. 5, (November 2010), pp. 980-912, ISNN 0326-2383

Marik, PF. (1993). Aminoglycoside volume of distribution and illness in critically ill septic patients. *Anaesth Intensive Care,* Vol. 21, No. 2, (April 1993), pp. 172-173, ISSN 0310-057X

Niederman, MS. (2006). Use of broad-spectrum antimicrobials for the treatment of pneumonia in seriously ill patients: maximizing clinical outcomes and minimizing selection of resistant organisms. *Clin Infect Dis,* Vol. 42, Suppl.2, pp. S72-S81, ISSN 1058-4838

Pea, F. & Viale, P. (2009). Bench-to-bedside review: appropriate antibiotic therapy in sever sepsis and septic shock-does the dose matter?. *Crit Care,* Vol. 13, No. 3, (June 2009), 214, ISSN 1364-8535

Petrosillo, N., Drapeau, CM., Agrafiotis, M. & Falagas ME. (2010). Some current issues in the pharmacokinetic/phramacodynamics of antimicrobials in intensive care. *Minerva Anestesiol* , Vol.76 , No.7, (July 2010), pp. 509-524, ISSN 0375-9393

Potschka, H., Fedrowitz, M. & Löscher, W. (2003). Multidrug resistance protein MRP2 contributes to blood-brain barrier function and restricts antiepileptic drug activity. *J Pharmacol Exp Ther,* Vol. 306, No.1, (March 2003), pp. 124-131, ISSN 0022-3565

Reddy, RC., Chen, GH., Tekchandani, PK. & Standiford, TJ. (2001). Sepsis-induced immunosuppression. From bad to worse. *Immunologic Research,* Vol. 24, No. 3, (December 2001), pp.273-288, ISSN 0257-277X

Roberts, JA., Kirkpatrick, CMJ., Roberts, MS., Robertson, TA., Dalley, AJ.& Lipman, J. (2009). Meropenem dosing in critically ill patients with sepsis and without renal dysfunction: intermittent bolus versus continuous administration? Monte Carlo dosing simulations and subcutaneous tissue distribution. *J Antimicrob Chemother,* Vol. 64, No.1, (July 2009), pp.142-150, ISSN 0066-4804

Slatter, JG., Stalker, DJ., Feenstra, KL., Welshman, IR., Bruss, JB., Sams, JP., Johnson, MG., Sanders, PE., Hauer, MJ., Fagerness, PE., Stryd, RP., Peng, GW. & Shobe, EM. (2001). Pharmacokinetics,metabolism, and excretion of linezolid following an oral dose of [^{14} C] linezolid to healthy human volunteers. *Drug Metab and Dispos,* Vol. 29, No.8, (April 2001), pp.1136-1145 ISSN 0090-9556

Taccone, FS., Laterre, PF., Dugernier, T., Spapen, H., Delattre I., Wittebole, X., De Backer, D., Layeux, B., Wallemacq, P., Vincent JL. & Jacobs, F. (2010a). Insufficient β-lactam concentrations in the early phase of severe sepsis and septic shock. *Crit Care,* Vol. 14, No.4, (July 2010), R126, ISSN 1364-8535

Taccone, FS., Laterre, PF., Spapen, H., Dugernier, T., Delattre I., Layeux, B., De Backer, D., Wittebole, X., Wallemacq, P., Vincent JL. & Jacobs, F. (2010b). Revisiting the loading dose of amikacin forpatients with sever sepsis and septic shock. *Crit Care,* Vol.14, No.2, (April 2010), R53, ISSN 1364-8535

Thallinger, C; Buerger, C., Plock, N., Kljucar, S., Wuenscher, S., Sauermann, R., Kloft, C. & Joukhadar, C. (2008). Effect of severity of sepsis on tissue concentrations of linezolid. *J Antimicrobial Chemother,* Vol. 61, No. 1, (January 2008), pp.173-176 ISSN 0305-7453

Vázquez, M., Fagiolino, P., Boronat, A., Buroni, M. & Maldonado, C. (2008). Therapeutic drug monitoring of vancomycin in severe sepsis and septic shock. *Int J Clin Pharmacol Ther,* Vol. 46, No. 3, (March 2008), pp. 140-145, ISSN 0946-1965.

Viaene, E., Chanteux, H., Servais, H., Mingeot-Leclercq, MP. & Tulkens, PM. (2002). Comparative stability studies of antipseudomonal beta-lactams for potential administration through portable elastomeric pumps (home therapy for cystic fibrosis patients) and motor-operated syringes (intensive care units). *Antimicrob Agents Chemother,* Vol. 46, No.8, (August 2002), pp. 2327-2332, ISSN 0066-4804

Wagenlehner, FME., Wydra, S., Onda, H., Kinzig-Schippers, M., Sörgel, F. & Naber KG. (2003). Concentrations in plasma, urinary excretion, and bactericidal activity of linezolid (600 milligrams) versus those of ciprofloxacin (500 milligrams) in healthy volunteers receiving a single oral dose. *Antimicrob Agents Chemother,*Vol. 47, No.12, (December 2003), pp. 3789-3794, ISSN 0066-4804

Zilberberg, MD., Shorr, AF., Micek, ST., Mody, SH. & Kollef, MH. (2008). Antimicrobial therapy escalation and hospital mortality among patients with health-care-associated pneumonia: a single center experience. *Chest,* Vol. 134, No. 5, (July 2008), pp. 963-68, ISSN 0012-3692

Part 5

Management

10

Management of Severe Sepsis and Septic Shock

Georges Samaha[1], Brian Casserly[2] and John-Michael Stevens[1]
[1]*University of Limerick*
[2]*Brown University - Rhode Island*
[1]*Ireland*
[2]*USA*

1. Introduction

Severe sepsis (systemic inflammation secondary to infection combined with acute organ dysfunction) and septic shock (severe sepsis combined with hypotension not rectified by fluid resuscitation) are complex multifactorial medical conditions with significant associated morbidity and mortality, and are among the leading causes of death in the intensive care unit (ICU). Even with aggressive treatment, the mortality has been shown to be around 40 percent (Bernard et al., 1997) and in some studies has been reported to be as high as 71.9 percent (Sasse et al., 1995).

In 2001, Angus et al conducted a study of the incidence, cost, and outcome of severe sepsis in the United States of America; the results showed an incidence of 3 cases per 1,000 population, a mortality rate of 28.6 percent, and a cost of $22,100 per case, giving an annual cost of $16.7 billion (Angus et al., 2001). The same study showed that the number of deaths per year associated with severe sepsis is equal to that of acute myocardial infarction, yet myocardial infarction has attracted far more attention and funding in terms of treatment and management research, leaving sepsis a relatively unacknowledged problem. With severe sepsis having such a high incidence, high and increasing mortality rate, and high annual cost, it is becoming a prime target for research into improving diagnosis, management, and survival.

Reducing morbidity and mortality in severe sepsis and septic shock has been the primary goal of the Surviving Sepsis Campaign (SSC) - a global initiative developed by the European Society of Intensive Care Medicine (ESICM), the International Sepsis Forum (ISF), and the Society of Critical Care Medicine (SCCM) to raise awareness of sepsis among healthcare professionals and to improve and standardize the early diagnosis and treatment of sepsis (Welcome To The Surviving Sepsis Campaign Website,n.d.). Containing a number of the world's experts on sepsis, this campaign attempts to tackle various challenges in the diagnosis and management of sepsis. Some of the challenges lie in the complexity of the condition and the variability in the presentation and course of sepsis, with many of the symptoms being of a general nature and easily attributable to a number of other conditions and etiologies. This makes it quite difficult to create a standard clinical definition of sepsis. This lack of definitive criteria for a diagnosis of sepsis makes it easily misdiagnosed, and consequently improperly treated. If, however, a diagnosis of sepsis is made, it is often still made late and treatment is less effective if delayed. As is discussed later in this chapter,

Disorder	Criteria
Systemic Inflammatory Response Syndrome (SIRS)	At least two of the following: • Body temperature >38.5°C or <35.0°C • Heart rate >90 beats per minute • Respiratory rate >20 breaths per minute or $PaCO_2$<32 mmHg or a need for mechanical ventilation • White blood cell count >12,000/mm^3 or <4,000/mm^3 or immature forms >10 percent
Sepsis	<u>SIRS</u> PLUS: documented infection based on either of the following: • Culture or Gram stain of blood, sputum, urine, or normally sterile body fluid positive for pathogenic microorganism • Focus of infection identified by visual inspection (e.g. a ruptured bowel with free air or bowel contents found in abdomen at surgery, or a wound with purulent discharge)
Severe Sepsis	<u>Sepsis</u> PLUS at least one of the following signs of organ hypoperfusion or organ dysfunction: • Areas of mottled skin • Capillary refill time ≥3s • Urinary output <0.5mL/kg for at least 1 hour or renal replacement therapy • Lactic acid levels >2mmol/L • Abrupt change in mental status or abnormal electroencephalogram (EEG) • Platelet counts <100,000/mL or disseminated intravascular coagulation (DIC) • Acute lung injury (ALI) or acute respiratory distress syndrome (ARDS) • Cardiac dysfunction (echocardiography)
Septic Shock	<u>Severe sepsis</u> PLUS at least one of the following: • Systemic mean blood pressure<60mmHg(<80mmHg if previous hypertension) after 20–30 mL/kg starch or 40–60 mL/kg serum saline, or pulmonary capillary wedge pressure between 12 and 20 mm Hg • Need for dopamine >5 μg/kg per minute or norepinephrine or epinephrine<0.25μg/kg per minute to maintain mean blood pressure above 60 mm Hg (80 mm Hg if previous hypertension)

Table 1. Definitions of diseases relevant to sepsis (adapted from Annane et al., 2005)

early diagnosis and early treatment are key to reducing morbidity and mortality in sepsis; and as such, it is advised to begin treatment while a diagnosis is being confirmed.

In 2004, the first set of SSC guidelines was published, providing clinicians with an internationally recognized bedside tool for diagnosing and treating sepsis. In 2008, an update to these guidelines was published, adding 33 new recommendations to the original 52 published in 2004 (Vincent, 2008). The updated recommendations were based on the results of a new method of assessing the quality of evidence and the strength of recommendations based on that evidence (Dellinger et al., 2008). The guidelines, however, are strictly guidelines, and as sepsis is so variable in etiology and presentation, these guidelines should not be seen to supersede the clinician's opinions or decisions when the entire patient's condition is taken into account.

2. Bundle treatment

The idea of bundled care has found its place in the management of severe sepsis and septic shock. Bundles are evidence-based collections of interventions that result in more favorable outcomes when administered together rather than separately. In severe sepsis and septic shock, two bundles are recommended by the SSC - a Sepsis Resuscitation Bundle (containing five elements) and a Sepsis Management Bundle (containing four elements) the first of which are intended to be completed 100 percent within the first six hours of treatment and the second is to be completed within the first 24 hours (Severe Sepsis Bundles, n.d.). The aim of the SSC to reduce mortality by 25 percent by 2009 has not been achieved but initial publications suggest significant improvements in mortality with increasing bundle compliance (Severe Sepsis Bundles, n.d.; Levy et al., 2010).

2.1 Sepsis resuscitation bundle

This bundle has 5 elements:

1. Measure Serum Lactate
2. Obtain blood cultures prior to antibiotic administration
3. Administer broad-spectrum antibiotic within 3 hours of Emergency Department (ED) admission and within 1 hour of non-ED admission
4. Treat hypotension and/or elevated lactate with fluids, and apply vasopressors for ongoing hypotension
5. Maintain adequate central venous pressure (CVP) and central venous oxygen saturation (ScvO2)

(Severe Sepsis Bundles, n.d.)

Each element is discussed in this chapter.

2.2 Sepsis management bundle

This bundle has 4 elements:

1. Administer low-dose steroids for septic shock
2. Administer recombinant human activated protein C (rhAPC)
3. Maintain glucose control with a goal blood glucose approximating 150 mg/dl with a recommendation against intravenous insulin therapy titrated to keep blood glucose in the normal range (80-110 mg/dl) in patients with severe sepsis. Clinicians should consider initiating insulin therapy when blood glucose levels exceed 180 mg/dL
4. Maintain a median inspiratory plateau pressure (IPP) <30 cm H20 for mechanically ventilated patients

(Severe Sepsis Bundles, n.d.)

Each element is discussed in this chapter.

3. Primary management of sepsis

Morbidity and mortality can be greatly reduced with prompt recognition, diagnosis, and treatment of severe sepsis and septic shock(Dellinger et al., 2008; Sessler et al., 2004). There is strong evidence that will be further discussed in detail, indicating that the onset of treatment has a direct affect on the outcome of disease. The initial goals are to stabilize any respiratory dysfunction and then to promptly assess and address deficits in tissue and organ perfusion in order to avoid or minimize multiple organ damage.

3.1 Stabilize respiration (mechanical ventilation)

As with any emergency, it is crucial to ensure there is sufficient respiration before addressing other issues. Oxygen should be administered early to patients with severe sepsis or septic shock, and it is often necessary to intubate and ventilate patients in the presence of significant CNS depression.

Investigations for acute lung injury (ALI) or acute respiratory distress syndrome (ARDS) should be performed once respiratory stabilization is established. In patients with ALI or ARDS, it is suggested that positive end-expiratory pressure ventilation be used to prevent lung collapse at end-expiration although evidence from randomized controlled trials (RCTs) for this recommendation is lacking (Villar et al., 2006).

During mechanical ventilation of patients with ARDS, traditional tidal volume targets (10 ml per kilogram of body weight to 15 ml per kilogram of body weight) have been implicated in potential stretch-induced lung injury, while targeting low tidal volumes has been shown to prevent further injury to the lungs (Acute Respiratory Distress Syndrome Network, 2000). The Acute Respiratory Distress Syndrome Network coordinated a large multicenter trial indicating that low tidal volume mechanical ventilation used in the presence of acute lung injury reduced mortality rates from 39.8 percent in the standard tidal volume group to 31 percent in the low tidal volume mechanical ventilation group (relative reduction in mortality rate of 22.1 percent; 95 percent CI for the absolute difference between groups 2.4 percent to 15.3 percent) (Acute Respiratory Distress Syndrome Network, 2000). This trial involved randomly allocating patients with acute lung injury into one of two groups: low mechanical ventilation tidal volumes (6 ml per kilogram of predicted body weight) or standard mechanical ventilation tidal volumes (12 ml per kilogram of predicted body weight). In the low tidal volume group, plateau airway pressures measured at the end of inspiration were kept to ≤30 cm of water, whereas the standard tidal volume group, airway plateau pressures were restricted to ≤50 cm of water (Acute Respiratory Distress Syndrome Network, 2000).

3.2 Assessment of perfusion

Hypoperfusion is a major contributing factor to the overall progression to multiple organ failure in septic shock (Casserly et al., 2009); therefore assessing perfusion is critical in management of severe sepsis and septic shock. Hypoperfusion often presents with cool extremities, oliguria, reduced pulse pressure, altered mental status, tachycardia, and high blood urea nitrogen to creatinine ratio; however these signs can be influenced by drugs and/or coincident disease, so their absence should not preclude perfusion assessment. In terms of assessment, blood pressure (BP) is a commonly used indicator of perfusion, however the sphygmomanometer has been shown to be potentially unreliable in hypotensive patients, and as such, arterial catheterization is recommended for assessment of perfusion (Hanna, 2003; Finnie et al., 1984; Cohn, 1967).

3.3 Restoration of perfusion

The inflammatory response associated with severe sepsis and septic shock is characterized by increased capillary permeability (resulting in leakage of plasma into the interstitial space) and decreased vasomotor tone, leading to decreased venous return to the heart (Snell and Parrillo, 1991) and ultimately a decreased cardiac output (Parrillo, 1993; Barochia et al., 2010). The consequence is hypoperfusion of organs and tissues. Typically, there is a sympathetic response - inducing tachycardia and increased arterial vasomotor tone; however, in severe sepsis and septic shock, there is often an attenuated vascular response (Parrillo, 1993). Since organ dysfunction or failure resulting from hypoperfusion is a major contributor to morbidity and mortality in severe sepsis and septic shock, prompt correction of hypoperfusion, once identified, is essential. The SSC guidelines "recommend... the protocolized resuscitation of a patient with sepsis-induced shock, defined as tissue hypoperfusion (hypotension persisting after initial fluid challenge or blood lactate concentration ≥4 mmol/L)... as soon as [it] is recognized" (Dellinger et al., 2008).

3.3.1 Central or mixed venous oxyhemoglobin saturation

Central or mixed venous oxyhemoglobin saturation (ScvO2 and SvO2, respectively) can be used as a measure to gauge perfusion restoration. Low mixed venous oxyhemoglobin saturation has linked to undesirable outcomes in patients with septic shock (Edwards, 1991). In 2004, Reinhart et al conducted a prospective descriptive study during which they compared the values of central and mixed venous oxygen saturations in critically ill patients. Their results showed that ScvO2 and ScO2 paralleled each other quite reliably, with ScvO2 measuring consistently about 7 saturation percent higher (Reinhart et al., 2004). Since SvO2 measurement requires the insertion of a Swan-Ganz catheter it is therefore a more invasive measurement than ScvO2. Therefore the fact that, in most cases of severe sepsis, these values change in parallel is a welcome discovery (Bauer et al., 2008). The SSC guidelines recommend an ScvO2 or ScO2 of ≥70 percent or ≥65 percent, respectively (Dellinger et al., 2008). Additionally, they recommend targeting a mean arterial pressure (MAP) of ≥65mm Hg and a urine output of ≥0.5 mL $\cdot kg^{-1} \cdot hr^{-1}$ (Dellinger et al., 2008).

In 2001, Rivers et al conducted a randomized controlled study of 263 patients to evaluate the efficacy, in terms of mortality reduction, of early goal-directed therapy (EGDT) administered prior to admission to the ICU. The aim of the study was to determine whether targeting a ScvO2 or SvO2 of ≥70 percent or ≥65 percent, respectively, in the first six hours post-admission would reduce mortality in patients presenting with severe sepsis and septic shock (Rivers et al., 2001). The results of this study showed a 30.5 percent in-hospital mortality in the early goal-directed therapy group as compared to an in-hospital mortality of 46.5 percent in the standard therapy group (Rivers et al., 2001), a 16 percent mortality reduction. In the time following the therapy up to three days post-presentation, the EGDT patients had a "higher mean (+/-SD) central venous oxygen saturation... lower lactate concentration... lower base deficit... and a higher pH" than the patients in the standard therapy group" (Rivers et al., 2001), indicating that the EGDT is significantly beneficial in the treatment of patients presenting with severe sepsis or septic shock.

As noted by Perel et al, many of the results obtained by Rivers at al, in their 2001 study, may not apply to patients in less severe sepsis. Perel states that "compared with other populations of septic patients, the patients of Rivers and colleagues had a higher incidence of severe comorbidities, a more severe hemodynamic status on admission (excessively low central venous oxygen saturation [ScvO2], low central venous pressure [CVP], and high lactate), and higher mortality rates" (Perel, 2008). Also, in sepsis, it has been shown that SvO2 may be raised even in the presence of tissue hypoxia. This implies that the ScvO2 may sometimes be unreliable in targeted resuscitation (Perel, 2008; Bellomo et al., 2008). Another concern, proposed by Reinhart and Bloos, is the reversal of the physiologic difference between ScvO2 and SvO2 that can be observed in the state of cardiocirculatory shock resulting from reduced mesenteric blood flow followed by an increase of O2 extraction in these organs. Consequently, this lowers venous saturation in the mesenteric circulation and, subsequently, the inferior vena cava. In healthy humans, the oxygen saturation in the inferior vena cava is higher than in the superior vena cava. But, in shock, when blood is diverted from the gut to other vital organs the oxygen saturation in the inferior vena may be substantially reduced. Since the pulmonary artery contains a mixture of blood from both the superior as well as the inferior vena cava, SvO2 is normally greater than the oxygen saturation in the superior vena cava but this can be reversed during shock due to venous desaturation in the mesenteric circulation and the inferior vena cava (Reinhart and Bloos, 2005).

3.3.2 Lactic acid clearance

Using lactic acid clearance has been proposed as an alternative to measuring ScvO2 and SvO2 for assessing restoration of perfusion where ScvO2/SvO2 monitoring may be unavailable; however, there is evidence that using both ScvO2/SvO2 and lactic acid clearance may be appropriate (Arnold et al., 2009). During sepsis, tissue hypoxia causes an increase in cellular lactic acid production that diffuses into the blood (Arnold et al., 2009). It has been shown that a rise in lactic acid levels in the blood is associated with increased morbidity and mortality, and a decrease in blood lactic acid is associated with better, in patients with septic shock (Bakker et al., 1991).

A recent multicenter randomized non-inferiority study by Jones et al was conducted to evaluate whether using lactic acid clearance as an EGDT target was as efficacious as using ScvO2. This study looked at 300 patients, where one randomly selected group was administered EGDT targeting a lactic acid clearance of 10 percent and the other was given EGDT targeting an ScvO2 of 70 percent (Jones et al., 2010). Both groups were resuscitated to normalize both CVP and MAP (Jones et al., 2010). The results showed the in-hospital mortality of the "ScvO2" group to be 23 % (95 % Confidence Interval [CI], 17 % - 30 %) and the "lactic acid clearance" group to be 17 percent (95 % CI, 11 % - 24 %) (Jones et al., 2010). This supported the non-inferiority hypothesis, as there was no significant difference in in-hospital mortality between the two groups.

In a 2004 prospective observational study by Nguyen et al, the clinical utility of lactic acid clearance was assessed. The researches observed the lactic acid clearance over the initial 6 hours of treatment and predicted that a high lactic acid clearance would correlate with higher in-hospital survival. They showed that "there was an approximately 11 percent decrease likelihood of mortality for each 10 percent increase in lactate clearance" (Nguyen et al., 2004).

A more recent study by Arnold et al investigated the association between early lactate clearance and severe sepsis patient survival (Arnold et al., 2009). Of the 166 patients, lactic acid non-clearance was evident in 15. The mortality rate for those 15 was 60 percent, whereas the mortality rate for the lactic acid clearance patients was 19 percent. Interestingly, this same study showed "discordance between ScvO2 optimization and lactate clearance; 79 percent of lactate non-clearance had concomitant ScvO2 of 70 percent or greater" (Arnold et al., 2009). They concluded that failing to clear lactic acid was associated with a high risk of death, and that attaining an ScvO2 of 70 percent or greater did not rule out lactic acid non-clearance, indicating that ScvO2 optimization alone may not be a sufficient target to reduce mortality in the early stages of severe sepsis and septic shock (Arnold et al., 2009).

3.3.3 Central venous pressure (CVP)

Central venous pressure has long been used as a determinant of central venous blood volume or right ventricular preload in critically ill patients requiring hemodynamic monitoring. The validity of these correlations, however, has been brought to question. In 2004, Kumar et al conducted a prospective, nonrandomized, non-blinded interventional study evaluating the correlation between pulmonary artery occlusion pressure (Ppao) and left ventricular preload and between CVP and right ventricular preload; the results of this study indicate that "neither central venous pressure nor pulmonary artery occlusion pressure appears to be a useful predictor of ventricular preload with respect to optimizing cardiac performance" (Kumar et al., 2004). The SSC guidelines, however, still recommend targeting resuscitation to a CVP of 8-12mm Hg (Dellinger et al., 2008).

3.3.4 Intravenous fluids

Hypovolemia is a commonly present in systemic inflammation, and is defined as an insufficient blood plasma volume. It is associated with tachycardia, hypotension, and hypoperfusion, and can further complicate severe sepsis and septic shock. Early and aggressive fluid resuscitation has been shown to greatly reduce morbidity and mortality in sepsis, and the evidence produced by Rivers et al in 2001 indicates that the administration of approximately 1.5L more fluids than standard treatments in the first 6 hours may confer benefit in the form of reduction of morbidity or mortality (Rivers et al., 2001). It is recommended that specific goals and endpoints bet set, treatment be titrated to these targets, and ongoing evaluations of the results be made by assessing perfusion (Hollenberg et al., 2004; Hollenberg, 2009). Worthy of note, is that CVP is not a good predictor of responsiveness to fluid resuscitation, and should not be used to guide treatment (Marik et al., 2008; Perel, 2008). Fluid resuscitation should be continued until hypotension and hypoperfusion are resolved, but should be discontinued or adjusted at the onset of pulmonary edema.

In term of the particular type of fluid used in resuscitation, a systematic review by Choi et al indicates that although resuscitation with crystalloids is associated with an overall lower mortality in trauma patients, there is no significant difference between crystalloid and colloid resuscitation in other patients (Choi et al., 1999). Also, in a multicenter, randomized, double blind trial comparing fluid resuscitation with albumin versus saline on patients in the ICU, Finfer et al found no difference in mortality (Finfer et al., 2004). In 2001, Wilkes and Navickis conducted a meta-analysis of randomized controlled trials to determine if human albumin administration was associated with increased mortality. Their findings were that there was no affect on mortality with the use of albumin, and therefor conclude that albumin use is safe (Wilkes et al., 2001). One recent multicenter two-by-two factorial trial evaluated the safety of pentastarch, a low-molecular-weight hydroxyethyl starch, in the fluid resuscitation of severe sepsis patients. Treatment of either pentastarch (a colloid) or Ringer's lactate (a crystalloid) was given to patients as fluid for resuscitation. In the HES group, there was a higher incidence of renal failure and a higher rate of renal-replacement therapy than in the group resuscitate with Ringer's lactate (Brunkhorst et al., 2008). So with the exception of pentastarch, it seems that thus far the choice of fluids, whether crystalloid or colloid is insignificant as far as safety and efficacy is concerned, and as far as fluid resuscitation is concerned, early and aggressive treatment is the key to reducing morbidity and mortality in severe sepsis and septic shock.

3.3.5 Vasopressors

Occasionally, fluid resuscitation does not sufficiently reverse the hemodynamic and metabolic abnormalities associated with septic shock, and intravenous vasopressor therapy can be used to augment treatment effectively. When the MAP falls low enough, auto-regulation can fail causing tissues to rely strictly on pressure for perfusion (Dellinger et al., 2008). Maintaining a minimum MAP of 65 mmHg has been shown to provide sufficient tissue perfusion (LeDoux et al., 2000). Ideally, *'fluid resuscitation'* alone is favorable over *'fluid resuscitation plus vasopressor therapy'*, so vasopressors should be utilized as second-line tools and used only when necessary. A true consensus has not been reached as to which specific vasopressor is most effective, and research into vasopressor therapy in severe sepsis and septic shock is ongoing (Hollenberg, 2009). As shown in Table 2, the various vasopressive agents have differing adrenergic affects (Schmidt, 2011b), and each case of severe sepsis or septic shock has its own characterisitics, it is difficult to determine which drug is most appropriate (Myburgh et al., 2008); however, De Backer et al, in a recent multicenter randomized trial, showed that norepinephrine and dopamine were equivalent in reducing mortality in patients suffering from shock, but treatment with dopamine was associated with a significantly increased incidence of cardiac arrhythmias (De Backer et al., 2010), hypercalcemia, and decreased splanchnic circulation (Agrawal et al., 2010). Russell et al performed a multicenter randomized double-blind trial to determine the value of treatment with vasopressin in septic shock as compared to treatment with norepinephrine. The results indicated that there was no difference in the 28-day post-initiation mortality

Drug	Effect on Heart Rate	Effect on Contractility	Effects on Arterial Constriction
Dobutamine	+	+++	- (dilates)
Dopamine	++	++	++
Epinephrine	+++	+++	++
Norepinephrine	++	++	+++
Phenylephrine	0	0	+++
Amrinone	+	+++	-- (dilates)

Table 2. Vasopressors used in the treatment of septic shock (adapted from Schmidt, 2011b)

or the 90-day post-initiation mortality between the two groups (Russell et al., 2008). Also, there was no statistically significant difference in the incidence of adverse events (Russell et al., 2008). It is recommend in the SSC guidelines that the MAP is maintained at a minimum of 65 mmHg and either intravenous norepinephrine or intravenous dopamine be administered as the initial vasopressor to combat hypotension in patients with septic shock–with epinephrine being the first choice alternative vasopressive agent in patients who do not respond to norepinephrine or dopamine (Dellinger et al., 2008). In a recent animal study by Boyd et al, however, it was shown that treatment with vasopressin could decrease sepsis-induced pulmonary inflammation. They showed that with the intraperitoneal introduction of lipopolysaccharide (LPS) there was consequent systemic and pulmonary inflammation - indicated by significant rises in both lung and serum interleukin-6 (IL-6; an inflammatory mediator) (Boyd et al., 2008). Two test groups were created - the test groups was treated with LPS and vasopressin, and the control group was treated with LPS and saline. With intraperitoneal LPS and vasopressin, the levels of both lung and serum IL-6 were reduced, whereas in the LPS and saline group, the LPS levels were raised as expected (Boyd et al., 2008). Pretreatment of the LPS and vasopressin group with V2R antagonists (agents which block the vasopressin receptor responsible for this protective effect) lead to similar rises in IL-6, as seen in the saline-treated mice (Boyd et al., 2008), indicating that vasopressin exerted its protective effects via the V2R receptor. These results suggest that vasopressin could have a potential future role as first line vasopressor in treating severe sepsis with acute lung injury.

3.3.6 Additional strategies

If all efforts with fluid resuscitation and vasopressor therapy fail to maintain a sufficient ScvO2, other strategies, such as inotrope therapy and transfusion of blood products, can be employed to attempt to reach acceptable pressure and perfusion targets. The SSC guidelines indicate that if the ScvO2 has not reached ≥70 percent (65 percent for SvO2) with fluid resuscitation to the CVP target, they recommend the administration of a dobutamine infusion and/or the transfusion of packed red blood cells to achieve a hematocrit of ≥30 percent to reach an acceptable ScvO2 or SvO2 (Dellinger, 2008).

3.3.6.1 Inotropes

Reserved for those patients not responding sufficiently to the above-mentioned interventions (attaining a ScvO2 of ≥70 mmHg via fluid resuscitation and vasopressor therapy), inotropes can be used to increase the force of cardiac contraction and consequently increase cardiac output, blood pressure, and tissue and organ perfusion. Dobutamine is the recommended inotrope for patients in septic shock with coexistent myocardial dysfunction (Dellinger et al., 2008). Dobutamine is a drug that was developed by modifying the structure of isoproterenol, another inotrope, to reduce its chronotropic, arrhythmogenic, and vascular side effects while maintaining its inotropic effects(Tuttle and Mills, 1975). It is often used in cardiogenic shock, acting on β1 and β2 adrenergic receptors, but minimally on α1 receptors. This profile accounts for its inotropic effects (β1 activity), its reduction of afterload (β2 activity), and its 'lack of vasoconstriction' or even 'mild vasodilation' effects (minimal α1 activity) allowing it to enhance flow and the distribution of flow (Shoemaker et al., 1991). Occasionally, at low doses, dobutamine can cause a drop in blood pressure due to the vasodilation, however increasing cardiac output at higher dobutamine doses tends to override the drop in vascular resistance and blood pressure rises.

In a trial performed by Gattinoni et al, it was shown that targeting a cardiac index of supranormal levels did not confer a lower mortality rate among patients (Gattinoni et al., 1995), and therefor it is advised against pursuing such targets (Dellinger et al., 2008). Further supporting this recommendation are the results from a randomized trial performed by Hayes et al to determine whether dobutamine infusion, targeting a cardiac index greater than 4.5 liters per minute per square meter of body-surface area, an oxygen delivery rate above 600 ml per minute per square meter of body-surface area, and an oxygen consumption rate of above 170 ml per minute per square meter of body-surface area, would be associated with improved outcome for a group of critically ill patients (Hayes et al., 1994).

In this study, the results indicated that boosting the cardiac index and systemic oxygen delivery with a dobutamine infusion was, in some cases, actually detrimental to the patients, based on the in-hospital mortality rate being 34 percent in the control group and 54 percent in the treatment group (an absolute mortality increase of 20 percent) (Hayes et al., 1994).

3.3.6.2 Blood product transfusions

There are conflicting data regarding the use of packed red blood cell transfusions used to raise the ScvO2 in septic shock (Vincent et al., 2008; Rivers et al., 2001; Fuller et al., 2010). The SSC guidelines recommend treatment with packed red blood cell transfusion and/or intravenous dobutamine to treat patients whose ScvO2 levels are inadequately responsive to fluid resuscitation and vasopressor therapy (Dellinger et al., 2008). This is based on the fact that the combination of fluid resuscitation, packed red blood cells, and intravenous dobutamine was associated with improved outcomes in severe sepsis and septic shock. It has been suggested, however, that the improved outcomes may be the result of the fluid resuscitation, dobutamine therapy, or other interventions included in the EGDT, and may have no link to the packed red blood cell transfusion itself.

In 2007, Sakr et al performed a prospective observational study to determine whether microvascular alterations participated in the development of multi-organ failure in severe sepsis. They set out to investigate the effect that red blood cell transfusions had on the microvascular perfusion of organs, using sublingual perfusion as their model. Their results showed that red blood cell transfusion had no significant effect on sublingual microcirculation in patients with severe sepsis, except for those with an altered baseline capillary perfusion (Sakr et al., 2007).

Recently, in a retrospective cohort study by Fuller et al, further evidence supports caution in the use of blood product transfusion in severe sepsis or septic shock. In this study, two groups were retrospectively compared - one treated with packed red blood cells and one treated without (Fuller et al., 2010). The pack red blood cell group produced a higher mortality (41.2 percent as compared to 33.9 percent in the group treated without red cells - an absolute mortality increase of 7.3 percent with red cell treatment) (Fuller et al., 2010). They also required more than double the mechanical ventilation days, more than double the hospital length of stay, and more than triple the ICU length of stay (Fuller et al., 2010).

4. Control of the septic focus

SSC recommends properly obtaining at least two sets of blood cultures, from two different sites, drawn prior to beginning antimicrobial therapy in order to aid treatment and to narrow antibiotic coverage (Dellinger et al., 2004; Dellinger et al., 2008). Cultures should also be taken from any other potential source of infection including body fluids, tissues, and indwelling catheters.

4.1 Identification of the septic focus

Cultures should be drawn prior to antimicrobial therapy so that to narrow antibiotic coverage and aid treatment. The SSC recommends proper identification of a pathogen, obtaining a least two sets of blood cultures from two different sites, as well as other potential source of infection (catheters, tissues, and body fluids). Patients presenting with severe sepsis should always be evaluated for the presence of a focus of infection, specifically the debridement of infected necrotic tissue, the drainage of an abscess or local focus of infection, the removal of a potentially infected device, or the definitive control of a source of ongoing microbial contamination (Jimenez and Marshall, 2001).

4.2 Eradication of infection

Since the infection is the main triggering event of sepsis, early identification and successful eradication of the responsible organism should be a prime focus.

4.2.1 Source control

Built on an understanding of the biology of inflammation and the natural history of infectious processes, a clinician can provide an adequate set of management options. Source control includes physical measures used to control a focus of invasive infection and to restore the optimal function of the affected area and quality of life. Table 3 illustrates many options for source control including debridement, drainage, device removal or more invasive steps. Studies supporting the various options for source control in reducing mortality would be difficult to conduce. Therefore, factors such as the current condition of the patient and past surgical and medical history should be taken into consideration when tailoring therapeutic and management options for source control to the individual patient (Houck et al., 2004). The present SSC guidelines recommend making a diagnosis in a septic patient requiring source control within six hours of presentation (Dellinger et al., 2008).

Source	Treatment
Sinusitis	Surgical decompression of the sinuses
Pneumonia	Chest physiotherapy, suctioning
Empyema thoracis	Drainage, decortication
Mediastinitis	Drainage, debridement, diversion
Peritonitis	Resection, repair, or diversion of ongoing sources of contamination, drainage of abscesses, debridement of necrotic tissue
Cholangitis	Bile duct decompression
Pancreatic infection	Drainage or debridement
Urinary tract	Drainage of abscesses, relief of obstruction, removal or changing of infected catheters
Catheter-related bacteremia	Removal of catheter
Endocarditis	Valve replacement
Septic arthritis	Joint drainage and debridement
Soft tissue infection	Debridement of necrotic tissue and drainage of discrete abscesses
Prosthetic device infection	Device removal

Table 3. Methods of source control for common ICU infections (adapted from Schmidt, 2011a)

4.2.2 Antimicrobial regimen

A retrospective study, of over 18,000 patient admitted with community acquired pneumonia, concluded that if antibiotics were given within 4 hours of arrival at the hospital, a significant reduction in in-hospital and 30 day mortality occurred (Houck et al., 2004). Another large multi-center retrospective cohort study reached the conclusion that in 2,731 patients with persistent or refractory hypotension, each hour of delay in the administration of appropriate antibiotics was associated with a 7.6 % mean decrease in survival. The same study found that if antibiotics were administered within 30 minutes of the first occurrence of hypotension, survival rate was 83 % but declined to 42 % when antibiotics were not administered until the sixth hour after first documentation of hypotension (Kumar et al., 2006). The relationship between the timing of administration of antibiotics, was further supported by Gaieski and colleagues who found that there was a 13.7 % decrease in mortality in 261 septic patients presenting to a single urban academic medical department, when appropriate antibiotics were given to septic patient within one hour of triage compared with more then 1 hour of triage (Gaieski et al., 2010;Zubert et al., 2010; Dellinger et al., 2008).

Appropriate initial choice of antibiotic coverage is an independent predictor of survival in patients with sepsis. Gaieski and Colleagues, used a recent retrospective cohort study to demonstrate that patients who received appropriate antibiotics, as prescribed by an institution specific antibiotic nomogram, compared to those who did not receive appropriate antibiotics, had a reduction of 17.5 % in mortality rates (Gaieski et al., 2010; Zubert et al., 2010). Other studies found a significantly increased relative risk of death of 2.18 if patients originally received inadequate antibiotic coverage in the UCU for bloodstream infections (Ibrahim et al., 2000). Another challenge to the appropriate and well-times administration of antimicrobial is the increasing drug resistant pathogens. In a 760 patients retrospective study, Micek et al found that patients who received initial combination therapy involving gram-negative bacteria had a significantly lower rates (36 %) as opposed to patients that did not (52 %) (Micek et al., 2010). Almost all evidence for timely and appropriate antibiotic use stem from cohort studies, it is therefore possible that the relationship with regards to mortality, timely and appropriate antibiotics management might be indirect and represent a surrogate marker for other components of quality care. The SSC recommends timely and appropriate empiric antibiotic therapy that has known susceptibility for all possible pathogens (Dellinger et al., 2008).

5. Additional therapies

Based on the personalized needs of the patient, several additional therapies, when appropriate, are considered for the management and treatment of a septic patient. These include therapies such as recombinant human activated protein C, steroids, nutrition and intensive insulin therapy. Strong evidence, discussed below, show benefits in improving patient outcomes and quality of life.

5.1 Recombinant human activated protein C (rhAPC)

Administration of Recombinant Human activated Protein C (rhAPC) has been linked to a significant reduction in mortality in patients with a relatively high likelihood of death (Fourrier, 2004). Produced by the liver and activated in the circulation, Protein C acts by cleavage and inhibition of factors Va and VIIIa therefore functioning as a natural anticoagulant. Activated protein C (APC) plays an essential role in inflammation by inhibiting thrombin generation and maintaining the permeability of blood vessel walls. Conversely, endogenous levels of activated protein C are markedly reduced in sepsis and are associated with poor outcome (Shorr et al., 2006; He et al., 2007; Fisher and Yan, 2000). The PROWESS study, where 1690 patients with severe sepsis were randomized to rhAPC infusion for 96 hours or placebo had to be aborted early for efficacy after an absolute risk reduction of death of 6.1 percent with the administration of rhAPC was demonstrated

(Bernard et al., 2001). Later sub-group analysis of the PROWESS study found that the highest reduction in mortality rate with the administration of rhAPC was in patients with multi-system organ failure or very high risk of death defined by Acute Physiology and Chronic Health Evaluation (APACHE) II score of 25 or greater (Beutler, 2004). Another safety study (ENHANCE) found a very similar reduction in mortality rate and that administration within the first twenty-four hours was indeed associated with a higher reduction in mortality (Levy et al., 2005). ADDRESS, another open-label safety study of 2640 patient with sepsis and a low risk of death were randomized to rhAPC or placebo. It was concluded that there were no reduction in mortality in patients with severe sepsis with a low likelihood of death (Abraham et al., 2005). A non-randomized propensity-matched analysis of 33,749 patients with severe sepsis, found a significant reduction in hospital mortality with the administration of rhAPC (Lindenauer et al., 2010). These findings led to the current recommendation from the SSC guidelines to use rhAPC for patients with sepsis with high risk of death if there are no contraindications (Dellinger et al., 2008). Although these are still the current SSC guidelines, recombinant human activated protein C has recently been withdrawn from the market due to lack of efficacy.

5.2 Steroids

Adrenal insufficiency is a common feature of sepsis. Adrenal dysfunction is found in about 30 percent of all critically ill patients, and this percentage rises to 50 to 60 percent in septic shock (Annane and Bellissant, 2000). The presence of adrenal insufficiency in septic shock patient has been associated with higher mortality rates (Annane and Bellissant, 2000). Nevertheless, the benefit of administering exogenous steroids in septic shock remains a controversy. Good evidence has shown that administration of high dose corticosteroids (>300 mg hydrocortisone per day) has no mortality benefit and in fact might even lead to increased mortality (Bone et al., 1987; Minneci et al., 2004). The utility of low dose corticosteroid in reducing mortality is however less controversial (<300 mg hydrocortisone per day). Annanne and colleagues randomized 300 septic patients in 19 French ICUs unresponsive to vasopressor therapy with a positive cosytropin stimulation test to low-dose hydrocortisone and fludrocotisone or placebo. They concluded that patients initially unresponsive to vasopressors with a positive cosytropin stimulation test randomized to low-dose hydrocortisone and fludrocotisone had a significantly lower mortality rate (Annane et al., 2002). According to the Corticosteroid Therapy for Septic Shock (CORTICUS) study, a subsequent multi-country trial of 499 patients showed no reduction in mortality in the group that received hydrocortisone compared to placebo. It is difficult to compare these two trials as the CORTICUS study included patients with septic shock irrespective of whether their blood pressure responded initially to vasopressors(Sprung et al., 2008). A recent randomized control trial found that adding fludrocotisone, when hydrocortisone is administered to patients with severe sepsis, showed no improvement in in-hospital mortality (Annane and Bellissant, 2000). Similarly, two recent systematic reviews found no overall survival benefit by administering low dose steroids (Annane et al., 2009; Sligl et al., 2009). The current SSC guidelines recommend using low dose hydrocortisone only when there is a poor initial response to vasopressors (Dellinger et al., 2008).

5.3 Nutrition

The primary aim of nutritional support is to supply the substrates essential to meet the metabolic needs of critically ill patients. The acute phase is characterized by catabolism exceeding anabolism where carbohydrates are used as the preferred energy source, since fat mobilization is impaired. Nutritional support would provide the necessary carbohydrates to meet this demand and therefore alleviate the usual metabolic response of an inflammatory state to break down muscle proteins into amino acids that will eventually serve as a substrate of gluconeogenesis. The recovery phase would shift the dominant response towards anabolism, in which the body corrects the hypoproteinemia, replenishes other nutritional stores, and repairs muscle loss (Dvir et al., 2006). Conflicting data with regards to route of delivery exist. Enteral nutrition, compared with parenteral nutrition, results in poorer achievement of nutritional goals but may be associated with fewer infections.

The mechanisms by which enteral nutrition decreases infectious complications are unknown. However, preservation of gut immune function and reduction of inflammation have been proposed (Alverdy et al., 2003; Clave and Heyland, 2009). It is uncertain whether nutritional support directly improves important clinical outcomes (e.g. duration of mechanical ventilation, length of stay, mortality), or when nutritional support should be initiated.

The goal of nutrition support has been to deliver 100% of nutrient requirements, calculated for the specific metabolic condition, and in the shortest time possible. Recently, clinical experts in intensive care medicine and nutrition, published studies that determined that for critically ill patients, administering nutrients at quantities less than the calculated metabolic expenditure may significantly improve outcomes (Dickerson et al., 2002). Conversely, in a prospective cohort study from Johns Hopkins Medical Center, ICU patients were divided into groups that received 0%-32% (group one) of recommended intake, groups that received 33%-65% (group two) and groups that received 66%-100% (group three) of caloric recommendations. Patients in group two showed the highest survival rate and experienced more sepsis free days as opposed to patients in group three who experienced the worst outcomes (Dickerson et al., 2002). In another retrospective analysis of obese critically ill patients, Dickerson et al. reported that patients receiving less than 20 kcal/kg adjusted weight/day compared with patients receiving greater than 20 kcal/kg adjusted weight/day experienced fewer days in the ICU, fewer days on mechanical ventilation, and fewer days of antibiotic use (Krishnan et al., 2003). However, definitive evidence for the optimal amount of nutritional support and the mode of delivery has yet to be determined in severe sepsis.

5.4 Intensive insulin therapy

Tight glucose control has showed early hopes of reducing mortality of critically ill patients. Indeed, Van den Berghe and colleagues studied 1548 cardiac surgery ICU patients who were randomized either to very tight glucose control (80-110mg per deciliter) through intensive insulin therapy (IIT) or to conventional treatment (280 to 200 mg per deciliter) (Van Den Berghe et al., 2001). The study showed a significant 3.4 percent absolute mortality reduction among all patients and a 9.6 percent absolute risk reduction in mortality for patients who remained in the ICU for greater than five days. However, the same authors showed that there was no reduction in mortality when the same procedure was applied in a medical ICU (Van den Berghe et al., 2006). Furthermore, accumulation of evidence through out recent years from RCTs show that tight glucose control in non-surgical ICU has no significant correlation in mortality benefit and could, in fact, be harmful. A meta-analysis of 29 randomized controlled trials involving 8432 patients found no reduction in mortality with IIT compared to standard treatment (Wiener et al., 2008). In one study, involving 532 patients with severe sepsis randomized to IIT or conventional insulin therapy (180 to 200 mg per deciliter) and various combinations of crystalloids or colloids, showed no difference in mortality with IIT or conventional therapy but a significant increase in severe hypoglycemia in the IIT group. The study had to be stopped earlier than predicted due to increased significant hypoglycemic events in the IIT group(Brunkhorst et al., 2008). The Normoglycemia in Intensive Care Evaluation-Survival Using Glucose Algorithm Regulation (NICE-SUGAR) study randomized 6104 medical and surgical patients within 24 hours of ICU admission to IIT or conventional therapy (180 mg per deciliter or less). A significant increased risk of death(odds ratio 1.14) was shown in both medical and surgical group of patients who received IIT. (Finfer et al., 2009). Current SSC guidelines recommend a glucose target of <180 mg/dl for patients with severe sepsis and septic shock (Dellinger et al., 2008).

6. Summary of SSC recommendations

The 2008 Surviving Sepsis Campaign Guidelines (Dellinger et al., 2008) contain 3 tables that are very useful in summarizing their recommendations for the management of severe sepsis and septic shock. The following recommendations are adapted from those three tables with the very kind permission of Dr. Phil Dellinger (chair of 2008 Surviving Sepsis Campaign Committee).

6.1 Initial resuscitation and infection issues (Dellinger, 2008)

Regular text represents "Strongly Recommended" and *italicized* text represents "Suggested".

6.1.1 Initial resuscitation (first 6 hours)

- Begin resuscitation immediately in patients with hypotension or elevated serum lactate >4 mmol/L; do not delay pending ICU admission
- Resuscitation goals
  - CVP 8–12 mm Hg (A higher target CVP of 12–15 mm Hg is recommended in the presence of mechanical ventilation or preexisting decreased ventricular compliance.)
  - Mean arterial pressure ≥ 65 mm Hg
  - Urine output ≥0.5 $mL \cdot kg^{-1} \cdot hr^{-1}$
  - Central venous (superior vena cava) oxygen saturation ≥70 percent or mixed venous ≥65 percent
- *If venous oxygen saturation target is not achieved*
  - *Consider further fluid Transfuse packed red blood cells if required to hematocrit of ≥30 percent and/or*
  - *Start dobutamine infusion, maximum 20* $\mu g \cdot kg^{-1} \cdot min^{-1}$

6.1.2 Diagnosis

- Obtain appropriate cultures before starting antibiotics provided this does not significantly delay antimicrobial administration
  - *Obtain two or more blood cultures*
  - *One or more blood cultures should be percutaneous*
  - *One blood culture from each vascular access device in place >48 hours*
  - *Culture other sites as clinically indicated*

- Perform imaging studies promptly to confirm and sample any source of infection, if safe to do so

6.1.3 Antibiotic therapy

- Begin intravenous antibiotics as early as possible and always within the first hour of recognizing severe sepsis and septic shock
- Broad-spectrum: one or more agents active against likely bacterial/fungal pathogens and with good penetration into presumed source
- Reassess antimicrobial regimen daily to optimize efficacy, prevent resistance, avoid toxicity, and minimize costs
- *Consider combination therapy in Pseudomonas infections*
- *Consider combination empiric therapy in neutropenic patients*
- *Combination therapy ≤3–5 days and de-escalation following susceptibilities*
- Duration of therapy typically limited to 7–10 days; longer if response is slow or there are undrainable foci of infection or immunologic deficiencies
- Stop antimicrobial therapy if cause is found to be noninfectious

6.1.4 Source identification and control

- A specific anatomic site of infection should be established as rapidly as possible and within first 6 hours of presentation
- Formally evaluate patient for a focus of infection amenable to source control measures (e.g. abscess drainage, tissue debridement)
- Implement source control measures as soon as possible following successful initial resuscitation (exception: infected pancreatic necrosis, where surgical intervention is best delayed)
- Choose source control measure with maximum efficacy and minimal physiologic upset
- Remove intravascular access devices if potentially infected

6.2 Hemodynamic support and adjunctive therapy (Dellinger, 2008)

Regular text represents "Strongly Recommended" and *italicized* text represents "Suggested".

6.2.1 Fluid therapy

- Fluid-resuscitate using crystalloids or colloids
- Target a CVP of ≥8 mm Hg (≥12 mm Hg if mechanically ventilated)
- Use a fluid challenge technique while associated with a hemodynamic improvement
- Give fluid challenges of 1,000 mL of crystalloids or 300–500 mL of colloids over 30 minutes. More rapid and larger volumes may be required in sepsis-induced tissue hypoperfusion
- Rate of fluid administration should be reduced if cardiac filling pressures increase without concurrent hemodynamic improvement

6.2.2 Vasopressors

- Maintain MAP ≥65 mm Hg
- Norepinephrine and dopamine centrally administered are the initial vasopressors of choice

- *Epinephrine, phenylephrine, or vasopressin should not be administered as the initial vasopressor in septic shock. Vasopressin 0.03 units/minute may be subsequently added to norepinephrine with anticipation of an effect equivalent to norepinephrine alone*
- *Use epinephrine as the first alternative agent in septic shock when blood pressure is poorly responsive to norepinephrine or dopamine.*
- Do not use low-dose dopamine for renal protection
- In patients requiring vasopressors, insert an arterial catheter as soon as practical

6.2.3 Inotropic therapy

- Use dobutamine in patients with myocardial dysfunction as supported by elevated cardiac filling pressures and low cardiac output
- Do not increase cardiac index to predetermined supranormal levels

6.2.4 Steroids

- *Consider intravenous hydrocortisone for adult septic shock when hypotension responds poorly to adequate fluid resuscitation and vasopressors*
- *ACTH stimulation test is not recommended to identify the subset of adults with septic shock who should receive hydrocortisone*
- *Hydrocortisone is preferred to dexamethasone*
- *Fludrocortisone (50 µg orally once a day) may be included if an alternative to hydrocortisone is being used that lacks significant mineralocorticoid activity. Fludrocortisone is optional if hydrocortisone is used*
- *Steroid therapy may be weaned once vasopressors are no longer required*
- Hydrocortisone dose should be ≤300 mg/day
- Do not use corticosteroids to treat sepsis in the absence of shock unless the patient's endocrine or corticosteroid history warrants it

6.2.5 Recombinant human activated protein C (rhAPC)

- *Consider rhAPC in adult patients with sepsis-induced organ dysfunction with clinical assessment of high risk of death (typically APACHE II ≥25 or multiple organ failure) if there are no contraindications.*
- Adult patients with severe sepsis and low risk of death (typically, APACHE II <20 or one organ failure) should not receive rhAPC

6.3 Other supportive therapy of severe sepsis (Dellinger, 2008)

Regular text represents "Strongly Recommended" and *italicized* text represents "Suggested".

6.3.1 Blood product administration

- Give red blood cells when hemoglobin decreases to <7.0 g/dL (<70 g/L) to target a hemoglobin concentration of 7.0–9.0 g/dL in adults. A higher hemoglobin level may be required in special circumstances (e.g., myocardial ischemia, severe hypoxemia, acute hemorrhage, cyanotic heart disease, or lactic acidosis)
- Do not use erythropoietin to treat sepsis-related anemia. Erythropoietin may be used for other accepted reasons
- *Do not use fresh frozen plasma to correct laboratory clotting abnormalities unless there is bleeding or planned invasive procedures*

- Do not use antithrombin therapy
- *Administer platelets when*
  - *Counts are <5,000/mm³ (5 •10⁹/L) regardless of bleeding*
  - *Counts are 5,000–30,000/mm³ (5–30 •10⁹/L) and there is significant bleeding risk*
  - *Higher platelet counts (≥50,000/mm³ [50 •10⁹/L]) are required for surgery or invasive procedures*

6.3.2 Mechanical ventilation of sepsis-induced ALI/ARDS

- Target a tidal volume of 6 mL/kg (predicted) body weight in patients with ALI/ARDS
- Target an initial upper limit plateau pressure ≤30 cm H2O. Consider chest wall compliance when assessing plateau pressure
- Allow PaCO2 to increase above normal, if needed, to minimize plateau pressures and tidal volumes
- Set PEEP to avoid extensive lung collapse at end-expiration
- *Consider using the prone position for ARDS patients requiring potentially injurious levels of FIO_2 or plateau pressure, provided they are not put at risk from positional changes*
- Maintain mechanically ventilated patients in a semirecumbent position (head of the bed raised to 45°) unless contraindicated, between 30° and 45°
- *Noninvasive ventilation may be considered in the minority of ALI/ARDS patients with mild to moderate hypoxemic respiratory failure. The patients need to be hemodynamically stable, comfortable, easily arousable, able to protect/clear their airway, and expected to recover rapidly*
- Use a weaning protocol and an SBT regularly to evaluate the potential for discontinuing mechanical ventilation
  - SBT options include a low level of pressure support with continuous positive airway pressure 5 cm H_2O or a T piece
  - Before the SBT, patients should:
    - Be arousable
    - Be hemodynamically stable without vasopressors
    - Have no new potentially serious conditions
    - Have low ventilatory and end-expiratory pressure requirement
    - Require FIO_2 levels that can be safely delivered with a face mask or nasal cannula
- Do not use a pulmonary artery catheter for the routine monitoring of patients with ALI/ARDS
- Use a conservative fluid strategy for patients with established ALI who do not have evidence of tissue hypoperfusion

6.3.3 Sedation, analgesia, and neuromuscular blockade in sepsis

- Use sedation protocols with a sedation goal for critically ill mechanically ventilated patients
- Use either intermittent bolus sedation or continuous infusion sedation to predetermined end points (sedation scales), with daily interruption/lightening to produce awakening. Re-titrate if necessary
  - Avoid neuromuscular blockers where possible. Monitor depth of block with train-of-four when using continuous infusions

6.3.4 Glucose control

- Use intravenous insulin to control hyperglycemia in patients with severe sepsis following stabilization in the ICU
- *Aim to keep blood glucose <150 mg/dL (8.3 mmol/L) using a validated protocol for insulin dose adjustment*
- Provide a glucose calorie source and monitor blood glucose values every 1-2 hours (4 hours when stable) in patients receiving intravenous insulin
- Interpret with caution low glucose levels obtained with point of care testing, as these techniques may overestimate arterial blood or plasma glucose values

6.3.5 Renal replacement

- *Intermittent hemodialysis and CVVH are considered equivalent*
- *CVVH offers easier management in hemodynamically unstable patients*

6.3.6 Bicarbonate therapy

- Do not use bicarbonate therapy for the purpose of improving hemodynamics or reducing vasopressor requirements when treating hypoperfusion- induced lactic acidemia with pH ≥7.15

6.3.7 Deep vein thrombosis prophylaxis

- Use either low-dose unfractionated heparin (UFH) or low molecular weight heparin (LMWH), unless contraindicated
- Use a mechanical prophylactic device, such as compression stockings or an intermittent compression device, when heparin is contraindicated
- *Use a combination of pharmacologic and mechanical therapy for patients who are at very high risk for deep vein thrombosis*
- *In patients at very high risk, LMWH should be used rather than UFH*

6.3.8 Stress ulcer prophylaxis

- Provide stress ulcer prophylaxis using H2 blocker or proton pump inhibitor. Benefits of prevention of upper gastrointestinal bleed must be weighed against the potential for development of ventilator-acquired pneumonia

6.3.9 Consideration for limitation of support

- Discuss advance care planning with patients and families. Describe likely outcomes and set realistic expectations

7. Novel and ongoing research

Severe sepsis and septic shock management is an evolving and still controversial subject. New research is ongoing, and various therapies are being proposed and investigated.

7.1 Recombinant Human Milk Fat Globule Epidermal Growth Factor 8 (rhMFG-E8)

A U.S. study is currently underway, and set for completion in on August 31st, 2012, investigating the benefits of rhMFG-E8 on the clearance of apoptotic cells in severe sepsis and septic shock. Apoptosis is an import any player in the pathobiology of sepsis, and the lack of clearance of apoptotic cells is partially responsible for some of the pathology. The basis of this study is that in a rat model, they demonstrated that down-regulating the MFG-E8 gene expression was associated with reduced apoptotic cell clearance during sepsis. The MFG-E8 protein acts as an opsonin, targeting apoptotic cells phagocytosis, and without this opsonization, proper cell clearance does not occur. They have created recombinant human MFG-E8 and propose to use it as an adjunctive treatment for sepsis with the goal of improving cardiovascular function, attenuating tissue injury and inflammation, and reducing mortality (2011a).

7.2 Magnesium sulphate does not improve microcirculatory alterations

It is well known that microcirculatory dysfunction is contributory to the pathology associated with severe sepsis and septic shock. Since magnesium sulphate has both endothelium-dependent and non-endothelium-dependent vasodilatory pathways, it has been proposed as a potential therapy for sepsis. Andrius et al conducted a single center open label clinical trial to assess the microcirculatory changes induced by infusion of magnesium sulphate. This trial failed to demonstrate any microcirculatory improvement with magnesium sulphate infusion (Pranskunas et al., 2011).

7.3 Targeting CCR2: A novel therapeutic strategy for septic shock

Since sepsis is an inflammation-mediated disease, and neutrophils are among the first cells recruited in the inflammatory process, Souto et al proposed that hyper-activation of neutrophils may contribute to tissue damage in sepsis. They studied the role of the chemokine receptor CCR2 in inappropriate neutrophil recruitment and tissue damage in remote organs of septic patients. CCR2 is a receptor for a chemotactic factor 'monocyte chemotattractant protein-1' (CCR2 chemokine (C-C motif) receptor 2 [Homo sapiens], 2011b). The receptor-ligand interaction mediates monocyte chemotaxis and monocyte infiltration in inflammation. In this study, the expression and responsiveness of CCR2 was induced in circulating neutrophils during induced sepsis in mice(Souto et al., 2011). Mortality was prevented in both genetically and pharmacologically CCR2-inhibited mice. Neutrophil infiltration into the lungs, heart, and kidneys was reduced in both models, and serum biochemical markers of organ injury and dysfunction were also reduced (Souto et al., 2011). These results implicate CCR2 as a potential target for antagonist pharmaceutical therapy in severe sepsis and septic shock to prevent 'multiple organ dysfunction syndrome'.

7.4 Targeting LPS to impair induction of inflammation

Lipopolysaccharide (LPS), a surface molecule of gram-negative bacteria, interacts with the Toll-like receptor 4 (TLR-4) in the induction of the inflammatory response, and the associated signal transduction pathway has been associated with the pathogenesis of sepsis. Neutralizing LPS before it can interact with TLR-4 has been proposed as an adjunctive therapy for sepsis (Wheeler et al., 2009). Lipid-binding protein (LBP) is a molecule that directs LPS to the TLR-4 receptor (Wheeler et al., 2009). Analogues of this molecule can block LPS-LBP interactions and inhibit LPS-induced inflammation. This may prove to be a promising novel therapy for sepsis.

8. Conclusion

It is evident that there is a great deal of research still needed to resolve many of the controversies around the management of sepsis and to discover the best management strategies for severe sepsis and septic shock. Sepsis management recommendations are clearly improving with each study performed, and efforts towards the standardization and universalization of protocols, is a great step in the right direction. The 2008 Surviving Sepsis Campaign guidelines are, pending an update, the most up-to-date complete set of evidence-based guidelines on the management of severe sepsis and septic shock that we have found.

9. References

A Novel Therapy for Septic Shock. (July 16, 2011a). Retrieved July 16th, 2011 from http://projectreporter.nih.gov/project_info_description.cfm?icde=0&aid=7921871

Abraham, E.; Laterre, P. F.; Garg, R.; Levy, H.; Talwar, D.; Trzaskoma, B. L.; Francois, B.; Guy, J. S.; Bruckmann, M.; Rea-Neto, A.; Rossaint, R.; Perrotin, D.; Sablotzki, A.; Arkins, N.; Utterback, B. G., & Macias, W. L. (2005 Sep 29). Drotrecogin alfa (activated) for adults with severe sepsis and a low risk of death. N Engl J Med, 353(13), 1332-1341. doi:10.1056/NEJMoa050935

Acute Respiratory Distress Syndrome Network. (2000 May 4). Ventilation with lower tidal volumes as compared with traditional tidal volumes for acute lung injury and the acute respiratory distress syndrome. The Acute Respiratory Distress Syndrome Network. N Engl J Med, 342(18), 1301-1308. doi:10.1056/NEJM200005043421801

Agrawal, R.; Al-Khafaji, A., & Yende, S. (2010). Epinephrine: is it really the black sheep of vasoactive agents? Crit Care, 14(3), 309. doi:10.1186/cc8998

Alverdy, J. C.; Laughlin, R. S., & Wu, L. (2003). Influence of the critically ill state on host-pathogen interactions within the intestine: gut-derived sepsis redefined. Critical Care MEdicine, 31, 598-607.

Angus, D. C.; Linde-Zwirble, W. T.; Lidicker, J.; Clermont, G.; Carcillo, J., & Pinsky, M. R. (2001 Jul). Epidemiology of severe sepsis in the United States: analysis of incidence, outcome, and associated costs of care. Crit Care Med, 29(7), 1303-1310. doi:10.1097/00003246-200107000-00002

Annane, D., & Bellissant, E. (2000 Jul 19). Prognostic value of cortisol response in septic shock. JAMA, 284(3), 308-309. doi:jlt0719-4 [pii]

Annane, D.; Bellissant, E.; Bollaert, P. E.; Briegel, J.; Confalonieri, M.; De Gaudio, R.; Keh, D.; Kupfer, Y.; Oppert, M., & Meduri, G. U. (2009 Jun 10). Corticosteroids in the treatment of severe sepsis and septic shock in adults: a systematic review. Jama, 301(22), 2362-2375. doi:10.1001/jama.2009.815

Annane, D.; Bellissant, E., & Cavaillon, J. M. (2005 Jan 1-7). Septic shock. Lancet, 365(9453), 63-78. doi:10.1016/S0140-6736(04)17667-8

Annane, D.; Sebille, V.; Charpentier, C.; Bollaert, P. E.; Francois, B.; Korach, J. M.; Capellier, G.; Cohen, Y.; Azoulay, E.; Troche, G.; Chaumet-Riffaud, P., & Bellissant, E. (2002 Aug 21). Effect of treatment with low doses of hydrocortisone and fludrocortisone on mortality in patients with septic shock. JAMA, 288(7), 862-871. doi:10.1001/jama.288.7.862

Arnold, R. C.; Shapiro, N. I.; Jones, A. E.; Schorr, C.; Pope, J.; Casner, E.; Parrillo, J. E.; Dellinger, R. P., & Trzeciak, S. (2009 Jul). Multicenter study of early lactate clearance as a determinant of survival in patients with presumed sepsis. Shock, 32(1), 35-39. doi:10.1097/SHK.0b013e3181971d47

Bakker, J.; Coffernils, M.; Leon, M.; Gris, P., & Vincent, J. L. (1991 Apr). Blood lactate levels are superior to oxygen-derived variables in predicting outcome in human septic shock. Chest, 99(4), 956-962. doi:10.1378/chest.99.4.956

Barochia, A. V.; Cui, X.; Vitberg, D.; Suffredini, A. F.; O'Grady, N. P.; Banks, S. M.; Minneci, P.; Kern, S. J.; Danner, R. L.; Natanson, C., & Eichacker, P. Q. (2010 Feb). Bundled care for septic shock: an analysis of clinical trials. Crit Care Med, 38(2), 668-678. doi:10.1097/CCM.0b013e3181cb0ddf

Bauer, P.; Reinhart, K., & Bauer, M. (2008 Apr). Significance of venous oximetry in the critically ill. Med Intensiva, 32(3), 134-142. doi:10.1016/S0210-5691(08)70923-9

Bellomo, R.; Reade, M. C., & Warrillow, S. J. (2008). The pursuit of a high central venous oxygen saturation in sepsis: growing concerns. Crit Care, 12(2), 130. doi:10.1186/cc6841

Bernard, G. R.; Vincent, J. L.; Laterre, P. F.; LaRosa, S. P.; Dhainaut, J. F.; Lopez-Rodriguez, A.; Steingrub, J. S.; Garber, G. E.; Helterbrand, J. D.; Ely, E. W., & Fisher, C. J. J. (2001 Mar 8). Efficacy and safety of recombinant human activated protein C for severe sepsis. N Engl J Med, 344(10), 699-709. doi:10.1056/NEJM200103083441001

Bernard, G. R.; Wheeler, A. P.; Russell, J. A.; Schein, R.; Summer, W. R.; Steinberg, K. P.; Fulkerson, W. J.; Wright, P. E.; Christman, B. W.; Dupont, W. D.; Higgins, S. B., & Swindell, B. B. (1997 Mar 27). The effects of ibuprofen on the physiology and survival of patients with sepsis. The Ibuprofen in Sepsis Study Group. N Engl J Med, 336(13), 912-918. doi:10.1056/NEJM199703273361303

Beutler, B. (2004 Feb). Innate immunity: an overview. Mol Immunol, 40(12), 845-859. doi:10.1016/j.molimm.2003.10.005

Boerma, E. C.; Koopmans, M.; Konijn, A.; Kaiferova, K.; Bakker, A. J.; van, R., Eric N.; Buter, H.; Bruins, N.; Egbers, P. H.; Gerritsen, R. T.; Koetsier, P. M.; Kingma, W. P.; Kuiper, M. A., & Ince, C. (2010///). Effects of nitroglycerin on sublingual microcirculatory blood flow in patients with severe sepsis/septic shock after a strict resuscitation protocol: A double-blind randomized placebo controlled trial. Critical Care Medicine, 38(1). Retrieved from http://journals.lww.com/ccmjournal/Fulltext/2010/01000/Effects_of_nitroglycerin_on_sublingual.15.aspx

Bone, R. C.; Fisher, C. J. J.; Clemmer, T. P.; Slotman, G. J.; Metz, C. A., & Balk, R. A. (1987 Sep 10). A controlled clinical trial of high-dose methylprednisolone in the treatment of severe sepsis and septic shock. N Engl J Med, 317(11), 653-658. doi:10.1056/NEJM198709103171101

Boyd, J. H.; Holmes, C. L.; Wang, Y.; Roberts, H., & Walley, K. R. (2008 Nov). Vasopressin decreases sepsis-induced pulmonary inflammation through the V2R. Resuscitation, 79(2), 325-331. doi:10.1016/j.resuscitation.2008.07.006

Brunkhorst, F. M.; Engel, C.; Bloos, F.; Meier-Hellmann, A.; Ragaller, M.; Weiler, N.; Moerer, O.; Gruendling, M.; Oppert, M.; Grond, S.; Olthoff, D.; Jaschinski, U.; John, S.; Rossaint, R.; Welte, T.; Schaefer, M.; Kern, P.; Kuhnt, E.; Kiehntopf, M.; Hartog, C.; Natanson, C.; Loeffler, M., & Reinhart, K. (2008 Jan 10). Intensive insulin therapy and pentastarch resuscitation in severe sepsis. N Engl J Med, 358(2), 125-139. doi:10.1056/NEJMoa070716

Casserly, B.; Read, R., & Levy, M. M. (2009 Oct). Hemodynamic monitoring in sepsis. Crit Care Clin, 25(4), 803-23, ix. doi:10.1016/j.ccc.2009.08.006

CCR2 chemokine (C-C motif) receptor 2 [Homo sapiens]. (July 17, 2011b). Retrieved from http://www.ncbi.nlm.nih.gov/gene/729230

Choi, P. T.; Yip, G.; Quinonez, L. G., & Cook, D. J. (1999 Jan). Crystalloids vs. colloids in fluid resuscitation: a systematic review. Crit Care Med, 27(1), 200-210. doi:10.1097/00003246-199901000-00053

Clave, S. A., & Heyland, D. K. (2009). The physiologic response and associated clinical benefits from provision of early enteral nutrition. Nutrition in Clinical Practice, 24, 305-315.

Cohn, J. N. (1967). Blood pressure measurement in shock. Mechanism of inaccuracy in ausculatory and palpatory methods. JAMA: The Journal of the American Medical Association, 199(13), 118-122. doi:10.1001/jama.199.13.118

De Backer, D.; Biston, P.; Devriendt, J.; Madl, C.; Chochrad, D.; Aldecoa, C.; Brasseur, A.; Defrance, P.; Gottignies, P., & Vincent, J. L. (2010 Mar 4). Comparison of dopamine and norepinephrine in the treatment of shock. N Engl J Med, 362(9), 779-789. doi:10.1056/NEJMoa0907118

Dellinger, R. P.; Carlet, J. M.; Masur, H.; Gerlach, H.; Calandra, T.; Cohen, J.; Gea-Banacloche, J.; Keh, D.; Marshall, J. C.; Parker, M. M.; Ramsay, G.; Zimmerman, J. L.; Vincent, J. L., & Levy, M. M. (2004 Mar). Surviving Sepsis Campaign guidelines for management of severe sepsis and septic shock. Crit Care Med, 32(3), 858-873. doi:10.1097/01.CCM.0000117317.18092.E4

Dellinger, R. P.; Levy, M. M.; Carlet, J. M.; Bion, J.; Parker, M. M.; Jaeschke, R.; Reinhart, K.; Angus, D. C.; Brun-Buisson, C.; Beale, R.; Calandra, T.; Dhainaut, J. F.; Gerlach, H.; Harvey, M.; Marini, J. J.; Marshall, J.; Ranieri, M.; Ramsay, G.; Sevransky, J.; Thompson, B. T.; Townsend, S.; Vender, J. S.; Zimmerman, J. L., & Vincent, J. L. (2008 Jan). Surviving Sepsis Campaign: international guidelines for management of severe sepsis and septic shock: 2008. Crit Care Med, 36(1), 296-327. doi:10.1097/01.CCM.0000298158.12101.41

Dickerson, R. N.; Boschert, K. J.; Kudsk, K. A., & Brown, R. O. (2002). Hypocaloric enteral tube feeding in critically ill obese patients. Nutrition, 18, 241-246.

Dvir, D.; Cohen, J., & Singer, P. (2006). Computerized energy balance and complications in critically ill patients: an observational study. Clinical Nutrition, 25(1), 37-44.

Edwards, J. D. (1991 May). Oxygen transport in cardiogenic and septic shock. Crit Care Med, 19(5), 658-663. doi:10.1097/00003246-199105000-00012

Finfer, S.; Bellomo, R.; Boyce, N.; French, J.; Myburgh, J., & Norton, R. (2004 May 27). A comparison of albumin and saline for fluid resuscitation in the intensive care unit. N Engl J Med, 350(22), 2247-2256. doi:10.1056/NEJMoa040232

Finfer, S.; Chittock, D. R.; Su, S. Y.; Blair, D.; Foster, D.; Dhingra, V.; Bellomo, R.; Cook, D.; Dodek, P.; Henderson, W. R.; Hebert, P. C.; Heritier, S.; Heyland, D. K.; McArthur, C.; McDonald, E.; Mitchell, I.; Myburgh, J. A.; Norton, R.; Potter, J.; Robinson, B. G., & Ronco, J. J. (2009 Mar 26). Intensive versus conventional glucose control in critically ill patients. N Engl J Med, 360(13), 1283-1297. doi:10.1056/NEJMoa0810625

Finnie, K. J.; Wattsam, D. G., & Armstrong, P. W. (1984). Biases in the measurement of arterial pressure. Critical Care Medicine, 12(11), 965-968. doi:10.1097/00003246-198411000-00009

Fisher, C. J. J., & Yan, S. B. (2000 Sep). Protein C levels as a prognostic indicator of outcome in sepsis and related diseases. Crit Care Med, 28(9 Suppl), S49-56. doi:10.1097/00003246-200009001-00011

Fourrier, F. (2004 Nov). Recombinant human activated protein C in the treatment of severe sepsis: an evidence-based review. Crit Care Med, 32(11 Suppl), S534-41. doi:10.1097/01.CCM.0000145944.64532.53

Fuller, B. M.; Gajera, M.; Schorr, C.; Gerber, D.; Dellinger, R. P.; Parrillo, J., & Zanotti, S. (2010 Oct). The impact of packed red blood cell transfusion on clinical outcomes in patients with septic shock treated with early goal directed therapy. Indian J Crit Care Med, 14(4), 165-169. doi:10.4103/0972-5229.76078

Gaieski, D. F.; Mikkelsen, M. E.; Band, R. A.; Pines, J. M.; Massone, R.; Furia, F. F.; Shofer, F. S., & Goyal, M. (2010 Apr). Impact of time to antibiotics on survival in patients with severe sepsis or septic shock in whom early goal-directed therapy was initiated in the emergency department. Crit Care Med, 38(4), 1045-1053. doi:10.1097/CCM.0b013e3181cc4824

Gattinoni, L.; Brazzi, L.; Pelosi, P.; Latini, R.; Tognoni, G.; Pesenti, A., & Fumagalli, R. (1995 Oct 19). A trial of goal-oriented hemodynamic therapy in critically ill patients. SvO2 Collaborative Group. N Engl J Med, 333(16), 1025-1032. doi:10.1056/NEJM199510193331601

Hanna, N. F. (2003). Sepsis and Septic Shock. Advanced Emergency Nursing Journal, 25(2), 158-165. Retrieved from http://journals.lww.com/aenjournal/Fulltext/2003/04000/Sepsis_and_Septic_Shock.10.aspx

Hayes, M. A.; Timmins, A. C.; Yau, E. H.; Palazzo, M.; Hinds, C. J., & Watson, D. (1994 Jun 16). Elevation of systemic oxygen delivery in the treatment of critically ill patients. N Engl J Med, 330(24), 1717-1722. doi:10.1056/NEJM199406163302404

He, Z. Y.; Gao, Y.; Wang, X. R., & Hang, Y. N. (2007 Jan). [Clinical evaluation of execution of early goal directed therapy in septic shock]. Zhongguo Wei Zhong Bing Ji Jiu Yi Xue, 19(1), 14-16. Retrieved from http://www.ncbi.nlm.nih.gov/entrez/query.fcgi?cmd=Retrieve&db=PubMed&dopt=Citation&list_uids=17207356

Hollenberg, S. M. (2009 Oct). Inotrope and vasopressor therapy of septic shock. Crit Care Clin, 25(4), 781-802, ix. doi:10.1016/j.ccc.2009.07.003

Hollenberg, S. M.; Ahrens, T. S.; Annane, D.; Astiz, M. E.; Chalfin, D. B.; Dasta, J. F.; Heard, S. O.; Martin, C.; Napolitano, L. M.; Susla, G. M.; Totaro, R.; Vincent, J.-L., & Zanotti-Cavazzoni, S. (2004). Practice parameters for hemodynamic support of sepsis in adult patients: 2004 update. Critical Care Medicine, 32(9), 1928-1948. doi:10.1097/01.CCM.0000139761.05492.D6

Houck, P. M.; Bratzler, D. W.; Nsa, W.; Ma, A., & Bartlett, J. G. (2004 Mar 22). Timing of antibiotic administration and outcomes for Medicare patients hospitalized with community-acquired pneumonia. Arch Intern Med, 164(6), 637-644. doi:10.1001/archinte.164.6.637

Ibrahim, E. H.; Sherman, G.; Ward, S.; Fraser, V. J., & Kollef, M. H. (2000 Jul). The influence of inadequate antimicrobial treatment of bloodstream infections on patient outcomes in the ICU setting. Chest, 118(1), 146-155. doi:10.1378/chest.118.1.146

Krishnan, J. A.; Parce, P. B.;,A. Martinez, Diette, G. B., & Brower, R. G. (2003). iette GB, Brower RG. Caloric intake in medical ICU patients: consistency of care with guidelines and relationship to clinical outcomes. Chest, 124, 297–305.

Jimenez, M. F. & Marshall, J. C. (2001). Source control in the management of sepsis. Intensive Care Med, 27(14), S49-S62. doi:10.1007/PL00003797

Jones, A. E.; Shapiro, N. I.; Trzeciak, S.; Arnold, R. C.; Claremont, H. A., & Kline, J. A. (2010 Feb 24). Lactate clearance vs central venous oxygen saturation as goals of early sepsis therapy: a randomized clinical trial. Jama, 303(8), 739-746. doi:10.1001/jama.2010.158

Kumar, A.; Anel, R.; Bunnell, E.; Habet, K.; Zanotti, S.; Marshall, S.; Neumann, A.; Ali, A.; Cheang, M.; Kavinsky, C., & Parrillo, J. E. (2004 Mar). Pulmonary artery occlusion pressure and central venous pressure fail to predict ventricular filling volume, cardiac performance, or the response to volume infusion in normal subjects. Crit Care Med, 32(3), 691-699. doi:10.1097/01.CCM.0000114996.68110.C9

Kumar, A.; Haery, C.; Paladugu, B.; Kumar, A.; Symeoneides, S.; Taiberg, L.; Osman, J.; Trenholme, G.; Opal, S. M.; Goldfarb, R., & Parrillo, J. E. (2006 Jan 15). The duration of hypotension before the initiation of antibiotic treatment is a critical determinant of survival in a murine model of Escherichia coli septic shock: association with serum lactate and inflammatory cytokine levels. J Infect Dis, 193(2), 251-258. doi:10.1086/498909

LeDoux, D.; Astiz, M. E.; Carpati, C. M., & Rackow, E. C. (2000 Aug). Effects of perfusion pressure on tissue perfusion in septic shock. Crit Care Med, 28(8), 2729-2732. doi:10.1097/00003246-200008000-00007

Levy, M. M.; Macias, W. L.; Vincent, J. L.; Russell, J. A.; Silva, E.; Trzaskoma, B., & Williams, M. D. (2005 Oct). Early changes in organ function predict eventual survival in severe sepsis. Crit Care Med, 33(10), 2194-2201. doi:10.1097/01.CCM.0000182798.39709.84

Levy, M. M.; Dellinger, R. P.; Townsend, S. R.; Linde-Zwirble, W. T.; Marshall, J. C.; Bion, J.; Schorr, C.; Artigas, A.; Ramsay, G.; Beale, R.; Parker, M. M.; Gerlach, H.; Reinhart, K.; Silva, E.; Harvey, M.; Regan, S. & Angus, D. C. (2010 Feb). The Surviving Sepsis Campaign: results of an international guideline-based performance improvement program targeting severe sepsis. Intensive Care Med, 36(2), 222-231. doi:10.1007/s00134-009-1738-3

Lindenauer, P. K.; Rothberg, M. B.; Nathanson, B. H.; Pekow, P. S., & Steingrub, J. S. (2010 Apr). Activated protein C and hospital mortality in septic shock: a propensity-matched analysis. Crit Care Med, 38(4), 1101-1107. doi:10.1097/CCM.0b013e3181d423b7

Marik, P. E.; Baram, M., & Vahid, B. (2008 Jul). Does central venous pressure predict fluid responsiveness? A systematic review of the literature and the tale of seven mares. Chest, 134(1), 172-178. doi:10.1378/chest.07-2331

Micek, S. T.; Welch, E. C.; Khan, J.; Pervez, M.; Doherty, J. A.; Reichley, R. M., & Kollef, M. H. (2010 May). Empiric combination antibiotic therapy is associated with improved outcome against sepsis due to Gram-negative bacteria: a retrospective analysis. Antimicrob Agents Chemother, 54(5), 1742-1748. doi:10.1128/AAC.01365-09

Minneci, P. C.; Deans, K. J.; Banks, S. M.; Eichacker, P. Q., & Natanson, C. (2004 Nov 2). Corticosteroids for septic shock. Ann Intern Med, 141(9), 742-743. Retrieved from http://www.ncbi.nlm.nih.gov/entrez/query.fcgi?cmd=Retrieve&db=PubMed&dopt=Citation&list_uids=15520444

Myburgh, J. A.; Higgins, A.; Jovanovska, A.; Lipman, J.; Ramakrishnan, N., & Santamaria, J. (2008 Dec). A comparison of epinephrine and norepinephrine in critically ill patients. Intensive Care Med, 34(12), 2226-2234. doi:10.1007/s00134-008-1219-0

Nguyen, H. B.; Rivers, E. P.; Knoblich, B. P.; Jacobsen, G.; Muzzin, A.; Ressler, J. A., & Tomlanovich, M. C. (2004 Aug). Early lactate clearance is associated with improved outcome in severe sepsis and septic shock. Crit Care Med, 32(8), 1637-1642. doi:10.1097/01.CCM.0000132904.35713.A7

Parrillo, J. E. (1993 May 20). Pathogenetic mechanisms of septic shock. N Engl J Med, 328(20), 1471-1477. doi:10.1056/NEJM199305203282008

Perel, A. (2008). Bench-to-bedside review: the initial hemodynamic resuscitation of the septic patient according to Surviving Sepsis Campaign guidelines--does one size fit all? Crit Care, 12(5), 223. doi:10.1186/cc6979

Pranskunas, A.; Vellinga, N. A. R.; Pilvinis, V.; Koopmans, M., & Boerma, E. C. (2011). Microcirculatory changes during open label magnesium sulphate infusion in patients with severe sepsis and septic shock. BMC Anesthesiology, 11(12).

Reinhart, K., & Bloos, F. (2005 Jun). The value of venous oximetry. Curr Opin Crit Care, 11(3), 259-263. doi:10.1097/01.ccx.0000158092.64795.cf

Reinhart, K.; Kuhn, H. J.; Hartog, C., & Bredle, D. L. (2004 Aug). Continuous central venous and pulmonary artery oxygen saturation monitoring in the critically ill. Intensive Care Med, 30(8), 1572-1578. doi:10.1007/s00134-004-2337-y

Rivers, E.; Nguyen, B.; Havstad, S.; Ressler, J.; Muzzin, A.; Knoblich, B.; Peterson, E., & Tomlanovich, M. (2001 Nov 8). Early goal-directed therapy in the treatment of severe sepsis and septic shock. N Engl J Med, 345(19), 1368-1377. doi:10.1056/NEJMoa010307

Russell, J. A.; Walley, K. R.; Singer, J.; Gordon, A. C.; Hebert, P. C.; Cooper, D. J.; Holmes, C. L.; Mehta, S.; Granton, J. T.; Storms, M. M.; Cook, D. J.; Presneill, J. J., & Ayers, D. (2008 Feb 28). Vasopressin versus norepinephrine infusion in patients with septic shock. N Engl J Med, 358(9), 877-887. doi:10.1056/NEJMoa067373

Sakr, Y.; Chierego, M.; Piagnerelli, M.; Verdant, C.; Dubois, M. J.; Koch, M.; Creteur, J.; Gullo, A.; Vincent, J. L., & De Backer, D. (2007 Jul). Microvascular response to red blood cell transfusion in patients with severe sepsis. Crit Care Med, 35(7), 1639-1644. doi:10.1097/01.CCM.0000269936.73788.32

Sasse, K. C.; Nauenberg, E.; Long, A.; Anton, B.; Tucker, H. J., & Hu, T. W. (1995 Jun). Long-term survival after intensive care unit admission with sepsis. Crit Care Med, 23(6), 1040-1047. doi:10.1097/00003246-199506000-00008

Schmidt, G. A., Mandel, J. (2011a). Source control methods for common ICU infections. In D. S. Basow (Ed.), UpToDate. Waltham, MA: UpToDate.

Schmidt, G. A., Mandel, J. (2011b). Vasoactive agents in septic shock. In D. S. Basow (Ed.), UpToDate. Waltham, MA: UpToDate.

Sessler, C. N.; Perry, J. C., & Varney, K. L. (2004). Management of severe sepsis and septic shock. Current Opinion in Critical Care, 10(5), 354-363. doi:10.1097/01.ccx.0000139363.76068.7b

Severe Sepsis Bundles. (n.d.). Retrieved June 6th, 2011 from http://www.survivingsepsis.org/Bundles/Pages/default.aspx

Shoemaker, W. C.; Appel, P. L., & Kram, H. B. (1991 May). Oxygen transport measurements to evaluate tissue perfusion and titrate therapy: dobutamine and dopamine effects. Crit Care Med, 19(5), 672-688. doi:10.1097/00003246-199105000-00014

Shorr, A. F.; Bernard, G. R.; Dhainaut, J. F.; Russell, J. R.; Macias, W. L.; Nelson, D. R., & Sundin, D. P. (2006). Protein C concentrations in severe sepsis: an early directional change in plasma levels predicts outcome. Crit Care, 10(3), R92. doi:10.1186/cc4946

Sligl, W. I.; Milner, D. A. J.; Sundar, S.; Mphatswe, W., & Majumdar, S. R. (2009 Jul 1). Safety and efficacy of corticosteroids for the treatment of septic shock: A systematic review and meta-analysis. Clin Infect Dis, 49(1), 93-101. doi:10.1086/599343

Snell, R. J., & Parrillo, J. E. (1991 Apr). Cardiovascular dysfunction in septic shock. Chest, 99(4), 1000-1009. doi:10.1378/chest.99.4.1000

Souto, F. O.; Alves-Filho, J. C.; Turato, W. M.; Auxiliadora-Martins, M.; Basile-Filho, A., & Cunha, F. Q. (2011 Jan 15). Essential role of CCR2 in neutrophil tissue infiltration and multiple organ dysfunction in sepsis. Am J Respir Crit Care Med, 183(2), 234-242. doi:10.1164/rccm.201003-0416OC

Sprung, C. L.; Annane, D.; Keh, D.; Moreno, R.; Singer, M.; Freivogel, K.; Weiss, Y. G.; Benbenishty, J.; Kalenka, A.; Forst, H.; Laterre, P. F.; Reinhart, K.; Cuthbertson, B. H.; Payen, D., & Briegel, J. (2008 Jan 10). Hydrocortisone therapy for patients with septic shock. N Engl J Med, 358(2), 111-124. doi:10.1056/NEJMoa071366

Tuttle, R. R., & Mills, J. (1975 Jan). Dobutamine: development of a new catecholamine to selectively increase cardiac contractility. Circ Res, 36(1), 185-196. Retrieved from http://www.ncbi.nlm.nih.gov/entrez/query.fcgi?cmd=Retrieve&db=PubMed&dopt=Citation&list_uids=234805

Van den Berghe, G.; Wilmer, A.; Hermans, G.; Meersseman, W.; Wouters, P. J.; Milants, I.; Van Wijngaerden, E.; Bobbaers, H., & Bouillon, R. (2006 Feb 2). Intensive insulin therapy in the medical ICU. N Engl J Med, 354(5), 449-461. doi:10.1056/NEJMoa052521

Van Den Berghe, G.; Wouters, P.; Weekers, F.; Verwaest, C.; Bruyninckx, F.; Schetz, M.; Vlasselaers, D.; Ferdinande, P.; Lauwers, P., & Bouillon, R. (2001 Nov 8). Intensive insulin therapy in the critically ill patients. N Engl J Med, 345(19), 1359-1367. doi:10.1056/NEJMoa011300

Villar, J.; Kacmarek, R. M.; Perez-Mendez, L., & Aguirre-Jaime, A. (2006 May). A high positive end-expiratory pressure, low tidal volume ventilatory strategy improves outcome in persistent acute respiratory distress syndrome: a randomized, controlled trial. Crit Care Med, 34(5), 1311-1318. doi:10.1097/01.CCM.0000215598.84885.01

Vincent, J. L. (2008). Update on sepsis guidelines: what has changed? International Journal of Intensive Care, 15(1), 18-21.

Vincent, J. L.; Sakr, Y.; Sprung, C.; Harboe, S., & Damas, P. (2008 Jan). Are blood transfusions associated with greater mortality rates? Results of the Sepsis Occurrence in Acutely Ill Patients study. Anesthesiology, 108(1), 31-39. doi:10.1097/01.anes.0000296070.75956.40

Welcome To The Surviving Sepsis Campaign Website. (n.d.). Retrieved June 6th, 2011 from http://www.survivingsepsis.org

Wheeler, D. S.; Zingarelli, B.; Wheeler, W. J. & Wong, H. R. (2009). Novel Pharmacologic Approaches to the Management of Sepsis: Targeting the Host Inflammatory Response. Recent Pat Inflamm Allergy Drug Discov., 3(2), 96-112.

Wiener, R. S.; Wiener, D. C., & Larson, R. J. (2008 Aug 27). Benefits and risks of tight glucose control in critically ill adults: a meta-analysis. Jama, 300(8), 933-944. doi:10.1001/jama.300.8.933

Wilkes, M. M.; Navickis, R. J., & Sibbald, W. J. (2001 Aug). Albumin versus hydroxyethyl starch in cardiopulmonary bypass surgery: a meta-analysis of postoperative bleeding. Ann Thorac Surg, 72(2), 527-33; discussion 534. Retrieved from http://www.ncbi.nlm.nih.gov/entrez/query.fcgi?cmd=Retrieve&db=PubMed&dopt=Citation&list_uids=11515893

Zubert, S.; Funk, D. J., & Kumar, A. (2010 Apr). Antibiotics in sepsis and septic shock: like everything else in life, timing is everything. Crit Care Med, 38(4), 1211-1212. doi:10.1097/CCM.0b013e3181d69db7

11

Update in the Treatment of Severe Sepsis and Septic Shock

D. Boodoosingh, C. Cruz, M. Egozcue,
R. Fernandez, V. Salinas and S. Valentin
Pulmonary Program Physicians
San Juan City Hospital
Puerto Rico

1. Introduction

The mortality rate of severe sepsis and septic shock has remain high and always has been recognized as one of the most common cause of death worldwide. On the other hand, new interventions has been shown to decrease the complications of this syndrome, even reducing the percent of deaths from over 50% to 30-40% in some studies.
In this chapter, we will discuss some of these therapies including the most important studies leading to better outcomes in the treatment of the above condition.

2. Diagnosis

So far there is no definitive test for the diagnosis of severe sepsis or septic shock. When the human body is exposed to an insult, whether caused by bacteria, trauma, burn, or drug overdose, the individual tends to respond differently depending on their health status and the presence or absence of co-morbidities. Despite no specific test available, there are certain findings that lead us to the diagnosis. These include tachycardia, tachypnea, leukocytosis or leucopenia, fever or hypothermia; all of them are basically criterias defining the Systemic Inflammatory Response Syndrome (SIRS). In addition, the presence of altered mental status, hyperbilirubinemia, metabolic acidosis or respiratory alkalosis and thrombocytopenia could also be useful.
Severe sepsis is known as an acute organ dysfunction secondary to infection. When evaluating a patient with this syndrome time becomes our worst enemy. The organism/s responsible for the acute illness should be identified within the first hours. Appropriate cultures should be obtained before antimicrobial therapy is initiated to confirm the presence of infection and proceed with de-escalation of antibiotic therapy after a susceptibility profile is available. Two quantitative blood cultures should be taken and in patients with indwelling catheters for more than 48 hours, at least one blood culture should be drawn through each lumen of the vascular access [1]. When the same organism is recovered from both cultures, the likelihood that the organism is causing the severe sepsis is enhanced. Quantitative cultures of other body sites, such as urine, cerebrospinal fluid, wounds and /or respiratory secretions should also be obtained if they are considered to be the source of infection. It is important to understand that obtaining cultures before the initiation of

therapy should only be done if not associated with significant delay in antibiotic administration.

Imaging studies might also be necessary to identify the source of infection, especially when the presence of foreign body or drainage is suspected to be the cause of severe sepsis. However, some patients may be too unstable to undergo invasive procedures or be transported outside the intensive care unit. In such cases bedside ultrasound can be useful.

The potential role of biomarkers in the diagnosis of severe sepsis remains unclear. The use of pro-calcitonin level has demonstrated controversial results since it can be altered in patients with an acute inflammatory process other than infection [2]. In the near future, it is expected that rapid diagnostic methods, such as polymerase chain reaction, be available for quicker identification of pathogens and antimicrobial resistance patterns [3].

3. Source control

Source control is known as the rapid diagnosis of the specific body site of infection amenable to proceed with control measures such as abscess drainage, debridement of infected necrotic tissue and removal of a potentially infected device. Possible infectious foci include: intra-abdominal abscess, intestinal infarction and/or gastrointestinal perforation, cholangitis, pyelonephritis, empyema and septic arthritis. Identification of these sites of infection should be within the first six hours of presentation [4,5].

When source control is required minimally invasive interventions should be employed. For example, performing percutaneous drainage rather than surgical intervention of an abscess [6]. If less invasive approaches are inadequate or there is uncertainty about the diagnosis, then more aggressive measures should be considered. When making such decisions the benefits versus risks as well as the patient's preferences and clinician's expertise must be considered [7].

When an intravascular access device has been identified as the possible cause of severe sepsis removal of the device should be done after other vascular access has been established [8,9]. Special attention should be given when the suspected source of infection is a peripancreatic necrosis. Definitive intervention should be delayed until adequate demarcation of viable and non-viable tissue has been made. In this case endoscopic rather than surgical drainage of biliary tree should be considered taking into consideration what represents the least physiologic insult for the patient [10].

4. Antibiotic therapy

Administration of antibiotics is considered as important as establishing a vascular access and giving fluid resuscitation. Therapy should be started within the first hour of recognition of septic shock. In some cases this may require additional vascular access, however this shouldn't represent a delay in the infusion of antibiotics since this has been associated with increased mortality [11, 12]. The choice of empirical antibiotics will depend on patient's history, including drug intolerance, co-morbidities, the clinical syndrome and susceptibility patterns of pathogens in the hospital, community and those that have previously infected the individual. Recently used antibiotics should definitely be avoided.

Another consideration is whether fungal infection with *Candida* species is the cause of sepsis. Risk factors for candidemia include: central venous catheters, total parenteral nutrition, broad- spectrum antibiotics, high APACHE scores (Acute Physiology and

Chronic Health Evaluation II), acute renal failure, prior surgery (particularly abdominal surgery), gastrointestinal perforations and anastomotic leaks [13, 14, 15]. Immunocompromised patients such as those with hematologic malignancies, recipients of solid organ or hematopoietic stem cell transplants and those receiving chemotherapy are also at increased risk of candidemia [16].

All patients with septic shock should be treated initially with broad-spectrum antibiotics to cover the most common or likely pathogens. It has been demonstrated that failure to initiate appropriate therapy against the pathogen that is later identified as the cause of infection is associated with increased morbidity and mortality [17, 18]. Therapy should be re-evaluated on a daily basis for four reasons: to optimize activity, to prevent the development of resistance, and, to reduce toxicity and costs.

Combination therapy should be given to those patients with risk factors for *Pseudomonas* infection and neutropenia, defined as an absolute neutrophil count (ANC) less than 1500. Although clinical evidence has failed to demonstrate that combination therapy produces superior clinical outcome for individual pathogens in a particular patient group, combination therapies do produce *in vitro* synergy against pathogens in some models [19, 20, 21, 22]. The rationale in administering combination therapy for suspected *Pseudomonas* infection is to increase the likelihood that at least one drug will be effective against that strain. This intervention has demonstrated to have a positive effect on outcome [23].

Duration of therapy should not exceed more than three to five days and de-escalation to single therapy should be performed as soon as susceptibility profiles are available. Narrowing the spectrum of antibiotic coverage and reducing the duration of therapy will decrease the possibility that the patient develops superinfections with pathogens or resistant organisms such as *Candida* species, *Clostridium dificile*, or vancomycin-resistant *Enterococcus faecium*. Therapy should be prolonged from seven to ten days in patients with slow clinical response and those who are immunocompromised or have a source of infection that cannot be controlled. If the cause of the clinical syndrome has been confirmed to be of noninfectious etiology, antibiotic therapy should discontinue immediately. This will decrease the likelihood that the patient becomes infected with drug resistant pathogens.

5. Hemodynamic management in severe sepsis and septic shock

Early sepsis signs are very difficult to diagnose,usually with nonspecific presentations. Patient who arrives with an unapparent infection can progress to a lethal form of disease.

In 1992 The Society of Critical Care Medicine Conference consensus defined sepsis as a systemic inflammatory response that includes 2 or more clinical findings: temperature, respiratory rate, heart rate and white blood cell count in the setting of presumed or a documented infection [24].

Severe sepsis is hallmarked by concomitant organ hypoperfusion or dysfunction [25,26,27].

Sepsis induced hypotension is defined as a systolic blood pressure (SBP) < 90mmhg or mean arterial pressure < 65mmhg or SBP decease >40mmhg or 2SD below normal for age in absence of other cause of hypotension. Septic shock is defined as sepsis induced hypotension persisting despite adequate fluid resuscitation basically requiring vasoactive drugs.

Early recognition of sepsis with integrated approach screening, triggering evidence-based protocolized care, is anticipated to reduce sepsis morbidity and mortality [28]. The Surviving Sepsis Campaign (SSC) provided some of the best clinical evidence for the management of severe sepsis and septic shock.

6. Initial resuscitation

Patients with septic shock often require early and vigorous resuscitation with an integrated approach directed to rapid restoring systemic oxygen delivery and improving tissue oxygenation.

The first priority involves stabilization of the airway and breathing,with supplemental oxygen and if necessary institution of mechanical ventilation.

Second assessment of perfusion should be done (hypotension persisting after initial fluid challenge, blood lactate ≥ 4mmmol/L). Once hypoperfusion is recognized, early restoration of perfusion is necessary to limit secondary organ dysfunction and reduce mortality. During the first 6 hours of resuscitation, the goals should include: Central venous pressure 8-12mm Hg with a Mean Arterial Pressure (MAP) over 65mmHg,a urine output ≥ 0.5ml/kg/hr and finally a Central venous (superior vena cava) or mixed venous oxygen saturation ≥70% or ≥ 65% respectively. If Svo2 is less than 70%, packed of red blood cells (PRBC) are transfuse to achieve an hematocrit level of 30%. If central venous pressure, MAP and hematocrit were optimized and Svo2/ScVo2 remained below 70% dobutamine is recommended to increase cardiac output and oxygen delivery.

The early goal directed therapy has been shown to improved survival for emergency department (ED) patients with severe sepsis and septic shock. This evidence comes from a randomized controlled single center trial that assigned 253 patients with severe sepsis or septic shock to receive protocolized early goal directed therapy during the first 6 hours in ED or to receive standard therapy before admission in ICU. These resuscitation goals reduced the in hospital mortality from 46.5% to 30.5% (P=. 009), a 28 days mortality rate (p=0.1) and at 60 day (p=0.3) [28].

In 2004 the international group experts published first internationally accepted guidelines [29].Eventually from 2006 to 2007 the group met again to update the guidelines using new evidence [30]. Central venous pressure is currently commonly used as guide for resuscitation, although there are recognized limitations to ventricular filling pressures estimated as surrogate for fluid resuscitations [31, 32]. In mechanical ventilated patient target CVP of 12 to 15 mmHg is recommended to account for impediment of filling due to increase intrathoracic pressure [33]. Other cases to consider higher CVP include increased abdominal pressure and diastolic dysfunction [34].

The MAP is the most powerful predictor of mortality, commonly used as an indicator of perfusion pressure [35]. Current recommended levels are between 60-65 mmHg in view of adequate autoregulation of blood flow to vital organs [36].

Oxygen is delivered to the tissues as a product of cardiac output (heart rate x stroke volume) and oxygen content (hemoglobin oxygen saturation x hemoglobin x 1.34) + (partial pressure of oxygen x .003). The tissues extract a percentage of the delivered for cellular respiration and the remaining returns to venous circulations. This amount can be measure from pulmonary artery (SvO2, mixed venous oxygen saturation) or by central venous circulation (central oxygen saturation). ScvO2 is only measure with a pulmonary catheter. However, the ScvO2 can be obtained by central insertion of the superior vena cava or right atrium. Pulmonary artery catheter for hemodynamic monitoring and mixed venous saturation has not shown any difference in outcome [37, 38] but it is used in selected cases.

The measurement of Scvo2 is 5-6% higher than Sv02, but some studies has shown excellent correlation [39, 40]. So basically a targeted SvO2 has demonstrated better outcome in this population.

7. Fluid therapy

Septic shock is associated with substantial volume depletion and myocardial dysfunction. The ventricular filling pressure is usually low due to an increase in external loses from gastrointestinal or urinary tracts, bleeding, skin surface or internal loses due to exudation or transudation of bloody fluids. This leads to a generalized vasodilatation and peripheral blood pooling, consequently decreasing the intravascular volume. Adequate fluid resuscitation therefore is one of the cornerstones of the management of septic shock. The aim is the restoration of intravascular fluid volume, reestablish effective tissue perfusion, increase cardiac output and systemic oxygen delivery.

The outcomes advantages between crystalloid and colloids solutions continue to remain unsolved. The recent sepsis campaign guidelines cannot recommend one type or another. The Saline versus Albumin Fluid Evaluation (SAFE),a multicenter randomized trial study showed no difference in 28 day all mortality cause, organ dysfunction, duration of mechanical ventilation, day of renal replacement, hospital or ICU length of stay [41].

However, other study compared 10% pentastarch (a low molecular weight hydroxyethyl starch) with ringer's lactate and the first therapy was associated with higher rates of renal replacement therapy [42].

As the volume of distribution is much large for crystalloids than for colloids, the use of crystalloids for resuscitation requires more fluid and infusion periods to achieve comparable hemodynamic endpoints. Though less colloid is requires, volume expansion with colloid is more expensive.The fluid challenge in patient with suspected hypovolemia may be give at rate of 500-1000ml of crystalloids or 300-500ml of colloids over 30 min and repeated on response (blood pressure, heart rate, urine output) and tolerance (evidence of intravascular fluid overload).

Since the validation of CVP measurements in patients with sepsis is widely debated, other methods has emerged to assess fluids responsiveness. Echocardiography can be use to estimate Left ventricular End Diastolic volume but it is skill operator dependant [43]. Pulse Pressure Variation (PPV) during pressure breath can be used to predict responsiveness cardiac output to change preload [44]. PPV in mechanical ventilated patient is useful for assessing preload responsiveness [45].

Other controversial topics are the fact that excessive amount of fluid may be harmful to the patients with septic shock. Multiple studies have correlated positive fluid balance with reduces survival in ARDS [46] and sepsis [47]. Other study of 87 patients in mechanical ventilation showed that positive fluid balance were associated with failure of spontaneous breathing trials [48].

A prospective study, The Fluid and Catheter Treatment Trial (FACTT) randomized 1,001 patients with acute lung injury or ARDS to conservative (CVP<4mm Hg or pulmonary artery occlusion pressure [PAOP], <8mm Hg) vs. liberal (CVP, 10 to 14 mmHg, or PAOP, 14 to 18mm Hg) fluid management and concluded that there was no mortality difference at 60 days, but the conservative fluid strategies improved lung function, ventilator free days and reduce ICU length of stay [49].

A new retrospective study review from the Vasopressin in Septic shock trial (VASST) in which was analyzed the positive fluid balance and determined correlation with CVP at 12hrs and during subsequent days. The study found increase mortality with positive fluid balance early in resuscitation and cumulative for 4 days. The CVP may be use as a gauge to fluid balance <12hrs, but becomes an unreliable marker of fluid balance thereafter. The overall data suggest

the optimal survival occurred at CVP of 8mmHg and positive fluid balance of 3 l during first 12hr; however a randomized control studies is necessary to prove this [50].
The approach of fluid resuscitation in sepsis shock patients suggest that should be liberal in the first 6h of acute resuscitation, guided by Svo2 or Scvo2. Once the patient is adequately resuscitated, fluids should be hold without the necessity of maintenance therapy. The intravascular status should be continuing monitoring with physical examination with observation of sign of hypoperfusion, weight, input and output chart and other measures [51].

8. Vasoactive therapy

When the fluid administration fails to restore an adequate arterial pressure and organ perfusion , a vasoactive agent should be started. The ultimate goals are to restore effective tissue perfusion and normalize cellular metabolism.
In shock state, the estimation of blood pressure using a cuff may be inaccurate and the use of arterial catheterization provides more precise and reproducible measurements of arterial pressure [52].
Most experts recommend a MAP ≥ 65 mm Hg.

9. Norepinephrine

Norepinephrine is the endogenous mediator of the sympathetic system having a strong α-adrenergic activity with less β-adrenergic effects.It increases MAP by vasoconstriction, with small (10-15%) increase in cardiac output and stroke volume [53-58] .Filling pressure is either unchanged[59] or modestly increased (1-3 mm Hg) [54-57].
In open labels trials, norepinephrine at doses ranges 0.01 to 3.3μg/kg/min has demonstrated to increase MAP in patients who remained hypotensive after fluid resuscitation and dopamine [54-56 , 58, 60, 64-65].
A randomized trial compared vasopressor agents in 32 resuscitated septic patients in which either dopamine or norepinephrine were given to keep homodynamic derangements. Dopamine was successful only in 31% vs. 93% treated with norepinephrine [63].
Another larger multicenter randomized trial study, which compared dopamine vs. norepinephrine for treatment for any kind of shock (cardiogenic, hypovolemic, septic), found no significant death rate at 28 days.However, there were more arrhythmic events among patients treated with dopamine.Also, patients who suffered cardiogenic shock and were managed with dopamine had an increase mortality rate at 28 days. This and other studies suggested that norepinephrine is a safer drug in cardiogenic shock and myocardial infarction patients due to tachyphylaxis [67].
Other important multivariate analysis included 97 septic shock patients and was statistically significant for a reduced mortality by the use of the norepinephrine. The use of high use dopamine, epinephrinephrine or dobutamine had no significant effect [68].
The studies of norepinephrine with splanchnic blood flow in septic patient have mixed results. A recent one compared norepinephrine, dopamine and epinephrine for septic shock and there was no significant difference between them [69].

10. Dopamine

Dopamine has predominantly β-adrenergic effects in low to moderate dose ranges (up to 10 μg/kg per minute). Higher doses cause α-adrenergic predominance leading to arterial vasoconstriction and increase blood pressure.

It may be useful in patients with decrease systolic dysfunction but causes more arrhythmias than norepinephrine [70]. Although is has shown diuretic properties,it is not recommended for above purposes [71] probably due to its neuroendocrine effects,which may interfere with prolactin, thyroid, pituitary function and some of the immunosuppressive functions [72-73]. Moreover, the use of Dopamine at "renal dose" has been discouraged due to ample evidence in meta-analysis and high quality prospective trial .An important one included 328 criticall ill patients with early renal dysfunction and were separated in groups for low dose dopamine or placebo. No difference was found in the primary outcome (peak serum creatinine level, need for renal replacement and urine output). Other variables such as survival or hospital length of stay were unremarkable as well.

Multiple recent studies has shown more detrimental effects with Dopamine.For example, the use of dopamine was associated with an increased mortality in patients with shock in a prospective multicenter observational study of 198 Europeans ICU [74].

In conclusion, many experts have recognized that Dopamine should not be the first vasoactive drug in patients in shock and some of them recommended that should not be used anymore in patients with septic shock.

11. Epinephrine

Epinephrine has potent β1-β2 and α1-adrenegic activity, although the elevated MAP in sepsis comes mainly form an increase in cardiac output [75].The major concerns in use of epinephrine are: higher myocardial oxygen demand, hyperglycemia,increased lactate levels and a reduction in regional blood flow[76-79].

Myburhg and colleagues performed a prospective multicenter, double blinded and randomized control trial in 280 ICU patients comparing epinephrine to norepinephrine founding no difference in the time to achieve arterial pressure goals, 28 day mortality, 90 day mortality.However, 13% of the patients in the epinephrine group were withdrawn from the study because lactic acidosis or tachycardia[84].

Another randomized control trial conducted by Annane and colleagues compared 330 patients with septic shock and evaluated the efficacy of norepinephrine with or without dobutamine against epinephrine alone [85]. They found that there was no difference in efficacy or safety between the two groups. For instance,epinephrine is not currently recommended as fist line vasopressor therapy in view of concerns about tachyarrhythmias and his effects on gastric perfusion.

12. Phenylephrine

Phenylephrine works at the α1 receptors causing increased blood pressure by vasoconstriction. Its use in septic shock has had controversial results but so far there has been only few related studies.

In comparison with norepinephrine, phenylephrine reduces splanchnic blood flow, oxygen delivery and lactate uptake [86].On the other hand,it may be a good option when tachyarrhythmias limit therapy with other vasopressors.

13. Vasopressin

Arginine-vasopressin is an endogenous hormone that is release in response to decrease intravascular volume and increase plasma osmolality. Vasopressin constrict vascular

smooth muscle though V1 receptors. It also increases the responsiveness of the vascular bed to catecholamines [87,88] . Vasopressin may also increase blood pressure by inhibiting vascular smooth muscle nitric oxide [89] production and K +-ATP channels [90].
A newer interest has emerged as an additive vasoconstrictor in patients with septic shock resistant to catecholamines [90]. Vasopressin have been found to be in lower levels than expected in patients with septic shock, suggesting relative deficiency. Its combination with norepinephrine increases the splanchnic flow and urinary output [91]. Several small-randomized studies comparing vasopressin with norepinephrine have demonstrated that initiation of it decreases catecholamine requirements [92].
A large, multicenter, randomized trial (VASST) [97] with 778 patients was done to determine whether norepinephrine and vasopressin decreases mortality compared with norepinephrine alone. No difference was found in mortality, ICU or hospital length of stay, discontinuation of vasopressors or organ dysfunction. The use of norepinephrine infusion was significantly lower in cases with vasopressin dose of 0.03U/min, but vasopressin seems to be better in less severe group. New retrospective analysis of the VASST suggests a beneficial effect between vasopressin and corticosteroid in patients with septic shock that were also treated with steroids. Patients with vasopressin with corticosteroids have significantly increased in plasma vasopressin levels. Vasopressin at 0.03u/min added to norepinephrine seems to be as safe as effective as norepinephrine in fluid resuscitated patients with septic shock.

14. Dobutamine

Is an inotrope that has variable effects on blood pressure due to β1 and β2 adrenergic agonist effect resulting in an increase heart rate and cardiac contractility. Dobutamine should be considered in patients who have low cardiac output in the presence of adequate ventricular filling pressures and appropriate mean arterial pressure [28-29] .
In septic patients, it increases oxygen delivery and consumption. As part the early goal directed therapy dobutamine was associated with significant absolute reduction in mortality [28].
An inotrope should be considered to maintain an adequate cardiac index, mean arterial pressure, mixed venous oxygen content and urine output . Other available agents includes phosphodisterase inhibitors such as milrinone and enoximone, and calcium sensitizers such as levosimedan. There are currently inadequate data to recommend them in septic shock.

15. Severe sepsis/septic shock and the use of steroids

Sepsis syndrome is characterized by having a disequilibrium between pro- inflammatory and anti-inflammatory cytokines leading to overproduction of IL-1, IL-6 and TNF-α from the lymphocytes, macrophages and endothelial cells [100] . It is known that TNF- alfa and IL-6 decreases cortisol levels from the adrenal gland and ACTH production from the pituitary gland resulting in secondary adrenal insufficiency in approximately 16.3 to 55% of patients [101] . Systemic steroids might then have a beneficial role by inhibiting pro-inflammatory cytokines, nitric oxide and phospholipase A2 [102] . They also enhance the activity of adrenergic receptors and increased myocardial contractility resulting in improvement of hemodynamics response.
Hydrocortisone is usually the steroid of choice because it is the synthetic derivative of cortisol and also has intrinsic mineralocorticoid activity. After the study by Schumer, a short

course of high- dose corticosteroids became an accepted therapy [103] . Subsequent studies, however, did not confirm a survival benefit with this regimen and suggested an increase in superinfection-related mortality were patients went from being immunomodulated to being immunosupressed.

Multiple randomized trials in patients with septic shock confirm that low-dose steroid therapy in these patients improves blood pressure, thereby, causing reduction in vasopressor support.

In 2002 Annane demonstrated a reduced mortality ($p=0.04$) in a subgroup of patients that were non responders to an adrenocorticotropic hormone tests (ACTH test) but the mortality rate was increased ($p=0.96$) in patients without evidence of relative adrenal insufficiency (responders) [104] . In 2008 Russell found out a reduced mortality in a subgroup of patients with severe septic shock in those receiving steroids and vasopressin versus norepinephrine and steroids raising the concern that vasopressin may increase the levels the intrinsic cortisol levels [105].

Bauer found a positive interaction of vasopressin and corticosteroids in a nonrandomized cohort study of patients with septic shock, all of whom received vasopressin. Patients who received corticosteroids and vasopressin had lower mortality rates (47.6% vs. 80.9%; $p = 0.02$) compared with patients who did not receive corticosteroids with vasopressin. Furthermore, a randomized, blinded, placebo-controlled trial ($n = 100$) of vasopressin plus corticosteroids or placebo in human cardiac arrest found a beneficial interaction of vasopressin and corticosteroids . Patients who received vasopressin plus corticosteroids had more frequent return of spontaneous circulation (81% vs. 52%; $p = .003$) and higher survival rates (19% vs. 4%, $p = .02$) than patients who received vasopressin plus placebo.

Finally a multicenter, randomized, double-blind, placebo-controlled study called Corticosteroid Therapy of Septic Shock (CORTICUS) study, evaluated the efficacy and safety of low-dose hydrocortisone therapy in a broad population of patients with septic shock[106] . The use of low-dose hydrocortisone had no significant effect on the rate of death in 251patients with septic shock versus placebo at 28 days, regardless of the patients' adrenal responsiveness to corticotropin. The proportion of patients in whom reversal of shock was achieved was similar in the two groups, though this goal was achieved earlier in patients who received hydrocortisone. On the basis of these findings, hydrocortisone cannot be recommended as general adjuvant therapy for septic shock (vasopressor responsive), nor can corticotropin testing be recommended to determine which patients should receive hydrocortisone therapy. Hydrocortisone may have a role among patients who are treated early after the onset of septic shock who remain hypotensive despite the administration of high-dose vasopressors and adequate fluid resuscitation.

16. Activated protein C and its role in severe sepsis/septic shock

Sepsis is associated with alterations in the blood coagulation, fibrinolytic systems and inflammatory pathway. This leads to disorders of tissue perfusion that generate multiple organ system failure with depletion of platelets and coagulation factors along with the activation of natural inhibitors of coagulation. Activated protein C (APC) , an endogenous protein that promotes fibrinolysis and inhibits thrombosis and inflammation, is an important modulator of the coagulation and inflammation associated with severe sepsis[107] . It is converted from its inactive precursor, protein C, by thrombin coupled to thrombomodulin. The conversion of protein C to activated protein C may be impaired during sepsis as a result of the down-regulation of thrombomodulin by inflammatory cytokines. Reduced levels of protein C are found in the majority of patients with sepsis and are associated with an increased risk of death.

A randomized, double-blind, placebo-controlled, multicenter trial was conducted with recombinant human activated protein C in 1998 in 1690 patients to evaluate mortality at 28 days [108]. The PROWESS (Protein C worldwide evaluation in severe sepsis) trial was completed in 2001 and statistical analysis indicated a decreased 28th mortality rate of 30.8% in the placebo group compared with 24.7% in the drotrecogin alfa group. The difference in the mortality was limited to patients with a higher risk of death, that is, APACHE II scores > 25. In these groups mortality was reduced from 44% in the placebo group to 31% in the treatment group. Efficacy was doubtful in patients with low risk for death and serious bleeding was higher in the APC group.

In 2005 the ADRESS trial evaluated the efficacy of APC in patients with APACHE score < 25 or single organ failure and there was no difference in mortality among both groups at 28 days [109].

There is increased risk for serious bleeding and no beneficial effect in those patients with low risk for death, such as those with single organ failure or an APACHE II score less than 25 [110].

More recently a Cochrane database submitted their review on APC and again no difference in mortality was observed in approximately 4434 adults with sepsis. Increased risk for serious bleeding was noted and for this reason a new trial was requested by the FDA that should be completed at the end of 2011.

On the basis of this findings APC is recommended for patients with severe sepsis and high risk for death if there is no contraindications.

17. Glucose control in ICU

Blood glucose control was originally investigated in the setting of diabetes because uncontrolled levels seemed to predisposed to multiple infections (e.g., cellulitis, postoperative wound infections). Although the exact pathogenesis was unknown, it was speculated that the increased risk of infection was related to decreased cellular immune function [111]. Later studies (both in animals and humans) demonstrated that the depressed ability to fight off infection was a result of impaired polymorphonuclear leukocyte function, chemotaxis, and phagocytosis.

Extensive observational data have shown a consistent, almost linear relationship between blood glucose levels in hospitalized patients and adverse clinical outcomes, even in patients without established diabetes [112].

Van den Berghe reported a dramatic 42% relative reduction in mortality in the surgical ICU when blood glucose was normalized to 80 to 110 mg per deciliter (4.4 to 6.1 mmol per liter) by means of insulin infusion in a prospective, randomized fashion [113]. Five years later, the same investigators reported findings from their medical ICU, revealing no mortality benefit from intensive glucose control, except in a subgroup requiring critical care for 3 or more days [114].

A parallel-group, randomized, controlled trial involving adult medical and surgical patients admitted to the ICUs of 42 hospitals was conducted from December 2004 through November 2008 to evaluate mortality in patients assigned to tight glucose control versus conventional glucose control (NICE SUGAR Trial)[115] . Ninety days after randomization,

829 of 3010 patients (27.5%) in the intensive-control group had died, as compared with 751 of 3012 patients (24.9%) in the conventional-control group. Severe hypoglycemia was significantly more common with intensive glucose control. In the basis of this findings, glucose control with intravenous insulin should be started in patients with severe sepsis upon stabilization at ICU when glucose levels are above 180 (1B) with a goal blood glucose target in the range of 150 mg/dL (2C). The American Association of Clinical Endocrinologists recommends a glucose range of 140 to 180 mg/dL for most hospitalized persons.

18. Mechanical ventilation in sepsis

The strategies to ventilate patients with severe sepsis have been changing for the last decades. Multiple studies demonstrated that ventilating with the usual tidal volume may have detrimental effects causing what is now recognized as ventilator induced lung injury. This complication have led to new forms of ventilation called lung protective management in which lower volumes are provided in order to prevent alveolar overdistention.

Sepsis itself can induce acute lung injury (ALI) in about 50% of the cases. ALI is defined as an acute onset insult resulting in bilateral radiographic infiltrates, pulmonary artery wedge pressure ≤ 18 mm Hg when measured by a pulmonary catheter, an echocardiogram showing no evidence of left atrial hypertension, and an arterial oxygen tension to fraction of inspired oxygen ratio (PaO_2/FiO_2) of 201 to 300 mmHg. The difference between ARDS is mainly the worsening of hypoxemia having above ratio less than 200 mmHg [116].

With conventional ventilation,patients with ARDS had higher mortality rate when used prior the new recommendations. Lung protective ventilation has shown a decrease mortality rate and ventilator-induce lung injury [117]. This intervention also know as low tidal volume ventilation involved an initial tidal volume of 6 ml/kilogram of predicted body weight (PBW) aiming for a plateau pressure of ≤ 30 cm H_2O. If plateau pressure remains > 30 after reduction of tidal volume, it should be reduced further to as low as 4 ml/kg PBW [118]. In contrast to the conventional ventilation that involved a tidal volume of 12 ml/kilogram of body weight with low positive end-expiratory pressure (PEEP), protective ventilation avoids alveolar overdistention and end-expiratory collapse [119]. The titration of the PEEP should approach a balance between lung recruitment and overdistention, barotrauma, and hypotension in order to maintain adequate oxygenation (arterial oxygen saturation over 88%). This permit lower FIO_2, decreasing the risk of oxygen toxicity. High PEEP level may increase airway pressures and lung volumes, which could contribute to ventilator induced lung injury from overdistention [120]. The optimal strategy to set PEEP has not been established [118,120,121].

The low tidal volume ventilation can result in respiratory acidosis which now is known as permissive hypercapnia. The respiratory rate is usually increased to keep adequate minute ventilation. The increase on carbon dioxide can cause vasodilation, increase in heart rate, cardiac output, blood pressure, pulmonary vascular resistance and decrease renal blood flow; but modest hypercapnia has been demonstrated to be safe in clinical trials. This ventilation is allowed in order to prevent pulmonary overdistention and consequently negative effect in ALI/ARDS [122].If severe respiratory acidosis, pH < 7.15, develops the infusion of sodium bicarbonate may be considered. These type of ventilation is contraindicated in patients with cerebral disorders such as cerebrovascular insults, trauma, or space-occupying intracranial lesions because it may increase the intracranial pressure.

In patients with refractory hypoxemia, prone position ventilation has been recommended despite no benefits in survival. Proper precautions should be taken to avoid complications like pressure sores, accidental dislodgment of the endotracheal tube and central venous catheters [118]. Same results has been noticed in studies with high frequency oscillatory ventilation and Extra Corporeal Membrane Oxygenation (ECMO).

Noninvasive ventilation (NIV) has been suggested in patients with ALI/ARDS since it allows better communication, reduces incidence of infection, requirements for sedation and duration of intensive care unit stay [124]. Its use should be considered only in hemodynamically stable patients who are cooperative, able to protect the airway and spontaneously clear the airway of secretions; and who are anticipated to recover rapidly from the precipitating insult [124]. Continuous positive airway pressure (CPAP) and noninvasive positive pressure ventilation (NIPPV) are the most commonly used modes. In NIPPV, two different pressures are used: inspiratory positive airway pressure (IPAP) and expiratory positive airway pressure (EPAP), whereas CPAP maintains a constant positive airway pressure throughout the respiratory cycle. NIPPV may confer an advantage over CPAP by reducing the work of breathing during inspiration by providing additional inspiratory pressure. The main goal of NIV in patients with ALI/ARDS includes improvement of hypoxemia, to unload the respiratory muscles and eventually relieve dyspnea. A practical approach has been postulated, it should be use judiciously in selected patients to prevent decrease in survival if intubation is delayed [124].

The discontinuation of mechanical ventilation crucial and should be base on weaning protocol to assess readiness of successful extubation, reducing the duration and the complications related to it [118].

19. Sedation, analgesia, and neuromuscular blocked in sepsis

Patients critically ill with sepsis usually require control of anxiety, agitation and pain, especially when they are with mechanical ventilation support.There are several options of sedative-analgesic medications including benzodiazepines,opioids and neuroleptics. The intention is to achieve adequate comfort and safety using protocols with a sedation goal [125].

This accomplishment should be use according to the patient clinical condition. Several scoring scale has been validated, none superior to the other; Riker Sedation-Agitation Scale (SAS), Motor Activity Assessment Scale (MAAS), Minnesota Sedation Assessment Tool (MSAT), and Richmond Agitation-Sedation Scale (RASS) and Ramsay Sedation Scale [126].

The use of protocol-directed sedation can reduce the duration of mechanical ventilation, the intensive care unit and hospital lengths of stay, and the need for tracheostomy [127]. The use of the combination of spontaneous awakening trials (SATs), daily interruption of sedatives, with spontaneous breathing trials (SBTs) for the management of mechanically ventilated patients in intensive care results in better outcomes. It can also decrease mechanical ventilation, intensive care and hospital stay with survival improvement [128].

The pain management should be assessed frequently using a pain scale appropriate to patient's condition. The numeric rating scale has been recommended in critical ill patients because it is easier to apply [126]. Patients who cannot communicate behavioral pain scale (BPS) may be used. The pain intensity is evaluated by facial expression, movement of the upper extremities and compliance with ventilation [129].

The neuromuscular blocking agents (NMBAs) are not recommended, when possible, in septic patients due to prolonged neuromuscular blocked following discontinuation [125].

They should be use when appropriate sedation and analgesia cannot be achieved. The indications are to facilitate mechanical ventilation, improving chest wall compliance, preventing respiratory dys-synchrony, reducing peak airway pressures and decrease oxygen consumption by reducing work of breathing (1, 6). Patients receiving NMBAs should be assessed both clinically and by train-of-four monitoring, a peripheral nerve stimulation test, with a goal of adjusting the degree of neuromuscular blockade to achieve one or two twitches from a scale of 0 to 4. This may reduce clinical recovery delay from NMBAs [125,130]. The administration of NMBAs in early ARDS was demonstrated to improve outcomes, it can decrease duration of mechanical ventilation, hospital stay and ventilation induce lung injury. Further studies are requiring before this clinical practice can be adopted [131].

The 'ABCDE' bundle has been proposed combining evidence-based interventions. It consist of A wakening and Breathing trial coordination, Choice of sedatives and analgesics, Daily delirium monitoring, Early mobility and exercise to improve the management of mechanically ventilated patients[132].

20. Acute kidney injury and sepsis

Acute kidney injury (AKI) is a common complication of sepsis and septic shock. Approximately 35 to 50% of the cases in the ICU can be attributed to sepsis [133] Patients with sepsis related AKI have higher hospital mortality, 74 % ,compared with a 45% due to other diagnosis [134]. If renal replacement therapy is required the mortality rate rises further to as high as 80% [135].

The diagnosis of acute kidney injury, previously termed acute renal failure, is based on an elevation in the serum creatinine (SCr) levels. Many definitions have been proposed throughout the years since there was no real consensus on the degree of elevation required for the diagnosis of AKI. Because of this variability there was the need to develop a classification system that could propose a uniform definition within the medical community.

The Acute Dialysis Quality Initiative's "RIFLE" (Risk, Injury, Failure, Loss, ESRD) criteria was first established and included five categories, the first three of which define AKI and its severity largely by percentage increases in SCr over baseline [136]. The Acute Kidney Injury Network (AKIN) criteria was then proposed and [137] includes three stages, the last two of which are identical to the RIFLE criteria. Both definitions also incorporate severity and duration of oliguria as alternative criteria.

An improvement in urine output is a sensitive indicator of AKI, with an oliguric AKI associated to a poorer prognosis. Documentation of urine volume should be of general practice in the management of any acutely ill patient, especially those with sepsis or septic shock.

21. Renal replacement therapy

The decision to start renal replacement therapy (RRT) in patients with AKI should be based on the clinical aspects after careful evaluation of fluid, electrolyte and metabolic status of each individual patient.

Currently there are no evidence-based guidelines to suggest an optimal time to initiate treatment; it continues to be a clinical decision after the diagnosis of AKI is confirmed and before overt complications develop.

22. Continuous Renal Replacement Therapy (CRRT) vs. Intermittent Hemodyalisis (IHD)

Intermittent hemodialysis-associated hypotension is estimated to occur in approximately 20-30% of treatments. Some of the causes are dialysis specific, such as excessive or rapid volume removal, changes in plasma osmolality, autonomic dysfunction, and anaphylactic membrane reactions [138]. CRRT is most frequently used in patients who are hemodynamically unstable, usually because of sepsis or severe cardiac dysfunction because it closely resembles normal physiologic renal function with slow correction of metabolic derangements and slow fluid removal. Despite this there is no clear evidence to support the superiority of either technique, regarding mortality in the ICU. Clinicians should choose a technique according to individual patient characteristics, nursing proficiency, and technical resources.

23. Sodium bicarbonate replacement in sepsis

Infusions of sodium bicarbonate long have been advocated to correct persistent metabolic acidosis. It was said to result in increased pH with less cellular dysfunction, improved cardiac contractility and the activity of vasopressor agents. However clinical studies suggest that this therapy should be tried as a last resort to improve the patient's clinical status.

In a recent review [139] the data supporting sodium bicarbonate infusion were evaluated. It seems clear from animal data that artificially increasing the pH does not improve such parameters as cardiac function or weaning of vassopressor agents. Further decrease in serum pH levels is possible since sodium bicarbonate is converted to carbon dioxide and water, which can also lead to sodium and fluid overload. Sodium bicarbonate replacement should be considered as a last resource and is not recommended in patients with hypoperfusion induced lactic acidema with pH _> 7.15.

24. Venous thromboembolic events prophylaxis

Patients with severe sepsis have higher risk of venous thromboembolic events (VTEs) due to one or more risk factors, including advanced age, chronic cardiopulmonary disease, recent surgery, immobilization, in-dwelling vascular catheters, and previous VTE history [140]. Sepsis is associated with systemic activation of coagulation and frequently results in disseminated intravascular coagulation (DIC) [141]. Also hypoperfusion and reperfusion seen in patients with shock has been associated with endothelial damage. Indeed, VTE prophylaxis using unfractionated heparin (UFH), low molecular weight heparin (LMWH), and/or mechanical methods has become standard of care in most institutions [142].

25. Stress ulcer prophylaxis

Stress ulcers are a common complication in ICU admissions and more importantly in those related to sepsis. A clear etiology has not been established but ischemia and reperfusion are thought to cause the mucosal defenses to break down, resulting in mucosal injury and ulceration [143]. During sepsis and septic shock, reduced blood flow, hypoperfusion, and reperfusion injury may be seen secondary to hypotension or hypovolemia. These are the most common risk factors contributing to mucosal injury, hence leading to development of stress ulcers.

Treatment options include H_2 receptor antagonists (H_2Ras) which act by decreasing gastric acid secretion through reversible, competitive inhibition of histamine-stimulated acid secretion and are effective in reducing basal acid production. However, because gastrin and acetylcholine provide alternative pathways to the stimulation of acid secretion, acid suppression with H_2RAs is incomplete.

Proton pump inhibitors (PPIs) inhibit the final step in acid production, the generation of gastric hydrogen ions via hydrogen potassium adenosinetriphosphatase; they provide long-lasting suppression of acid secretion.

Both H_2Ras and PPIs have been proved effective for prevention of stress ulcers and superiority of one treatment option over the other has not been clearly established in clinical trials. Careful considerations must be taken on greater incidence of ventilator associated pneumonias on patients with sepsis already placed on mechanical ventilation, due to an increase in stomach pH. Physicians most weight individual risk over benefits, especially in those patients at greater risks of developing gastrointestinal bleeding.

26. References

[1] Weinstein MP, Reller LP, Murphy JR, et al: the clinical significance of positive blood cultures: A comprehensive analysis of 500 episodes of bacteremia and fungemia in adults. Laboratory and epidemiologic observations. *Rev Infect Dis* 1983; 5: 35-53

[2] Giamarellos-Bourboulis EJ, Giannopoulou P, Grecka P, et al: Should procalcitonin be introduced in the diagnostic criteria for the systemic inflammatory response syndrome and sepsis? *J Crit Care* 200419:152-157

[3] Tenover FC: Rapid detection and identification of bacterial pathogens using novel molecular technologies: Infection control and beyond. *Clin Infect Dis* 2007; 44:418 - 423

[4] Jimenez MF, Marshall JC: Source control in the management of sepsis. *Intensive Care Med* 2001; 27:S49 -S62

[5] Moss RL, Musemeche CA, Kosloske AM: Necrotizing fascitis in children: Prompt recognition and aggressive therapy improve survival. *J Pediatr Surg* 1996; 31:1142–1146

[6] Bufalari A, Giustozzi G, Moggi L: Postoperative intraabdominal abscesses: Percutaneous versus surgical treatment. *Acta Chir Belg* 1996; 96:197–200

[7] Evans A, Winslow BH: Oxygen saturation and hemodynamic response in critically ill mechanically ventilated adults during intrahospital transport. *Am J Crit Care* 1995; 4:106 -111

[8] Centers for Disease Control and Prevention:Guidelines for the prevention of intravascular catheter-related infections. *MMWR Morbid Mortal Wkly Rep* 2002; 51(RR-10):1–29

[9] O'Grady NP, Alexander M, Dellinger EP, et al: Guidelines for the prevention of intravascular catheter-related infections. *Clin Infect Dis* 2002; 35:1281–1307

[10] Mier J, Leon EL, Castillo A, et al: Earlyversus late necrosectomy in severe necrotizing pancreatitis. *Am J Surg* 1997; 173:71–75

[11] Kumar A, Roberts D, Wood KE, et al: Duration of hypotension prior to initiation of effective antimicrobial therapy is the critical determinant of survival in human septic shock. *Crit Care Med* 2006; 34:1589 -1596

[12] Morrell M, Fraser VJ, Kollef MH: Delaying the empiric treatment of candida bloodstream infection until positive blood culture results are obtained: A potential risk factor for hospital mortality. *Antimicrob Agents Chemother* 2005; 49:3640 -3645

[13] Nguyen MH, Peacock JE Jr, Tanner DC, Morris AJ, Nguyen ML, Snydman DR, Wagener MM, Yu VL: Therapeutic approaches in patients with candidemia. Evaluation in a multicenter, prospective, observational study. *Arch Intern Med* 1995;155(22):2429

[14] Nucci M, Colombo AL, et al. Risk factors for death in patients with candidemia. *Infect Control Hosp Epidemiol* 1998;19(11):846.

[15] Lin MY et al.Prior antimicrobial therapy and risk of hospital- acquired Candida glabrata and Candida krusei fungemia; a case - control study. *Antimicrob Agents Chemother*.2005;49(11):4555.

[16] Chow JK, Golan Y et al. Risk factors for albicans and non-albicans candidemia in the intensive care unit. *Crit Care Med* 2008;3697):1993

[17] Leibovici L, Shraga I, Drucker M, et al: The benefit of appropriate empirical antibiotic treatment in patients with bloodstream infection. *J Intern Med* 1998; 244:379 -386

[18] Ibrahim EH, Sherman G, Ward S, et al: The influence of inadequate antimicrobial treatment of bloodstream infections on patient outcomes in the ICU setting. *Chest* 2000;118:146 -155

[19] herapy. *Crit Care Med* 2007; 25:1888 -1895Hughes WT, Armstrong D, Bodey GP, et al:2002 Guidelines for the use of antimicrobial agents in neutropenic patients with cancer.http://www.idsociety.org.

[20] Klastersky J: Management of fever in neutropenic patients with different risks of complications. *Clin Infect Dis* 2004 ;39 (Suppl 1):S32–S37

[21] Safdar N, Handelsman J, Maki DG: Does combination antimicrobial therapy reduce mortality in Gram-negative bacteraemia? A meta-analysis. *Lancet Infect Dis* 2004;4:519 -527

[22] Paul M, Silbiger I, Grozinsky S, et al: Beta lactam antibiotic monotherapy versus beta lactam-aminoglycoside antibiotic combination therapy for sepsis. *Cochrane Database Syst Rev* 2006; (1):CD003344

[23] Garnacho-Montero J, Sa-Borges M, SoleViolan J, et al: Optimal management therapy for Pseudomonas aeruginosa ventilator associated pneumonia: An observational,multicenter study comparing monotherapy with combination antibiotic . *Crit Care Med* 2007; 25:1888 -1895

[24] Bone RC, Balk RA, Cerra FB, et al. Definitions for sepsis and organ failure and guidelines for the use of none invasive therapies in sepsis. The ACCP/SCCM Consensus Conference committee. American Colleague of Chest Physician/Society Critical Care Medicine. *Chest* 1992; 1644-55.

[25] Marshall JC, Cook DJ, Christou NV, et al. Multiple organ dysfunction score: a reliable descriptor of complex clinical outcome. *Crit Care Med*.1995; 23:1638-52.

[26] Astiz ME, Rackow EC, Falk JL, Kaufman BS, Weil MH. Oxygen delivery and consumption in patients with hyperdynamic septic shock. Crit care Med 1987; 15:26-8.

[27] Ferreira FL, Bota DP, Bross A, et al. Serial evaluation of the SOFA score to predict outcome in critically ill patient. JAMA 2001; 286:174-1758.

[28] Rivers E, Nguyen B, Havstad S, et al; Early Goal Directed Therapy Collaborative group. Early Goal Directed Therapy in the treatment of severe sepsis and septic shock. *N Engl J Med.*2001; 345; 1368-77.

[29] Dellinger RP, Levy MM, Carlet JM, et al; Surviving Sepsis Campaign Guidelines for management of severe sepsis and septic shock: Crit Care med 2004; 32 859-873.

[30] Dellinger RP, Levy MM, Carlet JM, et al; International Surviving Sepsis Campaign Guidelines Committee, American Association Of Critical Care Nurses, American College Of Physician, et al. Surviving Sepsis Campaign: International guidelines of management of severe sepsis and septic shock: 2008 Crit Care med 2008;36;296-327.

[31] Magder S: Central venous pressure: A Useful but not so simple measurement. Crit Care Med 2206; 34:2222-2227.

[32] Bendjelid K: Right atrial pressure: Determinant or result of change in venous return? Chest 2005; 1283639-3640.

[33] Bendjelid K, Romand JA: Fluid responsiveness in mechanical ventilated patients: A review of indices used in intensive care. Intensive care Med 2033; 352-360.

[34] Malbrain ML, Deeren D, De Potter TJ: Intra-abdominal hypertension in the critically ill: It is time to pay attention. Curr Opin Crit care 2005; 11: 156-171.

[35] Varpula M, Tallgen M, Saukkonen K, et al: Hemodynamic variables related to outcome in septic shock. Intensive Care Med 2005; 31 1066-1071.

[36] Patton HD, Fuchs, AF, Hille B, Sacher AM, Steiner R (1989) Textbook of physiology, Sauders Phyladelphia.

[37] Harvey S, Harrison DA, Singer M, et al. Assessment of the clinical effectiveness or pulmonary artery catheters in management of patient in intensive care. (PAC-Man): a randomized controlled trial. Lancet 2005; 366: 472-477.

[38] Wheeler AP, Bernard GR, Thompson BT et al. Pulmonary artery versus central venous catheter to guide treatment of acute lung injury. N ENG J Med 2006; 354: 2213-2224.

[39] Supriya Maddirala, MD, Akram Kanm, MD. Optimizing hemodynamic support in septic shock using central and mixed venous oxygen saturation. Crit Care Clin 26 (2010) 323-333.

[40] Reinhart K, Kuhn HJ, Hartog C, Bredele DL. Continuous central venous and pulmonary artery oxygen saturation monitoring in the critically ill. Intensive Care Med 2004, 30:1572-8.

[41] Finfer S, Bellomo R, Boyce N, Et al. SAFE study investigators. A comparison of albumin and saline for fluid resuscitation in the intensive care unit. N Engl J med. 2004; 32, 2029-2038.

[42] Brunkhorst FM, Engel C, Bloos F, et al. German competence network Sepsis (SepNet). Intensive insulin therapy and pentastarch resuscitation in severe sepsis. N Engl J med. 2008; 358; 125-139.

[43] Smith MD, McPhail B, Harrison Mr, et al. Value and limitations of transesophageal echocardiography in determination of left ventricular volumes and ejection fraction. Jam Coll Cardiol 1992, 19:1213-1222.

[44] Michard F, Boussat S, Chemela D, Richard C, et al. Clinical use of respiratory changes in arterial pulse pressure to monitor the hyperdynamic effects of PEEP. Am J Resp Crit care Med 1999; 15:935-939.

[45] Gunn SR, Pinsky MR. Implications of arterial pressure variations in patients in the intensive care unit. Curr Opin Crit care 2001:7:212-217.

[46] Humprey H, Hall J, Szajder I et al. Improved survival in ARDS patient associated with reduction of in pulmonary capillary wedge pressure. Chest 1190, 97:1176-1180.

[47] Simmons RS, Berdine GC, Seidefeld JJ, et al. Fluid balance in the adult respiratory distress syndrome. Am Respir Dis 1987; 135:924-929.

[48] Updaya A. Tilluckdharry L, Muralidharam V, et al. Fluid balance and weaning outcomes. Intensive Care med 2005; 31:1643-1647.

[49] Wiedemann HP, Wheeler AP, Bernard GR, et al. Comparison of two fluid management strategies in acute lung injury. N Engl J Med 2006; 354:2564-2575.

[50] Boyd JH, Forbes J, Nakada TA, et al: fluid resuciatation in septic shock: a positive fluid balance and elevated central venous pressure are associated with increased mortality. Crit Care Med 2011, 39:259-265.

[51] Durairaj L, Schmidt GA. Fluid therapy in resuscitated sepsis: less is more. *Chest.* 2008; 133:252–263. doi: 10.1378/chest.07-1496.

[52] Hollenberg SM, Ahrens Ts, Annane D, et al. Practice parameters for hemodynamic support of sepsis in adult patients: 2004 update. Crit Care Med 2004:321928-1948.

[53] Desjars P, Pinaud M, Bugnon D, et al. Norepinephrine therapy has no deleterious renal effects in human septic shock. Crit Care Med 1989; 17:426–9.

[54] Desjars P, Pinaud M, Tasseau F, et al. A reappraisal of norepinephrine therapy inhuman septic shock. Crit Care Med 1987; 15:134–7.

[55] Hesselvik JF, Brodin B. Low dose norepinephrine in patients with septic shock and oliguria: effects on afterload, urine flow, and oxygen transport. Crit Care Med 1989; 17:179–80.

[56] Meadows D, Edwards JD, Wilkins RG, et al. Reversal of intractable septic shock with norepinephrine therapy. Crit Care Med 1988; 16:663–7.

[57] Martin C, Perrin G, Saux P, et al. Effects of norepinephrine on right ventricular function in septic shock patients. Intensive Care Med 1994; 20:444–7.

[58] Martin C, Saux P, Eon B, et al. Septic shock: a goal-directed therapy using volume loading, dobutamine and/or norepinephrine. Acta Anaesthesiol Scand 1990; 34:413–7.

[59] Martin C, Eon B, Saux P, et al. Renal effects of norepinephrine used to treat septic shock patients. Crit Care Med 1990; 18:282–5.

[60] Redl-Wenzl EM, Armbruster C, Edelmann G, et al. The effects of norepinephrine on hemodynamics and renal function in severe septic shock states. Intensive Care Med 1993; 19:151–4.
[61] Marik PE, Mohedin M. The contrasting effects of dopamine and norepinephrine on systemic and splanchnic oxygen utilization in hyperdynamic sepsis. JAMA 1994; 272:1354–7.
[62] Ruokonen E, Takala J, Kari A, et al. Regional blood flow and oxygen transport in septic shock. Crit Care Med 1993; 21:1296–303.
[63] Martin C, Papazian L, Perrin G, et al. Norepinephrine or dopamine for the treatment of hyperdynamic septic shock. Chest 1993; 103:1826–31.
[64] Levy B, Bollaert PE, Charpentier C, et al. Comparison of norepinephrine and dobutamine to epinephrine for hemodynamics, lactate metabolism, and gastric tonometric variables in septic shock: a prospective, randomized study. Intensive Care Med 1997; 23:282–7.
[65] Martin C, Viviand X, Arnaud S, et al. Effects of norepinephrine plus dobutamine or norepinephrine alone on left ventricular performance of septic shock patients. Crit Care Med 1999; 27:1708–13.
[66] Chernow B, Roth BL. Pharmacologic manipulation of the peripheral vasculature in shock: clinical and experimental approaches. Circ Shock 1986; 18:141–55.
[67] De Backer D, Briston P, Devereiendt J. et al. Comparison of dopamine and norepinephrine in the treatment of shock. N Engl J Med 2010; 362779-89.
[68] Martin C, Viviand X, Leone M, et al. Effect of norepinephrine on the outcome of septic shock. Crit Care Med 2000; 28:2758–65.
[69] De Backer D, Creteur J, Silva E, et al. Effects of dopamine, norepinephrine, and epinephrine on the splanchnic circulation in septic shock: which is best? Crit Care Med 2003; 31:1659–67.
[70] Regier B, Rapin M, Gory G, et al. Hemodynamic effects of dopamine in septic shock. Intensive Care Med. 1977,3: 47-53.
[71] Bellomo R, Chapman M, Finfer S, et al. Low dose dopamine in patents with early renal dysfunction: a placebo: A Placebo- controlled randomized trial. Australian and New Zealand Intensive Care Society (ANZICS) Clinical Trials Groups. Lancet. 2000; 356:2139-2143.
[72] Van den Berghe G, de Zegher F, Lauwers P. Dopamine suppress pituitary function in infants and children. Crit Care Med. 1994; 22:1747-1753.
[73] Oberbeck R, Schmitz D, Wilsnack K, et al. Dopamine affects cellular immune functions during polymicrobial sepsis. Intensive Care Med 2006; 32:32731-739.
[74] Sakr Y. Reinhart K, Vincent JL, et al. Does dopamine administration in shock influence outcome? Results of the Sepsis Occurrence in Acutely Ill Patients (SOAP) study. Crit Care Med 2006; 34: 589-597.
[75] Hannemann L, Reinhart K, Grenzer O. et al Comparison of dopamine to dobutamine and norepinephrine for oxygen delivery and uptake in septic shock . Crit Care Med.1995; 23:1962-1970.
[76] Meier-Hellman A, Reinhart K. Effects of catecholamines on regional perfusion and oxygenation in critically ill patients. Acta Anestesiol Scand Suppl 1995; 107:239-248.

[77] Bollart PE, Bauer P, Audibert G, et al. Effects of norepinephrine on hemodynamics and oxygen metabolism in dopamine- resistant septic shock. Chest 1990; 98:949-953.

[78] Wilson W, Lipman J, Scribante J, et al. Septic Shock: Does adrenaline have role as first line inotropic agent?. Anesth Intens Care 1992;20:470-4.

[79] Levy B., Bollaert P.E., Charpentier C., et al. Comparison of norepinephrine and dobutamine to epinephrine for hemodynamics,lactate metabolism and gastric tonometric variables in septic shock:A prospective,randomized study.*Intensive Care Med* 1997; 23:282-287.

[80] Zhou S.X., Qiu H.B., Huang Y.Z., et al: Effects of norepinephrine, epinephrine, and norepinephrine-dobutamine on systemic and gastric mucosal oxygenation in septic shock. *Acta Pharmacol Sin* 2002; 23:654-658.

[81] Meier-Hellmann A., Reinhart K., Bredle D.L., et al: Epinephrine impairs splanchnic perfusion in septic shock. *Crit Care Med* 1997; 25:399-404.

[82] Martikainen T.J., Tenhunen J.J., Giovannini I., et al: Epinephrine induces tissue perfusion deficit in porcine endotoxin shock: Evaluation by regional CO(2) content gradients and lactate-to-pyruvate ratios. *Am J Physiol Gastrointest Liver Physiol* 2005; 288:G586-G592.

[83] De Backer D, Cretaur J Silva E, et al. Effects of dopamine, norepinephrine, and epinephrine in the splenic circulation in septic shock: which are the best: Crit Care Med 2003; 31:1659.

[84] Myburgh J.A., Higgins A., Jovanovska A., et al:A comparison of epinephrine and norepinephrine in critically ill patients. *Intensive Care Med* 2008; 34:2226-2234.

[85] Annane D., Vignon P., Renault A., et al:Norepinephrine plus dobutamine versus epinephrine alone for management of septic shock:A randomized trial .*Lancet* 2007; 370:676-684.

[86] Reinelt H., Radermacher P., Kiefer P., et al:Impact of exogenous beta-adrenergic receptor stimulation on hepatosplanchnic oxygen kinetics and metabolic activity in septic shock. *Crit Care Med* 1999; 27:325-331.

[87] Holmes C.L., Patel B.M., Russell J.A., Walley K.R.: Physiology of vasopressin relevant to management of septic shock. *Chest* 2001; 120:989-1002.

[88] Barrett B.J., Parfrey P.S.: Clinical practice: Preventing nephropathy induced by contrast medium. *N Engl J Med* 2006; 354:379-386.

[89] Kusano E, TianS, UminoT, et al. Arginine-vasopressin inhibits interleukin-1beta-stimulated nitric oxide and cyclic guanosine monophosphate production via the V1 receptor in cultured rat vascular smooth muscle cells. J Hypertens 1997; 15:627–32.

[90] Wakatsuki T, Nakaya Y, Inoue I. Vasopressin modulates K (1)-channel activities of cultured smooth muscle cells from porcine coronary artery. Am J Physiol 1992; 263:H491–6.

[91] Malay M.B., Ashton Jr R.C., Landry D.W, Townsend R.N.:Low dose vasopressin in the treatment of vasodilatory septic shock. *J Trauma* 1999; 47:699-703.discussion 705.

[92] Buijk S.E., Bruining H.A.: Vasopressin deficiency contributes to the vasodilation of septic shock. *Circulation* 1998; 98:187.

[93] Goldsmith S. R.: Vasopressin deficiency and vasodilation of septic shock. *Circulation* 1998; 97:292-293.

[94] Reid I. A.: Role of vasopressin deficiency in the vasodilation of septic shock. *Circulation* 1997; 95:1108-1110.

[95] Patel B. M., Chittock D.R., Russell J.A., Walley K. R.: Beneficial effects of short term vasopressin infusion during severe septic shock. *Anesthesiology* 2002; 96: 576-582.

[96] Dunser MW, Mayr AJ, Ulmer H, et al. Arginine vasopressin in advanced vasodilatory shock: a prospective, randomized, controlled study. Circulation 2003; 107:2313–9.

[97] Russell JA, Walley KR, Singer J, et al. Vasopressin versus norepinephrine infusion in patients with septic shock. N Engl J Med 2008; 358:877–87.

[98] Russell J.A., Walley K.R., Gordon A.C., et al: Interaction of vasopressin infusion,corticosteroid treatment and mortality of septic shock. *Crit Care Med* 2009; 37:811-818.

[99] Meier-Hellmann A, Bredle DL, Specht M, et al. The effects of low-dose dopamine on splanchnic blood flow and oxygen utilization in patients with septic shock. Intensive Care Med 1997; 23:31–7.

[100] Marshall JC. Inflammation, coagulopathy, and the pathogenesis of multiple organ dysfunction syndrome Crit Care Med 2001;29:S99-106.

[101] Soni A, Pepper GM, Wyrwinski PM, Ramirez NE, Simon R, Pina T, et al. Adrenal insufficiency occurring during septic shock: Incidence, outcome, and relationship to peripheral cytokine levels. Am J Med 1995;98:266-71.

[102] Szabo C, Thiemermann C, Wu CC, Perretti M, Vane JR. Attenuation of the induction of nitric oxide synthetase by endogenous glucocorticoids accounts for endotoxin tolerance in vivo. Proc Nati Acad Sci U S A 1994;91:271-5.

[103] Schumer W: Steroids in the treatment of clinical septic shock. Ann Surg 1976; 184:333-341

[104] Annane D. Corticosteroids for septic shock. Crit Care Med 2001;29:S117-20

[105] Russell JA, Walley KR, Gordon AC, et al: Interaction of vasopressin infusion, corticosteroid treatment, and mortality of septic shock. CritCare Med 2009; 37:811- 818

[106] Sprung, CL MD., Annane D MD., et al: Hydrocortisone Therapy for Patients with Septic Shock. N Engl J Med 2008;358:111-24.

[107] Esmon CT. The protein C anticoagulant pathway. Arterioscler Thromb 1992;12:135-45.

[108] Bernard GR, Vincent JL, Laterre PF, et al.Efficacy and safety of recombinant human activated protein C for severe sepsis. New England Journal Medicine 2001;344(10):699–709.

[109] Laterre PF, Abraham E, Janes JM, Trzaskoma BL, Correl NL, Booth F. ADDRESS (ADministration of DRotrecogin alfa[activated] in Early stage Severe sepsis) long-term follow-up: one year safety and efficacy evaluation. Critical Care Medicine 2007;35(6):1457–63.

[110] Laterre PF Abraham, Garg R, Levy H, Talwar D, Trzaskoma BL, et al.Drotrecogin alfa (activated) for adults with severe sepsis and a low risk of death. New England Journal of Medicine 2005;353 (13):1332–41.

[111] Tan JS. Infectious complications in patients with diabetes mellitus. Int Diabetes Monitor. 2000;12:1-7.

[112] Inzucchi SE. Management of hyperglycemia in the hospital setting. N Engl J Med 2006; 355:1903-11.

[113] Van den Berghe G, Wouters P, Weekers F, et al. Intensive insulin therapy in critically ill patients. N Engl J Med 2001; 345:1359-67.

[114] Van den Berghe G, Wilmer A, Hermans G, et al. Intensive insulin therapy in the medical ICU. N Engl J Med 2006; 354:449-61.

[115] The NICE-SUGAR Study investigators. Intensive versus Conventional Glucose Control in Critically Ill Patients N Engl J Med 2009; 360:13.

[116] Bernard GR, Artigas A, Brigham KL, Carlet J, Falke K, Hudson L, et al. The American- European Consensus Conferences on ARDS. Definitions, mechanisms, relevant outcomes, and clinical trial coordination. Am J Respir Crit Care Med 1994;149:818-24

[117] Ventilation with lower tidal volumes as compared with traditional tidal volumes for acute lung injury and acute respiratory distress syndrome. Acute Respiratory Distress Syndrome Network. N Engl J Med 2000;342 (18):1301-8

[118] Dellinger RP,Levy MM,Carlet JM,Bion J,Parker MM,Jaeschke R et al. Surviving Sepsis Campaign: International guidelines for management of severe sepsis and septic shock: 2008. Crit Care Med. 2008; 36(1):296-327.

[119] Malhotra A. Low-tidal-volume ventilation in the acute respiratory distress syndrome. N Engl J Med 2007;357(11):1113-20

[120] Brower RG,Lanken PN,MacIntyre N,Mathay MA,Morris A,Ancukiewicz M,et al.National Heart,Lung and Blood Institute ARDS Clinical Trials Network.Higher versus lower positive end-expiratory pressures in patients with the acute respiratory distress syndrome.N Engl J Med 2004;351(4):327-36

[121] Esan A,Hess DR,Raoof S,George L,Sessler CN. Severe hypoxemic respiratory failure: part 1-ventilatory strategies Chest 2010;137(5);1203-1216

[122] Esan A,Hess DR,Raoof S,George L,Sessler CN,Feihl F,Perret C.Permissive hypercapnia. How permissive should we be? Am J Resp Crit Care Med 1994;150:1722-37

[123] Raoof S,Goulet K,Esan A,Hess DR,Sessler CN. Severe hypoxemic respiratory failure: part 2-nonventilatory strategies. Chest 2010;137(6);1437-1448

[124] Agarwal R. Non invasive ventilation in Acute Lung Injury/ Acute respiratory Distress Syndrome. In: Esquinas AM. Noninvasive Mechanical Ventilation: Theory, Equipment and Clinical applications. Springer-Verlag Berlin Heidelberg 2010: 241-248

[125] Dellinger P,Levy MM,Carlet JM,Bion J,Parker MM,Jaeschke R et al. Surviving Sepsis Campaign: International guidelines for management of severe sepsis and septic shock: 2008. Crit Care Med. 2008; 36 (1):296-327.

[126] Jacob J, Fraser GL, Coursin DB, Riker RR, Fontaine D, Wittbrodt ET, et al. Clinical practice guidelines for the sustained use of sedatives and analgesics in the critically ill adult. Crit Care Med. 2002;30 (1):119-41.

[127] Brook AD, Ahrens TS, Schaiff R,Prentice D,Sherman G,Shannon W et al: Effect of a nursing-implemented sedation protocol on the duration of mechanical ventilation. Crit Care Med 1999; 27(12):2609–15

[128] Girard TD, Kress JP, Fuchs BD, Thomason JW, Schweickert WD, Pun BT, et al. Efficacy and safety of a paired sedation and ventilator weaning protocol for mechanically ventilated patients in intensive care (Awakening and Breathing Controlled trial): a randomised controlled trial. Lancet. 2008;371 (9607):126-34.

[129] Payen JF, Bru O, Bosson JL, Lagrasta A, Novel E, Deschaux I, et al. Assessing pain in critically ill sedated patients by using a behavioral pain scale. Crit Care Med. 2001;29 (12):2258-63.

[130] Murray MJ, Cowen J, DeBlock H, Erstad B, Gray AW Jr, Tescher AN, et al. Clinical practice guidelines for sustained neuromuscular blockade in the adult critically ill patient. Crit Care Med. 2002;30 (1):142-56.

[131] Papazian L.Foerl Jm,Gacouin A,Penot-Rangon C,Perrin G,Loundou A,et al. Neuromuscular blockers in early acute respiratory distress syndrome. N Engl J Med. 2010;363 (12):1107-16.

[132] Morandi A, Brummel NE, Ely EW. Sedation, delirium and mechanical ventilation: the 'ABCDE' approach. Curr Opin Crit Care. 2011;17(1):43-9

[133] Uchino S, Kellum JA, Bellomo R, Doig GS, Morimatsu H, Morgera S, Schetz M, Tan I, Bouman C, Macedo E, Gibney N, Tolwani A,Ronco C: Acute renal failure in critically ill patients: A multinational, multicenter study. *JAMA 2005*;294:813-818

[134] Robert W. Schrier, M.D., and Wei Wang, M.D. Acute Renal Failure and Sepsis. N Engl J Med 2004; 351:159-169

[135] Liaño F, Junco E, Pascual J, Madero R, Verde E. The spectrum of acute renal failure in the intensive care unit compared with that seen in other settings. The Madrid Acute Renal Failure Study Group. Kidney Int 1998; 53:S16-24

[136] Bellomo R, Ronco C, Kellum JA, Mehta RL, Palevsky P, Acute Dialysis Quality Initiative workgroup.Acute renal failure - definition, outcome measures, animal models, fluid therapy and information technology needs: the Second International Consensus Conference of the Acute Dialysis Quality Initiative (ADQI). Group Crit Care. 2004;8(4):R204.

[137] Mehta RL, Kellum JA, Shah SV, Molitoris BA, Ronco C, Warnock DG, Levin A, Acute Kidney Injury Network.. Acute Kidney Injury Network: report of an initiative to improve outcomes in acute kidney injury. Crit Care. 2007;11(2):R31.

[138] Emili, S., N. A. Black, R. V. Paul, C. J. Rexing, and M. E. Ullian. 1999. A protocol-based treatment for intradialytic hypotension in hospitalized hemodialysis patients. *Am. J. Kidney Dis.* 33:1107–1114.

[139] Cooper DJ, Walley KR, Wiggs BR, et al: Bicarbonate does not improve hemodynamics in critically ill patients who have lactic acidosis: A prospective, controlled clinical study. *Ann Intern Med* 1990; 112:492–498

[140] Cook DJ, Crowther MA, Meade MO, Douketis J, for the VTE in the ICU Workshop Participants. Prevalence, incidence, and risk factors for venous thromboembolism in medical-surgical intensive care unit patients. *J Crit Care* 2005;20:309–313

[141] Sacha Zeerleder, MD, C. Erik Hack, MD, PhD, Walter A. Wuillemin, MD; PhD. Disseminated Intravascular Coagulation in Sepsis· CHEST October 2005 vol. 128 no. 4 2864-2875

[142] Perez J, Dellinger RP, and International Sepsis Forum. Other supportive therapies in sepsis. *Intensive Care Med* 2001;27(Suppl 1):S116–S127

[143] Spirt MJ. Stress-related mucosal disease. Curr Treat Options Gastroenterol. 2003;6: 135-145.

12

Applied Physiology and the Hemodynamic Management of Septic Shock Utilizing the Physiologic Optimization Program

William McGee and Patrick Mailloux
Baystate Medical Center, Tufts University School of Medicine
United States

1. Introduction

Volume management is an important aspect of caring for patients with sepsis. Multiple factors contribute to the challenge of resuscitating septic patients, including volume depletion, a decrease in vascular tone and myocardial depression. Goal directed therapy incorporates the use of physiologic targets to guide fluid resuscitation in this population, taking into account the changes in physiology of a patient with sepsis. Further, evolving technology and knowledge is allowing for a better understanding of endpoints when managing fluids in this critically ill patient group.

Patient's presenting with hypo-perfusion secondary to septic shock benefit from early, aggressive resuscitation in a protocolized manner (Rivers, 2001). The goals of initial resuscitation, to be achieved within 6 hours of presentation, include a central venous pressure of 8 - 12 mmHg, mean arterial pressure (MAP) of ≥ 65 mmHg, urine output > 0.5 mL/kg/hr and a central venous ($ScvO_2$) or mixed venous oxygen saturation ≥ 70% or 65%, respectively (Rivers 2001, Dellinger, 2008). This concept is known as early goal directed therapy (EGDT) (Rivers, 2001).

1.1 Oxygen delivery

The ultimate goal of early resuscitation is to achieve adequate oxygen delivery so the balance between supply and demand to vital organs is maintained. A critical level of oxygen delivery (DO_2) exists for septic patients and increasing the DO_2 above that level does not further increase oxygen consumption. (Ronco, 1993; Shibutani, 1983;, Danek, 1980; Nelson, 1987, 1988) When below critical DO_2, oxygen utilization is dependent upon DO_2 (Figure 1), compensation via increased oxygen extraction is no longer sufficient, oxygen debt develops and anaerobic metabolism ensues. (Pieracci, 2011) One accepted method to measure whether DO_2 is above this threshold involves determining the oxygen saturation of venous blood returning to the heart (McGee & Jodka, 2002; Krafft, 1993). $ScvO_2$ as a proxy for SVO_2 is reasonable (Lee, 1972; Reinhart, 2004; Ladakis, 2001) and reflects the oxygen saturation of SVC blood. As the saturation of venous blood (Figure 2) declines, oxygen consumption is increasing for a constant value of oxygen delivery, or oxygen delivery itself may be declining. In either circumstance assessment of $ScVO_2$ represents the balance between delivery and consumption simultaneously and can be measured continuously alerting the clinician to reassess the components of both delivery and consumption. Critical imbalances often require acute intervention to assure survival and prevent organ dysfunction. Lower values are the result of increased oxygen extraction at the tissue level typically due to decreased oxygen delivery (DO_2) and values <70% suggest tissue hypoperfusion. If the $ScVO_2$ drops below 50% there is an increased risk of developing anaerobic metabolism and lactic acidosis. (Simmons, 1978) Low or declining $ScVO_2$ indicates further manipulation of DO_2 or less commonly VO_2 may be necessary to assure adequate cellular oxygenation. (Rivers, 2001; Lee, 1972; Kasnitz, 1976; Reinhart, 1989)

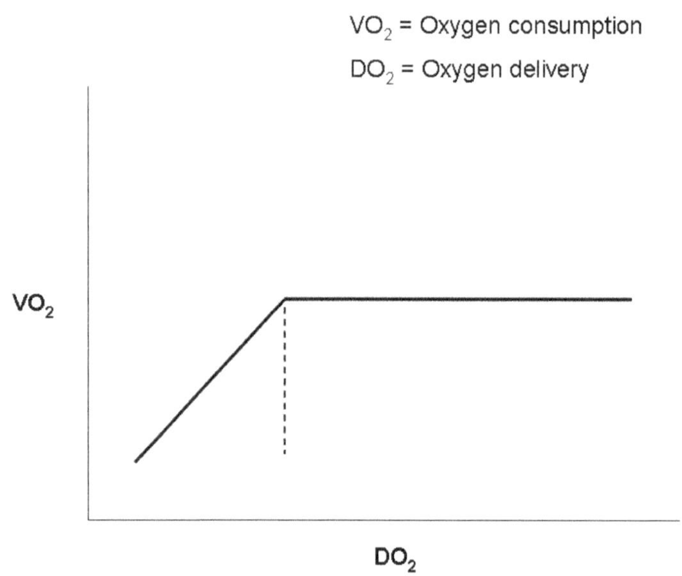

Provided an individual at rest is above the critical DO_2 threshold (dashed vertical line), VO_2 does not change as DO_2 increases. If below the critical threshold, VO_2 becomes dependent on DO_2.

Fig. 1.

1.2 Therapeutic targets

Multiple studies demonstrated the survivors of high stress situations induced by surgery, sepsis, trauma or cardiac insults achieved a higher cardiac index, oxygen delivery (DO2) and oxygen consumption (VO2) as compared to non-survivors (Heyland, 1996; Shoemaker, 1993, Bishop, 1993; Shoemaker, 1993; Edwards, 1989; Gilbert, 1986; Shoemaker, 1993; Creamer, 1990; Hankein, 1991; Hayes, 1993; Kankein, 1987; Cryer, 1989). As a result of these findings, efforts were made to target these variables in an effort to improve outcomes of the critically ill. The first randomized, controlled trial (Shoemaker, 1988) implemented protocols to generate supraphysiologic values as therapeutic goals in high risk surgical patients.

Patients with oxygen transport maximized by a PA catheter protocol had a lower mortality, reduced duration of mechanical ventilation and ICU stay. Study limitations in baseline characteristics of the various groups along with an unblinded design raise the question of bias versus an actual treatment impact (Shoemaker, 1988; Heyland, 1996).

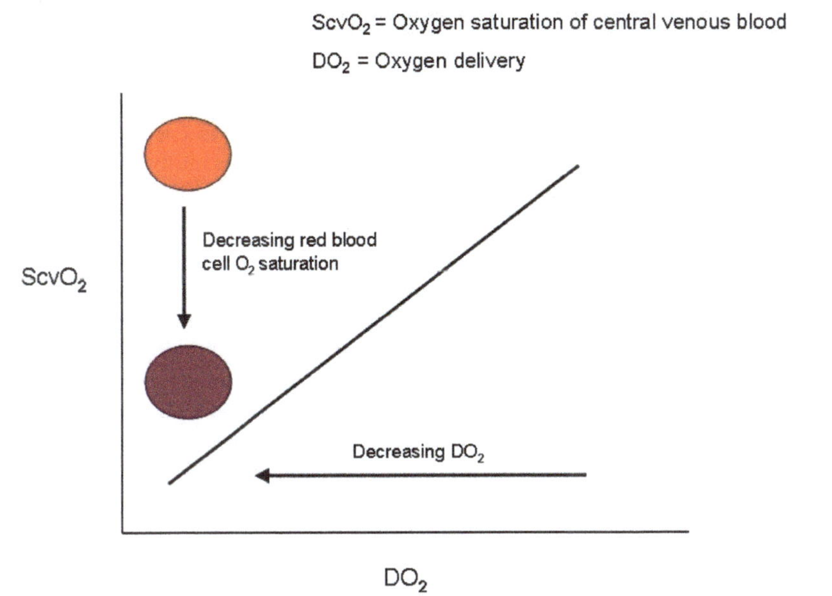

As DO_2 decreases for a given degree of oxygen consumption, the tissues increase the amount of oxygen extracted from red blood cells as they transit the capillary beds, manifest as a drop in $ScvO_2$

Fig. 2.

Hayes et al (Hayes, 1994) randomly assigned patients failing to reach established therapeutic goals following volume resuscitation alone to continue with standard care or receive dobutamine to increase cardiac index, oxygen delivery and oxygen consumption. The treatment group had a higher mortality, suggesting efforts to achieve supranormal physiologic targets may result in more risk than benefit. In addition, Gattinoni et al (Gattinoni, 1995) failed to demonstrate a favorable impact on morbidity or mortality when targeting hemodynamic therapy to achieve supranormal values for cardiac index or normal values for mixed venous oxygen saturation.

In 2001, Rivers et al (Rivers, 2001) published the results of a randomized trial of EGDT in the treatment of patients with severe sepsis and septic shock. By instituting a multi-faceted protocol targeted to increase oxygen delivery they were able to demonstrate significant benefits to outcome in this patient population. The main components of this approach included continuous monitoring of central venous oxygen saturation ($ScvO_2$), treatment in a dedicated area of the emergency department for the first six hours and fluid boluses to achieve a central venous pressure (CVP) of 8 to 12 mmHg. If the MAP remained < 65 mmHg following fluid resuscitation to a CVP of 8 - 12 mmHg, vasopressor therapy began, red blood cells were transfused to achieve a hematocrit of at least 30% if the $ScvO_2$ was less than 70% and dobutamine administration titrated to achieve an $ScvO_2$ of at least 70% despite the other interventions. (Rivers, 2001) The intervention group was more likely to achieve the $ScvO_2$, CVP, MAP and urine output goals along with an improvement in mortality. 46.5% in those receiving standard therapy died compared to 30.5% in the EGDT cohort ($p=0.009$). The EGDT group also received significantly more fluid (4981 mL vs. 3499 mL), red blood cells (64.1% transfused vs. 18.5%), and inotropic support (13.7% vs. 0.8%) during the first 6 hours. The difference in fluid balance did not persist at 72 hours (13,443 mL in EGDT vs. 13,358 in standard therapy) emphasizing the importance of rapid volume optimization for septic shock. (Rivers, 2001) This study demonstrated for the first time the importance of an aggressive, early, protocolized, goal directed treatment regimen in caring for patients with severe sepsis and septic shock. This protocol has been adopted in multiple guidelines as the standard of care for treating septic patients (Dellinger, 2008). Table 1 summarizes the findings of the above trials.

Study	Intervention	Results
Shoemaker, 1988	Supraphysiologic values as therapeutic goals in high risk surgical patients	Oxygen transport maximized by a PA catheter protocol lead to lower mortality, reduced duration of mechanical ventilation and shorter ICU stay
Hayes, 1994	Dobutamine to increase cardiac index, oxygen delivery and oxygen consumption	Higher mortality in patients treated with dobutamine compared to standard care
Gattinoni, 1995	Achieving supranormal values for cardiac index or normal values for mixed venous oxygen saturation	No improvement on morbidity or mortality
Rivers, 2001	Early goal directed therapy with CVP of 8 - 12 mmHg, vasopressors if MAP < 65 mmHg following fluid resuscitation, $ScvO_2 \geq 70\%$, dobutamine and red blood cells to keep hematocrit at least 30% if $ScvO_2$ < 70%	Improved mortality with intervention compared to standard care. More fluid, red blood cells and inotropic support during first 6 hours in intervention group.

Table 1. Summary of Studies on Goal Directed Therapy

1.3 Physiological derangements

Aggressive fluid resuscitation is a mainstay of therapy for septic patients as this population tends to be severely hypovolemic related to multiple mechanisms, venodilation from altered vascular tone leads to pooling of blood in the capacitance vessels. (McGee & Jodka. 2002; Kumar, 2009, Teule 1984) Septic patients also have extravasation of fluid into the interstitium related to increased permeability of the capillary endothelium (Rivers 2008;

Pieracci 2011). These phenomena result in decreased preload, cardiac output and inadequate oxygen delivery. It remains essential to restore volume status and improve cardiac performance. Additionally, the body's inflammatory response is further modulated by cellular hypoxia brought about by the decline in bulk oxygen delivery (Rivers, 2007) may compound the physiologic derangement.

Concurrent with the needs to restore adequate preload and circulating blood volume, septic patients often demonstrate myocardial depression. This dysfunction is related to the presence of myocardial depressant factors early in the septic process, not decreased myocardial perfusion, and include cytokines, tumor necrosis factor alpha (TNF-α) and interleukin one beta (IL-1β) acting synergistically. (Court, 2002; Pathan, 2002) Additionally, nitric oxide generation, interstitial myocarditis, calcium trafficking, endothelin receptor antagonists and apoptosis likely all contribute to the ongoing process of myocardial depression. (Fernandes, 2008). This is manifest as a low cardiac output concurrent with a decrease in ejection fraction and oxygen delivery despite adequate filling pressures. Ventricular interdependence and impairment of left ventricular filling may be an important concern especially with concomitant ARDS and RV dysfunction/dilatation. (Michard, 2010; von Ballmoos, 2010)

The use of echocardiogram plays an important role in quantifying the degree of dysfunction as it is used to assess biventricular contractility and identifies hemodynamically unstable patients who will benefit from either inotropic support or further volume expansion (Griffee, 2010; Beaulieu, 2007). Dobutamine is a typical first line inotropic agent when myocardial depression of sepsis is confirmed and the goal is to establish adequate oxygen delivery or tissue perfusion as measured by $ScvO_2$. No benefit is seen using inotropes to create a supra-physiologic state though studies achieving this did not have echocardiogram data to determine what proportion of subjects had impaired contractility (Hayes, 1994; Gattinoni, 1995). Sepsis induced myocardial depression usually resolves completely over the course of the illness for survivors. (Griffee, 2010; Parker, 1984).

1.4 Role of red blood cells

Controversy exists as to the ideal hemoglobin concentration for septic patients undergoing EGDT as the risks of transfusion often outweigh the benefits. (Hebert, 1999; Marik, 2008; Fuller, 2010) The goal of transfusion of red blood cells is to improve DO_2. There is no impact on the sublingual microcirculation as detected by an orthogonal polarization spectral device in septic patients receiving a red blood cell transfusion (Sakr, 2007). Further, transfusing anemic, septic patients does not improve either regional or global oxygen utilization as determined by either the Fick equation or indirect calorimetry and may increase pulmonary vascular resistance, further hindering right ventricular function. (Fernandes, 2001; Bone, 1993) At this time unless there is active myocardial ischemia, it is difficult to define exact triggers for transfusion of red blood cells in septic patients undergoing active resuscitation. (Pieracci, 2011)

1.5 Avoiding volume overload

An aggressive, early intervention targeted at improving hemodynamic performance in septic patients improves outcomes and is now recognized as the standard of care. The trigger to transfuse red blood cells during the early resuscitation of septic patients remains controversial and is a major criticism of EGDT, especially given the known complications of providing transfusions to critically ill patients. Critical care practitioners need to recognize both the importance of implementing EGDT and avoiding the deleterious effects of fluid overload. When septic patients have a more positive fluid balance both early in the resuscitation process and cumulatively over 4 days there is an associated increased risk of mortality (Boyd, 2011). The importance of carefully managing fluids is further illustrated in patients with acute lung injury or ARDS as those with a lower cumulative fluid balance demonstrate improved outcomes. (Murphy, 2009; the NHLBI ARDSNet, 2006) When complicated by acute kidney injury, fluid overload further impacts mortality in critically ill patients (Payen, 2008; Bouchard, 2009)

2. Applied physiology for the management of severe sepsis/septic shock

The foundation of all resuscitation strategies for severe sepsis and septic shock is volume therapy. Early goal directed therapy is complicated by the requirement for central venous access which is not always available especially during the initial patient evaluation, and the use of a CVP target which has been called in to question as a meaningful measure of preload responsiveness. (Michard, 2002; Marik, 2008;Osman, 2007) Additionally although rapid resuscitation is important excess volume that does not improve cardiac performance is potentially contributing to complications; excess length of stay (Wiedemann, 2006) and mortality (Murphy, 2009). Generally as the goal of any volume therapy in the critically ill is to improve cardiac performance, we propose physiology based hemodynamic therapy for the severely septic patient that considers the pathophysiology already described.

2.1 Physiologic optimization program for sepsis resuscitation, dynamic variables of volume responsiveness

Utilizing dynamic variables of volume responsiveness to guide resuscitation allows precise titration of preload with clear endpoints for fluid resuscitation to minimize the risk of inappropriate fluid overload. Dynamic variables of volume responsiveness, stroke volume variation (SVV) and pulse pressure variations (PPV) exploit the physiology of the heart/lung interaction during positive pressure ventilation that relates the variation of stroke volume or pulse pressure to the degree of volume responsiveness. The respirophasic change in blood pressure (commonly observed in the arterial pressure tracing) of hypovolemic patients is a well known example. (McGee, 2009) (Figure 3).

The available devices quantify the variability and display the variation as a primary output. This variation is highly correlated with the degree of volume responsiveness, i.e., the greater the variation, the greater the expected response to a volume challenge. (Figure 4).

This approach is available only for patients with controlled positive pressure ventilation without a significant dysrhythmia as the utility of SVV or PPV to assess volume responsiveness is not valid beyond these conditions. The use of the dynamic variables SVV and PPV, especially during early resuscitation prior to intubation is generally not possible. Resuscitation of these patients, however, is straight forward and relies on titration of volume against cardiac performance measured by SV and CO. This approach provides assurance that preload optimization has occurred prior to implementation of pharmacotherapy. Our preference is to use the indexed values in an attempt to normalize targets across variability in body surface area. This may be problematic in the super obese (McGee, 2006). (Figure 5).

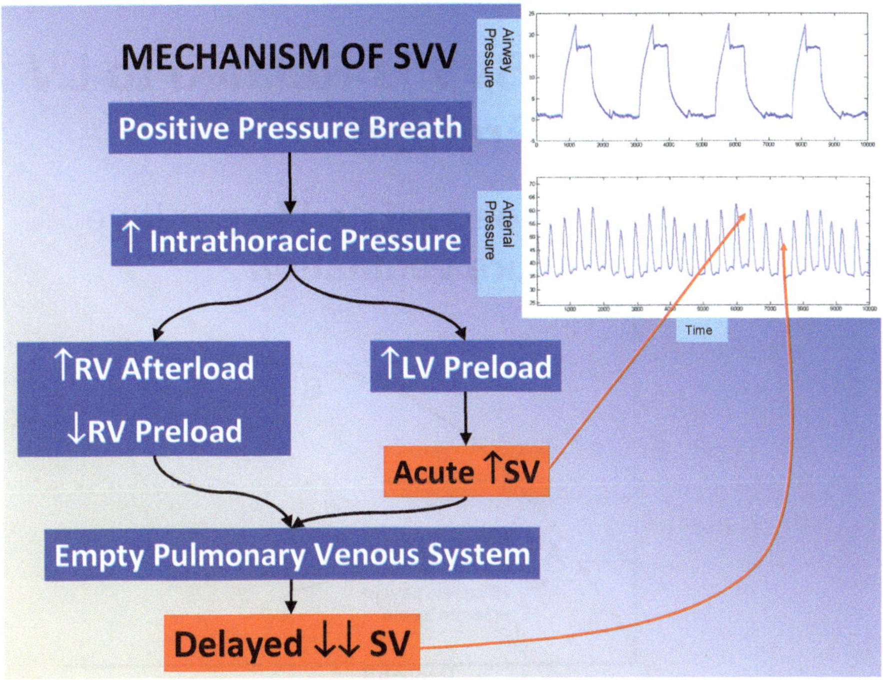

Fig. 3. The phasic change in blood pressure and its timing to the ventilatory cycle is illustrated with four positive pressure breaths and the simultaneously displayed arterial waveform directly below it. Blood pressure goes up during the inspiratory phase of mechanical ventilation and decreases during expiration. The swings in blood pressure (pulse pressure variation, PPV) are generated by the change in stroke volume SV (stroke volume variation, SVV) effected by positive pressure ventilation. The variability is respirophasic as this figure illustrates. The impact on right (RV) and left ventricular (LV) pre and afterload induced by positive pressure ventilation is shown.

In those clinical settings where SVV or PPV does not predict volume responsiveness how can this be determined? As long as stroke volume can be measured this question can be answered. This represents a huge advantage of the technologies that allow measurement of stroke volume and cardiac output, FloTrac/Vigileo, PICCO, and LiDCO, over those that simply provide pulse pressure variation, which is now readily available on bedside monitors that display an arterial waveform (IntelliVue MP90, 2006). This physiology also explains why this literature has been primarily developed in the operating room where ideal conditions often exist for the measurement and application of dynamic parameters, namely controlled mechanical ventilation with a large enough tidal volume to induce a significant change in pleural pressure to impact venous return. A threshold value for tidal volume of 8 cc per kilogram ideal body weight has been determined in several studies that evaluated the tidal volume necessary to meaningfully impact venous return. (Feissel, 2001; Tavernier, 1998; Michard, 2000; Perel, 1987) Across a heterogeneous population, this may be true, although there will be specific examples depending on the patient's lung compliance and intravascular volume status where it may not be.

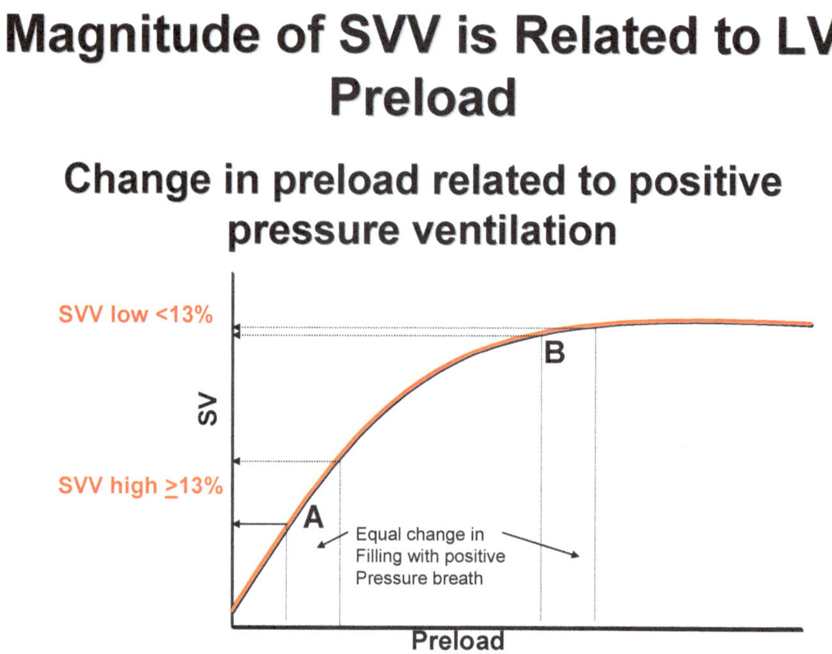

Fig. 4. Legend: A and B represent different locations on the Starling Curve. The change in preload induced by the ventilator is identical. The impact on SV is not. The change in SV induced by one positive pressure breath is proportional to SVV. SVV determines the magnitude of preload dependency. Patients with higher SVV are more volume responsive (A - preload dependent) functioning on the steeper portion of the Frank Starling curve. SVV decreases as preload dependent LV function is optimized (B - preload independent). In these patients (B) volume can be safely removed as cardiac performance is not influenced by changes in preload. SVV/SVI pairs allow individual discrimination of a patient's Starling curve that can determine when volume is required to improve cardiac performance and conversely when volume can be safely removed. SV (stroke volume) SVV (stroke volume variation)

At lower tidal volumes, false negatives where stroke volume variation is low, and the patient is still significantly volume responsive occur. Extreme examples of this were encountered during the H1N1 flu epidemic in the fall of 2009, where many patients were being oscillated at very high frequencies but with minimal tidal volume and hence pleural pressure change. These patients could be significantly volume responsive with essentially no stroke volume or pulse pressure variation because of the very small change in pleural pressure induced with this strategy of ventilation. Similarly, patients being ventilated using a low tidal volume strategy for ALI/ARDS may manifest a similar phenomenon. In those patients, teasing out volume responsiveness utilizing physiology is fairly simple. Listed below are three possible strategies to ascertain volume responsiveness when SVV is unable to provide direction: (DeBacker, 2005)

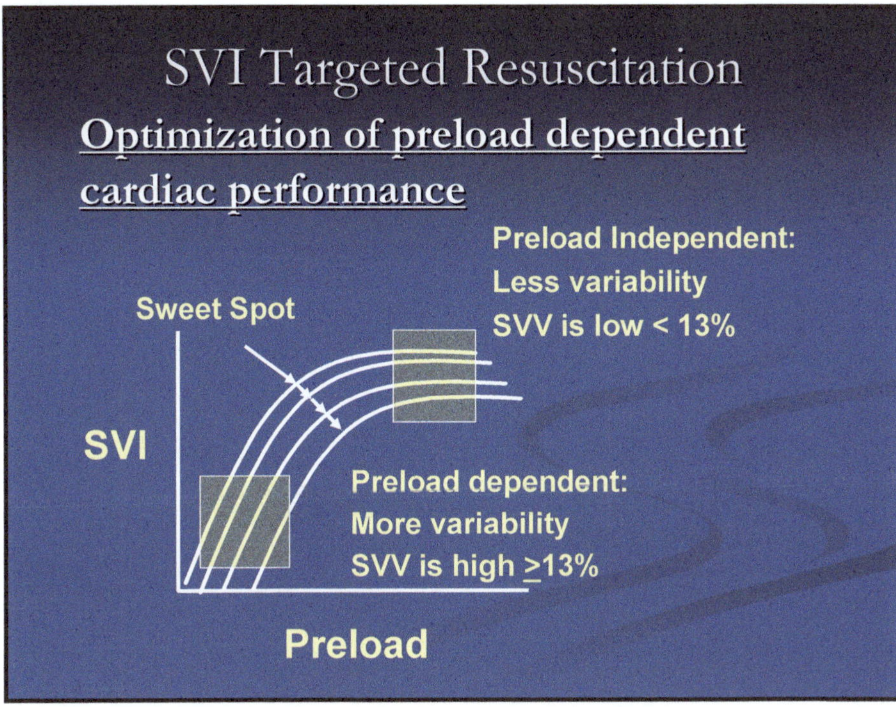

Fig. 5. The goal of volume therapy during resuscitation is to optimize the use of preload augmentation of cardiac function. Stroke volume variation is a very useful parameter to allow rapid safe resuscitation. When this parameter is not useful (dysrhythmia, small tidal volume, spontaneous breathing), simply targeting the maximum stroke volume index (SVI), is another means to guide volume therapy. Independent of which Frank-Starling Curve the patient is on ,the goal of volume therapy is always the same during resuscitation; to obtain the most benefit from the preload dependent portion of the Frank-Starling Curve. These techniques have the additional benefit of more precisely targeting the "sweet spot" of the Frank-Starling Curve without excessive volume overload.

2.2 Stroke volume index targeted resuscitation: Obtaining the sweet spot on the Frank-Starling curve (figure 5)

1. Recruitable stroke volume:

Increase the tidal volume to at least 8-10 cc/kg and look for the change in SVV. For volume responsive patients, once beyond a threshold value for tidal volume, volume responsiveness becomes apparent as the SVV will increase to greater than 10-13%, a reliable cutoff above which patients are generally volume responsive. The time responsiveness of these technologies is fairly rapid and tidal volume needs to be increased for only a short period of time, typically less than 5 minutes. Physician presence at the bedside during this maneuver is important to:

a. View the change; and
b. Assure that the pressure encountered with the ventilation change is not harmful to the patients. If this change in tidal volume results in SVV becoming greater than 10-13%, a

fluid bolus is then given after the patient has been returned to the initial ventilator settings.

Two additional strategies are also useful for non-ventilated patients or those with significant dysrhythmias.

2. The passive leg raising maneuver (PLR) ((Cavallaro, 2010, Monnet, 2006) (Figure 6.)

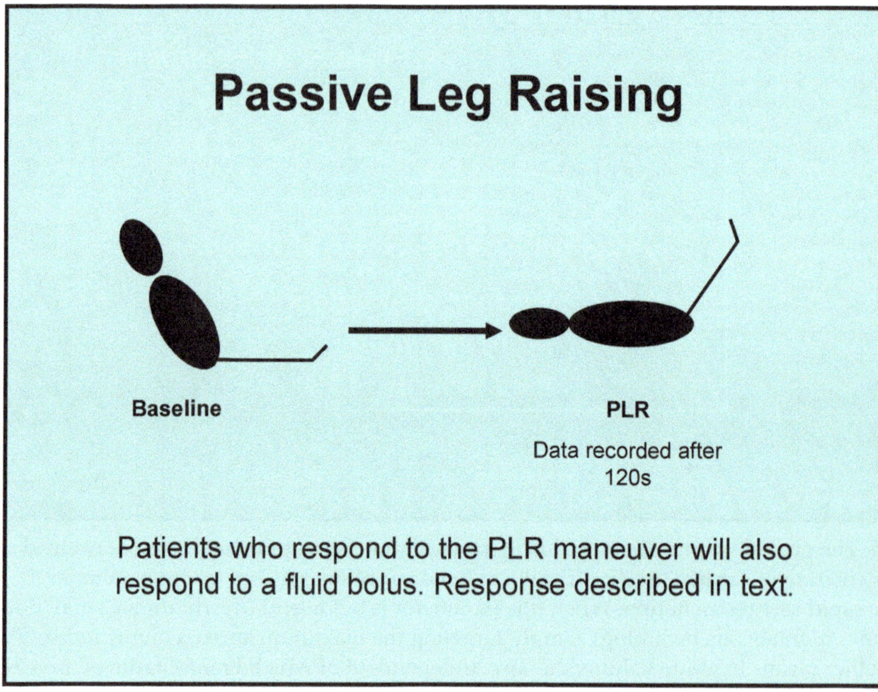

Fig. 6.

The patient is placed flat and the legs are elevated to 45 degrees and the change in stroke volume and cardiac output is recorded. Those patients that have a positive response usually defined as greater than 12-15% increase in cardiac output are then given a fluid challenge, typically 250-500 cc of colloid or crystalloid. This can be done numerous times until the indicator of volume responsiveness disappears or an adequate stroke volume/cardiac output is reached. Although the change in SV using aortic flow is fully apparent within 30 seconds, the increase in venous return that this maneuver induces in cardiac performance requires the legs be elevated for roughly 120 seconds to allow for the time constraints of the pulse contour technology. (Teboul, 2009; Biais, 2009) In numerous studies, this has been shown to be essentially a perfect test as a measure of volume responsiveness as long as the improvement in stroke volume/cardiac output is the cardiac performance parameter of interest. (Cavallaro, 2010) Simply looking at the change in blood pressure is not helpful. (Monnet, 2006) This technique works well especially in those patients who are either spontaneously breathing or have a significant dysrhythmia. This reversible volume challenge is most useful in patients with acute lung injury or ARDS or those with either acute or chronic renal failure, where giving a volume challenge that does not result in improvement in cardiac performance may in fact be detrimental to the patient. (Cavallaro, 2010; McGee, 2009)

3. Volume challenges: As long as there is a cardiac performance measure, stroke volume or cardiac output, simply giving a fluid bolus and assessing its impact on cardiac performance is a reasonable way to assess volume responsiveness for patients where we suspect that additional volume will not be injurious, i.e. clear lungs and without renal failure. If cardiac performance does not improve, volume is not the correct therapy (Figure 5).

It is important to recognize when the patient is on the flat part of the Frank-Starling Curve and not responding to volume. Excess volume therapy has been associated with increased length of stay, increased time on mechanical ventilation, and mortality. (Boyd, 2011; Murphy, 2009; the NHLBI ARDSNet, 2006; Payen, 2008;Bouchard, 2009; Maitland, 2011) The major impact of using these technologies well is that we now have the ability for precise titration of volume management in the majority of critically ill patients. The simple premise underlying volume therapy in the ICU or OR is to affect a change in cardiac performance. This simply is not possible without a cardiac performance measure.

2.3 Physiologic optimization program (figure 7)

Figure 7 illustrates the use of dynamic parameters of volume responsiveness for the hemodynamic management of patients with severe sepsis or septic shock. Volume responsive patients SVV $\geq$ 13% receive volume therapy titrated against both SVV and SVI. For non-volume responsive patients, the physiology is interrogated at the level of cardiac performance on a beat to beat basis. Ultimately and with this approach rapidly a majority of patients will develop a SVI $\geq$ normal (pathway 1). This represents resuscitated septic shock and these patients may be safely placed on a vasopressor, knowing that volume resuscitation has been accomplished. Precise volume titration can be maintained but once SVI is supraphysiologic (pathway 3) volume therapy is stopped and diuretics might be warranted for that population who go on to develop ALI/ARDS typically after the initial resuscitation phase. Approaches to the patient in pathway 2 will be discussed in the text (McGee, 2009).

2.4 Assessment of oxygen delivery

Non-volume responsive patients (SVV < 13%) with low SVI or CO are a particularly challenging population. DO_2 adequacy must be determined on an individual basis. This will also apply to some patients with normal SVI or CO. O_2 extraction is particularly useful in this regard facilitating determination of the adequacy of bulk oxygen transport. When extraction is low or normal (<33%) augmentation of DO_2 has not been shown to be helpful. (Gattinoni, 1995, Hayes 1994) Alternatively, high extraction (>40%) usually precipitates some attempt at DO_2 optimization, although this approach has not been rigorously evaluated, it remains the basis of all resuscitation strategies. It is clear that as O_2 extraction increases, physiologic reserve is compromised, lactic acidosis ensues, and mortality results. Using O_2 extraction as an endpoint further refines hemodynamic care of this severely ill group of patients and is the physiologic foundation of early goal directed therapy.

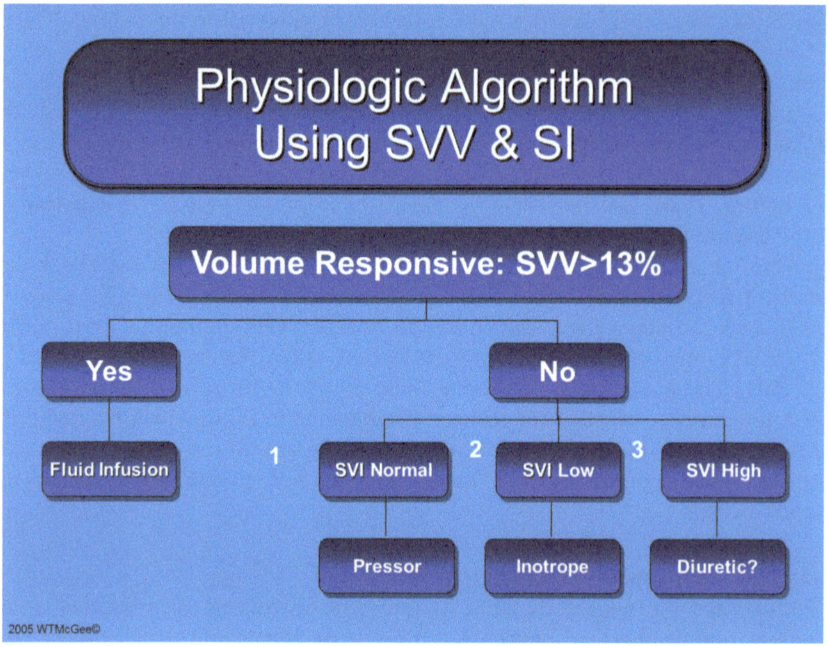
Physiologic Algorithm
Using SVV & SI
Volume Responsive: SVV>13%
Yes
No
Fluid Infusion
1
SVI Normal
2
SVI Low
3
SVI High
Pressor
Inotrope
Diuretic?
2005 WTMcGee©

Fig. 7.

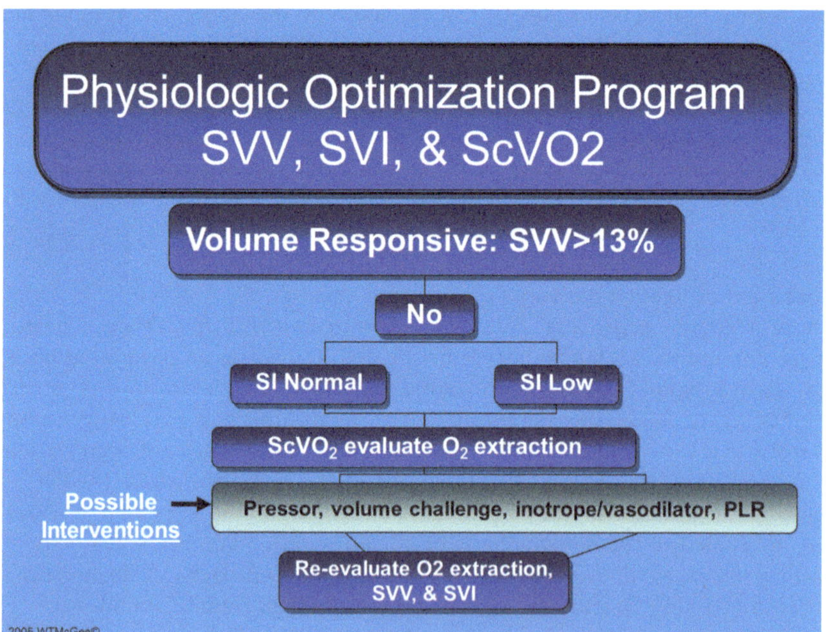
Physiologic Optimization Program
SVV, SVI, & ScVO2
Volume Responsive: SVV>13%
No
SI Normal
SI Low
ScVO2 evaluate O2 extraction
Possible Interventions
Pressor, volume challenge, inotrope/vasodilator, PLR
Re-evaluate O2 extraction, SVV, & SVI
2005 WTMcGee©

Fig. 8.

For those patients with extraction greater than normal but not excessively elevated (>33% to < 40%). Best clinical management remains unclear. DO_2 should be determined as a first step. Clinical assessment of physiology as it relates to the individual patient along with frequent reassessment of other clinical parameters would typically lead to a watchful waiting approach or more aggressive resuscitation. (Figure 8)

O_2 extraction data helps assess the adequacy of O_2 delivery. If adequate (extraction <33%) a vasopressor depending on the blood pressure or no further therapy is generally appropriate. Other possible interventions are shown in Figure 8, all titrated against a change in SVI/cardiac output and ultimately oxygen delivery.

In applying these algorithms at the bedside, the use of sound physiologic principles guides management in a group of patients in whom advanced hemodynamic monitoring can be easily and safely obtained (McGee, 2009).

2.5 Total physiologic assessment for septic shock

When possible but especially for those patients in whom we desire a more complete picture of cardiac performance typically those with normal or decreased stroke volume/cardiac output; echocardiography with assessment of biventricular function and ventricular interdependence along with pulmonary artery pressure allows for a complete description of cardiac performance and suggests possible therapies for augmentation if necessary. Inotropes for pure left ventricular failure or diagnosis and treatment of impairment of left ventricular filling from right ventricular distension as two common examples of how this additional cardiac functional anatomic data refines clinical care. Numerous other etiologies are possible and beyond the scope of this manuscript, but functional biventricular assessment is perhaps the final piece to a complete hemodynamic assessment of the critically ill septic shock patient. Flow (SV/CO and DO_2), preload responsiveness (SVV/PPV), perfusion ($ScVO_2$ and calculation of O_2 extraction) along with biventricular function (echo) can all be obtained reasonably safely for a majority of critically ill patients who routinely have arterial and central venous catheters and often have echocardiography performed.

Goal directed therapy saves lives of patients with severe sepsis. Application of physiology based volume management for the care of these patients further refines therapy while providing assurance that preload optimization is accomplished while minimizing the impact of excess volume. Titrated hemodynamic management using applied physiology has further potential to improve outcomes over more traditional approaches to the management of severe sepsis and septic shock.

3. References

Beaulieu Y. (2007) Bedside echocardiography in the assessment of the critically ill. Crit Care Med 35, No. 5 Suppl: S235 - S249.

Biais M, Vidil L, Sarrabay P et al: (2009) Changes in stroke volume induced by passive leg raising in spontaneously breathing patients: comparison between echocardiography and Vigileo/FloTrac device. Crit Care 13(6):R195.

Bishop MH, Shoemaker WC, Appel PL et al: (1993) Relationship between supranormal circulatory values, time delays, and outcome in severely traumatized patients. Crit Care Med 21:56-63.

Bone R, Marik P, Sibbald WJ. (1993) Effect of stored-blood transfusion on oxygen delivery in patients with sepsis. JAMA 269(23):3024 - 3029.

Bouchard J, Soroko SB, Chertow GM, et al. (2009) Fluid accumulation, survival and recovery of kidney function in critically ill patients with acute kidney injury. Kidney International 76:422 - 427.

Boyd JH, Forbes J, Nakada T, et al. (2011) Fluid resuscitation in septic shock: A positive fluid balance and elevated central venous pressure are associated with increased mortality. Crit Care Med 39:259 - 265.

Cavallaro F, Sandroni C, Marano C et al: Diagnostic accuracy of passive leg raising for prediction of fluid responsiveness in adults: systematic review and meta-analysis of clinical studies. Intensive Care Med 2010, 36(9):1475-1483.

Court O, Kumar A, Parrillo JE, et al. (2002) Clinical Review : Myocardial depression in sepsis and septic shock. Critical Care 6:500 - 508.

Creamer JE, Edwards JD, Nightingale P: (1990) Hemodynamic and oxygen transport variables in cardiogenic shock secondary to acute myocardial infarction and response to treatment. Am J Cardiol 65:1297-1300.

Cryer HG, Richardson JD, Longmire-Cook S, et al: (1989) Oxygen delivery in patients with adult respiratory distress syndrome who undergo surgery. Correlation with multiple system organ failure. Arch Surg 124:1378-1384.

Danek SJ, Lynch JP, Wegg JG, et al. (1980) The dependence of oxygen uptake on oxygen delivery in the adult respiratory distress syndrome. Am Rev Respir Dis. 122: 387 - 395.

DeBacker D, Heenen S, Piagnerelli M et al: (2005)Pulse pressure variations to predict fluid responsiveness: influence of tidal volume. Intensive Care Med 31(4):517-523.

Dellinger RP, Levy M, Carlet JM, et al. (2008) Surviving Sepsis Campaign: International guidelines for management of severe sepsis and septic shock: 2008. Intensive Care Med 34:17 - 61.

Edwards JD, Brown GCS, Nightingale P, et al: (1989) Use of survivors' cardiorespiratory values as therapeutic goals in septic shock. Crit Care Med 17:1098-1103.

Feissel M, Michard F, Mangin I, et al: (2001) Respiratory changes in aortic blood velocity as an indicator of fluid responsiveness in ventilated patients with septic shock. Chest 119(3):867-873.

Fernandes CJ, Akamine N, De Marco F, et al. (2001) Red blood cell transfusion does not increase oxygen consumption in critically ill septic patients. Critical Care 5:362 - 367.

Fernandes CJ, Akamine N, Knobel E. (2008) Myocardial depression in sepsis. Shock 30; Suppl 1:14 - 17.

Fuller BM, Gajera M, Schorr C, et al. (2010) The impact of packed red blood cell transfusion on clinical outcomes in patients with septic shock treated with early goal directed therapy. Indian J Crit Care Med 14(4):165 - 169.

Gattinoni L, Brazzi L, Pelosi P, et al. (1995) A trial of goal-oriented hemodynamic therapy in critically ill patients. N Engl J Med 333:1025 - 1032.

Gilbert EM, Haupt MT, Mandanas RY et al: (1986) The effect of fluid loading, blood transfusion, and catecholamine infusion on oxygen delivery and consumption in patients with sepsis. Am Rev Respir Dis 134:873-878.

Griffee MJ, Merkel MJ, Wei KS. (2010) The role of echocardiography in hemodynamic assessment of septic shock. Crit Care Clin 26:365 - 382.

Hankein KB, Gronemeyer R, Held A et al: (1991) Use of continuous noninvasive measurement of oxygen consumption in patients with adult respiratory distress syndrome following shock of various etiologies. Crit Care Med 19:642-649.

Hankein KB, Senker R, Schwarten JU et al: (1987) Evaluation of prognostic indices based on hemodynamic and oxygen transport variables in shock patients with adult respiratory distress syndrome. Crit Care Med 15:1-7.

Hayes MA, Timmins AC, Yau E, et al. (1994) Elevation of systemic oxygen delivery in the treatment of critically ill patients. N Engl J Med 330:1717 - 1722.

Hayes MA, Yau EHS, Timmins AC et al: (1993) Response of critically ill patients to treatment aimed at achieving supranormal oxygen delivery and consumption. Chest 103:886-895.

Hebert PC, Wells G, Blajchman MA, et al. (1999) A multicenter, randomized, controlled clinical trial of transfusion requirements in critical care. N Engl J Med 340:409 - 417.

Heyland DK, Cook DJ, King D, et al. (1996) Maximizing oxygen delivery in critically ill patients: A methodologic appraisal of the evidence. Crit Care Med 24(3): 517 - 524

IntelliVue M90: (2006) Networked patient monitors with portal technology for highest intensity care. Philips Medical Systems Brochure; Accessed on September 30, 2008, from www.medical.philips.com

Kasnitz P, Druger GL, Torra F, Simmons DH: (1976) Mixed venous oxygen tension and hyperlactatemia. Survival in severe cardiopulmonary disease. JAMA 236(6):570-574.

Krafft P, Steltzer H, Hiesmayr M, et al. (1993) Mixed venous oxygen saturation in critically ill septic shock patients. The role of defined events. Chest 103:900 - 906)

Kumar A, Kumar A. (2009) Sepsis and Septic Shock. Chapter 57. Civetta, Taylor and Kirby's Critical Care, Fourth Edition. Lippincott, Williams and Wilkins 2009.

Ladakis C, Myrianthefs P, Karabinis A, et al. (2001) Central venous and mixed venous oxygen saturation in critically ill patients. Respiration 68(3):279 - 285

Lee J, Wright F, Barber R, Stanley L: (1972) Central venous oxygen saturation in shock: a study in man. Anesthesiology 36(5):472.

Magder S, Vanelli G. (1996) Circuit factors in the high cardiac output of sepsis. J Crit Care 11(4):155 - 166.

Maitland K, Kiguli S, Opoka RO et al: (2011) Mortality after fluid bolus in African children with severe infection. New England J Med 364(26):2483-2495.

Marik PE, Baram M, Vahid B: (2008) Does trhe central venous pressure predict fluid responsiveness? A systemicatic review of the literature and the tale of severe mares. Chest 134(1):172-178.

Marik PE, Corwin HL. (2008) Efficacy of red blood cell transfusion in the critically ill: A systematic review of the literature. Crit Care Med 36:2667 - 2674.

McGee WT, Jodka P. (2002) Oxygen transport and tissue oxygenation. Chapter 3. Cardiopulmonary Critical Care BIOS Scientific Publishers, LTD. 2002.

McGee WT: (2009) A simple physiologic algorithm for managing hemodynamics using stroke volume and stroke volume variation: physiologic optimization program. J Inten Care Med;24(6):352-360.

Michard F, Boussat S, Chemla D et al: (2000) Relation between respiratory changes in arterial pulse pressure and fluid responsiveness in septic patients with acute circulatory failure. Am J Respir Crit Care Med 162(1):134-138.

Michard F, Richards G, Biais M et al: (2010) Using pulse pressure variation or stroke volume variation to diagnose right ventricular failure? Critical Care 14:451.

Michard F, Teboul JL: (2002) Predicting fluid responsiveness in ICU patients: a critical analysis of the evidence. Chest 121(6):2000-2008.

Monnet X, Rienzo M, Osman D et al: (2006) Passive leg raising predicts fluid responsiveness in the critically ill. Crit Care Med 34(5):1402-1407.

Murphy CV, Schramm GE, Doherty JA, et al. (2009) The importance of fluid management in acute lung injury secondary to septic shock. Chest 136:102 - 109.

Natanson C, Fink MP, Ballantyne HK, et al. (1986) Gram-negative bacteremia produces both severe systolic and diastolic cardiac dysfunction in a canine model that simulates human septic shock. J Clin Invest 78:259 - 270.

Nelson DP, Beyer C, Samsel RW, et al. (1987) Pathological supply dependence of O_2 uptake during bacteremia in dogs. J Appl Physiol. 63: 1487 - 1492.

Nelson DP, Samsel RW, Wood LDH, et al. (1988) Pathological supply dependence of systemic and intestinal O2 uptake during endotoxemia. J Appl Physiol. 64: 2410 - 2419

Osman D, Ridel C, Ray P et al: (2007) Cardiac filling pressures are not appropriate to predict hemodynamic response to volume challenge. Crit Care Med 35(1): 64-68.

Parker MM, Shelhamer JH, Bacharach SL, et al. (1984) Profound but reversible myocardial depression in patients with septic shock. Ann of Intern Med 100:483 - 490.

Pathan N, Sandiford C, Harding SE, et al. (2002) Characterization of a myocardial depressant factor in meningococcal septicemia. Crit Care Med 30:2191 - 2198.

Payen D, Cornelie de Pont A, Sakr Y, et al. (2008) A positive fluid balance is associated with a worse outcome in patients with acute renal failure. Critical Care 12:R74

Perel A, Pizov R, Cotev S: (1987) Systolic blood pressure variation is a sensitive indicator of hypovolemia in ventilated dogs subjected to graded hemorrhage. Anesthesiology 67(4):498-502.

Pieracci FM, Biffl WL, Moore EE. (2011) Current concepts in resuscitation. J Intensive Care Med published online 7 February 2011

Reinhart K: (1989) Monitoring O_2 transport and tissue oxygenation in critically ill patients. In: Reinhart K, Eyrich K eds. Clinical Aspects of O2 Transport and Tissue Oxygenation. Berlin, Germany: Springer; 195-211.

Reinhart K, Kuhn HU, Hartog C, Bredle DL: (2004) Continuous central venous and pulmonary artery oxygen saturation monitoring in the critically ill. Intensive Care Med 30(8):1572-1578.

Rivers EP, Coba V, Visbal A, et al. (2008) Management of Sepsis: Early resuscitation. Clin Chest Med 689 - 704.

Rivers EP, Kruse JA, Jacobsen G, et al. (2007) The influence of early hemodynamic optimization on biomarker patterns of severe sepsis and septic shock. Crit Care Med 35(9):2016 - 2024

Rivers E, Nguyen B, Havstad S, et al.(2001) Early goal-directed therapy in the treatment of severe sepsis and septic shock. N Engl J Med 345:1368 - 77.

Ronco JJ, Fenwick JC, Tweeddale MG, et al. (1993) Identification of the critical oxygen delivery for anaerobic metabolism in critically ill septic and non-septic humans. JAMA 270(14): 1724 - 1730.

Sakr Y, Chierego M, Piagnerelli M, et al. (2007) Microvascular response to red blood cell transfusion in patients with severe sepsis. Crit Care Med 35:1639 - 1644.

Shibutani k, Komatsu T, Kubal K, et al. (1983) Critical level of oxygen delivery in man. Crit Care Med. 11:640 - 643

Shoemaker WC, Appel PL, Kram HB: (1993) Hemodynamic and oxygen transport responses in survivors and non-survivors of high-risk surgery. Crit Care Med 21:977-1097.

Shoemaker WC, Appel PL, Kram HB et al: (1993) Temporal hemodynamic and oxygen patterns in medical patients. Chest 104:1529-1536.

Shoemaker WC, Appel PL, Kram HB et al: (1993) Sequence of physiologic patterns in surgical septic shock. Crit Care Med 21:1876-1889.

Simmons DH, Alpas AP, Tashkin DP, Coulson A: (1978) Hyperlactatemia due to arterial hypoxemia or reduced cardiac output, or both. Am Phys Soc 45(2):195.

Shoemaker WC, Appel PL, Kram HB, et al. (1988) Prospective trial of supranormal values of survivors as therapeutic goals in high risk surgical patients. Chest 94:1176 - 1186.

Tavernier B, Makhotine O, Lebuffe G et al: (1998) Systolic pressure variation as a guide to fluid therapy in patients with sepsis-induced hypotension. Anesthesiology 89(6):1313-1321.

Teule Gjj, Van Lingen A, Verweij-van Vught MA, et al. (1984) Role of peripheral pooling in porcine Escherichia coli sepsis. Circ Shock 12:115 - 123.

The National Heart, Lung and Blood Institute Acute Respiratory Distress Syndrome (ARDS) Clinical Trials Network. (2006) Comparison of two fluid-management strategies in acute lung injury. N Engl J Med 354:2564 - 2575.

Von Ballmoos MW, Takala J, Roeck M et al: (2010) Pulse-pressure variation and hemodynamic response in patients with elevated pulmonary artery pressure: a clinical study. Critical Care 14:R111.

Part 6

Pediatric Sepsis

13

Septic Shock in Neonates

Lidia Decembrino[1] ,Giulia Ruffinazzi[1],
Armando D'Angelo[2], Nunzia Decembrino[3], Paolo Manzoni[4],
Agata Boncimino[1] and Mauro Stronati[1]
[1]Neonatology and Neonatal Intensive Care Unit
Fondazione IRCCS Policlinico San Matteo, Pavia
[2]Coagulation Sevice & Thrombosis Research Unit, Scientific Institute HS. S. Raffaele Milan
[3]Neonatal Intensive Care Unit Fondazione MBBM San Gerardo Monza, Neonatology
[4]Neonatal Intensive Care Unit. S.Anna Hospital Torino
Italy

1. Introduction

Every year 1.6 million of newborn infants die from sepsis (Lawn et al 2000). The prevalence of sepsis, meningitis, and other confirmed bacterial infections has been estimated to range between 1 to 5/1000 live births. Preterm infants are 20 times more likely to get infection than term infants with a prevalence of 1/230 (Haque KN 2003). Very low birth weight infants, evaluated and treated for infections are around 50% of all admissions to neonatal intensive care (Stoll et al 2003).

Sepsis is responsible for 30-80% increased risk of neuro-developmental impairment and 30-100% increase in odds for poor head growth and long term morbidity (Stoll et al 2004). 45% of late deaths in the Neonatal Intensive Care Unit (NICU) are caused by an infectiouse disease (Ince 2005). Despite assistance progress, mortality rates from sepsis have not declined over the last three decades (Haque 2003).

While the incidence of sepsis is known, the true incidence of septic shock in neonates has not been well documented. It is estimated to be around 1-5% of all infants with proven severe sepsis (Haque 2004). Kermorvant-Duchemin E. et al.(2008) reported septic shock in 1.3% of extremely low birth weight newborns with an associated mortality peaking at 71%.

2. Definition and risk factors

Infection, far from being a homogeneous condition, reflects a continuum from fetal inflammatory response syndrome to sepsis, severe sepsis, septic shock, multiorgan failure, and death. The difficulty for the clinician is to define precisely the phase in which his/her patient is at any given moment as the patient may move from one phase to another imperceptibly (Haque 2007).

Definition of sepsis derives from the international consensus definitions that have been adapted for pediatric and neonatal use, including term neonates (0-7 days) and newborns (1 week to 1 month) (Carcillo et al 2002, Goldestein et al 2005) (tab 1 and 2). Sepsis is a complex entity, with wide variations in clinical, laboratory parameters and outcome. Septic shock is a condition of inadequate tissue perfusion secondary to cardiovascular dysfunction occurring in the course of suspected or certain systemic infection, requiring fluid resuscitation or inotropic support (Goldstein et al 2005, Haque 2007). This definition, valid for newborns born > 37 weeks gestation, is problematic for preterms due to immaturity of organ systems and transitional physiology (Jones 2008). For these reasons, the hemodynamic response to septic shock and optimum clinical interventions in preterm neonates are not well understood.

Risk factors for a neonate to develop septic shock have not been described in detail, but they overlap those for sepsis. Prenatal risk factors include maternal intrapartum fever, chorioamnionitis or prolonged rupture of membranes, treatment with steroids, group B *Streptoccocci* recto-vaginal colonization. A few days after aspiration of infected amniotic fluid during the birth, the neonate may manifest with signs and symptoms of neonatal shock. Gram-positive germs as group B *Streptococci* are those most frequently described as causative agents in early neonatal sepsis, even if, more recently, some gram-negative agents have been frequently described (*Escherichia coli, Klebsiella spp., Enterobacter spp.*). This probably is due to the intrapartum use of antibiotics directed against gram-positive pathogens that allows gram-negative flora's outbreak (Schrag et al 2007). Other microbes include *Listeria monocytogenes, coagulase-negative staphylococci* (ConS) (22%) and *nonpyogenic streptococci* (9%) (Muller-Pebody et al. 2011).

Post-natal risk factors include: male gender, birth weight less than 1000 g, hypogammaglobulinemia, parenteral nutrition, central venous catheters, steroids or drugs that decrease gastric acidity, prolonged duration of mechanical ventilation, hand contamination of health care personnel, mother and other family members, aspiration of feeds, and disruption of skin integrity. *Staphylococcus aureus* is the most frequent germ in late sepsis. Gram negative and ConS, almost half the isolates (45%), are the predominant pathogens associated with late severe sepsis or septic shock ((Muller-Pebody et al. 2011).). Also viruses (*herpes simplex, enteroviruses*) or fungi (*candida albicans*) have been associated with fulminant neonatal sepsis. Compared with ConS, Gram-negative infections are associated with a higher mortality: one-fifth of those infected by gram negatives die. (Stoll et al 2002, Gordon et al 2006).

3. Pathophysiology

The development of septic shock is associated with elevated levels of proinflammatory cytokines including IL-1β, IL-6, IL-8 and TNFα (Lynch et al 2008). The inflammatory cytokine response to sepsis in neonates is more pronounced and faster than in adults and associated with an increase in early mortality (<48 hours), while the compensatory anti-inflammatory response system appears to be immature, with both term and preterm infants demonstrating profoundly decreased IL-10 production and a lower amount of transforming growth factor beta-positive lymphocytes, than do adults, after lipopolysaccharide (LPS) stimulation (Langer et al 2006). In addition, in the neonate eosinophils, macrophages and polymorphonuclear neutrophils have reduced surface binding components and have defective opsonization, phagocytosis and antigen-processing capabilities, leading to a generally less robust response to pathogen exposure (Urlichs et al 2006, Marodi et al 2006).

Several studies indicate that the mechanisms of sepsis include excessive activation of the coagulation cascade, inhibition of endogenous natural anticoagulants, and impaired fibrinolysis (Short 2004). Within the microcirculation, this leads to fibrin deposition, contributing to hypoperfusion that eventually results in tissue damage and organ dysfunction. On the other hand, consumption of coagulation factors and platelets promotes a bleeding tendency that may clinically manifest as petechiae, ecchymoses, and sometimes hemorrhages, all of which are associated to increased mortality. (Fourrier et al 1992, Kenet et l 2008, Levi 2010). The immune system and coagulation are closely related. Cytokines mediating neutrophils activation and migration to the tissues and extravascular compartment, generate the thrombin and fibrin deposit formation, triggering tissue factor, that is considered the main both septic shock and diffuse tissue injury mediator. That's why, disseminated intravascular coagulation (DIC) is not so rare in septic shock, resulting from the sustained thrombin generation. Thrombin, in turn, stimulates more inflammatory mediators' formation. Fibrin formation stabilizes platelet plugs, in addition to its important role in pathogens' adhesion to the leukocyte surface, facilitating phagocytosis (Levi et 2010).

The Toll-like receptors (TLRs), found in immune system cells, have a fundamental role in the septic shock pathophysiology. They can interfere with the cardiovascular system depending on the systemic inflammatory response to pathogen. They are able to detect pathogens-associated molecular patterns (PAMPs), causing the induction of pro-inflammatory and anti-inflammatory mediators, particularly cytokines.(Gao et al 2008Gao et al 2005, Fleer et al 2007). TLRs, present in endothelial cells, alveolar epithelium cells, and cardiomyocytes, may induced TNFα and IL-1β production, responsible for the early myocardial dysfunction in gram-negative (TLR4) and gram-positive (TLR2) germs severe sepsis.(Zhang et al 2007). Unlike in adults, TLRs genetic polymorphisms and signaling proteins (MYD88) regulating the host response to infection and different septic shock patterns, are less characterized in neonates. (Zhang et al 2007, Cornell et al 2010).

In septic shock the action of inflammatory mediators leads to damage of the capillary wall with loss of vascular tone, resulting in vasodilatation and reduction of systemic vascular resistance with low to normal blood pressure and increased systemic blood flow. Thanks to the compensatory heart rate increase, skin is well perfused and warm (warm shock). In the late phase of shock there is a reduction of myocardial contractility that leads to vasoconstriction, decreased systemic blood flow, decreased pulse volume, cold periphery, prolonged capillary refill time, and increased vascular tone in an attempt to centralize the circulation (cold shock). Shock, that is not recognized and treated, progresses from early to late stages, referred to as compensated, uncompensated, and irreversible shock. (Jones et al 2008).

The hemodynamic response to sepsis of a newborn is markedly different from that of an adults or an older child with relevant difference between the preterm and the term newborn owing to the different anatomical structure, the functional activity and excitation-contraction (Brierley et al 2008).

In the neonates, the absence of hypotension does not precludes shock that is mainly related with blood flow rather than blood pressure as the mean blood pressure may be in the normal range due to compensatory mechanisms (Cayabyab et al 2009).

In the evaluation of blood pressure, the physiological variability with age and gestational age should be taken in account (Silveira et al 2010). Despite this, 30 mmHg should be considered the absolute minimum tolerable of in the extremely premature infants. (Munro et al 2004). Furthermore in critically ill prematures, refractory hypotension may be related to patent ductus arteriosus, intraventricular hemorrhage and poor prognosis. (Carcillo et al 2002). While in healthy prematures lower mean blood pressure levels may be accepted being associated with appropriate cerebral perfusion and normal cardiac output (30), in septic shock hypotension is not permissive and need a therapeutical intervent.

The neonate is enable to increase the stroke volume or myocardial contractility in case of sepsis, due to different physiologic abnormalities: a relatively decreased left ventricular muscle mass (Joyce et al 2004), an impaired left ventricular diastolic function and alterations in mid-wall left ventricular fractional shortening (Kozak-Barany et al 2001). These differences may be mediated by alterations in calcium channel expression and activity, in ATP-sensitive potassium channel function and in β-receptor coupling (Huang et al 2006, Morrissey et al 2005).

These developmental alterations make the neonates critically dependent on increasing the heart rate to generate increased cardiac output, but unable to compensate in this manner because of their relatively higher baseline heart rate (Carcillo et al 2009).

The development of cardiovascular disfunction and septic shock make newborn infants susceptible to sudden cardiac deterioration, also because left ventricular sistolic performance is highly dependent on afterload. So the reopening of a patent ductus arteriosus and the development of persistent pulmonary hypertension (Carcillo et al 2002) may complicate the cardiovascular response to sepsis.

4. Clinical features

Septic shock should be suspected in any newborn with tachycardia, respiratory distress, poor feeding, poor tone, poor color, tachypnea, diarrhea or reduced perfusion particularly in the presence of prenatal risk factors like chorionamnionitis or prolonged rupture of membranes. (Kisson et al 2010)

The predominant clinical sign is circulatory failure that can coexist with multiple organ damage, severe coagulopathy, metabolic acidosis and electrolyte alterations. During the compensated stage blood pressure remains normal and cardiac output is maintained. Clinical signs are pallor, increased capillary refill time (refill> 2''), tachycardia, decreased urine output, mild agitation and confusion, signs of cerebral hypoperfusion. When compensatory mechanisms fail, cardiac output falls resulting in a reduction of oxygenation and increase of anaerobic metabolic mechanisms. The toe/core temperature gap widens, and the peripheries become cool and mottled, the pulse becomes small and weak, oliguria worsens to the point of anuria. The further deterioration of cerebral perfusion leads to irritability, sleepiness and impairment of conscious state. Despite intense peripheral vasoconstriction, hypotension occurs. In the meantime, the clinical condition of the newborn becomes critical. The lack of adequate resuscitation leads to a state of irreversible shock which causes the death of the baby. Furthermore, in newborn babies septic shock may be complicated by the physiological transition from fetal to neonatal circulation. Newborn septic shock is tipically accompanied by, acidosis and hypoxia that can lead to an increase in pulmonary resistance and persistence of the patent ductus Botallo, resulting in persistent fetal circulation which will result in right ventricle failure with right to left shunting at the atrial and ductus arteriosus levels causing cyanosis, hepatomegaly and tricuspid regurgitation. (Brierley et al 2009)

5. Diagnosis

Early recognition of neonatal shock allows to establish an adequate therapy and save lives (Han et al 2003). Ideally shock should be clinically diagnosed before hypotension occurs. Laboratory diagnosis is mainly based on controlling the blood gases, complete blood count with differential, glucose, electrolytes, albumin, creatinine, urea, lactate, blood pyruvate, coagulationparameters, serum and urine osmolarity, cultures with susceptibility testing (blood culture, urine culture, culture catheters or drainage).

Research offers an increasing number of biological markers for early detection of sepsis, but many of them failed to differentiate between sepsis and other non septic critical illness. The most commonly available and used markers are shown in table 3 (Haque 2005).

Procalcitonine (PCT) revealed superior to C reactive protein (CRP) to differentiate children with sepsis from those with septic shock (Simon et al 2006), mainly at admission and 12 h later (Fioretto et al 2010). Baruti Garufi et al. (2010) found that the increase of PCT levels was related to the severity, course and prognosis of disease. Procalcitonin values were significantly increased in neonates with septic shock (92.5 ng/mL) compared to those with systemic inflammatory response syndrome- SIRS (41 ng/mL), neonatal sepsis (10,26 ng/mL) and purulent meningitis (9,80 ng/mL). CRP was increased without statistical differences in all stages. Casado-Flores et al. (2006) observed a stronger correlation between PCT and PRISM score in septic shock than RCP, possibly due to the kinetics of this mediator that after an approximately 2 h latency period from initial stimulus, rises to a plateau within 12–48 h and then slowly declines.

Serum lactate level is considered an important biomarker to distinguish sepsis from septic shock. Normally a small amount of lactate is produced and all healthy tissue have the capacity to convert it, in aerobic condition, to pyruvate, used for cellular metabolism. When sepsis-associated multisystem organ failure occurs, this metabolic capacity, in anaerobic condition, is decreased and lactate levels rise. In the past the lactate levels were used to distinguish between state of adeguate perfusion and poor oxygen delivery. At present, as has been that lactate could be increased by others factors like adrenergic stimuli and lung injury, it became important to consider the increase lactate levels in the general clinical context while a reduction of serum lactate is still advocated as a target for treatment (Arnold et al 2009, Jones et al 2010).

Among imaging techniques: chest X-ray, ECG, ultrasound scans of brain, heart and kidney are proposed.

Minimally invasive monitoring like central vein access and arterial presuure monitoring, and non invasive tools like echocardiography are considered necessary in septic neonates.

Hemodynamic variables including (perfusion pressure mean arterial pressure [MAP], minus central venous pressure [CVP]), and cardiac output (CO) should guide resuscitation treatment.

The systemic circulation is represented by CO = (MAP - CVP)/SVR (systemic vascular resistance). This relationship is important for organ perfusion.

Measurement of urine output and creatinine clearance can be also used as an indicator of adequate blood flow and perfusion pressure. Because blood pressure does not necessarily reflect CO, it is recommended that normal CO and/or SVC (superior vena cava) flow, measured by Doppler echocardiography, be a primary goal as well. (Carcillo et al 2002, Brieley et al 2009, Kluckow 2001, Kluckow et al 2000, Kluckow et al 2000)

Measurement of CO and O_2 consumption were proposed as being of benefit in patients with persistent shock because a cardiac index (CI) between 3.3 and 6.0 $L/min/m^2$ and O_2 consumption >200 $mL/min/m^2$ are associated with improved survival (Pollack et al 1985). Because low CO is associated with increased O2 extraction, ScvO2 saturation can be used as an indirect indicator of whether CO is adequate to meet tissue metabolic demand. If tissue oxygen delivery is adequate, then assuming a normal arterial oxygen saturation of 100%, mixed venous saturation is >70% .

In VLBW infants, SVC blood flow measurement was reportedly useful in assessing the effectiveness of shock therapies and prognostic value because approximates blood flow from the brain. It has been observed that a value > 40 mL/kg/min is associated with improved neurologic outcome and survival. ScvO2 saturation can be used in low birth weight infants, but may be misleading in the presence of left to right shunting through the patent ductus arteriosus. (Kluckow 2001, Kluckow et al 2000, Kluckow et al 2000)

Shock should be diagnosed before blood pressure decrease by clinical signs like hypothermia, hyperthermia, vascular alterations, tachycardia, bradycardia. Blood pressure should not be used as a marker of systemic blood flow in neonates because oxygen delivery to cells is dependent upon cardiac output and systemic blood flow than on blood pressure and a neonate may be hypotenisve but still have adequate oxygen delivery.

E-selectin, a protein expressed by the endothelium after activation at sites of acute inflammation, taking part in the first step of the adhesion cascade, shows plasma levels higher in nonsurvivors than in survivors (*P*= .01) and in patients with hemodynamic dysfunction than in those without hemodynamic dysfunction (*P* _.001). (El Sayed Zaki et al 2009)

6. Management

In spite there are extensively studied multiple organ dysfunction scores and well-defined algorhythmic guidelines for treatment, there is a large amount of practice variability in neonatal septic shock.

In the onset of septic shock an early and aggressive management of septic shock is needed because for each hour of delay the risk of death increases by 2 times. The immediate objective is to optimize the perfusion and delivery of oxygen and nutrients to tissues.

According to the guidelines of the American College of Critical Care Medicine, 60 min is the average time needed to provide adequate circulatory support and block the development of shock. (Brierley et al 2009). Recognize decreased perfusion, cyanosis and respiratory distress syndrome (RDS), establishing an airway for adequate ventilation and oxygenation and obtaining rapid peripheral or central venous access or intraosseus access are the first steps in managing a newborn in shock (0-5 min) (7).

It is important to rember that all babies with shock and hepatomegaly, cyanosis or pressure gap between upper and lower limbs should begin treatment with prostaglandin within 10 min, until congenital heart disease is excluded (Carcillo et al 2002, Brieley et al 2009).

A key element in the therapeutic management of septic shock is the early recognition of infection. One of the most important factors in progression from infection to septic shock is the use of inappropriate or delayed antibiotic therapy (Kumar et al 2006).

6.1 Antibiotics

After appropriate blood cultures, tests for biomarkers of sepsis, glucose and ionized calcium are made, the empirical antibiotic therapy must be established.

A term neonate or a late pre-term infant ≤7 days of age with sepsis should be treated with ampicillin and gentamicin within 60 min. from the suspected diagnosis (Rao et al 2006). Many NICU use Cefotaxime, as a first-line agent, but neonates treated with ampicillin/cefotaxime were more likely to die, and less likely to be discharged to home as compared to neonates treated with ampicillin/gentamicin (Clark et al 2006).

The empiric therapy for late onset sepsis (LOS) in term or late preterm infants admitted from the community after 7 days, is a combination of ampicillin and gentamicin too. In case of meningitis, cefotaxime is administered every 8 h instead of gentamicin. If there is history of prolonged hospitalization or the newborn infant has a central venous catheter (CVC) vancomycin is preferable to ampicillin. In this case, vancomycin and gentamicin/cefotaxime is preferable empiric coverage because provides additional coverage for *S. aureus* and CONS. Clindamycin is now recommended for susceptible MRSA isolates in term infants (Aneja et al 2011).

Afetrwards, once the causative organism has been identified, antibiotics can be targeted only against that organism. As Herpes simplex virus Type I is one of the causes of intractable 'shock', anti-viral (acyclovir) medication, should be initiated, even in the absence of history of maternal infection with herpes virus, in infants who either does not respond. to standard therapy or has persistent signs and symptoms of infection with negative bacterial or fungal cultures or present in septic shock. (Haque 2007).

Therapeutic plasma levels should be monitored because renal and hepatic dysfunction may lead to abnormal volumes and levels of distribution of drugs. The duration of antibiotic therapy is debatable. Serial measurements of CRP or preferably IL-6 or IL-8 are desiderable to minimize resistance, super-infection, and other complications from prolonged use of antibiotics. The decision to continue or stop antibiotic therapy must be based on clinical signs plus biomarkers of sepsis and not only on negative blood culture results, that are frequently negative. Intravascular access devices potential source of severe sepsis or septic shock should be promptly removed after establishing other vascular access.

6.2 Mechanical ventilation

Respiratory failure in severe sepsis and septic shock, due to low functional residual capacity may require elective intubation and ventilation to garantee oxygenation and tissue perfusion, trying to avoid hyperoxemia and over distention of alveoli, which is a potent inducer of IL-6 release.

6.3 Hypoglycemia and hypocalcemia

Correction of hypoglycemia and hypocalcemia should be done if needed. Hypoglicemia can cause neurological damage, if non corrected. Hyperglycemia, particularly cortisol-induced hyperglycemia, is immunosuppressive and prothrombotic. Being due to insulin resistance, which prevents glucose entering into the Krebs cycle, early institution of insulin therapy in hyperglycemic states ensures that glucose is delivered into the Krebs cycle, in particular to the cardiac muscles.

There is no consensus as to what is the ideal blood glucose level, anyhow there is consensus that it should not be lower than 30 mg/dl. Similarly, there is no agreement as to what is the upper limit of blood sugar when insulin therapy should be initiated. In pediatric patients, a glucose level of 178 mg/dL or more was associated with a 2.59 increased risk of mortality (Branco et al 2005). Other researchers noted a similar outcome in extremely low-birth-weight-infants who had glucose levels greater than 150 mg/dL.

Solutions containing 10% dextrose as maintenance fluid are adequate to provide energy (glucose 4 to 8 mg/kg/minute).

In septic shock strict glycemic controls are needed to avoid marked blood glucose levels changes, therefore it is advisable to prevent rapid fluctuation in blood glucose levels by

giving boluses or high concentration glucose infusion. Hyperglycemia peaks appear to be related with the disease severity.
Since insulin hyperglycemia control in parenteral nutrition preterms has been responsible for hypoglycemic episodes effects,(Beardsall et al 2008) until better evidence is available, insulin is indicated in the newborn only when marked hyperglycemia is seen (> 180 mg/dL), in refractory shock and unfavorable response newborns. (Vlasselaers et al 2009)
Normalization of ionized calcium concentration should be the goal of calcium replacement, because hypocalcemia may be a reversible cause of cardiac disfunction.

6.4 Bicarbonate therapy

There is no evidence to support the use of bicarbonate therapy in the treatment of hypoperfusion induced acidemia, during sepsis. Bicarbonate solutions are very hyperosmolar even when diluted and if infused rapidly may increase the risk of ventricular hemorrhage in the newborn, particularly the preterm infants.

6.5 Volume replacement

Septic prematures microcirculation evaluation shows that changes are already detectable 24 hours before the systemic sepsis parameters are apparent. (Weidlich et al 2009). The damage of vascular endothelium, caused by inflammatory mediators, results in vasodilation and fluid shifts into the interstitial space resulting in intravascular volume decrease. So neonates in shock often require volume replacement to maintain and/or restore adequate tissue perfusion. A significant reduction in mortality has been obtained if hemodynamic function is optimized in a few time (Rivers et al 2001). The underlying importance is the maintenance of preload and tissue perfusion.
Volume expansion could be carried with crystalloids, colloid or blood products, if hemorrhage. Actually there is a lack of consensus in the literature regarding which product is most effective than the other. In clinical practice, crystalloids have been used more extensively because they are inexpensive and fluid retention and the incidence of adverse effects (eg, intraventricular hemorrhage and infection transmission) may be lower (Lynch et al 2008, Oca et al 2003). Normal saline and lactated ringers are 2 examples of crystalloid solutions used for volume expansion. Colloid solutions contain minerals and electrolytes. They increase oncotic pressure, do not easily cross semipermeable membranes, may remain in the intravascular space longer than crystalloids and allow to use small volumes with less incidence of pulmonary edema. The colloid most commonly used for volume expansion is 5% albumin.
In term infants or older preterm infants, aggressive volume expansion (push boluses of 10-40 mL/kg up to 60mL/kg over 20 to 30 minutes should be considered (Carcillo et al 2002). To prevent reperfusion injury it is preferable to increase the total volume and rate of fluid infusion rather than give repeated boluses of fluids.
Those infants who after adequate fluid resuscitation do not self-diurese may need diuretics to prevent fluid overload. For very preterm neonates there is insufficient evidence to support early volume expansion because of a significant risk of intracranial hemorrhage associated with rapid volume expansion from fluctuations in cerebral perfusion and developing heart failure and/or pulmonary overcirculation from resultant left to right flow through a patent ductus arteriosus, specially in case of anemia. In the septic shock, when hemoglobin levels are below 12 g/dL (Hb < 12 g/dL), packed red blood cells transfusion is recommended.

6.6 Cardiovascular agents

Inotropes are indicated when myocardial contractility remains compromised despite adequate volume replacement (Irazuzta et al 2007). They should be administered through a peripheral or intraosseous line before central access is available. A delay in administration of inotropes was associated with a 20-fold increased mortality risk (Kisson et al 2010). Medications in this group include dopamine, dobutamine, epinephrine, and norepinephrine. During neonatal sepsis can be established a hypodynamic state with vasoconstriction that may respond better to inotrope and vasodilator therapy than adults. Both dopamine and epinephrine were found to be efficacious in improving the mean arterial blood pressure but epinephrine was associated with more short-term adverse effects such as enhanced chronotropic response, hyperglycemia requiring insulin treatment, increased plasma lactate levels and inadequate gastric mucosa perfusion (Valverde et al 2006, Levy et al 2011). Recently, a randomized controlled trial showed that dobutamine increased systemic blood flow more effectively than dopamine (Osborn et al 2002). Anyhow Dopamine remains the first-line agent in neonates, and epinephrine may be used in dopamine-resistant septic shock (Carcillo et al 2002). Dopamine: is a natural precursor of both epinephrine and norepinephrine, stimulates the dopaminergic receptors β and α, in this order, with increasing dose. The initial dose of 5-10 mcg/kg/min is recommended and incremented by 2.5 mcg/kg/min steps every 10-15 minutes (Pellicer et al 2009). The prematures may be resistant to its action due to deficient deposit of norepinephrine. A dose ≥ 10 mcg/kg/min dopamine may reduce TSH release, making difficult hypothyroidism diagnosis and producing relevant adverse effects such as tachycardia, arrhythmias, bradycardia, nausea and vomiting. If low cardiac output and high systemic vascular resistance persist, dobutamine and/or a type III phosphodiesterase inhibitor may be indicated. Dobutamine is frequently associated to dopamine in the newborn septic shock; Trough β-adrenergic effects determines vasodilation, through α-adrenergic myocardial receptors stimulation, increases heart contractility and frequency. As reduces after-load, it is particularly useful for septic shock characterized by myocardial dysfunction and high peripheral resistance. In the premature, improves the systemic blood flow, however is not superior to dopamine for septic shock hypotension reversion. Dobutamine may reduce pulmonary vascular resistance, with additional benefit for PPH. Caution is advised when using dobutamine for LV flow obstruction patients. It may cause hypotension if the infant remains hypovolemic, and in higher doses causes tachyarrhythmia.(Dempsey et al 2009) . In the term or near-to-term newborn, once assured previous losses replacement and started volume resuscitation, β-adrenergic (inotropic) dose dopamine is indicated between 5-9 mcg/kg/min associated with dobutamine 2.5-10 mcg/kg/min, already during the first management hour (Brierley et al 2009, Pellicer et al 2009). If the patient does not adequately respond to these interventions, then epinephrine (0.05– 0.3 μg/kg/min) can be infused. For extreme premature transition period shock, the best starting vasoactive drugs schedule was not yet established.(Noori et al 2009) It is very important to have service procedures standardized to control for the results. Dopamine use is safe in these patients. A combination of dopamine at low dosage and dobutamine is initially recommended. *Epinephrine* At a low dose < 0.03 mg/kg/min acts as a potent inotrope (β1), chronotrope (α1), and both systemic and pulmonary vasodilatator (β2). At higher doses, has systemic and pulmonary circulation vasopressor effect (α-adrenergic). The use of ***Norepinephrine*** is limited in neonatal shock. It is indicated for "warm" shock (doses 0.05 to 0.5 mcg/kg/min), an uncommon condition in the newborn. Tourneux et al.obtained improved blood pressure and PPH-related hemodynamic values and positive effects on the heart and cerebral flow (Tourneux et al 2008).

6.7 Corticosteroids

Corticosteroids are often used to treat shock when volume expansion and inotropes are ineffective to raise blood pressure. They may act by improving the vessel wall sensitivity to circulating cathecolamines or to exogenous vasoactive drugs, inhibiting the nitric oxide synthase enzyme expression, or suppressing immune responses. Additionally, septic newborns may develop relative adrenal insufficiency, manifested by low stress cortisol levels.(Fernandez et al 2008) Despite this, the use of corticosteroids remains relatively untested. A recent large cohort study of steroid administration to children and infants with severe sepsis showed no improvement in outcome and an increase in mortality in a subset of patients (Markovitz et al 2005).

Hydrocotisone and dexamethasone are the most used steroids. There are no specific recommendations for neonates regarding the use of dexametasone, conversely Hydrocotison is life saving and should be reserved for refractory shock patients, or in services missing inodilators (milrinone), in epinephrine-resistant shock, when adrenal insufficiency is suspected (Vincent 2008). The dose of hydrocortisone ranged from the "stress-dose" used in adrenal insufficiency of 1-2 mg/kg to the empirical shock dose of 50 mg/kg. (Parker et al 2004). Higher mean arterial blood pressures and less vasopressor support and volume expanders use were observed in neonates treated with low-dose hydrocortisone (NG et al 2006).

6.8 Nutrition

Severe illness causes a catabolic process, increases an infant's metabolic requirements, specially in preterm infants owing to poor muscle mass and energy reserves. Appropriate quantities of energy, minerals, and vitamins can be provided rather by enteral feedings to reduce bacterial translocation from the gut mucosa into the circulation and preserve gut mucosal function.

7. Adjuntive treatments

7.1 Nitric oxide (iNO)

Infants with sepsis and persistent pulmonary hypertension (PPHN) may require **iNO** to reduce pulmonary vascular resistance and off-load the right ventricle (Roberts et al 1997). The dose of NO with the best results is generally 20 ppm.

7.2 Triiodothyronine

Is an effective inotrope in newborns in case of thyroid insufficiency (Carcillo et al 2002, Carcillo et al 2009).

7.3 Phosphodiesterase inhibitors

Phosphodiesterase inhibitors are indicated if cardiac output does not improve and high systemic vascular resistance persists.

7.4 Milrinone

Milrinone is an inodilator (inotrope/vasodilator) that exerting the selective phosphodiesterase type III inhibition, improves myocardial contractility and relaxation by effects on calcium influx, efflux, and myofilament calcium binding. In the vasculature relaxes arterial and venous smooth muscle. These properties have led to increased use of Milrinone in shocked newborns with high peripheral vascular resistance ("cold" shock), ventricular dysfunction and normal pressure, specially with PPH, epinephrine-resistant shock with the aim to increase cardiac contractility and cardiac output (Paradisis et al 2006, Paradisis et al 2007). Milrinone due to its sistemic and pulmonary vasodilatator effects may need volume expansion or inotropic support during the therapy. The recommended dose is 0.75 mcg/kg/min for 3 hours, followed by 0.2 mcg/kg/min. Limited data are available about the use of milrinone in preterm infants. Milrinone failed to show significant effects in extreme low systemic flow prematures within their first 24 hours of life. In these subjects it should be used under hemodynamic control. It is also important to consider that this subjects have a glomerular filtration rate riduced by half compared to term infants in the first 2 weeks of life and that the velocity of improvement over the first several weeks of life is riduced. (Paradisis et al 2009). These differences among varying gestational age newborns make that dosing should be often renally adjusted. Lindsay et al used a loading doses of 75 g/kg and a start infusion rates of 0.75 to 1.0 g/kg/min for patients with normal renal function. The authors recommanded for every increase of 0.25 g/kg/min, a 25 g/kg bolus dose be given. Because the median half-life is 1.47 hours, immediate hemodynamic effects may not be seen unless appropriate loading doses and infusion adjustments are made. (Lindasy et al 1998)

7.5 Arginine-vasopressin (AVP)

AVP and TP are 2 forms of vasopressin indicated for rescue therapy in neonates and pediatric patients in case of catecholamine-refractory shock, able to determine an increase in arterial pressure within 1 hour after administration. The meta-analysis conducted by Meyer et al. did not demonstrate a clear advantage of one drug over the other (Vincent.et al 2006, Meyer et al 2008).

Endogenous AVP, released in response to hypovolemia and hypotension, shows a biphasic response in septic shock, with initial high levels followed by inappropriately low levels, that more likely occurs after 36 hours from the onset of shock in approximately one third of late septic shock patients.(Sharshar et al 2008) This justifies exogenous administration to correct hypotension in vasodilatory shock in children and also in extremely-low-birth weight infants.

The best dosages of vasopressin remain controversial. Dosages of 0.067 IU/min seem to be more effective to reverse cardiovascular failure in vasodilatory shock requiring high norepinephrine dosages than 0.033 IU/min. (Luckner et al 2007)

Low-dose vasopressin (0.04 IU/min) infusion has been shown to be effective in reversing catecholamine-resistant hypotension in adult septic shock patients. (Klinzing et al 2007). However, one should keep in mind that the pressor activity of vasopressin in the absence of shock, is minimal.

A study suggested that vasopressin is more efficient to increase urine output than norepinephrine. (Patel et al 2002). However, use of vasopressin instead of norepinephrine cannot be recommended.

7.6 Terlipressin (TP)

A synthetic AVP analogue with prolonged action and a higher affinity for vascular receptors than vasopressin. Recently resulted effective in rescue treatment of refractory vasodilatory septic shock, although few data are available. Its use has been promoted because vasopressin is not available in most European countries. It is considered as a last resort when septic patients remain hypotensive despite fluid resuscitation and high doses of cathecolamine.

As a prodrug, TP is continuously converted by endopeptidases to vasoactive lysine-vasopressin with a peak level approximately 10 minutes after intravenous administration.

Accordingly, despite low plasma levels it has a prolonged action. In fact, half-life is 6 h for TP versus 6 min for VP and duration of action is 2–10 h versus 30–60 min, respectively (Kam et al 2004). This allows TP intermittent administration without hypotension rebound at drug withdrawal. An intermittent intravenous dosing schedule of approximately every 4 to 6 hours would be appropriate (Pesaturo et al 2006). Matok et al administered TP in an 8-day-old neonate with refractory septic shock to dopamine, milrinone and adrenaline, as rescue therapy (0.07 mg/kg twice a day). Rapid BP improvement and tissue perfusion without side effects, followed (Matok et al 2004). Similarly Filippi et al. used TP because of refractory hypotension in a shocked but not septic neonate, at dose of (0.02 mg/kg every 4 h) with a maximum duration of therapy of 60h. BP dramatically increased 30 min after the first bolus and diuresis was promptly re-established, indicating improvement of tissue perfusion. MAP rapidly increased so that adrenaline and norepinephrine, dopamine and dobutamine were reduced and stopped so TP was administered as the only vasopressor. No rebound hypotension occurred (Filippi et al 2008).

No evidence exists at present on the appropriate timing of TP initiation. Some data suggest that in infants TP should be administered when norepinephrine need is 0.5-2.5 μg/kg/min, probably a precocious administration may be beneficial in order to avoid episodes of severe hypotension (Filippi et al 2008, Zeballos et al 2006, Rodríguez-Núñez et al 2010). In adult preliminary clinical data on ultra low dose terlipressin infusion as first line agent, suggest that "the earlier may be the better" (Morelli et al 2008). However, the level of evidence based on the data available in the literature is very low.

Low-dose continuous infusion has also been described. (Leone et al 2008). Nunez et al obtained an increase of median MAP 30 minutes after administration and a norepinephrine infusion reduction through continuous terlipressin infusion in pediatric refractory septic shock. After a loading dose of (20 μg/kg) was administered a continuous infusion at a rate of 4–20 μg/kg/h (Rodrı´guez-Nu´n˜ez et al 2008).

Terlipressin experimental studies showed a protective effect from capillary leakage, less rebound hypotension during weaning (Westphal Westphal et al 2009, Rehberg et al 2009, Morelli et al 2009).

Ischaemic adverse effects secondary to local vasoconstriction, as in the skin and gut were reported in children above all if TP was administered as intermittent bolus. A fact that promoted in adults the TERLIVAP study based on TP continuous infusion and significantly lower dose (1.3 μg/kg/h) to limit this adverse effects (Morelli et al 2009).

7.7 Levosimendan

Levosimendan is an extensively investigated inodilator showing cardioprotective and antiinflammatory effects. Levosimendan is a calcium-sensitizing agent acting by binding to myocardial troponin C in a calcium-dependant manner, causing a configuration change in tropomyosin. This exposes actin and myosin elements, allowing more efficient contraction. In peripheral vascular beds, levosimendan opens adenosine triphosphate–sensitive vascular potassium channels, causing hyperpolarization and vascular relaxation. This effect reduces cardiac afterload and promotes coronary vasodilation. In adults has been demonstrated benefits in low cardiac output states (Moiseyev et al 2002, Slawsky et al 2000).

Levosimendan potential utility is due to a number of reasons; it can be used with conventional inotropic agents, has a simple dosing regimen, and does not worsen the diastolic dysfunction often present in structural heart disease. Levosimendan has received little attention in the pediatric field other than 2 case reports. In both case with clinical improvement (Luther et al 2004, Braun et al 2004). Egan et al (2006) in their experience with 19 cardiac surgical infants and children documented the improvement of myocardial contractility and perfusion, particularly when used early in the evolution of the low cardiac output syndrome, without increasing myocardial oxygen consumption and negative events. Recently Hasslacher et al (2011) showed that levosimendan reduces oxidative burst activity of PMN both in vitro and in patients with acute heart failure or septic shock with septic myocardial depression. This may contribute to the anticipated cardioprotective effects of the drug. It has a half life of 1 hour and a duration of action of 4 days. The recommended dose is 6-12 mcg over 60 min, followed by continuous infusion at 0.05 to 1 mcg / kg / min for 24 hours.

7.8 Granulocyte and granulocyte-macrophage colony stimulating factors (G-CSF, GM-CSF)

The use of G-CSF, GM-CSF has been shown to increase the number of circulating white cells but don't reduce mortality from neonatal sepsis or septic shock (Carr et al 2003).

7.9 Pentoxifylline

Pentoxifylline is a carbonic anhydrase inhibitor that has been shown to improve white cell function. In one randomized controlled trial in prematures infants, was shown to significantly reduce the development of multiorgan failure, mortality and coagulopathy with improvement of blood pressure (Lauterbach et al 1999). This is currently a promising option for refractory shock dosed at 5 mg/kg/hour for 6 hours for next 5 days.

7.10 Intravenous immunoglobulin (IVIG)

Polyclonal and IgM-enriched IVIG have been shown to reduce mortality from sepsis in newborn infants. The activity of Tumour necrosis factor (TNF), a major pro-inflammatory cytokine, can be blocked by various antagonists. In a search was designed a single-domain monoclonal antibody (V_HH), which recognizes TNF biologically active *in vivo*. Therefore, therapeutic application of **TNF-V_HH-ELP** fusion protein was tested in humanized TNF mice and was shown to be effective in preventing death caused by septic shock. Immunomodulator agents have shown frustrating results in newborn septic shock management. (Conrad et al 2011)

7.11 Protein C (PC)

The strong activation of coagulation occurring during sepsis may cause the depletion of PC, a vitamin K dependent natural anticoagulant, which exerts a crucial role in the modulation of coagulation, fibrinolysis, and inflammation. Low PC plasma activity correlates with adverse outcomes, such as multiple organ failure and mortality. It has been considered a useful predictor of organ failure in severe sepsis and an important factor of high diagnostic and negative prognostic significance. (Shaw et al 2011, Lauterbach et al 2006, Venkataseshan et al 2007).

Recently in an animal newborn model, was demonstrated impairment of intestinal microcirculation early after induction of endotoxic shock, and its prevention through to continuous infusion of 24 µg/kg/h activated PC (aPC). This underlines that the use of PC results in an improvement of sepsis-induced microcirculatory dysfunction. (Fischer et al 2009) and underlines the warrants of its supplementation. Whereas several studies, in adults and children, has shown some significant reduction in septic shock mortality thanks to aPC supplementation, a large clinical trial was stopped early, due the finding of an increased incidence of intracranial bleeding in children younger than 60 days (Nadel et al 2007). In addition, the efficacy of aPC may also be different in neonates due to underlying developmental differences in the coagulation pathway. The anticoagulant effect of aPC has been shown to be decreased in neonatal cord plasma, which is due, in part, to the lower levels of tissue factor pathway inhibitor, antithrombin and protein S in neonatal versus adult plasma (Bernard et al 2001, Cvirn et al 2005). In contrast, non-activated plasma-derived human protein concentrate (PCConc) has been successfully used in paediatric, neonatal and adult patients at high-risk of haemorrhage, especially in those suffering from meningococcal septic Shock (de Kleijn et al 2003). PCConc has been successfully used in term neonates and preterms at high-risk of haemorrhage with sepsis-induced coagulopathy (Fischer et al 2009, Decembrino et al 2010). Supplementation was followed by micro- and macrocirculatory, haemodinamic parameters and coagulation, improvement, increased levels of PC activity. PCConc was given intravenously as bolus administration of 200 IU / kg / day or 100 IU / kg/ day followed by a daily bolus administration of 50 IU / kg every 6 h for 72 h. No adverse events were observed.

When enough prothromotic factors are consumed, spontaneous bleeding occurs. It is important, therefore, to determine early whether the infant is in a prothrombotic or fibrinolytic phase. Appropriate coagulation studies should be undertaken. If the baby has a prolonged prothrombin time/partial thromboplastin time and low fibrinogen then it is likely to be DIC. If, however, fibrinogen levels are normal or high then it is likely to be thrombotic thrombocytopenic purpura. Even if routine use of fresh frozen plasma to correct laboratory clotting abnormalities is not recommended, some professional bodies find it useful. The transfusion of platelets is recommended when platelets are between 5000 and 30,000 × 109/l.

8. Septic shock in preterms

The therapeutic approach of very low birth weight is affected by specific hemodynamic response and multiple factors. The echocardiographic evidence of a reduction of the right and left ventricular function, leads to the use of volume expanders and inotropic to improve cardiac output, contractility and blood pressure. Parathyroid, adrenal and thyroid hormone deficit may require therapy with thyroid hormones, calcium or hydrocortisone. Immaturity of thermogenic mechanisms needs special heating measures.

During the first three days of life the extremely very low birth weight (BW < 1,000 g) frequently with maternal chorioamnionitis history, metabolic acidosis and altered perfusion in the first 24 hours of life, often present progressive respiratory worsening, tachycardia, silent ductus arteriousus. In this case, a rapid infusion of fluid above 30 mL/kg during the first 48 hours of life is responsible for left-right shunt, congestive heart failure and ventricular overload and increased mortality (Ewer et al 2003, Hamrick et al 2010) The failure to close the patent ductus is associated with increased mortality, intraventricular hemorrhage, and poor neurodevelopmental outcome.(Noori et al 2009). Ultrasonography techniques to estimate superior vena cava flow and heart output are effective to replace MBP as an evaluation tool, although not widely available.

The optimal shock oxygenation for extreme prematures it is not yet determined. If under too restricted saturation control (between 83% - 89%), they have increased patent ductus arteriosus incidence. (Noori et al 2009) On the other hand, the harmful hyperoxia effects on ischemic tissues reperfusion are also feared. In extreme prematures, saturation > 94% should be avoided. PaO2 should not be kept in supra-systemic levels. (Hamrick et al 2010, Weindling et al 2007)

9. Conclusion

Despite major improvements in the management of severe sepsis, neonates can develop septic shock, a critical condition associated with high morbidity and mortality. For these reasons neonatal septic shock requires emergency treatment with antibiotics, appropriate fluid resuscitation and vasoactive drugs. Knowledge of risk factors will help to identify those neonates at greatest risk for development of septic shock. In the future genomic and proteomic approaches may be helpful in early diagnosis. Although at present antimicrobial therapy and supportive care remain the foundation of treatment, it is desirable that future agents may improve outcomes, specially for particularly vulnerable premature neonates. It is estimated that intra-uterine infection, a risk factor for developing severe infection, is present in up to 35% of preterm deliveries [2].

SIRS: presence of at least 2 of the following 4 criteria, 1 of which must be abnormal temperature or leukocyte count: • Core temperature of >38.5°C or <36°C • Tachycardia, defined as a mean heart rate >2SD more than normal for age in the absence of external stimulus, chronic drugs, or painful stimuli; or otherwise unexplained persistent increase in a 0.5- to 4-h time period OR for children <1 y old: bradycardia, defined as a mean heart rate <10th percentile for age in the absence of external vagal stimulus, b-blocker drugs, or congenital heart disease; or otherwise unexplained persistent depression in a 0.5-h time period • Mean respiratory rate >2SD more than normal for age or mechanical ventilation for an acute process not related to underlying neuromuscular disease or the receipt of general anesthesia • Leukocyte count increased or decreased for age (not secondary to chemotherapy-induced leukopenia) or >10% immature neutrophils
Infection: a suspected or proven (by positive culture, tissue stain, or polymerase chain reaction test) infection caused by any pathogen OR a clinical syndrome associated with a high probability of infection. Evidence of infection includes positive findings on clinical examination, imaging, or laboratory tests (eg, white blood cells in a normally sterile body fluid, perforated viscus, chest radiograph consistent with pneumonia, petechial or purpuric rash, or purpura fulminans).
Sepsis: SIRS in the presence of or as a result of suspected or proven infection.
Severe sepsis: sepsis plus 1 of the following: cardiovascular organ dysfunction OR ARDS OR 2 or more other organ dysfunctions.
Septic shock: sepsis and cardiovascular organ dysfunction.

From Goldstein B, Giroir B, Randolph A. International pediatric sepsis consensus conference: definitions for sepsis and organ dysfunction in pediatrics. Pediatr Crit Care Med 2005;6(1):2–8.
Fleer A, Krediet TG. Innate immunity: toll-like receptors and some more. A brief history, basic organization and relevance for the human newborn. Neonatology. 2007;92(3):145-57.

Table 1. Definition of systemic inflammatory response syndrome (SIRS), infection, sepsis, severe sepsis, septic shock

Cardiovascular dysfunction:
Despite administration of isotonic intravenous fluid bolus >40 mL/kg in 1h
- Decrease in BP (hypotension) <5th percentile for age or systolic BP >2SD less than normal for age

OR
- Need for vasoactive drug to maintain BP in normal range (dopamine >5 mg/kg/min or dobutamine, epinephrine, or norepinephrine at any dose)

OR
- Two of the following:

Unexplained metabolic acidosis: base deficit >5.0 mEq/L
Increased arterial lactate >2 times upper limit of normal
Oliguria: urine output <0.5 mL/kg/h
Prolonged capillary refill >5 s
Core to peripheral temperature gap >3°C

Pulmonary:
- PaO2/FIO2 <300 in absence of cyanotic heart disease or preexisting lung disease

OR
- PaCO2 >65 torr or 20 mm Hg more than baseline PaCO2

OR
- Proven need for >50% FIO2 to maintain saturation >92%

OR
- Need for nonelective invasive or noninvasive mechanical ventilation

Neurologic:
- Glasgow Coma Score >11

OR
- Acute change in mental status with a decrease in Glasgow Coma Score >3 points from abnormal baseline

Hematologic:
- Platelet count <80,000/mm3 or a decline of 50% in platelet count from highest value recorded in the past 3 days (for chronic hematology/oncology patients)

OR
- International normalized ratio >2

Renal:
- Serum creatinine >2 times upper limit of normal for age or 2-fold increase in baseline creatinine

Hepatic:
- Total bilirubin >4 mg/dL (not applicable for newborn)

OR
- ALT 2 times upper limit of normal for age

From Goldstein B, Giroir B, Randolph A. International pediatric sepsis consensus conference: definitions for sepsis and organ dysfunction in pediatrics. Pediatr Crit Care Med 2005;6(1):2–8.

Table 2. Organ disfunction criteria

- Infant 72 hours or less in age.
- Tachypnea (Respiratory rate > 60 bpm) plus either grunting/retraction or desaturations.
- Temperature instability (<36°C or > 37-9 °C)
- Capillary refill time > 3 seconds
- WBC count (‹ 4000 × 109/L or 8 34,000 × 109/l)
- CRP > 10 mg/dl
- IL-6 or IL-8 > 70 pg/ml
- 16S rRNA gene PCR: Positive.
- WBC: white blood cell; CRP: C-reactive protein; IL: interlukin; rRNA: recombinant RNA; PCR: polymerase chain reaction.

From Haque KN (2005) Definitions of blood stream infection in the newborn. Pediatr Crit Care Med 6 (Suppl):545–549

Table 3. Two or more of the following are required to diagnose the fetal inflammatory response syndrome (FIRS)

10. References

Aneja RK, Varughese-Aneja R, Vetterly CG. Et al. (2011) Antibiotic therapy in neonatal and pediatric septic shock. Curr Infect Dis Rep. Published online 6 July

Arnold RC, Shapiro NI, Jones AF et al.(2009) Multicenter study of early lactate clearance as a determinant of survival in patients with presumed sepsis. Shock; 32 (1): 35 - 39.

Baruti Gafurri Z, Pacarizi H, Zhubi B et al. (2010) The importance of determining procalcitonin and C reactive protein in different stages of sepsis Bosnian J Basic Medical Scences. 10 (1): 6.

Beardsall K, Vanhaesebrouck S, Ogilvy-Stuart AL, et al. (2008) Early insulin therapy in very-low-birth-weight infants. N Engl J Med. 359(18):1873-84

Bernard GR, Vincent JL, Laterre PF, et al.: (2001) Efficacy and safety of recombinant human activated protein C for severe sepsis. N Engl J Med 344:699-709

Branco RG, Garcia PC, Piva JP, et al. (2005) Glucose level and risk of mortality in pediatric septic shock. Pediatr Crit Care Med. 6(4):470-2.

Brierley J, Peters MJ. (2008) Distinct hemodynamic patterns of septic shock at presentation to pediatric intensive care. Pediatrics.122(4):752-9.

Brierley J, Carcillo JA, Choong K et al. (2009) Clinical practice parameters for hemodynamic support of pediatric and neonatal septic shock: 2007 update from the American College of Critical Care Medicine. Crit Care Med; 37: 2.

Braun JP, Schneider M, Kastrup M, et al. (2004) Treatment of acute heart failure in an infant after cardiac surgery using levosimendan. Eur J Cardiothorac Surg. 26: 228-230.

Carcillo JA, Fields AI (2002): Clinical practice parameters for hemodynamic support of pediatric and neonatal patients in septic shock. Crit Care Med; 30:1365-1378.

Carcillo JA, Kuch BA, Han YY, et al. (2009)Mortality and functional morbidity after use of PALS/APLS by community physicians. Pediatrics. 124 (2): 500 - 508.

Carr, R, Modi N (2003) G-CSF and GM-CSF for treating or preventing neonatal infections. Cochrane Database Syst Rev CD003066

Casado-Flores J, Blanco-Quirós A, Nieto M, et al. (2006) Prognostic utility of the semi-quantitative procalcitonin test, neutrophil count and C-reactive protein in meningococcal infection in children. Eur J Pediatr. 165(1):26-9.

Cayabyab R, McLean CW, Seri I. (2009) Definition of hypotension and assessment of hemodynamics in the preterm neonate. J Perinatol. 29 Suppl 2: 58-62.

Clark RH, Bloom BT, Spitzer AR. (2006) Empiric use if ampicillin and cefotaxime, compared to ampicillin and gentamicin, for neonates at risk for sepsis is associated with an increased risk of neonatal death. Pediatrics 117 (1): 67-74.

Conrad U, Plagmann I, Malchow S et al. (2011) ELPylated anti-human TNF therapeutic single-domain antibodies for prevention of lethal septic shock. Plant Biotechnology Journal 9 (1): 22–31

Cornell TT, Wynn J, Shaney TP et al. (2010) Mechanisms and regulation of the gene-expression response to sepsis. Pediatrics 125 (6): 1248-58.

Cvirn G, Koestenberger M, Leschnik B et al (2005): Protein S modulates the anticoagulant action of recombinant human activated protein C: a comparison between neonates and adults. Br J Pharmacol 146:1082-1086.

Decembrino L, D'Angelo A,. Manzato F. et al. (2010) Protein C concentrate as adjuvant treatment in neonates with sepsis-induced coagulopathy: a pilot study. SHOCK. 34 (4): 341-345.

de Kleijn ED, de GR, Hack CE, Mulder PG et al.(2003) Activation of protein C following infusion of protein C concentrate in children with severe meningococcal sepsis and purpura fulminans: a randomized, double-blinded, placebocontrolled, dose-finding study. Crit Care Med. 31:1839–47

Dempsey EM, Barrington KJ. (2009) Evaluation and treatment of hypotension in the preterm infant. Clin Perinatol. 36(1):75-85. Review.

Egan JR, Clarke AJB, Williams S et al (2006) Levosimendan for Low Cardiac Output: A Pediatric Experience. J Intensive Care Med 21: 183

El Sayed Zaki M, El Sayed H. (2009) Evaluation of Microbiologic and Hematologic parameters and E-Selectin as early predictors for outcome of neonatal sepsis. Arch Pathol Lab Med. (133): 1291-96.

Ewer AK, Tyler W, Francis A, et al. (2003) Excessive volume expansion and neonatal death in preterm infants born at 27-28 weeks gestation. Paediatr Perinat Epidemiol. 17(2):180-6.

Fernandez EF, Montman R, Watterberg KL. (2008) ACTH and cortisol response to critical illness in term and late preterm newborns. J Perinatol. 28(12): 797-802.

Fischer D, Schloesser RL, Nold-Petry CA et al (2009) Protein C concentrate in preterm neonates with sepsis Acta Pædiatrica 98, pp. 1526–1529

Fischer D, Nold MF, Nold-Petry CA et al (2009) Protein C preserves microcirculation in a model of neonatal septic shock. Vascular Health and Risk Management 5,775-781.

Fioretto JR, Martin JG, Kurokawa CS et al.(2010) Comparison between procalcitonin and C-reactive protein for early diagnosis of children with sepsis or septic shock. Inflamm. Res. 59: 581 –586.

Fleer A, Krediet TG. (2007) Innate immunity: toll-like receptors and some more. A brief history, basic organization and relevance for the human newborn. Neonatology. 92(3): 145 - 57.

Fourrier F, Chopin C, Goudemand J, et al. (1992) Septic shock, multiple organ failure, and disseminated intravascular coagulation. Compared patterns of antithrombin III, protein C, and protein S deficiencies. Chest ; 101:816Y823,.

Gao H, Leaver SK, Burke-Gaffney A, et al. (2008) Severe sepsis and Toll-like receptors. Semin Immunopathol. 30(1): 29 - 40. Review.

Goldstein B, Giroir B, Randolph A. (2005) International Consensus Conference on Pediatric Sepsis. International pediatric sepsis consensus conference: definitions for sepsis and organ dysfunction in pediatrics. Pediatr Crit Care Med. 6 (1): 2-8.

Gordon A, Isaacs D. (2006) Late onset neonatal Gram-negative bacillary infection in Australia and New Zealand: 1992–2002. Pediatr Infect Dis J. 25(1): 25 - 9.

Filippi L, Poggi C, Serafini L et al (2008) Terlipressin as rescue treatment of refractory shock in a neonate. Acta Pædiatrica; 97: 500–512

Hamrick SE, Hansmann G. Patent ductus arteriosus of the preterm infant. Pediatrics. 2010;125(5):1020-30.

Han YY, Carcillo JA, Dragotta MA et al. (2003) Early reversal of pediatric-neonatal septic shock by community physicians is associated with improved outcome. Pediatrics 112 (4): 793-799

Haque KN. (2003) Infection and immunity in the newborn. In: McIntosh N, Helms P (eds) Textbook of Pediatrics, 6th edn. Churchill Livingstone, Edinburgh, 273–290.

Haque KN, Khan A, Kerry S et al. (2004) Pattern of neonatal sepsis in a District General Hospital in United Kingdom. Infect Control Hosp Epidemiol; 25:759–764

Haque KN (2005) Definitions of blood stream infection in the newborn. Pediatr Crit Care Med 6 (Suppl):545–549

Haque KN. (2007) Understanding and optimizing outcome in neonates with sepsis and septic shock. In Yearbook of intensive care and emergency medicine. 55-68.

Haque KN (2007) Defining common infections in children and neonates. J Hosp Infect. 2007; 65 Suppl 2: 110 - 4.

Hasslacher J, Bijuklic K, Bertocchi C et al. (2011) Levosimendan inhibits release of reactive oxygen species in polymorphonuclear leukocytes in vitro and in patients with acute heart failure and septic shock: a prospective observational study. Critical Care 15:R166

Huang J, Xu L, Thomas M, Whitaker K, et al (2006) L-type Ca2+ channel function and expression in neonatal rabbit ventricular myocytes. Am J Physiol Heart Circ Physiol 290: 2267 - 2276.

Kenet G, Strauss T, Kaplinsky C, et al. (2008) Hemostasis and thrombosis in critically ill children. Semin Thromb Hemost. 34(5): 451 - 8.

Kermorvant-Duchemin E, S. Laborie, M. Rabilloud, et al. (2008). Outcome and prognostic factors in neonates with septic shock. Pediatr Crit Care Med; 9(2):186–91.

Kissoon N, Orr RA, Carcillo J. (2010) Updated American College of Critical Care Medicine Pediatric Advanced Life Support Guidelines for Management of Pediatric and Neonatal Septic Shock. Relevance to the Emergency Care Clinician. Pediatr Emer Care 26: 867-869.

Kluckow M (2001) Low systemic blood flow in the preterm infant. Semin Neonatol 6:75–84

Kluckow M, Evans N (2000) Ductal shunting, high pulmonary blood flow, and pulmonary hemorrhage. J Pediatr 137:68–72

Kluckow M, Evans N (2000) Low superior vena cava flow and intraventricular haemorrhage in preterm infants. Arch Dis Child Fetal Neonatal 82:F188–F194

Ince C. (2005). The microcirculation is the motor of sepsis. Crit Care; 9 (Suppl 4): 13-9.

Irazuzta j, Sullivan KJ, Garcia PC et al. (2007) Pharmacologic support of infants and children in septic shock. J Pediatr (Rio J). 83(2)(Suppl):S36–S45.

Jones JG, S. Smith L. (2008) Shock in the Critically Ill Neonate. J Perinat Neonat Nurs. 23 (4): 346–354.

Jones AE, Shapiro NI, Trzeciak S et al.(2010) Lactate clearance vs central venous oxygen saturation as golas of early sepsis therapy: a randomized clnical trial. JAMA 303 (8): 2010

Joyce JJ, Dickson PI, Qi N, Noble JE, et al (2004) Normal right and left ventricular mass development during early infancy. Am J Cardiol 93: 797 - 801.

Kam PCA, Williams S, Yoong FFY. (2004) Vasopressin and terlipressin: pharmacology and its clinical relevance. Anesthesia 59: 993–1001

Klinzing S, Simon M, Reinhart K et al. (2003) High-dose vasopressin is not superior to norepinephrine in septic shock. Critical Care Medicine 31: 2646–2650

Kozak-Barany A, Jokinen E, Saraste M, et al (2001) Development of left ventricular systolic and diastolic function in preterm infants during the first month of life: a prospective follow-up study. J Pediatr 139: 539 - 545.

Kumar A, Roberts D, Wood KE, et al (2006) Duration of hypotension before initiation of effective antimicrobial therapy is the critical determinant of survival is human septic shock. Crit Care Med. 34:1589–1596.

Langer M, Modi BP, Agus M. (2006) Adrenal insufficiency in the critically ill neonate and child. Curr Opin Pediatr. 18(4): 448 - 453.

Lauterbach R, Pawlik D, Kowalczyk D,et al. (1999) Effect of the immunomodulating agent, pentoxifylline, in the treatment of sepsis in prematurely delivered infants: a placebo-controlled, double-blind trial. Crit Care Med 27:807-814.

Lauterbach R, Pawlik D, Radziszewska R et al (2006) Plasma antitrombin III and protein C levels in early recognition of late onset sepsis in newborns. Eur J Pediatr 165:585Y589

Lawn JE, Wilczynska-Ketende K, Cousens SN. Et al (2006).Estimating the cause of 4 million neonatal deaths in the year 2000. Int J Epidermiol; 35:706–718.

Leone M, Martin C. (2008) Role of terlipressin in the treatment of infants and neonates with catecholamine-resistant septic shock. Best Practice & Research Clinical Anaesthesiology. 22: (2) 323–333

Levi M. (2010) The coagulant response in sepsis and inflammation. Hamostaseologie. 30(1): 14 - 6. Review.

Levy B, Perez P, Perny J et al (2011) Comparison of norepinephrine-dobutamine to epinephrine for hemodynamics, lactate metabolism, and organ function variables in cardiogenic shock. A prospective, randomized pilot study Critical Care Medicine. 39 (3): 450 - 455

Lindsay CA, Barton P, Lawless S, et al. (1998) Pharmacokinetics and pharmacodynamics of milrinone lactate in pediatric patients with septic shock. J Ped. 132 (2): 329-334.

Luckner G, Mayr VD, Jochberger S et al. (2007) Comparison of two dose regimens of arginine vaopressin in advanced dilatory shock. Critical Care Medicine. 35: 2280-2285.

Luther YC, Schulze-Neick I, Stiller B, et al. (2004) Levosimendan long-term inodilation in an infant with myocardial infarction. Z Kardiol. 93:234-239.

Lynch SK, Mullett MD, Graeber JE et al (2008) . A comparison of albumin-bolus therapy versus normal salinebolus therapy for hypotension in neonates. J Perinatol. 28(1): 29 - 33.

Markovitz BP, Goodman DM, Watson RS, et al (2005) A retrospective cohort study of prognostic factors associated with outcome in pediatric severe sepsis: what is the role of steroids? Pediatr Crit Care Med. 6:270-274.

Marodi L. (2006) Innate cellular immune responses in newborns. Clin Immunol. 118 (2-3): 137 - 44

Matok I, Leibovitch L, Vardi A, et al. (2004) Terlipressin as rescue therapy for intractable hypotension during neonatal septic shock. Pediatr Crit CareMed. 5: 116–8.

Matok I, Vard A, Efrati O et al. (2005) Terlipressin as rescue therapy for intractable hypotension duc to septic shock in children. Shock 23: 305–310.

Meyer S, Gortner L, McGuire W, et al. (2008) Vasopressin in catecholamine-refractory shock in children. Anaesthesia. 63(3):228–234.

Moiseyev VS, Poder P, Andrejevs N, et al.(2002) Safety and efficacy of a novel calcium sensitizer, levosimendan, in patients with left ventricular failure due to an acute myocardial infarction. A randomized, placebo-controlled, double-blind study (RUSSLAN).Eur Heart J. 23:1422-1432.

Morelli A, Ertmer C, Westphal M. (2008) Terlipressin in the treatment of septic shock: the earlier the better?'' Best Practice & Research Clinical Anaesthesiology 22 (2): 317-321

Morelli A, Ertmer C, Rehberg S, et al. (2009) Continuous terlipressin versus vasopressin infusion in septic shock (TERLIVAP): a randomized, controller pilot study. Crit Care 13:R130.

Morrissey A, Parachuru L, Leung M et al. (2005) et al.: Expression of ATP-sensitive K+ channel subunits during perinatal maturation in the mouse heart. Pediatr Res. 58: 185 - 192.

Muller-Pebody B, Johnson AP, Heath PT, et al. (2011) Empirical treatment of neonatal sepsis: are the current guidelines adequate? Arch Dis Child Fetal Neonatal. 96 (1): F4 - 8.

Munro MJ, A.M. Walke, C.P. Barfield. (2004) Hypotensive extremely low birth weight infants have reduced cerebral blood flow. Pediatrics; 114:1591–1596.

Nadel S, Goldstein B, Williams MD, et al (2007) Drotrecogin alfa (activated) in children with severe sepsis: a multicentre phase III randomised controlled trial. Lancet. 369:836-843

Ng PC, Lee CH, Bnur FL, et al. (2006) A double-blind, randomized, controlled study of a "stress dose" of hydrocortisone for rescue treatment of refractory hypotension in preterm infants. Pediatrics. 117(2):367–375.

Noori S, McCoy M, Friedlich P et al. (2009) Failure of ductus arteriosus closure is associated with increased mortality in preterm infants. Pediatrics. 123(1):e138-44.

Osborn D, Evans N, Kluckow M. (2002) Randomized trial of dobutamine versus dopamine in preterm infants with low systemic blood flow. J Pediatr. 140:183-191.

Oca MJ, Nelson M, Donn SM. (2003) Randomized trial of normal saline versus 5% albumin for the treatment of neonatal hypotension. J Perinatol. 23(6):473–476.

Paradisis M, Evans N, Kluckow M, et al. (2009) Randomized trial of milrinone versus placebo for prevention of low systemic blood flow in very preterm infants. J Pediatr. 154(2):189-95.

M. Paradisis, N. Evans, M. Kluckow et al.(2006) Pilot study of milrinone for low systemic blood flow in very preterm infants. J Pediatr. 148 (3): 306–313.

M. Paradisis, X. Jiang, AJ. McLachlan et al. (2007) Population pharmacokinetics and dosing regimen design of milrinone in preterm infants. Arch Dis Child Fetal Neonatal 92(3):F204–F209.

Parker MM, Hazelzet JA, Carcillo JA. (2004) Pediatric considerations.

Crit Care Med. 32(11)(Suppl):S591–S594.

Patel BM, Chittock DR, Russell JA & Walley KR. (2002) Beneficial effects of short-term vasopressin infusion during severe septic shock. Anesthesiology; 96: 576–582

Pellicer A, Bravo MC, Madero R et al. (2009) Early systemic hypotension and vasopressor support in low birth weight infants: impact on neurodevelopment. Pediatrics. 123(5):1369-7666.

Pesaturo AB, Jennings HR & Voils SA. (2006) Terlipressin: vasopressin analog and novel drug for septic shock. Annals of Pharmacotherapy. 40: 2170–2177

Pollack MM, Fields AI, Ruttimann UE (1985) Distributions of cardiopulmonary variables in pediatric survivors and nonsurvivors of septic shock. Crit Care Med. 13:454–459

Rao SC, Ahmed M, Hagan R. (2006) One dose per day compared to mulptiple doses per day of gentamicine for treatment of suspected or proven sepsis in neonates. Cochrane database Syst Rev (1): CD005091

Rehberg S, Ertmer C, Köhler G, et al. (2009) Role of arginine vasopressin and terlipressin as first-line vasopressor agents in fulminant ovine septic shock. Intensive Care Med.35:1286-96.

Rivers E, Nguyen B, Havstad S, et al.(2001) : Early goal-directed therapy in the treatment of severe sepsis and septic shock. N Engl J Med. 345:1368-1377.

Roberts JD, Fineman JR, Morin FC et al. (1997) Inhaled nitric oxide and persistent pulmonary hypertension of the newborn. The Inhaled Nitric Oxide Study Group. N Engl J Med. 336 (9): 605–10.

Rodrı´guez-Nu´n˜ez A, Lo´pez-Herce J, Gil-Anto´n J et al. (2006) Rescue treatment with terlipressin in children with refractory septic shock: a clinical study. Critical Care. 10. R20.

Rodríguez-Núñez A, Oulego-Erroz I, Gil-Antón J et al. (2010) Continuous Terlipressin Infusion as Rescue Treatment in a Case Series of Children with Refractory Septic Shock. The Annals of Pharmacotherapy. 44:1545-1543.

Schrag SJ, Stoll BJ. (2006) Early-onset neonatal sepsis in the era of widespread intrapartum chemoprophylaxis. Pediatr Infect Dis J. 25 (10): 939 - 40. Review

Sharshar T, Blanchard A, Paillard M et al. (2003) Circulating vasopressin levels in septic shock. Critical Care Medicine. 31: 1752–1758.

Shaw AD, Vail GM, Haney DJ et al. (2011) Severe protein C deficiency is associated with organ dysfunction in patients with severe sepsis. J of Critical Care. Article in press

Short MA (2004) Linking the sepsis triad of inflammation, coagulation, and suppressed fibrinolysis to infants. Adv Neonatal Care 4(5): 258Y273,.

Silveira RC, Giacomini C, Soibelmann Procianoy R. (2010) Neonatal sepsis and septic shock: concepts update and review. Rev Bras Ter Intensiva. 22(3): 280-290.

Simon L, Saint-Louis P, Amre DK et al. (2006) Procalcitonin and C-reactive protein as markers of bacterial infection in critically ill children at onset of systemic inflammatory response syndrome. Pediatr Crit Care Med. 8 (9): 407–13.

Slawsky MT, Colucci WS, Gottlieb SS, et al. (2000) Acute hemodynamic and clinical effects of levosimendan in patients with severe heart failure. Study Investigators. Circulation. 102:2222-2227.

Stoll BJ, Hansen N. (2003) Infection in very-low-birth-weight-infants. Studies from NICHD Neonatal Network. Semin Perinatol; 27:293–301.

Stoll BJ, Hansen N, Fanaroff AA, et al.(2002) Late-onset sepsis in very low birth weight neonates: the experience of the NICHD Neonatal Research Network. Pediatrics. 110 (2 Pt 1): 285 - 91.

Stoll BJ, Hansen N, Adams-Chapman I, et al (2004). Neuro-development and growth impairment among extremely low birth weight infants with neonatal infections. JAMA; 292:2357- 2365.

Tourneux P, Rakza T, Abazine A, et al.(2008) Noradrenaline for management of septic shock refractory to fluid loading and dopamine or dobutamine in full-term newborn infants. Acta Paediatr. 97(2):177-80.

Urlichs F, Speer C. (2004) Neutrophil function in preterm and term infants. Neoreviews 5: 417 - 30.

Valverde E, Pellicer A, Madero R et al. (2006) Dopamine versus epinephrine for cardiovascular support in low birth weight infants: analysis of systemic effects and neonatal clinical outcomes. Pediatrics 117:1213-1222.

Venkataseshan S, Dutta S, Ahluwalia J, Narang A. (2007) Low plasma protein C values predict mortality in low birth weight neonates with septicemia. Pediatr Infect Dis J 26: 684–8

Vincent. JL (2006) Vasopressin in hypotensive and shock states. Crit Care Clin. 22(2):187–197.

Vincent JL. (2008) Clinical sepsis and septic shock--definition, diagnosis and management principles. Langenbecks Arch Surg. 393(6):817-24. Review.

Vlasselaers D, Milants I, Desmet L, et al. (2009) Intensive insulin therapy for patients in paediatric intensive care: a prospective, randomised controlled study. Lancet. 373(9663):547-56.

Weidlich K, Kroth J, Nussbaum C et al. (2009) Changes in microcirculation as early markers for infection in preterm infants-- an observational prospective study. Pediatr Res. 66(4):461

Weindling AM, Subhedar NV. (2007) The definition of hypotension in very low-birthweight infants during the immediate neonatal period. NeoReviews. 8(1):e32-43.

Westphal M, Rehberg S, Ertmer C, Morelli A. (2009) Terlipressin—more than just a prodrug of lysine vasopressin? Crit Care Med. 37:1135-6.

Zeballos G, Lopez-Herce J, Fernandez C, et al. (2006) Rescue therapy with terlipressin by continuous infusion in a child with catecholamine-resistant septic shock. Resuscitation 68: 151–3

Zhang JP, Chen C, Yang Y. (2007) Changes and clinical significance of Toll-like receptor 2 and 4 expression in neonatal infections. Zhonghua Er Ke Za Zhi 45(2):130–3 [in Chinese].

14

Management of Septic Shock in Children

Martin C. J. Kneyber
Department of Paediatric Intensive Care, Beatrix Children's Hospital
University Medical Center Groningen, University of Groningen, Groningen
The Netherlands

1. Introduction

Paediatric septic shock is a frequently occurring disease condition that is associated with high morbidity and mortality (Watson et al, 2003). Shock is an acute, complex state of circulatory dysfunction resulting in failure to deliver oxygen (DO_2) and nutrients to meet metabolic demands (VO_2) which are usually increased during shock. If left untreated, multiple organ failure and ultimately death will occur (Smith et al, 2006). This strongly points out the importance of early recognition and aggressive treatment of children with shock. Comparable to adults, such an approach - termed early-goal directed therapy (EGDT) - has been shown to significantly reduce mortality in paediatric septic shock. Paediatric studies have pointed out that the risk of death showed a two-fold increase with each hour delay in the reversal of shock (Carcillo et al, 2009; Han et al, 2003; Inwald et al, 2009; Rivers et al, 2001).

Hypovolaemic shock and septic shock are the most common forms of shock in children. Hypovolaemic shock is characterized by a decrease in intravascular blood volume to such an extent that effective tissue perfusion cannot be maintained. In children hypovolaemic shock is mainly caused by fluid and electrolyte loss due to vomiting and diarrhea or acute haemorrhage. Septic shock is actually a combination of distributive shock (i.e. a decreased total vascular resistance and maldistribution of blood flow in the microcirculation) and relative as well as a absolute hypovolaemia. Furthermore, impairment of myocardial fuction may occur with symptoms of cardiogenic shock.

The great majority of children with septic shock will not be presented in hospitals with PICU facilities. Furthermore, from a pathophysiologic perspective paediatric shock does not resemble adult septic shock. This strongly suggests that every physician that could be faced with these children needs to understand how to recognize paediatric shock and have basic knowledge of the principles of primary management. This chapter summarizes the pathophysiology, clinical manifestations and primary management of paediatric septic shock.

2. Pathophysiology of paediatric shock

The balance between DO_2 and VO_2 is the key factor in the pathophysiology of shock. DO_2 is also in children determined by the cardiac output (CO) and arterial oxygen content (CaO_2) according to the formula

$$DO_2 = CO * (Haemoglobin * 1.36 * SaO_2) + (0.003 * PaO_2) \quad (1)$$

The CO is determined by the heart rate (HR) and stroke volume (SV), the latter is determined by the pre-load, afterload and contractility of the heart.

The VO_2 is increased in septic shock. Hence, the body will try to compensate for this by increasing the DO_2 through various mechanisms including increasing the HR and the venous vascular tone to optimize cardiac pre-load. Tachycardia is one of the earliest compensatory mechanisms. If this compensation is inadequate to meet cellular oxygen demands, the systemic vascular resistance (SVR) will be increased allowing perfusion of vital organs such as the heart and brain. In addition, oxygen extraction will be increased. Of importance, children are able to maintain normal blood pressure. This phase of shock is termed *compensated shock*.

Oxygen debt will occur if these mechanisms fail when the shock is not reversed. Under normal conditions oxygen debt will occur when the ratio $DO_2 : VO_2$ is 3 : 1. However, as a result of the increase in VO_2 during septic shock oxygen debt will occur already at $DO_2 : VO_2$ 2 : 1. Microvascular perfusion becomes marginal and cellular function deteriorates, affecting all organ systems (*uncompensated shock*). If not adequately managed, *irreversible shock* will occur. Vital organs will be damaged to such an extent that death is inevitable.

There are considerable differences in the pathophyiology of septic shock between children and adults. Vasomotor paralysis is the predominant cause of mortality in adults (Parker et al, 1987). Myocardial dysfunction in adult septic shock manifests mainly as decreased ejection fraction with either normal or increased CO. This is because adults are capable of increasing their CO by tachycardia in combination with ventricular dilatation allowing an increase in SV (Parker et al, 1984). In contrast, paediatric septic shock is mainly characterized by severe hypovolaemia; the decrease in CO and not SVR is associated with mortality (Carcillo et al, 2002). This is because especially younger children have higher baseline HR's compared to adults; hence they cannot increase their HR without impairing CO. Furthermore, children are not capable of increasing their SV (Feltes et al, 1994). This means that children need to be resuscitated with fluids aggressively. Nevertheless, the haemodynamic response of fluid-resuscitated children is different from adults. Ceneviva and co-workers evaluated 50 children with fluid-refractory, dopamine resistant septic shock (Ceneviva et al, 1998). The majority had low CO in combination with high SVR, but 22% had low CO and low SVR. Furthermore, haemodynamic profiles changed frequently during the first 48 hours.

Another interesting difference between children and adults relates to the VO_2. The VO_2 is mainly determined by oxygen extraction in adults, whereas in children is it mainly determined by the DO_2 (Carcillo et al, 1989). This indicates that all efforts must be made to maintain adequate DO_2.

3. Symptoms of paediatric shock

The early diagnosis of paediatric shock warrants a high index of suspicion and knowledge of disease conditions that predispose children to shock. It is imperative to understand the reference values for vital parameters in children.

Early signs of septic shock may be subtle and easily missed. Tachycardia is the earliest presenting symptom. Blood pressure will be normal during compensated shock, but the pulse pressure is widened. Children will have plethora, warm extremities and bounding pulses ("warm shock". If the shock is not reversed, signs of failure of the compensatory mechanisms can be noted including cold extremities and prolonged capillary refill time ("cold shock"). Of note, the capillary refill time has little discriminative value in paediatric shock. Hypovolaemic children may still have a capillary refill time that is within the normal limit (2 seconds).

Age	Heart rate / min (95th percentile)	Respiratory rate / min (95th percentile)	Systolic blood pressure mmHg (5th percentile)
0 - 7 days	180	50	59
8 - 28 days	180	40	69
1 - 12 months	180	34	74
1 - 5 years	140	22	75
6 - 12 years	130	18	83
13 - 18 years	110	14	90

Table 1. Age-related reference values for vital parameters in children (derived from reference values by age, height and weight). Values above the 95th percentile (for heart rate and respiratory rate), and below the 5th percentile (for systolic blood pressure) are abnormal. Adapted from (Anonymous, 2004).

Symptoms of septic shock
General symptoms
Tachycardia
Hypothermia or fever
Decreased consciousness
Decreased urinary output
"Warm shock"
Shortened capillary refill time
Bounding pulses
Widened blood pressure
"Cold shock"
Capillary refill time > 2 secons
Weak pulses
Cold extremities, mottled skin
Hypotension (not necessarily)

Table 2. Symptoms of paediatric septic shock

Many children with fever have tachycardia and warm extremities on physical examination. Not all of these children are in shock. For early recognition of shock it is then absolute necessary to evaluate the mental state of the child. In general, children in shock are lethargic and have decreased consciousness, but the opposite (i.e. agitation, restless, anxious) also occurs. Underlying mechanisms include most likely a combination of cerebral hypoperfusion, metabolic alterations and production of cytotoxic substances.

Oxygen debt will occur when the shock is not recognized and thus not treated properly. Clinically, the child suffers from depressed consciousness, poor skin perfusion, decreased urinary output and hyperventilation to compensate for the metabolic acidosis.

The contribution of laboratory tests is limited. In contrast with adult septic shock, blood gasses and serum lactate levels are not diagnostic for paediatric shock but may be used for monitoring the effectiveness of treatment (Brierley et al, 2009). Repeated evaluation and monitoring of the patient remains the most effective physiologic monitor.

4. Management of paediatric shock

The American College of Critical Care Medicine (ACCM) has published clinical guidelines for the haemodynamic support of neonates and children with septic shock in 2002 and revised them in 2009 (Brierley et al, 2009; Carcillo et al, 2002). These guidelines advocate amongst others early recognition, adequate fluid resuscitation and timely and appropriate antibiotic therapy. Notwithstanding the fact that the efficacy of these guidelines has not been confirmed in a randomized clinical trial, data strongly suggests that adherence to these guidelines results in improved survival (de Oliveira et al, 2008; Dellinger et al, 2008; Han et al, 2003). Han and co-workers evaluated 91 patients with septic shock who were referred to their PICU (Han et al, 2003). Shock reversal within 75 minutes and adherence with the ACCM guidelines was associated with > 90% survival. Worrisome however was that adherence to these guidelines was only achieved in < 30% of all patients. A study of 200 children with severe sepsis in the United Kingdom showed a drop from 25% to 6% in mortality when shock was reversed, although only 8% of patients were managed according to the ACCM guidelines (Inwald et al, 2009).

The primary goal of the primary management of paediatric shock is to prevent organ failure caused by oxygen debt through optimalisation of and balancing DO_2 and VO_2. This means that is important to maintain blood pressure above the critical point which below flow cannot be effectively maintained. Thus, shock should be clinically diagnosed before hypotension occurs. Clinical targets include age-appropriate HR and blood pressure, normalisation of the capillary refill time, normal consciousness and adequate urinary output (> 1 mL/kg/hour) (Figure 1) (Brierley et al, 2009). After each intervention it is evaluated whether or not these clinical targets have been achieved.

4.1 Recognition and management during the first 15 minutes

Within the first five minutes the child is evaluated according to the Paediatric Advanced Life Support approach - i.e. a structural approach examining Airway, Breathing and Circulation (Figure 1). The diagnosis septic shock is confirmed when tachycardia, fever and symptoms of inadequate tissue perfusion are present. These symptoms include altered consciousness, as well as shortened capillary refill time, bounding pulses and widened pulse pressure (in case of "warm shock") or prolonged capillary refill time, weak pulses, mottled skin and decreased urinary output (in case of "cold shock").

The next step then is to administer 100% oxygen via a non-rebreathing mask (flow 10 - 15 L/min) and to insert two peripheral lines. Blood is drawn for haematological, biochemical studies and blood culture. Subsequently, aggressive fluid resuscitation is mandated (Carcillo et al, 1991). This means that within 15 minutes three fluid boluses of 20 mL/kg (max 500 mL) are administered. Crystalloid fluids are the first choice. After each bolus the child is evaluated if the clinical targets have been met. Rapid and sufficient fluid administration is significantly associated with improved survival (Ceneviva et al, 1998).

Of importance, antibiotics must be administered within the first 15 minutes. Although not confirmed in paediatric studies, adult data indicated that mortality doubled for each hour delay in administration of antibiotic treatment (Kumar et al, 2006). Electrolyte disturbances or hypoglycaemia is corrected in this first phase of primary management.

4.2 Management after the first 15 minutes

After 15 minutes it is evaluated if the clinical targets have been met. If not, the shock is classified as "fluid-resistant". The next step then would be to refer the patient to a PICU facility. It now depends upon the haemodynamic profile of the child what the next therapeutic intervention would be. If the child has a haemodynamic profile that is compatible with "cold shock", fluid administration is continued and dopamine 10 microgram/kg/minute is started via a peripheral line while in the mean time a central venous line is inserted. If the child has a haemodynamic profile that is compatible with "warm shock", fluid administration is continued and norepinephrine 0.1 microgram/kg/minute is started. Fluid administration will be continued until the liver becomes palpable enlarged or crackles are noted at pulmonary auscultation. Nevertheless, cumulative fluid administration up to 200 mL/kg may be necessary (Maar, 2004). Fluid administration should not be discontinued because of assumed possible development of pulmonary oedema, acute respiratory distress syndrome (ARDS) or cerebral oedema (Brierley et al, 2009). As an alternative to crystalloids, colloids such as albumin may be considered at this stage (Boluyt et al, 2006).

Also, endotracheal intubation and initiation of mechanical ventilation should be strongly considered in order to optimize DO_2. As discussed, in paediatric shock VO_2 is dependent upon DO_2. Furthermore, especially small children have a small functional residual capacity (FRC) that is easily compromised by pulmonary capillary leakage or if the child gets fatigued. Also, VO_2 may rise with 15 - 30% due to increased work of breathing during septic shock (Butt, 2001; Carcillo et al, 1989). Last, but not less important, sedation and mechanical ventilation may be needed to facilitate invasive procedures such as insertion of central lines. Also, increased intrathoracic pressure reduces left ventricular afterload that may be beneficial when there is a low CI/high SVR state. Nevertheless, early intubation may still be subject of debate. One of the arguments often used is the vasodilatory effect of agents used for induction. This effect may further compromise DO_2 in the septic child. We advocate the use of ketamine as induction agent (Yamamoto, 2000). Ketamine is a centrally acting N-methyl-D-aspartate (NMDA) receptor antagonist allowing cardiovascular stability. We would also advocate refraining from the use of etomidate because of its negative effects on adrenal gland function (Brierley et al, 2009).

The use of corticosteroids and sodium bicarbonate during the first hour of primary management of paediatric shock is also subject of heavy scientific debate. Corticosteroids are definitely indicated for children with purpura fulminans, or children with a recent history of prolonged corticosteroid use of proven abnormalities in the hypothalamic-pituitary-adrenal gland axis (Langer et al, 2006). In addition, the use of corticosteroids may be considered when children do not respond to infusion of vaso-active drugs (*"catecholamine-resistant shock"*) (Brierley et al, 2009). Sodium bicarbonate is usually administered to correct metabolic acidosis as it is presumed that vaso-active drugs function less well in an acidic environment (Tabbutt, 2001). However, the metabolic acidosis is caused by insufficient tissue perfusion. This indicates that is necessary to optimize tissue perfusion rather than correcting the acidosis with sodium bicarbonate (Dellinger et al, 2008). Also, two studies performed in critically ill adults with septic shock and $pH \geq 7.15$ have shown no beneficial effect on haemodynamic variables when patients were treated with

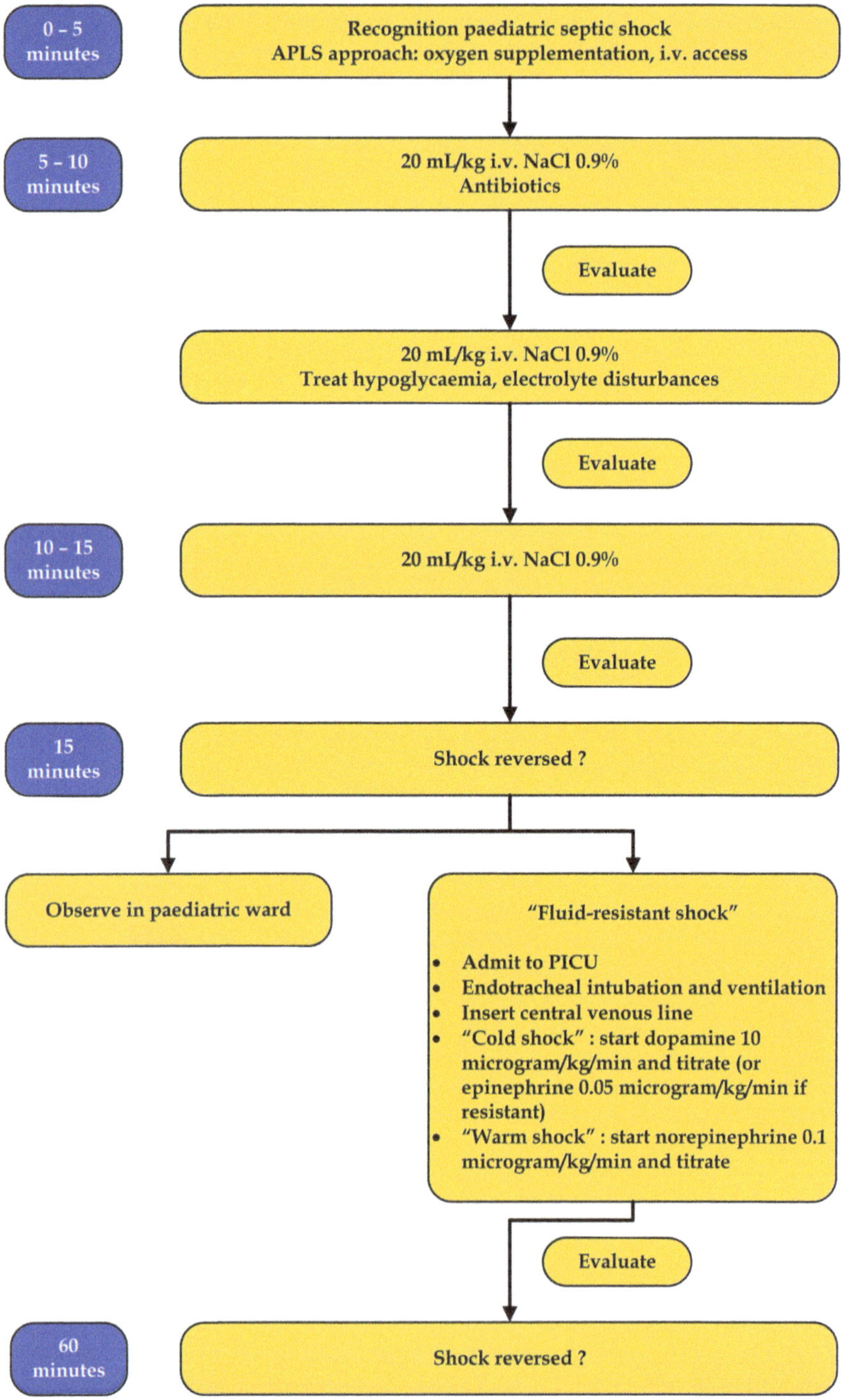
0 – 5
minutes
Recognition paediatric septic shock
APLS approach: oxygen supplementation, i.v. access
5 - 10
minutes
20 mL/kg i.v. NaCl 0.9%
Antibiotics
Evaluate
20 mL/kg i.v. NaCl 0.9%
Treat hypoglycaemia, electrolyte disturbances
Evaluate
10 – 15
minutes
20 mL/kg i.v. NaCl 0.9%
Evaluate
15
minutes
Shock reversed ?
Observe in paediatric ward
"Fluid-resistant shock"
• Admit to PICU
• Endotracheal intubation and ventilation
• Insert central venous line
• "Cold shock" : start dopamine 10 microgram/kg/min and titrate (or epinephrine 0.05 microgram/kg/min if resistant)
• "Warm shock" : start norepinephrine 0.1 microgram/kg/min and titrate
Evaluate
60
minutes
Shock reversed ?

sodium bicarbonate. Recent adult recommendations indicate to use sodium bicarbonate when pH < 7.00 (Boyd et al, 2008).

It is unclear if optimizing haemoglobin (Hb) levels through transfusion of red blood cells (RBC) is beneficial. One group of investigators could not confirm a beneficial effect on VO_2 despite optimalisation of CaO_2 in paediatric shock (Mink et al, 1990). Nevertheless, it is currently recommended to maintain Hb > 10 g/dL (Brierley et al, 2009). Fresh Frozen Plasma (FFP) is indicated for active haemorrhage or a prolonged activated partial thromboplastin time (APTT); in clinical practice usually twice the age-dependent reference value (Brierley et al, 2009).

4.3 Management after the first hour

One hour after presentation it is determined whether or not the shock has been reversed. If not, then the patient is recognized as having a fluid refractory dopamine-resistant shock. The patient is managed in the PICU. Treatment goals in this phase are similar to the golden hour (i.e. age-appropriate HR and blood pressure, normalisation of the capillary refill time, normal consciousness and urinary output > 1 mL/kg/hour), but now also include maintainance of age-appropriate perfusion pressure (mean airway pressure minus central venous pressure), cardiac index (CI) between 3.3 and 6.0 L/min/m^2, central venous oxygen saturation (SvO_2) > 70%, normal anion gap and normal lactate. Fluid replacement should be continued and directed at these endpoints.

The type of haemodynamic support depends upon the haemodyamic profile of the child (i.e. low CO/high SVR, high CO/low SVR, or low CO/low SVR) (Figure 2). It seems therefore rational to use haemodynamic monitoring devices such as pulse contour analysis or Doppler ultrasound to assess the haemodynamic profile especially since frequently change. Irrespective of haemodynamic profile, support should be targeted at a CI between 3.3 and 6.0 L/min/m^2. Pollack and co-workers have shown that a CI within this range was associated with the best outcome in paediatric shock (Pollack et al, 1985). Also, SvO_2 should be maintained > 70%. The SvO_2 can be used as a surrogate marker of the CO. Oliveira and co-workers randomized 102 children with septic shock to be managed using the ACCM guidelines with or without monitoring the SvO_2 (de Oliveira et al, 2008). Their SvO_2 goal-directed therapy resulted in less mortality (28-day mortality 11.8% vs. 39.2%, p = 0.002), and fewer new organ dysfunctions (p = 0.03). However, this strategy was associated with more crystalloid (28 (20-40) vs. 5 (0-20 ml/kg, p<0.0001), blood transfusion (45.1% vs. 15.7%, p =0.002) and inotropic (29.4% vs. 7.8%, p = 0.01) support in the first 6 hours of admission.

For patients with low CI, normal blood pressure and high SVR (i.e. "cold shock" with normal blood pressure), it is recommended to reduce ventricular afterload. This can be achieved using either epinephrine or dobutamine. Some have argued to additionally use a short-acting vasodilator such as nitroprusside or nitroglycerin to recruit the microcirculation. Alternatively, the use of type III phosphor-diesterase inhibitors such as milrinone may be considered (Barton et al, 1996). These agents have a synergistic effect with beta-adrenergic agents because they stimule intracellular cyclic adenosine monophosphate.

Patients with low CI, low blood pressure and low SVR (i.e. "cold shock with low blood pressure) it is recommended to titrate vasopressor therapy. In general, dopamine is the first-line vasopressor therapy. At high infusion rates, the alpha-adrenergic effects of dopamine predominate. Alternatively, norepinephrine or high dosage epinephrine may be considered. Once adequate blood pressure is achieved, a vasodilator can be added to improve the SvO_2 by recruiting the microcirculation.

Finally, patients with persisting high CI and low SVR despite fluid administration and norepinephrine may benefit of agents such as vasopressin or phenylephrine. Of importance, CO may be reduced when these agents are used so close monitoring of the CO and/or SvO_2 is mandated.

When the shock cannot be reversed and co-morbidities that fuel the shock (such as pericardial effusion, pneumothorax, hypoadrenalism, ongoing blood loss, increased intra-abdominal pressure, or necrotic tissue) high-flow veno-arterial extra-corporeal membrane oxygenation (ECMO) or high-flux continues renal replacement therapy (CRRT) with flows > 35 mL/kg/hour may be considered. Yet, these modalities may be qualified as last resort and their effects on final outcome need to be established.

5. Conclusion

Early recognition and aggressive primary management of paediatric septic shock is significantly associated with improved patient survival. Tachycardia, fever and altered consciousness are the first clinical manifestations of paediatric septic shock. Primary management includes aggressive fluid resuscitation, adequate oxygen delivery through early intubation and mechanical ventilation, and early referral to a paediatric intensive care unit. Future research should be directed towards obtaining stronger scientific evidence to confirm the components of the ACCM guidelines.

6. References

Anonymous. (2004) The fourth report on the diagnosis, evaluation, and treatment of high blood pressure in children and adolescents. *Pediatrics*. Vol. 114, issue 2 Suppl 4th Report, pp. 555-576,

Barton P, Garcia J, Kouatli A, Kitchen L, Zorka A, Lindsay C, Lawless S & Giroir B. (1996) Hemodynamic effects of i.v. milrinone lactate in pediatric patients with septic shock. A prospective, double-blinded, randomized, placebo-controlled, interventional study. *Chest*. Vol. 109, issue 5, pp. 1302-1312,

Boluyt N, Bollen CW, Bos AP, Kok JH & Offringa M. (2006) Fluid resuscitation in neonatal and pediatric hypovolemic shock: a Dutch Pediatric Society evidence-based clinical practice guideline. *Intensive Care Med*. Vol. 32, issue 7, pp. 995-1003,

Boyd JH & Walley KR. (2008) Is there a role for sodium bicarbonate in treating lactic acidosis from shock? *Curr.Opin.Crit Care*. Vol. 14, issue 4, pp. 379-383,

Brierley J, Carcillo JA, Choong K, Cornell T, Decaen A, Deymann A, Doctor A, Davis A, Duff J, Dugas MA, Duncan A, Evans B, Feldman J, Felmet K, Fisher G, Frankel L, Jeffries H, Greenwald B, Gutierrez J, Hall M, Han YY, Hanson J, Hazelzet J, Hernan L, Kiff J, Kissoon N, Kon A, Irazuzta J, Lin J, Lorts A, Mariscalco M, Mehta R, Nadel S, Nguyen T, Nicholson C, Peters M, Okhuysen-Cawley R, Poulton T, Relves M, Rodriguez A, Rozenfeld R, Schnitzler E, Shanley T, Kache S, Skippen P, Torres A, von Dessauer B, Weingarten J, Yeh T, Zaritsky A, Stojadinovic B, Zimmerman J & Zuckerberg A. (2009) Clinical practice parameters for hemodynamic support of pediatric and neonatal septic shock: 2007 update from the American College of Critical Care Medicine. *Crit Care Med*. Vol. 37, issue 2, pp. 666-688,

Butt W. (2001) Septic shock. *Pediatr.Clin.North Am*. Vol. 48, issue 3, pp. 601-25, viii,

Carcillo JA, Davis AL & Zaritsky A. (1991) Role of early fluid resuscitation in pediatric septic shock. *JAMA*. Vol. 266, issue 9, pp. 1242-1245,

Carcillo JA & Fields AI. (2002) Clinical practice parameters for hemodynamic support of pediatric and neonatal patients in septic shock. *Crit Care Med.* Vol. 30, issue 6, pp. 1365-1378,

Carcillo JA, Kuch BA, Han YY, Day S, Greenwald BM, McCloskey KA, Pearson-Shaver AL & Orr RA. (2009) Mortality and functional morbidity after use of PALS/APLS by community physicians. *Pediatrics*. Vol. 124, issue 2, pp. 500-508,

Carcillo JA, Pollack MM, Ruttimann UE & Fields AI. (1989) Sequential physiologic interactions in pediatric cardiogenic and septic shock. *Crit Care Med.* Vol. 17, issue 1, pp. 12-16,

Ceneviva G, Paschall JA, Maffei F & Carcillo JA. (1998) Hemodynamic support in fluid-refractory pediatric septic shock. *Pediatrics*. Vol. 102, issue 2, pp. e19-

de Oliveira CF, de Oliveira DS, Gottschald AF, Moura JD, Costa GA, Ventura AC, Fernandes JC, Vaz FA, Carcillo JA, Rivers EP & Troster EJ. (2008) ACCM/PALS haemodynamic support guidelines for paediatric septic shock: an outcomes comparison with and without monitoring central venous oxygen saturation. *Intensive Care Med.* Vol. 34, issue 6, pp. 1065-1075,

Dellinger RP, Levy MM, Carlet JM, Bion J, Parker MM, Jaeschke R, Reinhart K, Angus DC, Brun-Buisson C, Beale R, Calandra T, Dhainaut JF, Gerlach H, Harvey M, Marini JJ, Marshall J, Ranieri M, Ramsay G, Sevransky J, Thompson BT, Townsend S, Vender JS, Zimmerman JL & Vincent JL. (2008) Surviving Sepsis Campaign: international guidelines for management of severe sepsis and septic shock: 2008. *Crit Care Med.* Vol. 36, issue 1, pp. 296-327,

Feltes TF, Pignatelli R, Kleinert S & Mariscalco MM. (1994) Quantitated left ventricular systolic mechanics in children with septic shock utilizing noninvasive wall-stress analysis. *Crit Care Med.* Vol. 22, issue 10, pp. 1647-1658,

Han YY, Carcillo JA, Dragotta MA, Bills DM, Watson RS, Westerman ME & Orr RA. (2003) Early reversal of pediatric-neonatal septic shock by community physicians is associated with improved outcome. *Pediatrics*. Vol. 112, issue 4, pp. 793-799,

Inwald DP, Tasker RC, Peters MJ & Nadel S. (2009) Emergency management of children with severe sepsis in the United Kingdom: the results of the Paediatric Intensive Care Society sepsis audit. *Arch.Dis.Child*. Vol. 94, issue 5, pp. 348-353,

Kumar A, Roberts D, Wood KE, Light B, Parrillo JE, Sharma S, Suppes R, Feinstein D, Zanotti S, Taiberg L, Gurka D, Kumar A & Cheang M. (2006) Duration of hypotension before initiation of effective antimicrobial therapy is the critical determinant of survival in human septic shock. *Crit Care Med.* Vol. 34, issue 6, pp. 1589-1596,

Langer M, Modi BP & Agus M. (2006) Adrenal insufficiency in the critically ill neonate and child. *Curr.Opin.Pediatr.* Vol. 18, issue 4, pp. 448-453,

Maar SP. (2004) Emergency care in pediatric septic shock. *Pediatr.Emerg.Care*. Vol. 20, issue 9, pp. 617-624,

Mink RB & Pollack MM. (1990) Effect of blood transfusion on oxygen consumption in pediatric septic shock. *Crit Care Med.* Vol. 18, issue 10, pp. 1087-1091,

Parker MM, Shelhamer JH, Bacharach SL, Green MV, Natanson C, Frederick TM, Damske BA & Parrillo JE. (1984) Profound but reversible myocardial depression in patients with septic shock. *Ann.Intern.Med.* Vol. 100, issue 4, pp. 483-490,

Parker MM, Shelhamer JH, Natanson C, Alling DW & Parrillo JE. (1987) Serial cardiovascular variables in survivors and nonsurvivors of human septic shock: heart rate as an early predictor of prognosis. *Crit Care Med.* Vol. 15, issue 10, pp. 923-929,

Pollack MM, Fields AI & Ruttimann UE. (1985) Distributions of cardiopulmonary variables in pediatric survivors and nonsurvivors of septic shock. *Crit Care Med.* Vol. 13, issue 6, pp. 454-459,

Rivers E, Nguyen B, Havstad S, Ressler J, Muzzin A, Knoblich B, Peterson E & Tomlanovich M. (2001) Early goal-directed therapy in the treatment of severe sepsis and septic shock. *N.Engl.J.Med.* Vol. 345, issue 19, pp. 1368-1377,

Smith L & Hernan L. (2006) Shock states. Third, issue 27, pp. 394-410,

Tabbutt S. (2001) Heart failure in pediatric septic shock: utilizing inotropic support. *Crit Care Med.* Vol. 29, issue 10 Suppl, pp. S231-S236,

Watson RS, Carcillo JA, Linde-Zwirble WT, Clermont G, Lidicker J & Angus DC. (2003) The epidemiology of severe sepsis in children in the United States. *Am.J.Respir.Crit Care Med.* Vol. 167, issue 5, pp. 695-701,

Yamamoto LG. (2000) Rapid sequence intubation. Fourth, issue 5, pp. 81-92.

Part 7

Septic Shock in Obstetrics and Gynecology

15

Septic Shock in Obstetrics and Gynecology

Apostolos Kaponis, Theodoros Filindris and George Decavalas
Department of Obstetrics & Gynecology
Patra University School of Medicine, Patra
Greece

1. Introduction

Septic shock is a life-threatening clinical syndrome caused by decreased tissue perfusion and oxygen delivery, as a result of severe infection and sepsis. The insertion of bacteria or viruses into the blood stream produces a condition called bacteremia or viremia. Sepsis is the systemic inflammatory response due to bacteremia. When sepsis worsen to the point where blood pressure cannot be maintained with intravenous fluid alone, then the condition is called septic shock and may be accompanied with multiple organ dysfunction (liver, kidney, heart, brain). The mortality rate remains high, range between 25 and 50%[1]. Septic shock is the first cause of deaths in intensive care units patients[2].

1.1 Causes of septic shock

Most episodes of septic shock are caused by gram negative and gram positive organisms. Bacteremia is not necessary to develop sepsis, since patients with septic shock have a positive blood culture only in 40% to 70% of the cases[3]. A number of organisms may produce exotoxins or endotoxins that also initiate a systemic response. Gram negative bacteria contain endotoxin, a complex lipopolysaccharide, in the cell membrane. Lysis of them leads to the release of endotoxin. Some gram positive organisms produce also an exotoxin and "toxic shock syndrome" toxin; their release produces a similar response to lipopolysaccharides. Most cases of septic shock (approximately 70%) are caused by endotoxin-producing Gram negative bacteria. However, 5% to 10% have a fungal cause, and 15% to 20% are polymicrobial[4]. In emergency patients and the increased use of arterial and venous catheters, Gram positive cocci are implicated, as well.

Invasion of the microorganism into soft tissue leads in a complex cascade of events involving monocyte, macrophage and neutrophil recognition, activation, and initial release of inflammatory mediators. This constitutes a hyper-inflammatory state5,6. The release of inflammatory cytokines, chemokines, prostanoids, reactive oxygen, and nitrogen species leads to endothelial dysfunction and increased vascular permeability, myocardial suppression, and activation of the coagulation cascade. Patient's survival correlates with the recovery of the inflammatory responses[7].

The response to a microorganism depends on its virulence, size of the inoculum, co-morbid conditions, age, nutritional status and genetic polymorphisms in immune related genes[6].

Early recognition, prompt diagnostic workup and immediate initiation of therapy improve the prognosis of patients with septic shock syndrome.
Shock associated with sepsis can be caused by a variety of pathologic phenomena. It needs to be recalled that other mechanisms can be responsible. Hypovolemic shock can occur under conditions of sepsis due to massive fluid accumulation at the local site of infection. Other non-immunogenic causes of shock during sepsis that require consideration are cardiogenic causes.

1.2 Differential diagnosis of septic shock

Septic shock must be differentiated between systemic inflammatory response syndrome, sepsis, severe sepsis, hypotension, and multiple organ dysfunction syndrome as definitions were set in 1991 by the American College of Chest Physicians and the Society of Critical Care Medicine[8,9].
The phrase "systemic inflammatory response syndrome" describes the inflammatory process that can be generated by infection or by noninfectious causes such as pancreatitis, burns, and trauma. The response is manifested by two or more of the following conditions: 1) temperature greater than 38°C or less than 36°C, 2) heart rate greater than 90 beats per minute, 3) respiratory rate greater than 20 breaths per minute or arterial carbon dioxide pressure less than 32 mmHg, and 4) white blood cell count greater than 12000/mm^3 or less than 4000/ mm^3 or greater than 10% band forms. Sepsis as was described above is systemic inflammatory response syndrome due to infection. Severe sepsis is sepsis associated with organ dysfunction, hypoperfusion, or hypotension. Hypotension is defined as a systolic blood pressure <90 mmHg or a reduction of greater than or equal to 40 mmHg from baseline. Finally multiple organ dysfunction syndrome is the presence of altered organ function in an acutely ill patient such that homeostasis cannot be maintained without intervention.

2. Incidence of sepsis and septic shock

An accurate estimation of the incidence of sepsis and septic shock is hampered by the lack of reliable case definition. Inconsistent application of sepsis definition criteria contributes to confusion and variability in the literature[10]. The Centers for Disease Control estimated an incidence of 73.6 per 100,000 population in 1979, rising to 175.9 per 100,000 in 1989[11]. The rates have been probably increased because of more immuno-suppressed patients, new immunomodulating therapy, increased use of invasive devices (e.g., central venous catheters), and an increase in antibiotic resistance[5,6,12]. A review of discharge data on approximately 750 million hospitalizations in U.S.A. over a 22-year period (1979-2000) identified 10,319,418 cases of sepsis[5]. Sepsis was more common among men than among women (mean annual relative risk, 1.28; 95% CI: 1.24-1.32) and among non-white persons (mean annual relative risk 1.90; 95%CI: 1.81-2.00)[5]. However, these data is hampered due to the broad definition of sepsis and may be overestimate the accurate incidence of sepsis and septic shock since include all the ICD-9-CM* codes for definition of sepsis (038 [septicemia], 020.0 [septicemic], 790.7 [bacteremia], 117.9 [disseminated fungal infection], 112.5 [disseminated candida infection], and 112.81 [disseminated fungal endocarditis]. Organ

* ICD-9 CM denotes International Classification of Diseases, Ninth Revision, Clinical Modification

failure was defined by a combination of ICD-9 CM and CPT† codes. In general, there are few population-based prospective cohort studies that allow us to accurately delineate the incidence of sepsis and septic shock.
The mortality rate from sepsis is approximately 40% in adults, and 25% in children. It is significantly greater when sepsis left untreated for more than seven days[13].

3. Sepsis and septic shock during pregnancy

3.1 Prevalence and mortality rate in pregnancy

Septic shock in obstetric patients is rare because pregnant women are younger and have less co-morbid conditions. The common area of infection is the pelvis and the responsible microorganisms are sensitive in most of the broad spectrum antibiotics. Specific data on serious acute maternal morbidity due to sepsis are scarce, partly because of lack of a uniform definition of sepsis, but reported incidences in western countries vary from 0.1 to 0.6 per 1000 deliveries[14]. Although the incidence of septic shock in obstetric patients is low and has been decreased throughout the years it remains a significant factor of maternal morbidity and mortality related with pregnancy. Sepsis continues to account for approximately 7.6% of maternal deaths in the United States[15].
WHO defines puerperal sepsis as infection of the genital tract occurring at any time between the onset of the rupture of membranes or labour and the 42nd day postpartum in which fever and one or more of the following are present: pelvic pain, abnormal vaginal discharge, abnormal odour of discharge, and delay in the rate of reduction of size of the uterus[16]. It is estimated that puerperal sepsis causes at least 75,000 maternal deaths every year, mostly in low-income countries[17]. Studies from high-income countries report incidence of maternal morbidity due to sepsis of 0.1-0.6 per 1000 deliveries[17].

3.2 Are pregnant women more prone to infections and sepsis?

The concept that pregnancy is associated with immune suppression has created a myth of pregnancy as a state of immunological weakness and therefore, of increased susceptibility to infectious disease. Pregnancy represents the most important period for the conservation of the species, thus, it is fundamental to strengthen all the means to protect the mother and the fetus. The maternal immune system is characterized by a reinforced network of recognition, communication, trafficking and repair, in order to maintain the well-being of the mother and the fetus[18]. The fetus provides a developing active immune system that will modify the way the mother responds to antigens[18]. Therefore, it is appropriate to refer to pregnancy as a unique immune condition that is modulated but not suppressed[19].
Pregnancy has three distinct immunological phases that are characterized by distinct biological processes[20,21]. The first stage of implantation is a pro-inflammatory condition that the blastocyst has to invade the endometrial tissue in order to implant; the endometrium has to be replaced by trophoblast and new vessels in order to secure an adequate placental-fetal blood supply[22]. The placentation phase of pregnancy characterized by an anti-inflammatory state, where, the mother, the placenta, and the fetus are symbiotic[18]. Finally, during the last immunological phase, the mother needs to deliver the baby, and this can only be achieved through renewed inflammation. Parturition is characterized by an influx of immune cells

† CPT Current Procedural Terminology

into the myometrium in order to promote recrudescense of an inflammatory process[23,24]. A recent longitudinal study during uncomplicated pregnancies revealed a general trend toward enhanced counter-regulatory cytokine expression (IL-10), and an overall decrease of pro-inflammatory (Th1; TNFa, IL-1β, and IL-6) cytokines expression[25]. Pregnancy itself does not impair the woman's immunological system and other risk factors have to be implemented to develop infections in pregnant women.

3.3 Risk factors and routes of infection in pregnancy

Sepsis during pregnancy usually is the result of invasion of the uterine cavity with bacterial pathogens. Although transplacental spread of infection can occur in women with bacteremia that doesn't correlate with pregnancy, the most common route is an ascending infection from bacteria colonize the vagina and/or the cervix[15]. Pelvic infections in pregnant women have their microbiologic origin in one of three sources: the endogenous vaginal microflora, the intestinal microflora, and sexual transmission[26]. The infection occurs via migration of the organisms from the vagina through the endocervix into the uterus. Some organisms may traverse the columnar epithelium, as is the case with infection caused by Neisseria gonorrhoeae and Chlamydia trachomatis[26]. Bacteria such as Streptococcus agalactiae may gain entrance to the uterus and fallopian tubes via the lymphatics[26]. A third route of migration is by ascending into the pregnant uterus and colonizing amniotic fluid. Then bacteria are able to reproduce and reach numbers in excess of 10^5 per milliliter of amniotic fluid[27].

Risk factors for the development of maternal sepsis include home birth in unhygienic conditions, low socioeconomic status, poor nutrition, primiparity, anaemia, prolonged rupture of membranes, prolonged labour, multiple vaginal examinations in labour (more than five), caesarean section, multiple pregnancy, artificial reproductive techniques, overweight and obstetrical manoeuvres[14,28].

3.4 Reasons for infection and sepsis during pregnancy

Physiologic changes in the lower genital tract, such as a decreased in pH and increased glycogen in the vaginal epithelium, place the pregnant woman at risk for intra-amniotic infection. Pregnant women, with the enlargement of uterus, especially during the 3rd trimester, may cause stricture or even obstruction of the ureter, predisposing for the development of pyelonephritis. In addition, normal pregnancy is characterized by numerous changes in the hemostatic system, creating the hypercoagulable state which increases the risk of venous thromboembolic event occurrence[29]. An elevated leukocyte count, associated with a slightly increased c-reacting protein, and increased heart rate of 15-20 bpm, may mask early signs and symptoms of infection favouring the dissemination of bacteria into the blood-stream. Conditions that predispose pregnant women to septic shock syndrome can be intra-amniotic infection, septic abortion, septic pelvis thrombophlebitis, postpartum endometritis, pyelonephritis, wound infection, necrotizing fasciitis, appendiceal abscess, cholecystitis and invasive procedures like amniocentesis, chorionic villus sampling, and cervical cerclage placement.

Moreover, septic shock in pregnancy can be due to reasons that don't correlate with pregnancy. Non-obstetric septic shock can be caused by pneumonia and peritonitis with origin in colon, gastro-duodenum, post-duodenal small bowel, biliary tract and appendix. (Table 1)

Obstetrics	Non-obstetrics
Intra-amniotic infections	Pyelonephritis
Chorioamnionitis	Septic pelvic thrombophlebitis
Septic abortion	Abscess of the appendix
Invasive procedures for prenatal diagnosis (amniocentesis, chorionic villous sampling)	Cholecystitis
Cervical cerclage placement	Pneumonia
Post-partum endometritis	Peritonitis (colon, small bowel, gastro-duodenum, biliary tract)
Wound infection	
Necrotizing fasciitis	

Table 1. Conditions that predispose women to sepsis and septic shock syndrome during pregnancy

3.5 Chorioamnionitis and intra-amniotic infection

Intra-amniotic infections before 1970 was a major cause of maternal mortality because of patient delays in seeking treatment, unavailability of intensive care, and the absence of broad spectrum antibiotics[30]. Nowadays, the association of intraamniotic infections with septic shock, coagulopathy, and adult respiratory syndrome (ARDS) is rare, accounting for less than 1% in cases of intraamniotic infections[30,31].

It is important to note that intraamniotic infections in pregnancy usually are polymicrobial in nature. The most common route is an ascending infection from one or more of the endogenous flora of the cervix or vagina. The most frequent causative pathogens are Aerobic Bacteria (group B *β-hemolitic Streptoccocus, Enteroccocus*, other *Streptoccocus* species, *Escherichia coli, Hemophilus Influenzae, Pseudomonas species, Staphylococcus aureus, Klebsiella-Enterobacter* species, *Proteus* species), Anaerobic Bacteria (*Peptococcus* species, *Peptostreptococcus* species, *Clostridium* species, *Bacteroides* species, *Fusobacterium* species) and other (*Gardnerella vaginalis, Mycoplasme Hominis, Ureaplasma Ureulyticum, Chlamydia Trachomatis*) (Table 2). It is important to note when group B β-Streptococcus or Escherichia coli are the causative pathogens, the incidence of bacteremia is higher (18% and 15%, respectively)[30].

As a consequence of intraamniotic infection is the spontaneous rupture of membranes by weakening the membranes, either by a direct effect of microorganisms on the membranes or indirectly by activation of the host defense mechanisms. However, there is not an absolute and exclusive correlation between intra-amniotic infection and spontaneous rupture of membranes. Rupture of membranes predispose but not secure the development of intra-amniotic infection. This is especially true, after the administration of broad spectrum antibiotics.

An estimated 5-10% of women with intraamniotic infections have bacteremia[30]. Almost half of the patients with bacteremia will demonstrate signs and symptoms of sepsis[32]. Approximately 40% of patients with sepsis have the condition progress to septic shock[33]. Progression from intraamniotic infections to bacteremia, sepsis, and septic shock can occur in a few days or several hours. Typical clinical manifestations of septic shock appeared additionally to the signs of intraamniotic infections and include altered mental status, peripheral vasodilation, tachypnea, tachycardia, temperature instability, hypotension, increased cardiac output, and decreased peripheral resistance[31,34]. If the condition is not promptly identified and aggressively treated, progressive symptoms of peripheral vasoconstriction, oliguria, cyanosis, ARDS, disseminated intravascular coagulation, decreased cardiac output, and decreased peripheral resistance may occur[34].

Aerobic bacteria	
	Group B β-hemolytic Streptococcus
	Streptococcus species
	Enterococcus
	Escherichia coli
	Haemophilus influenza
	Staphylococcus aureus
	Pseudomonas species
	Klebsiella species
	Proteus species
	Enterobacter species
Anaerobic bacteria	
	Peptococcus species
	Peptostreptococcus species
	Clostridium species
	Bacteroides species
	Fusobacterium species
Other	
	Gardnerella vaginalis
	Mycoplasma Hominis
	Ureaplasma urealyticum
	Chlamydia trachomatis

Table 2. Common causative pathogens of ascending infection in pregnant women.

Chorioamnionitis is an acute inflammation of the membranes and chorion of the placenta. Typically is the result of ascending polymicrobial bacterial infection in the setting of membrane rupture. It can also occurs with intact membranes after infection with *Ureaplasma* species and *Mycoplasma hominis*, found in the lower genital tract[35]. Only rarely is hematogenous spread implicated in chorioamnionitis, as occurs with *Listeria monocytogenes*[36].Overall, 1-4% of all births in the U.S.A. are complicated by chorioamnionitis[36]; however, the frequency varies markedly by diagnostic criteria, specific risk factors, and gestational age[37,38]. The key clinical findings include fever, uterine fundal tenderness, maternal tachycardia (>100/min), fetal tachycardia (>160/min), and purulent or foul amniotic fluid[36,39]. The most common organisms isolated in up to 47% and 30% respectively, in cases of culture confirmed chorioamnionitis are *Ureaplasma urealyticum* and *Mycoplasma hominis*[40,41].

Chrorioamnionitis leads to a 2 to 3-fold increased risk for caesarean delivery and to 2 to 4-fold increase in endomyometritis, would infection, pelvic abscess, bacteremia, and post-partum hemorrhage[42-44]. Women with chorioamnionitis in 10% have positive blood cultures (bacteremia)[36]. Fortunately, septic shock, disseminated intravascular coagulation, adult respiratory distress syndrome, and maternal death are only rarely encountered[44,45]. In contrast, fetal exposure to infection may lead to fetal death, neonatal sepsis, and septic shock. In one study, neonatal pneumonia, sepsis, and perinatal death occurred respectively,

in 4%, 8%, and 2% of term deliveries associated with chorioamnionitis[46]. The frequency of neonatal sepsis is reduced by 80% with intrapartum antibiotic treatment[47].
Prompt initiation of antibiotic therapy is essential to prevent both maternal and fetal complications in the setting of clinical chorioamnionitis[44]. Time-to-delivery after institution of antibiotic therapy has been shown to not affect morbidities; therefore caesarean section to expedite delivery is not indicated for chorioamnionitis unless there are other obstetric indications[44,48].

3.6 Does the mode of delivery affect the incidence of sepsis and septic shock?

Nowadays, rates of caesarean section (CS) are progressively increasing in many parts of the world. There has been an increasing tendency for pregnant women without justifiable medical indications for CS to ask for this procedure. Despite the World Health Organization's estimate that CS rates should not be >15%, in the developed world, CS rates are already above 30%[49,50]. Following CS, maternal mortality and morbidity may result from a number of infections including endometritis, urinary tract infection and surgical site infection, which if deep rather than superficial, increase hospital stay and cost per case[51-53]. The most common infection-related complication following CS is endometritis[53]. A major risk factor for post-CS infection is emergency CS (compared with elective).
The rate of infection following CS is 1.1-25% compared with 0.2–5.5% following vaginal birth[54-56]. In antepartum patients the most common infection is asymptomatic bacteriuria with an incidence estimated at 4-7%. However, with the use of prophylactic antibiotic treatment is extremely rare these infections to become sepsis and septic shock, regardless of the mode of delivery. Recent evidence suggests that pre-incision broad spectrum antibiotics are more effective in preventing post-CS infections than post-clamping of the cord narrow-range antibiotics, without prejudice to neonatal infectious morbidity[57]. Prophylactic antibiotics can reduce the incidence of endometritis following CS by two thirds to three quarters[53].
Data from Europe for the years 2003–2004 showed a range of maternal mortality ratio from 2/100,000 live births in Sweden, to 29.6/100,000 in Estonia[58]. Direct maternal mortality associated with CS was about 0.06‰[59]. However, very few women are dying from primary infection and sepsis. Haemorrhage is the main cause of death following by thromboembolism and preeclampsia. Even though the majority of women are dying during puerperium (60%), the infection mostly started during pregnancy or delivery and only in rare cases after delivery and subsequently was not correlated with the mode of delivery. Collectively, we can suggest that CS affects the incidence of infection and hospitalization of women but is not correlated with severe sepsis and septic shock.

3.7 Amniocentesis, chorionic villous sampling (CVS): Routine procedures but invasive?

Although amniocentesis and CVS are routine procedures in prenatal diagnosis and are nowadays performed in most clinics under continuous ultrasonographic vision and aseptic conditions, they are invasive procedures carrying potential risks of serious complications for both the mother and the fetus. Intrauterine infection is a rare event after invasive prenatal diagnostic procedures[60]. According to data from large studies, the incidence of chorioamnionitis is 5 per 1,000 cases after CVS; 3.7 per 1,000 cases after amniocentesis; and 8.8 per 1000 cases after cordocentesis, compared with 3 per 1,000 cases in non-exposed women[61,62]. Infection is usually mild to moderate. There are, however, sporadic reports in the literature describing cases of post-procedure sepsis with devastating results60. Deterioration to septic shock may develop in 0.03% to 0.19% of intra-amniotic infection cases[63].

Contamination of the uterine cavity after amniocentesis or CVS may occur through ascending infection, direct inoculation of intestinal germs, and rarely, after use of deficiently sterilized equipment and direct spread of the infection from the vagina to the blood stream, by-passing the uterus[64]. Direct inoculation of vaginal or cervical pathogens into the uterine cavity may underlie the development of sepsis after trans-cervical CVS[65-67]. The reported rate of transient post-procedure bacteremia is 4.1% for transcervical CVS and nearly zero for transabdominal procedure[64,68]. Inoculation of intestinal germs has been implicated in cases of sepsis after transabdominal procedures. In such cases, peritoneal signs are expected to predominate[69].

Incubation time is usually short, and the onset of symptoms is usually manifested within 24 hours after the procedure. The onset can be insidious, but the clinical and laboratory indicators deteriorate quickly, and the progress can be fulminant[60]. *Clostridium perfrigens,* together with *Escherihia coli,* are the most common pathogens encountered in cases of sepsis after prenatal diagnosis and they are associated with severe and serious complications. Other pathogens isolated from endometrial remnants or blood cultures after amniocentesis or CVS include *Klebsiella pneumoniae, Enterobacter, Staphylococcus aureus, Serratia rubidaea, Citrobacter, Clostridium welchii, group B β-hemolytic streptococcus,* and *Candida albicans* (Table 3).

Administration of prophylactic antibiosis is not recommended since most retrospective studies failed to prove a direct association between needle insertion and maternal or fetal complications[70-72]. Prospective, double-blind studies in this topic are lacking. In cases of sepsis, evacuation of the uterine cavity and suction curettage can be performed. In severe cases prompt hysterectomy with the dead fetus in situ may be advisable if there is evidence of sepsis with hemolysis, multiple organ failure and rapid progress of infection. However, the decision to perform hysterectomy is difficult, especially in a case of a young nulliparous woman or a woman with an affected child and should be performed only in cases where woman's life is at risk. Although very rare, potentially fatal sepsis can occur after invasive prenatal diagnostic procedures. Sepsis can begin with very subtle clinical signs and symptoms, but quickly develop complications, which can become irreversible if intervention is delayed.

3.8 Septic abortion

Septic abortion, an abortion related with infection and complicated by fever, endometritis, and parametritis, remains one of the most serious threats to the health of women throughout the world[85]. More than 95% of the septic abortion and septic shock cases are synonymous with illegal, criminal or non-medical abortions[86]. The most important effect of the legalization of abortion on public health in the U.S.A. was the almost elimination of deaths due to infection from illegal abortion[87,88]. The mortality rate after septic abortion has been decreased dramatically after the introduction of broad spectrum antibiotics. In the U.S.A., is 0.4 cases per 100,000 legal abortions, whereas, in Europe is 1 case per 100,000 legal abortions[89,90]. Abortion remains a primary cause of maternal death in Third World countries. W.H.O. estimates that 25-50% of the 500,000 maternal deaths that occurs every year result from illegal abortion[91]. Abortion-related deaths result primarily from sepsis[92].

Author	Procedure	Management	Complications	Outcome	Culture
Wurster et al.[63]	Amniocentesis	Hysterectomy	NA	Recovery	*C. welchii*
Fray et al.[73]	Amniocentesis	Hysterectomy	NA	Recovery	*Clostridium+S. rubidaea+Citrobacter*
Muggah et al.[74]	CVS	Hysterectomy	DIC-ARDS	Recovery	*E. coli*
Hovav et al.[75]	Amniocentesis	D&C	ARDS-ARF	Recovery	*C. perfrigens+E.coli*
Ayadi et al.[76]	Amniocentesis	D&C	DIC-ARDS-cardiac arrest	Deceased	*C. perfrigens+E.coli*
Thabet et al.[77]	Amniocentesis	Expulsion	DIC-MOF	Recovery	*Klebsiella+Enterobacter*
Winer et al. (2 cases)[78]	Amniocentesis	Induction of abortion	DIC-cardiorespiratory arrest	Recovery	*E.coli*
Lau Tze Kin et al.[79]	Amniocentesis	Abortion+antibiotic	DIC-hypoxemia	Recovery	*E. coli*
Paz et al.[80]	CVS	Antibiotic	-		*Candida albicans*
Hamanishi et al.[69]	Amniocentesis	Abortion+hysterectomy	DIC-MOF	Recovery	*E.coli*
Li Kim Mui et al.[81]	Cordocentesis	Abortion	-	Recovery	*C. perfrigens+S. aureus*
Plachouras et al.[60]	Amniocentesis+ Cordocentesis	Hysterectomy	DIC-MOF	Recovery	*C. perfrigens*
Oron et al.[64]	CVS	Antibiotic	-	Recovery	*Group B β-hemolytic Streptococcus*
Kye Hun Kim et al.[82]	Amniocentesis	Conservative	DIC-AMI	Recovery	*E.coli*
Thorp et al.[83]	Amniocentesis	Conservative	DIC	Deceased	*E.coli*
Elchalal et al. (2 cases)[84]	Amniocentesis	Antibiotic+D&C	DIC-MOF	Deceased	*E.coli*

NA: not available; CVS: chorionic villous sampling; DIC: disseminated intravascular coagulation; ARDS: adult respiratory distress syndrome; D&C: dilation and curettage; ARF: acute renal failure; MOF: multiple organ failure; AMI: acute myocardial infarction

Table 3. Case report of sepsis after invasive prenatal diagnosis

The risk of sepsis from abortion rises from the first trimester of pregnancy to the second[89]. In the first trimester, abortion is readily performed by vacuum curettage, usually in an outpatient setting. Incomplete abortions produced by incompetent physicians represent another risk factor. Insertion of rigid foreign objects into the uterus or cervix increases the risk of perforation and infection[93]. Intrauterine instillation of soap solution containing cresol and phenol has been abandoned, due to the risk of uterine necrosis, renal failure, toxicity to the central nervous system, cardiac depression, and respiratory arrest[94].

The bacteria associated with septic abortion are usually polymicrobial, derived from the normal flora of the vagina and endocervix, with the important addition of sexually transmitted pathogens[95,96]. Septic shock complicates approximately 0.7% of septic abortions and the offending organisms are Gram-negative bacteria (*Escherichia coli, Aerobacter aerogenes, Proteus mirabilis* or *vulgaris* and *Pseudomonas aeruginosa*) which produce an endotoxin[86]. However, Gram-positive bacteria (*Clostridium welchii or perfrigens, Neisseria gonorrhoae, Staphylococcus epidermisis, Streptococcus agalactiae*), anaerobic bacteria and

Chlamydia trachomatis are all possible pathogens[86, 97]. Because of the variety of bacterial agents that can be associated with septic abortion, no-one antibiotic agent is ideal. The regimens recommended for outpatient management of pelvic inflammatory disease (PID) are appropriate for early post-abortion infection limited to the uterine cavity[95].

The diagnosis of septic abortion must be considered when any woman of reproductive age presents with vaginal bleeding, lower abdominal pain, and fever. If the woman has had symptoms for several days, a generalized, serious illness may be present. Bacteremia, which is more common with septic abortion than with other pelvic infection, may result in septic shock and the adult respiratory distress syndrome[98]. Management of severe sepsis requires eradication of the infection and supportive care for the cardiovascular system and other involved organ systems. Any tissue remaining from the pregnancy must be evacuated without delay as soon as antibiotic therapy and fluid resuscitation have been started. In critically ill women with severe sepsis, a hysterectomy will probably be needed. Other indications of laparotomy are uterine perforation with a suspected bowel injury, a pelvic abscess, and clostridial myometritis[98].

Cervical dilation with laminaria placement has been also associated rarely, with septic abortion and septic shock[99]. Laminarias are sea plant with hydroscopic properties that enable their expansion up to five times in diameter over 12-24 hours, thereby gradually dilating the cervix. The potential of laminarias to harbor pathogens led some investigators to speculate that colonization of laminaria tents may lead to post-abortion infection. However, with modern sterilization techniques, the associated infection rates are similar to those achieved with standard methods for cervical dilation[99].

Nowadays, medical termination of pregnancy using mifepristone and/or misoprostol doesn't require admission to the hospital or anesthesia and is alternative to surgical termination[100]. The incidence of uterine infection after medical termination of pregnancy is very low. However, severe and fatal infections have been reported in certain cases; most of them were associated with *Clostridium* infections and development of toxic shock syndrome[101-103]. Klebsiella pneumoniae has also been reported as the cause of septic shock after medical termination of pregnancy with misoprostol-only regimen[100]. Although a direct association of these drugs and septic shock has established, it was postulated that mifepristone blocks both progesterone and glucocorticoid receptors and affects the innate immune system[104]. However, most of these severe and occasionally fatal complications are the result from inappropriate usage of drugs without any medical monitoring and consultation.

3.9 Non-obstetric causes of septic shock

Septic shock in the pregnant woman usually results from an infection in the urinary or genital tract. Pyelonephritis is the most frequent cause of bacterial shock associated with pregnancy[105]. Enlargement of the uterus during the 2nd and 3rd trimester of pregnancy may cause stricture and/or obstruction of the ureters, a condition that predisposes to urinary infections and pyelonephritis. Escherichia coli is responsible for most of the cases. *Klebsiella pneumoniae, Proteus species*, and *Enterobacter-Citrobacter* are less common pathogens.

All pregnant women should be screened for the presence of bacteriuria at their first prenatal visit. Failure to treat bacteriuria during pregnancy may result in as many as 25% of women experiencing acute pyelonephritis106. Acute pyelonephritis has an incidence of approximately 0.1-1% in pregnancy; most occurs at second trimester107. It is associated with multiple complications, including fetal growth restriction, preterm labour, cerebral palsy and septicemia, although the underlying mechanisms are poorly understood[108]. One mechanism could be the alteration in the profile of angiogenic and anti-angiogenic factors (increased expression of vascular endothelial growth factor [VEGF], decreased expression of PIGF and sVEGFR-2) observed in cases with acute pyelonephritis that resembles the one observed in sepsis[109]. In most reports of acute pyelonephritis the incidence of bacteremia is not stated. However, 20% of women with severe pyelonephritis will develop complications that include septic shock syndrome or its presumed variants[110]. These latter include renal dysfunction, hemolysis and thrombocytopenia, and pulmonary capillary injury. In another series of 55,621 pregnant women with acute pyelonephritis, the incidence of septic shock in pregnancy was 3.77%[111]. The first fatal case of gestational interstitial tubulonephritis and chronic pyelitis caused by *Escherichia coli* has been recently described [112]. In the great majority of cases, continued fluid and antimicrobial therapy result in a salutary outcome, but there is still an occasional maternal morbidity.

Post-partum endometritis (PE) can also result to septic shock. Patients with PE may show a delayed response to antibiotic treatment because of the development of septic pelvic vein thrombosis26. In these cases heparin should be administered. Patients who do not respond to antibiotics and heparin should be considered to have thrombosis of the vasculature of the uterus or an abscess26. Decreased perfusion of the myometrium does not permit adequate antibiotic levels to be established in the myometrium and uterine necrosis could be observed. In such occasions, hysterectomy should be performed.

Various other conditions have been reported to predispose the pregnant woman to sepsis and septic shock including pelvic abscess, wound infection, necrotizing fasciitis, appendiceal abscess, acute cholecystitis, septic pelvic vein thrombosis, pneumonia, pancreatitis, and lupus.

4. Septic shock in gynecologic patients

In Gynecology, incidence of sepsis have been increased during the last 15 years, presumably due to an aging population, an increase in the number of invasive procedures performed, and possibly due to a resistance to the current antibiotic treatment appeared in the infecting pathogens. Sepsis-related situations in Gynecology can be found, in women using intra uterine devices (IUD), after untreated pelvic inflammatory disease (PID), after toxic shock syndrome provoked mainly by the use of tampons during menstrual period, and in patients with gynecological cancer. The above causes will be discussed explicitly, thereafter.

4.1 Toxic shock syndrome

Toxic shock syndrome (TSS), is a rare, life-threatening, multiorgan illness that is caused by toxins that circulate in the bloodstream. Development of TSS involves three distinct stages: local proliferation of toxin-producing bacteria at the site of infection, production of toxin, and exposure of this toxin to the immune system with resultant immune response[113,114].

Toxic shock syndrome was initially identified as a pediatric infection in 1978[115]. Subsequent reports identified an association with tampon use by menstruating women.[116-118]. Menstrual TSS is more likely in women using highly absorbent tampons, using tampons for more days of their cycle, and keeping a single tampon in place for a longer period of time. Over the past two decades, the number of cases of menstrual TSS (1 case per 100,000) has steadily declined; this is thought to be due to the withdrawal of highly absorbent tampons from the market[116].

In the most typical form of toxic shock syndrome, the bacteria, most commonly, group A *Streptococcus, Staphylococcus aureus* and *Clostridium sordellii* produce an enterotoxin that transfers into the bloodstream, provoking the overstimulation of the immune system. This, in turn, causes the severe symptoms of TSS, such as: fever, rash, myalgias, diarrhea, vomiting, headache, sore throat, vaginal discharge, rigors, desquamation (typically of the palms and soles), hypotension, and multi-organ failure (involving at least 3 or more organ systems[116,119,120]. The mortality rate of toxic shock syndrome is approximately 5-15%, and recurrences have been reported in as many as 30-40% of cases[121,122].

The role of tampons in the pathogenesis of TSS is incompletely understood. Although tampons are not a source for toxigenic *S.aureus* and do not appear to increase the *S. aureus* cell density vaginally, studies have shown that tampons used during menstruation often colonized with this pathogen[123,124]. Vaginal conditions during menses and tampon use, contribute to the proliferation of toxin-producing *S.aureus*. An elevated vaginal temperature and neutral pH, both of which occur during menses are enhanced by tampon use, allowing bacterial proliferation[125]. Endometrial blood can serve as a medium for bacterial growth; persistence of this blood in the cervical and vaginal canal with tampon use has been also shown to increase the proliferation of *S.aureus*[126]. In addition, synthetic fibers are thought to alter the availability of certain substrates to lactobacilli, a normal vaginal colonist that limits the proliferation of *S.aureus*. The same conditions also aid in the production of TSS Toxin-1. Menses and tampon use increase the partial pressure of both oxygen and carbon dioxide, which also stimulate toxin production[127]. In addition, tampons obstruct the flow of endometrial blood and may even cause the reflux of blood and bacteria into the uterus.

Toxic shock syndrome is the typical example of a systemic inflammatory response syndrome, with virtually all of the effects derived from immune mediators rather than as a direct result of infection. The diagnosis of TSS should be considered in a patient who presents with septic shock but without any obvious source of infection. The case fatality rates for menstrual-related STSS have declined from 5.5% in 1980 to 1.8% in 1996[121,122]. Organ supportive therapy remains the standard of care with antibiotics used to prevent recurrence, although newer immune-based therapies are being developed that may help in the treatment of TSS and other inflammatory syndromes in the future.

4.2 Pelvic inflammatory disease (PID)

Pelvic inflammatory disease (PID) refers to acute infection of the upper genital tract structures in women, involving any or all of the cervix, uterus, fallopian tubes, ovaries and surrounding structures. By definition, PID is a community-acquired infection, initiated by a sexually transmitted agent, distinguishing it from pelvic infections due to medical procedures, pregnancy and other primary abdominal processes. Pelvic inflammatory disease in the United States annually accounts for about 2,5 million outpatient visits, 200,000 hospitalizations and 100,000 surgical procedures[128]. It is the most frequent gynecologic cause for emergency department visits (350,000/year)[128,129].

PID is most frequently caused by bacteria that are transmitted through sexual contact and other bodily secretions. Bacteria that cause gonorrhea and additionally the *Chlamydia trachomatis* cause more than half of cases. Many studies suggest that a number of patients with PID and other sexually transmitted diseases are often infected with two or more infectious agents and commonly these are *Chlamydia trachomatis, Neisseria gonorrhoeae* and *Mycoplasma genitalium*[130]. Sexually active adolescent females and women younger than 25 years are at greatest risk, although PID can occur at any age. Abdominal pain (usually lower) or tenderness, fever, nausea, vomiting, back pain, unusual or heavy vaginal discharge, abdominal uterine bleeding, painful urination, painful sexual intercourse are some of the symptoms of PID[131].

The vaginal flora of most normal, healthy women includes a variety of potentially pathogenic bacteria[132]. Among these are species of streptococci, staphylococci, Enterobacteriaceae (most commonly, *Klebsiella* spp, *Escherichia coli*, and *Proteus* spp), and a variety of anaerobes. Compared with the dominant hydrogen peroxide-producing Lactobacillus, these organisms are present in low numbers, and ebb and flow under the influence of hormonal changes, contraceptive method, sexual activity, and other as yet unknown forces. Complete disruption of the vaginal ecosystem can occur, in which anaerobic bacteria assume predominance over the desirable strains of lactobacilli[133]. Then an ascending infection occurs causing: cervicitis, endometritis, salpingitis or hydro-, pyo-salpinx. In tubes and ovaries, salpingo-oophoritis (acute, subacute and chronic) or a tubo-ovarian abscess may also occur. In the peritoneal cavity spreading of the infection causes pelvic and/or generalized peritonitis or a pelvic abscess. Infection may be also spread through the uterine wall into broad ligaments to cause pelvic cellulitis (parametritis), a broad ligament abscess or septic thrombophlebitis of the ovarian or uterine veins, leading to septicemia with few local signs[134].

Bacteremia is an unusual condition and is not correlated with PID. Blood cultures for women hospitalized with acute PID showed negative results in 97% of the cases[135]. The results of blood culture are not affect the clinical management of PID and routine specimens may not be needed from patients hospitalized for acute PID[135]. However, if diagnosis and treatment are not performed in a timely manner, PID may cause sepsis, septic shock and even death. Even if they survive, as many as 15% to 20% of these women experience long-term sequelae of PID, such as ectopic pregnancy, tubo-ovarian abscess, infertility, dyspareunia and chronic pelvic pain. The best treatments for PID are interventions that lead to prevention and early detection[136].

4.3 Intrauterine devices (IUD)

Intrauterine contraceptive devices (IUDs) are highly effective, long-term methods of contraception. It is also one of the most cost-effective method available, providing long-term protection[137]. Most modern IUDs are medicated; they contain either copper or a progestin to enhance the contraceptive action of the device. The total number of current IUD users is estimated at over 150 million women worldwide[138]. Infection risk is a relative contraindication to fitting any woman with an IUD, it is only present for a few weeks after insertion and probably arises from an undiagnosed cervical infection at the time of insertion. Although evidence of a direct association between IUD use and PID is scarce, concerns about PID related to IUDs use has limited their use throughout the world. On the other hand, bacteriologic cultures of removed IUDs have shown that the bacterial flora of the removed IUDs consisted of common aerobic and anaerobic microorganisms that do not account for PID[139]. In a study with 200 subjects, the most common bacteria identified from removed IUDs were *Staphylococcus* coagulase negative, *Esherichia coli*, and *Enterococcus faecalis*[139]. The authors concluded that culture of the removed IUDs and therapeutic management of women with positive cultures are not recommended when women are asymptomatic for PID[139]. A systematic review reported the risks of PID with insertion of an

IUD in the presence of existing infection. With IUD insertion in the presence of Chlamydia infection or gonorrhoea, subsequent PID rates were 0-5%, compared to insertion in the absence of infection (0-2%)[140]. Although trial results do not indicate the need to screen for and treat sexually transmitted diseases before inserting and IUD[141], it is rationale to suggest that the insertion of an IUD is indicated only in women with negative vaginal cultures (Table 4)[142].

NOT contraindicated	Contraindicated
Increased risk of STI or HIV	Current PID
Continuation after STI diagnosed	Current purulent cervicitis
Past PID	Chlamydial infection
Past ectopic pregnancy	Gonorrheal infection
HIV or AIDS	Pelvic tuberculosis
Diabetes	Puerperal sepsis
Menorrhagia	Septic abortion
Fibroids	
Age<20	

STI: sexually transmitted infection; PID: pelvic inflammatory disease

Table 4. Conditions in which intrauterine contraception is and is NOT contraindicated (WHO, 2004)

In cases of vaginal infection, it is possible that the insertion of an IUD carries bacteria into the uterus and traumatizing the endometrium causes several infections. Cases of vaginitis[143], transfer of actinomyces into the uterine cavity[144], PID[145], and even toxic shock syndrome[146], and sepsis[147], have occasionally been reported. Three cases of streptococcal toxic shock syndrome following insertion of an IUD have been reported, recently[146,148,149]. This pathogen is not normally found in the vaginal flora or after an intrauterine device is inserted[150]. However, an association between the use of IUD and the risk for infection and sepsis does not exist. Conditions which represent an unacceptable health risk if an IUD is inserted are: current PID, current purulent cervicitis, chlamydial or gonorrheal infection, as well as, pelvic tuberculosis, puerperal sepsis, and septic abortion (Table 4)[151].

4.4 Gynecologic cancer

Sepsis and septic shock are not directly associated with gynecologic cancer. The female cancer patient is a vulnerable patient. Usually after having undergone a difficult operation, followed up by several chemotherapy cycles, has reduced defenses against infection due to: a) reduced antibody formation; b) deficient cell immunity; c) reduced or abnormal granulocytes; d) damaged mucocutaneous barriers, such as, ulceration of the oropharynx due to methotrexate toxicity; e) obstruction of biliary and urinary tracts. Thus, myelosuppression may also give rise to an acute septic problem associated with neutropenia, granulocytopenia. In these patients, any infection may have an acute form leading to rapid septicemia and severe shock developing rapidly.
The frequency of patients with gynecologic cancer and septic shock is not seen very often. In a recent study, the mortality rate was 33% (of 6 reported cases, 2 died)[152]. Sepsis can occur independently of the optimal management of cancer. Among 74 women with gynecologic cancer, there was one death due to the development of septic shock in a patient with

optimal cytoreductive operation[153]. Toxic shock syndrome has been developed in a patient with a metastatic cervical cancer[154]. In advanced operations (pelvic exenterosis) where a colostomy has been performed, there is also a possibility of sepsis due to spillage of stool upon maturing the colostomy[155]. When operations for gynecologic cancer involve the intestine there is increased possibility for sepsis. In a series of 113 patients three died due to sepsis post-operatively[156]. Early diagnosis, careful monitoring, prompt removal of septic foci, and appropriate antibiotic and supportive treatment are the most important factors influencing prognosis in these patients.

5. Conclusion

Sepsis and septic shock are not specifically correlated with obstetrics or gynecologic conditions. Risk factors that may predispose an Ob/Gyn patient to infectious agents are essentially the same risk factors that place any patient in harm's way. In Obstetrics, a prior history of peripatum infection, prolonged rupture of membranes, or genitourinary instrumentation associated with cardiovascular instability and fever should raise the possibility of septic shock.

Patients with obstetrics or gynecologic problems are not different in the management of septic shock with other patients that sepsis results from other organs. Management of a patient with septic shock requires simultaneous administration of agents to reverse the pathophysiologic processes set in motion. It is important to treat patients with sepsis early and vigorously. Volume expansion and correction of hypovolemia are critical. Understanding the pathways, mediators, feedback loops and interactions involved in the pathogenesis of sepsis and organ failure has advanced profoundly, giving us the opportunity to treat sepsis-related multiple organ failure, and therefore, improve both survival rates and quality of life of women patients.

6. Acknowledgments

The authors want to thank very much Dr. Antonis Andriotis for his valuable assistance to gather the literature for the current chapter.

7. References

[1] Kumar, Vinay, Abbas, Abul K; Fausto, Nelson, & Mitchell, Richard N (2007). Robbins Basic Pathology (8th ed.). Saunders Elsevier, pp. 102-103 ISBN 978-1-4160-2973-1.

[2] Levinson AT, Casserly BP, Levy MM. Reducing mortality in severe sepsis and septic shock. Semin Respir Crit Care Med 2011; 32: 195-205.

[3] Sheffield JS. Sepsis and septic shock in pregnancy. Crit Care Clin 2004; 20: 651-660.

[4] Sands KE, Bates DW, Lanken PN, Gramam PS, Hibberd PL, Kahn KL, Parsonnet J, Panzer R, Orav EJ, Snydman DR, Black E, Schwartz JS, Moore R, Johnson BL Jr, Platt R; Epidemiology of sepsis syndrome in 8 academic medical centers: Academic Medical Center Consortium Sepsis Project Working Group. JAMA 1997; 278: 234-240.

[5] Martin GS, Mannino DM,Easton S, Moss M. The epidemiology of sepsis in the United States from 1979-2000. N Engl J Med 2003; 348: 1546-1554.

[6] Hotchkiss RS, Karl IE. The pathophysiology and treatment of sepsis. N Engl J Med 2003; 348: 138-150.
[7] Munford RS, Pugin J. The crucial role of systemic responses in the innate (non-adaptive) host defense. J Endotoxin Res 2001; 7:327-232.
[8] Bone RC, Balk RA, Cerra FB, Dellinger RP, Fein AM, Knaus WA, et al. Definitions for sepsis and organ failure and guidelines for the use of innovative therapies in sepsis. Chest 1992; 101: 1644-1655.
[9] American College of Obstetricians and Gynecologists. Septic shock. ACOG technical bulletin no. 204. Washington DC: American College of Obstetricians and Gynecologists, 1995.
[10] Angus DC, Wax RX. Epidemiology of sepsis: an update. Crit Care Med 2001; 29 (Suppl. 7): 109-116.
[11] Center for Disease Control: Increase in national hospital discharge survey rates for septicemia: United States, 1979-1987. MMWR Morb Mortal Wkly Rep 1990; 39: 31-34.
[12] Angus DC, Linde-Zwirble WT, Lidicker J, Clermont G, Carcillo J, Pinsky MR. Epidemiology of severe sepsis in the United States: analysis of incidence, outcome and associated costs of care. Crit Care Med 2001; 29:1303-1310.
[13] Huether SE, & McCance KL. Understanding Pathophysiology (4th ed.), 2008.
[14] Kramer HMC, Schutte JM, Zwart JJ, Schuitemaker NW, Steegers EA, van Roosmalen J. Maternal mortality and severe morbidity from sepsis in the Netherlands. Acta Obstet Gynecol 2009; 88:647–653.
[15] Simpson KR. Sepsis during pregnancy. JOGNN 1995; 24: 550-556.
[16] WHO. Mother-baby package: implementing safe motherhood in countries. Geneva: World Health Organization, 1994. http://www.who.int/reproductive-health/publications/MSM_94_11/mother_baby_package_safe_motherhood.
[17] van Dillen J, Zwart J, Schutte J, van Roosmalen J. Maternal sepsis: epidemiology, etiology and outcome. Curr Opin Infect Dis. 2010; 23: 249-254.
[18] Mor G, Cardenas I, Abrahams V, Guller S. Inflammation and pregnancy: the role of the immune system at the implantation site. Ann NY Acad Sci 2011; 1221: 80-87.
[19] Cardenas I, Means RE, Aldo P, Koga K, Lang SM, Booth C, Manzur A, Oyarzun E, Romero R, Mor G. Viral infection of the placenta leads to fetal inflammation and sensitization to bacterial products predisposing to preterm labor. J Immunol 2010; 185: 1248-1257.
[20] Mor G. Pregnancy reconceived. Nat History 2007; 116: 36-41.
[21] Mor G, Koga K. Macrophages and pregnancy. Reprod Sci 2008; 15: 435-436.
[22] Dekel N, Gnainsky Y, Granot I, Mor G. Inflammation and implantation. Am J Reprod Immunol 2010; 63: 17-21.
[23] Romero R, Espinoza J, Kusanovic JP, Gotsch F, Hassan S, Erez O, Chaiworapongza T, Mazor M. The preterm parturition syndrome. BJOG 2006; 113: 17-42.
[24] Romero R, Espinoza J, Goncalves LF, Kusanovic JP, Friel LA, Nien JK. Inflammation in preterm and term labour and delivery. Semin Fetal Neonat Med 2006; 11: 317-326.
[25] Denney JM, Nelson EL, Wadhwa PD, Waters TP, Mathew L, Chung EK, Goldenberg RL, Culhane JF. Longitudinal modulation of immune system cytokine profile during pregnancy. Cytokine 2011; 53: 170-177.

[26] Faro S. Sepsis in obstetric and gynecologic patients. Curr Clin Topics Infect Disease 1999; 19: 60-82.
[27] Pinell P, Faro S, Roberts S, Le S, Maccato M, Hammill H. Intrauterine pressure catheter in labor: associated microbiology. Infect Dis Obstet Gynecol 1993; 1: 60-64.
[28] Maharaj D. Puerperal pyrexia: a review. Part I. Obstet Gynecol Surv 2007; 62:393–399.
[29] Mitic G, Kovac M, Jurisic D, Djordjevic V, Ilic V, Salatic I, Spacic D, Novakov Mikic A. Clinical characteristics and type of thrombophilia in women with pregnancy-related thromboembolic disease. Gynecol Obstet Invest 2011; (in press).
[30] Newton E. Chorioamnionitis and intraamniotic infection, Clin Obstet Gynecol 1993; 36: 795-808.
[31] Gonik B. Septic shock in obstetrics. In S. Clark, D. Cotton, G Hankins, J. Phelan. Critical care obsterics 1991, (pp.289-306).
[32] Iverson R. Septic shock: a clinical perspective. Critical Care Clinics 1988; 4: 215-228.
[33] Bone R. Sepsis, the sepsis syndrome, multi organ failure: The plea for comparable definitions. Annals of Internal Medicine 1991; 115: 332-333.
[34] Pearlman M, Faro S. Obstetric septic shock. Clinical Obstetrics and Gynecology 1990; 33: 482-492.
[35] Eschenbach DA. Ureaplasma urealiticum and preterm birth. Clin Infect Dis 1993; 17(Suppl. 1): S100-S106.
[36] Gibbs RS, Duff P. Progress in pathogenesis and management of clinical intraamniotic infection. Am J Obstet Gynecol 1991; 164: 1317-1326.
[37] Piper JM, Newton ER, Berkus MD, Peairs WA. Meconium: a marker for peripartum infection. Obstet Gynecol 1998; 91: 741-745.
[38] Tran SH, Caughey AB, Musci TJ. Meconium-stained amniotic fluid is associated with puerperal infections. Am J Obstet Gynecol 2003; 189: 746-750.
[39] Newton ER. Chorioamnionitis and intraamniotic infection. Clin Obstet Gynecol 1993; 36: 795-808.
[40] Sperling RS, Newton E, Gibbs RS. Intraamniotic infection in low-birth-weight infants. J Infect Dis 1988; 157: 113-117.
[41] Waites KB, Katz B, Schelonka RL. Mycoplasmas and ureaplasmas as neonatal pathogens. Clin Microbiol Rev 2005; 18: 757-789.
[42] Mark SP, Croughan-Minihane MS, Kilpatrick SJ. Chorioamnionitis and uterine function. Obstet Gynecol 2000; 95: 909-912.
[43] Satin AJ, Maberry MC, Leveno KJ, Sherman ML. Chorioamnionitis: a harbinger of dystocia. Obstet Gynecol 1992; 79: 913-915.
[44] Tita AT, Andrews WW. Diagnosis and management of clinical chorioamnionitis. Clin Perinatol 2010; 37: 339-354.
[45] Moretti M, Sibai BM. Maternal and perinatal outcome of expectant management of premature rupture of membranes in the midtrimester. Am J Obstet Gynecol 1988; 159: 390-396.
[46] Yoder PR, Gibbs RS, Blanco JD, Castaneda YS. A prospective, controlled study of maternal and perinatal outcome after intra-amniotic infection at term. Am J Obstet Gynecol 1983; 145: 695-701.

[47] Gilstrap LC 3rd, Leveno KJ, Cox SM, Burris JS. Intrapartum treatment of acute chorioamnionitis: impact on neonatal sepsis. Am J Obstet Gynecol 1988; 159: 579-583.
[48] Gilstrap LC 3rd, Cox SM. Acute chorioamnionitis. Obstet Gynecol Clin North Am 1989; 16: 373-379. Althabe F, Belizan JM. Caesarean section: the paradox. Lancet 2006; 368:1472–1473.
[49] Brennan DJ, Robson MS, Murphy M, O'Herlihy C. Comparative analysis of international cesarean delivery rates using 10-group classification identifies significant variation in spontaneous labor. Am J Obstet Gynecol 2009; 201: 308.
[50] Lamont RF, Sobel JD, Kusanovic JP, Vaisbuch E, Mazaki-Tovi S, Kim SK, Uldbjerg N, Romero R. Current debate on the use of antibiotic prophylaxis for caesarean section.BJOG 2011; 118: 193-201.
[51] Vegas AA, Jodra VM, Garcia ML. Nosocomial infection in surgery wards: a controlled study of increased duration of hospital stays and direct cost of hospitalization. Eur J Epidemiol 1993; 9:504–510.
[52] Martone WJ, Jarvis WR, Culver DH, Haley RW. Incidence and nature of endemic and epidemic nosocomial infections. In: Bennett JV, Brachman PS, editors. Hospital Infections. Boston: Little, Brown and Co; 1992. pp. 577–596.
[53] Smaill F, Hofmeyr GJ. Antibiotic prophylaxis for cesarean section. Cochrane Database Syst Rev 2002; (3): CD000933.
[54] Tran TS, Jamulitrat S, Chongsuvivatwong V, Geater A. Risk factors for post-cesarean surgical site infection. Obstet Gynecol 2000; 95: 367–371.
[55] Yokoe DS, Christiansen CL, Johnson R, Sands KE, Livingston J, Shtatland ES, Platt R. Epidemiology of and surveillance for postpartum infections. Emerg Infect Dis 2001; 7: 837–841.
[56] Hebert PR, Reed G, Entman SS, Mitchel EF Jr, Berg C, Griffin MR. Serious maternal morbidity after childbirth: prolonged hospital stays and readmissions. Obstet Gynecol 1999; 94: 942–947.
[57] American Academy of Pediatrics and American College of Obstetricians and Gynecologists. Guidelines for Perinatal Care, 6th edn. Washington DC: American College of Obstetricians and Gynecologists, 2007.
[58] EURO-PERISTAT. European Perinatal Health Report 2008.
[59] Fässler M, Zimmermann R, Quack Lötscher KC. Maternal mortality in Switzerland 1995–2004. Swiss Med Weekly 2010; 140: 25-30.
[60] Plachouras N, Sotiriadis A, Dalkalitsis N, Kontostolis E, Xiropotamos N, Paraskevaidis E. Fulminant sepsis after invasive prenatal diagnosis. Obstet Gynecol 2004; 104: 1244-1247.
[61] Cederholm M, Haglund B, Axelsson O. Maternal complications following amniocentesis and chorionic villous sampling for prenatal karyotyping. BJOG 2003; 110: 392-399.
[62] Tongsong T, Wanapirak C, Kunavikatikul C, Sirirchotiyakul S, Piyamongkol W, Chanprapaph P. Fetal loss rate associated with cordocentesis at midgestation. Am J Obstet Gynecol 2001; 184: 719-723.
[63] Wurster KG, Roemer VM, Decker K, Hirsch HA. Amniotic infection syndrome after amniocentesis-a case report. Geburtshilfe Frauenheilkd 1982; 42: 676-679.

[64] Oron G, Krissi H, Peled Y. A successful pregnancy following transcervical CVS related GBS sepsis. Prenat Diagn 2010; 30: 380-381.
[65] Barela AI, Kleinman GE, Golditch IM, Menke DJ, Hogge WA, Globus MS. Septic shock with renal failure after chorionic villous sampling. Am J Obstet Gynecol 1986; 154: 1100-1102.
[66] Fejgin M, Amiel A, Kaneti H, Ben-Nun I, Beyth Y. Fulminant sepsis due to group B beta-hemolytic streptococci following transcervical chorionic villous sampling. Clin Infect Dis 1993; 17: 142-143.
[67] Paz A, Gonen R, Potasman I. Candida sepsis following transcervical chorionic villous sampling. Infect Dis Obstet Gynecol 2001; 9: 147-148.
[68] Silverman N, Sullivan MW, Jungkind DL, Weinblatt V, Beavis K, Wapner RJ. Incidence of bacteremia associated with chorionic villous sampling. Obstet Gynecol 1994; 84: 1021-1024.
[69] Hamanishi J, Itoh H, Sagawa N, Nakayama T, Yamada S, Nakamura K, Saito A, Kumakura E, Yura S, Fujii S. A case of successful management of maternal septic shock with multiple organ failure following amniocentesis at midgestation. J Obstet Gynaecol Res 2002; 28: 258-261.
[70] Poutamo J, Keski-Nisula L, Kuopio T, Heinonen S. Amniocentesis-a routine procedure, but invasive. Prenat Diagn 2003; 23: 762-770.
[71] Hill JA, Reindollar RH, McDonough PG. Ultrasonic placental localization in relation to spontaneous abortion after mid-trimester amniocentesis. Prenat Diagn 1982; 2: 289-295.
[72] Hanson FW, Zorn EM, Tennant FR, Marianos S, Samuel S. Amniocentesis before 15 weeks' gestation: outcome, risks, and technical problems. Am J Obstet Gynecol 1987; 156: 1524-1531.
[73] Fray RE, Davis TP, Brown EA. Clostridium welchii infection after amniocentesis. BMJ 1984; 288: 901-902.
[74] Muggah HF, D'Alton ME, Hunter AG. Chrionic villous sampling followed by genetic amniocentesis and septic shock. Lancet 1987; 1: 867-868.
[75] Hovav Y, Hornstein E, Pollack RN, Yaffe C. Sepsis due to Clostridium perfrigens after second trimester amniocentesis. Clin Infect Dis 1995; 21: 235-236.
[76] Ayadi S, Carbillon S, Varlet C, Uzan M, Pourriat JL. Fatal sepsis due to Escherichia coli after second-trimester amniocentesis. Fetal Diagn Ther 1998; 13: 98-99.
[77] Thabet NP, Thabet H, Zaghdoudi I, Brahmi N, Chelli H, Amamou M. Septic shock complicating amniocentesis. Gynecol Obstet Fertil 2000; 28: 832-834.
[78] Winer M, David A, Leconte P, Aubron F, Rogez JM, Rival JM, Pinaud M, Roze JC, Boog G. Amniocentesis and amnioinfusion during pregnancy: report of four complicated cases. Eur J Obstet Gynecol Reprod Biol 2001; 100: 108-111.
[79] Kin LT, Ngong LT, Yeung LT, Wah SP, Hung TW. Rare major maternal complications after second trimester amniocentesis: sequelae of avoiding a transplacental approach. Aust N Z Obstet Gynecol 2001; 41: 472-473.
[80] Paz A, Gonen R, Potasman I. Candida sepsis following transcervical chorionic villi sampling. Infect Dis Obstet gynecol 2001; 9: 147-148.
[81] Li Kim Mui SV, Chitrit Y, Boulanger MC, Maisonneuve L, Choudat L, de Bievre P. Sepsis due to Clostridium perfrigens after pregnancy termination with feticide by cordocentesis : a case report. Fetal Diagn Ther 2002; 17: 124-126.

[82] Kim KH, Jeong MH, Chung IJ, Cho JG, Song TB, Park JC, Kang JC. A case of septic shock and disseminated intravascular coagulation complicated by acute myocardial infarction following amniocentesis. Korean J Intern Med 2005; 20: 325-329.
[83] Thorp JA, Helfgott AW, King EA, King AA, Minyard AN. Maternal death after second-trimester genetic amniocentesis. Obstet Gynecol 2005; 105: 1213-1215.
[84] Elchalal U, Shachar IB, Peleg D, Schenker JG. Maternal mortality following 2nd-trimester genetic amniocentesis. Fetal Diagn Ther 2004; 19: 195-198.
[85] Stedman TL. Stedman's medical dictionary. 21st ed. Baltimore: Williams & Wilkins, 1966:4.
[86] Santamarina BA, Smith SA. Septic abortion and septic shock. Clin Obstet Gynecol 1970; 13: 291-304.
[87] Jewett JF. Septic induced abortion. N Engl J Med 1973; 289: 748-749.
[88] Cates W Jr, Rochat RW. Illegal abortions in the United States: 1972-1974. Fam Plann Perspect 1976; 8: 86-92.
[89] Atrash HK, Lawson HW, Smith JC. Legal abortion in the US: trends and mortality. Contemp Ob/Gyn 1990; 35: 58-69.
[90] Henshaw HK. How safe is therapeutic abortion? In: Teoh ES, Ratnam SS, Macnaughton M, eds. Pregnancy termination and labour. Lancaster, United Kingdom: Parthenon, 1993: 31-41.
[91] Mahler H. The save motherhood initiative: a call to action. Lancet 1987; 1: 668-670.
[92] Fauveau V, Koenig MA, Chakraborty J, Chowdhury AI. Causes of maternal mortality in rural Baglandesh, 1976-85. Bull World Health Organ 1988; 66: 643-651.
[93] Polgar S, Fried ES. The bad old days: clandestine abortion among the poor in New York City before liberalization of the abortion law. Fam Plan Perspect 1976; 8: 125-127.
[94] Burnhill MS. Treatment of women who have undergone chemically induced abortion. J Reprod Med 1985; 30: 610-614.
[95] Stubblefield PG, Grimes DA. Septic abortion. New Engl J Med 1994; 331: 310-314.
[96] Burkman RT, Atienza MF, King TM. Culture and treatment results in endometritis following elective abortion. Am J Obstet Gynecol 1977; 128: 556-559.
[97] Faro S, Pearlman M. Infections and abortion. New York: Elsevier, 1992: 41-50.
[98] Postabortion infection and septic shock. In: Sweet RL, Gibbs RS. Infectious diseases of the female genital tract. 2nd ed. Baltimore: Williams & Wilkins 1990: 229-240.
[99] Lin SY, Cheng WF, Su YN, Chen CA, Lee CN. Septic shock after intracervical laminaria insertion. Taiwanese Obstet Gynecol 2006; 45: 76-78.
[100] Kaponis A, Papatheodorou S, Makrydimas G. Septic shock due to Klebsiella pneumoniae after medical abortion with misoprostol-only regimen. Fertil Steril. 2010 Sep;94(4):1529.e3-5.
[101] Fisher M, Bhatnagar J, Guarner J, Reagan S, Hacker JK, Van Meter SH, Poukens V, Whiteman DB, Iton A, Cheung M, Dassey DE, Shieh WH, Zaki SR. Fatal toxic shock syndrome associated with *Clostridium sordelii* after medical abortion. N Engl J Med 2005; 353: 2352-2360.
[102] Cohen AL, Bhatnagar J, Reagan S, Zane SB, D'Angeli MA, Fisher M, Killgore G, Kwan-Gett TS, Blossom DB, Shieh WJ, Guarner J, Jernigan J, Duchin JS, Zaki SR, McDonald LC. Toxic shock associated with *Clostridium sordelii* and *Clostridium*

perfrigens after medical and spontaneous abortion. Obstet Gynecol 2007; 110: 1027-1033.

[103] Sivave C, Le Templier G, Blouin D, Leveille F, Deland E. Toxic shock syndrome due to *Clostridium sordelii*: a dramatic postpartum and postabortion disease. Clin Infec Dis 2002; 35: 1441-1443.

[104] Miech RP. Pathophysiology of mifepristone-induced septic shock due to Clostridium sordelii. Ann Pharmacother 2005; 39: 1483-1488.

[105] Adams RH, Pritchard JA. Bacterial shock in obtetrics and gynecology. Obstet Gynecol 1960; 16: 387-397.

[106] Gilstrap LC 3rd, Ramin SM. Urinary tract infections during pregnancy. Obstet Gynecol Clin North Am 2001; 28: 581-591.

[107] Cunningham FG, Gant NF, Leveno KJ, Gitstrap LC, Hauth JC, Wenstrom KD. Renal and urinary tract disorders. Williams obstetrics, New York: McGraw-Hill; 2001. p. 1251-71.

[108] Nowicki B. Urinary tract infection in pregnant women: old dogmas and current concepts. Curr Infect Dis Rep 2002; 4: 529-535.

[109] Chaiworapongsa T, Roero R, Gotsch F, Kusanovic JP, Mittal P, Kim SK, Erez O, Vaisbuch E, Mazaki-Tovi S, Kim CJ, Dong Z, Yeo L, Hassan SS. Acute pyelonephritis during pregnancy changes the balance of angiogenic and anti-angiogenic factors in maternal plasma. J Matern Fetal Neonatal Med 2010; 23: 167-178.

[110] Cunningham FG, Lucas MJ. Urinary tract infections complicating pregnancy. Bailliers Clin Obstet Gynecol 1994; 8: 353-373.

[111] Pitukkijronnakorn S, Chittacharoen A, Herabutya Y. Maternal and perinatal outcomes in pregnancy with acute pyelonephritis. Int J Gynaecol Obstet. 2005 Jun;89(3):286-7

[112] Sledzinska A, Mielech A, Krawczyk B, Samet A, Nowicki B, Nowicki S, Jankowski Z, Kur J. Fatal sepsis in a pregnant woman with pyelonephritis caused by Escherichia coli bearing Dr and P adhesins: diagnosis based on post-mortem strain genotyping. BJOG 2011; 118: 266-269.

[113] Bennett JV. Toxins and toxic-shock syndrome. J Infect Dis. 1981; 143: 631-632.

[114] Crass BA, Bergdoll MS. Toxin involvement in toxic shock syndrome. J Infect Dis. 1986; 153:918-926.

[115] Todd J, Fishaut M, Kapral F, Welch T. Toxic-shock syndrome associated with phage-Group 1 staphylococci. Lancet. 1978; 2: 1116-1118.

[116] Shands KN, Schmid GP, Dan BB. Toxic-shock syndrome in menstruating women: association with tampon use and Staphylococcus aureus and clinical features in 52 cases. N Engl J Med 1980; 303: 1436-1442.

[117] Davis JP, Chesney PJ, Wand PJ. Toxic-shock syndrome: epidemiologic features, recurrence, risk factors, and prevention. N Engl J Med 1980; 303: 1429-1435.

[118] Ellies E, Vallée F, Mari A, Silva S, Bauriaud R, Fourcade O, Genestal M. [Toxic shock syndrome consecutive to the presence of vaginal tampon for menstruation regressive after early haemodynamic optimization and activated protein C infusion]. Ann Fr Anesth Reanim 2009; 28: 91-95.

[119] Sweet RL. Toxic shock syndrome. In: Sweet RL, Gibbs RS, eds. Infectious diseases of the genital tract. Baltimore. Williams & Wilkins, 1900: 202-215.

[120] Centers for Disease Control. Toxic shock syndrome United States, 1970-1982. MMWR.1982; 31: 201.

[121] Stevens DL. Invasive group A streptococcus infections. Clin Infect Dis 1992; 14: 2-11.

[122] Demers B, Simor AE, Vellend H. Severe invasive group A streptococcal infections in Ontario, Canada: 1987-1991. Clin Infect Dis 1993; 16: 792-800.

[123] Onderdonk AB, Zamarchi GR, Rodriguez ML, Hirsch MI, Munoz A, Kass EH. Quantitative assessment of vaginal microflora during use of tampons of various compositions. Appl.Environ.Microbiol 1987; 53: 2774-2778.

[124] Schlievert PM, Case LC, Strandberg KL, Tripp TJ, Lin YC, Peterson ML. Vaginal Staphylococcus aureus superantigen profile shift from 1980 and 1981 to 2003,2004 and 2005. J.Clin.Microbiol.2007; 45: 2704-2707.

[125] Noble VS, Jacobson JA, Smith CB. The effect of menses and use of catamenial products on cervical carriage of S.aureus. Am J Obstet Gynecol. 1982; 144: 186-189.

[126] Berkley SF, Hightower AW, Broome CV, Reingold AL. The relationship of tampon characteristics to menstrual toxic shock syndrome. JAMA 1987; 258: 917-920.

[127] Wagner G, Bohr L, Wagner P, Petersen LN. Tampon induced changes in vaginal oxygen and carbon dioxide tensions. Am J Obset Gynecol. 1984; 148: 147-150.

[128] Washington AE, Katz P. Cost of and payment source of PID. Trends and projections, 1983 through 2000. JAMA 1991; 226: 2565-2569.

[129] Curtis KM, Hillis SD, Kieke BA Jr, Brett KM, Marchbanks PA, Peterson HB. Visits to emergency departments for gynecologic disorders in the United States, 1992-1994. Obstet Gynecol 1998; 91: 1007-1012.

[130] Ness RB, Soper DE, Richter HE, Randal H, Peipert JF, Nelson DB, Schubeck D, McNeeley SG, Trout W, Bass DC, Hutchison K, Kip K, Brunham RC. Chlamydia antibodies, Chlamydia heat shock protein and adverse sequelse after pelvic inflammatory disease: the PID Evaluation and Clinical Health (PEACH) study. Sex Transm Dis 2008; 35: 129-135.

[131] U.S. Department of Health and Human Services Centers for Disease Control and Prevention. Sexually Transmitted Disease Surveillance, 2006. Atlanta, GA. U.S. Department of Health and Human Services, November 2007. Available at: www.cdc.gov/std/stats/default.htm.

[132] Galask RP, Larsen B, Ohm MJ. Vaginal flora and its role in disease entities. Clin Obstet Gynecol. 1976; 19: 61-81.

[133] Platz-Christensen JJ, Mattsby-Baltzer I, Thomsen P, Wiqvist N. Endotoxin and interleukin-1 alpha in the cervical mucus and vaginal fluid of pregnant women with bacterial vaginosis. Am J Obstet Gynecol. 1993;169(5):1161.

[134] Infection of the female genital tract; pelvic inflammatory disease PID. Primary surgery: Volume One: Non-Trauma, Chapter 4. The surgery of sepsis.

[135] Apuzzio JJ, Hessami S, Rodriguez P. Blood cultures for women hospitalized with acute pelvic inflammatory disease. Are they necessary? J Reprod Med 2001; 46: 815-818.

[136] Dulin JD, Akers MC. Pelvic inflammatory disease and sepsis. Crit Care Nurs Clin North Am. 2003 mar;15(1):63-70.

[137] An extremely low-cost option: IUCD Method Brief No 3. Nairobi: Kenya Ministry of Health 2003.

[138] The ESHRE Capri Workshop Group. Intrauterine devices and intrauterine systems. Hum Reprod Update 2008; 14: 197-208.

[139] Tsanadis G, Kalantaridou SN, Kaponis A, Paraskevaidis E, Zikopoulos K, Gesouli E, Dalkalitsis N, Korkontzelos I, Mouzakioti E, Lolis DE. Bacteriological cultures of removed intrauterine devices and pelvic inflammatory disease. Contraception 2002; 339-342.

[140] Mohllajee AP, Curtis KM, Peterson HB. Does insertion and use of an intrauterine device increase the risk of pelvic inflammatory disease among women with sexually transmitted infections? A systematic review. Contraception 2006; 73: 145-153.

[141] Grimes DA, Lopez LM, Manion C, Schoulz KF. Cochrane systematic reviews of IUD trials: lessons learned. Contraception 2007; 75: S55-S59.

[142] World Health Organization, Reproductive Health and Research. *Medical Eligibility Criteria for Contraceptive* use, 3rd ed. Geneva: World Health Organization, 2004. http://www.who.int/reproductive_health/publications/mec/index.htm.

[143] Shoubnikova M, Hellberg D, Nilsson S, Mardh PA. Contraceptive use in women with bacterial vaginosis. Contraception 1997; 55: 355-358.

[144] Keebler C, Chatwani A, Schwartz R. Actinomycosis infection associated with intrauterine contraceptive devices. Am J Obstet Gynecol 1983; 145: 596-599.

[145] Farley TM, Rosenberg MJ, Rowe PJ, Chen JH, Meirik O.. Intrauterine devices and pelvic inflammatory disease: an international perspective. Lancet 1992; 339: 785-788.

[146] Klug CD, Keay CR, Ginde AA. Fatal toxic shock syndrome from an intrauterine device. Ann Emerg Med 2009; 54: 701-703.

[147] Ledger WJ, Schhrader FJ : Death from septicemia following insertion of an intrauterine device. Obstet. Gynecol 1968; 31: 845-848,

[148] Venkataramanasetty R, Aburawi A, Phillip H. Streptococcal toxic shock syndrome following insertion of an intrauterine device-a case report. Eur J Contracept Reprod Health Care 2009; 14: 379-382.

[149] Ottander U, Backstrom T, Hogberg U, Lofgren M. A case report. Sepsis in connection with levonorgestrel IUD. Lakartidningen 1995; 92: 4555-4557.

[150] Ledger WJ, Headington JJ : Group A β-hemolytic streptococcus. An important cause of serious infections in obstetrics and gynecology. Obstet Gynecol 1972; 39: 474-482.

[151] Martinez F, Lopez-Arrequi E. Infection risk and intrauterine device. Acta Obstet Gynecol Scand 2009; 88: 246-250.

[152] Denis Cavanagh, MD, Robert A. Knuppel, MD, John H. Shepherd, MD, Richard Anderson, MD, and Papineni S. Rao, PhD, Tampa, Fla. Septic shock and the Obstetrician/Gynecologist. Section on Gynecology Southern Medical association, 75th Annual Scientific Assembly, New Orleans, La, Nov 15-18, 1981.

[153] Kuyumcuoglu U, Kale A. Tragic results of suboptimal gynaecologic cancer operations. Eur J Gynaecol Oncol 2008; 29: 620-627.

[154] Rose PG, Wilson G. Advanced cervical carcinoma presenting with toxic shock syndrome. Gynecol Oncol 1994; 52: 264-266.

[155] Hoffman MS, Barton DP, Gates J, Roberts WS, Fiorica JV, Finan MA, Cavanagh D. Complications of colostomy performed on gynaecologic cancer patients. Gynecol Oncol 1992; 44: 231-234.

[156] Barnhill D, Doering D, Remmenga S, Bosscher J, Nash J, Park R. Intestinal surgery performed on gynaecologic cancer patients. Gynecol Oncol 1991; 40: 38-41.

Part 8

Novel and Alternative Therapies

16

Hormonal Therapies in Severe Sepsis

Karen Choong
McMaster University, Hamilton, Ontario
Canada

1. Introduction

Endocrine dysfunction is common in severe sepsis and is associated with increased morbidity and mortality risk. Clinical detection of this heterogenous disorder is challenging, and the accuracy of laboratory diagnosis is complicated by the limitations in methods of hormonal assays and the variable definitions used in its diagnosis. This chapter will review the pathophysiology of neuroendocrine dysfunction during sepsis, the current evidence for hormone supplementation, and the use of hormonal markers and predictors of outcome following severe sepsis. The three hormones that have been most extensively researched and therefore most commonly considered for use in septic shock are corticosteroids, vasopressin, and insulin. We will describe the rationale, explore the controversies and provide recommendations for their use based on the available evidence. We present current recommendations for hormone therapy in adults and children, but caution that further research is needed to better understand the dynamic and complex endocrine responses during septic shock, and to develop improved methods for diagnosis and monitoring of patient response, so that we can determine not only which therapies to use, but how, when, and in which patients.

2. Neuroendocrine dysfunction in severe sepsis

Severe sepsis is characterized by a complex cascade involving widespread inflammation, enhanced coagulation, diminished fibrinolysis, immunomodulation, and release of stress hormones including adrenocorticotropic hormone, cortisol, vasopressin, glucagon and growth hormone[1]. Endocrine dysfunction plays an important role in the pathogenesis of multiple organ dysfunction that occurs in septic shock, and several studies have correlated the degree of neuroendocrine dysfunction with severity of illness[2]. Neuroendocrine dysfunction is common during critically illness, and can affect multiple neurohormonal pathways in an individual patient[3]. The hypothalamic-pituitary-adrenal (HPA) axis is a key coordinator of the stress response, and involves a series of complex central and peripheral adaptations essential for survival. The HPA axis is functionally related to the sympathoadrenal system, which is responsible for endogenous catecholamine secretion and inflammatory cytokine activation, as well as the neurohypophyseal system, which is responsible for vasopressin release; all pivotal integrative components in the stress response. The response of the anterior pituitary during severe sepsis consists of two distinct phases -

an acute phase, which is likely adaptive and beneficial, and a more prolonged or chronic phase characterized by suppression of the neuroendocrine axes resulting in hypoactivity or hyporesponsiveness of target hormones, which may no longer be beneficial[4]. Disruption of these axes, as we will discuss subsequently, compromises the adaptive response, and potentially survival. Differentiation between beneficial and harmful endocrine responses to septic shock is difficult. Nevertheless, the association between endocrine dysfunction and increased morbidity and mortality risk has fueled investigators to examine the role of hormonal therapy during sepsis. There are numerous adult studies in this area, some of which have revealed conflicting results. Pediatric data is much more limited. The results of these studies have arguably sparked more debate than provided definitive conclusions in the current management of sepsis.

3. Hormonal therapies in severe sepsis

3.1 Corticosteroids

The normal response of the HPA axis to the stress of illness results in the release of cortisol from the adrenal cortex[5, 6]. This activation is crucial for the general adaptation to illness and the physiological response of multiple organs. The mechanism for HPA axis dysfunction in severe sepsis are complex and multifactorial, but can result in decreased production of corticotropin-releasing hormone, adrenocorticotropic hormone (ACTH), and cortisol, as well as dysfunction of their receptors even in the presence of "adequate" measured serum hormone levels. Inhibition of hormone production by cytokines and other peptides derived from blood cells (known as corticostatins) may compete with corticotropin and its receptor[7]. Septicemia itself and the medications used in its treatment may result in decreased corticosteroid production and increased metabolism, interfere with receptor signaling, as well as enzymatic and mitochondrial function that are critical in steroidogenesis. Furthermore, hypothalamic, pituitary or adrenal destruction by hemorrhage or ischemia, and the accumulation of nitric oxide, superoxide, or central neuropeptides can contribute to receptor down regulation of HPA hormones in patients with severe sepsis and septic shock[8]. The end-result of this disruption in the HPA axis is a syndrome of adrenal insufficiency.

It has been suggested by the expert panels and consensus from the American College of Critical Care Medicine International Task Force, that the terms absolute or relative adrenal insufficiency be replaced by "critical illness-related corticosteroid insufficiency" (CIRCI)[5]. CIRCI has been defined as inadequate glucocorticoid activity in relation to the severity of the patient's illness and has been most prominently investigated in cases of sepsis and septic shock[9-11]. It is a heterogeneous disorder that can occur as a result of dysfunction at any point in the HPA axis. CIRCI has been recognized in both adult and pediatric patients with severe sepsis, with an incidence as wide ranging from 10% up to 70% depending on the definition used and the study[3, 12-14]. The diagnosis of CIRCI carries with it prognostic implications. These patients are more likely to require vasopressor support, be refractory to fluid and catecholamine therapy, and are more likely to die[15]. There are several proposed definitions for CIRCI, but the most widely accepted definition in adults and pediatrics is an increment in cortisol of less than 9 μg/dL (250 nmol/L), 30-60 minutes after a 1μg ACTH stimulation test[5, 14]. The traditional dose of 250 μg of ACTH is a very large, supraphysiologic adrenal stimulus, and it is suggested that a low dose (1μg) ACTH stimulation is more appropriate and sensitive in distinguishing primary vs. secondary adrenal failure[14, 16]. The diagnosis of CIRCI in severe sepsis is challenging for the following reasons: firstly, there is debate with respect to the ACTH stimulation test itself. While there is more evidence on the use of the 250μg stimulation test, expert panels agree that the 1μg stimulation test may be more physiologic, although they concede that there is a moderate grade of evidence supporting this recommendation[5, 17]. Secondly, confounding factors such as variability in sampling and cortisol assays need to be considered. Commercially available assays measure total cortisol, not the biologically active free fraction of the hormone[18]. Circulating cortisol is 90% bound to albumin and cortisol binding globulin, which may be decreased in severe sepsis. Hypoabuminemic septic patients may therefore have subnormal total cortisol levels but normal free cortisol levels[19]. Defining normal adrenal function can therefore be extremely challenging in the setting of severe sepsis and septic shock, as it needs to consider numerous variables such as the physiologic variation among individuals, the performance of commercially available cortisol assays, levels of free versus bound cortisol, and medications that may interfere with cortisol secretion or regulation.

3.1.1 The evidence for corticosteroid supplementation in severe sepsis

Corticosteroids have been studied extensively as an adjunctive therapy in septic patients for over 40 years and has been a subject of controversy for decades. As corticosteroid insufficiency can occur in severe sepsis, the rationale for steroid use in this setting is to attenuate the exaggerated systemic inflammatory response and cytokine activation, improve hemodynamic function, and reverse the HPA axis suppression and subsequent adrenal insufficiency. Corticosteroids have been shown to improve the vascular response to exogenous catecholamines in the septic state through its up-regulation of adrenergic receptors, and inhibition of vasodilatory stimulants such as nitric oxide synthase, prostaglandin E_1 and prostacyclin[20]. Corticosteroids may also reverse vascular hyporesponsiveness to vasopressin[21].

Clinical trials of corticosteroids date back as far as 1963, and although it may now be recognized that CIRCI is common in septic shock, consensus on how best to treat this phenomenon is yet to be reached. This stems from several challenges - the difficulties in establishing its diagnosis as described above, the controversies on appropriate dosing of corticosteroids and contradictory results from numerous trials on the efficacy of steroid replacement in this setting, and finally, the identification of CIRCI is not predictive of a favourable response to corticosteroids. Nevertheless, meta-analyses, reviews and guidelines have advocated the use of low-dose hydrocortisone in patients with septic shock[9-11, 22]. Arguments in favor of steroid replacement are that CIRCI is common in this population, steroids may results in a more rapid shock reversal and therefore improve survival, and steroids may be have additional advantages when septic shock is complicated by acute respiratory distress syndrome. Arguments against its use include the increased risk of adverse effects such as superinfection, critical illness myopathy, hyperglycemia and ultimately increased mortality[11, 23]. Hence, there are multiple questions with respect to CIRCI that pertain not only to should we treat, but who to treat and how to treat.

The earlier sepsis trials of the 1980's evaluated high-dose corticosteroids and found no mortality reduction, but a trend towards harm[24]. Further analyses suggested an inverse relationship with steroid dose and survival - the higher the dose the lower the survival rate. Subsequent trials performed in the 1990's in which lower, more physiologic doses of glucocorticoids were administered for longer courses demonstrated improved shock reversal, but a more heterogenous beneficial effect on mortality[22]. The largest of these trials, conducted by Annane et al. demonstrated improved survival with 7 days of 200 mg hydrocortisone and 50 mg fludrocortisone per day when compared to placebo, in patients with evidence of CIRCI (ACTH nonresponders)[25]. There was no significant difference in mortality between groups amongst responders. A criticism of this trial is that 72 of 229 nonresponders received etomidate, an inhibitor of 11 β-hydroxylase and hence cortisol production[26]. 94% of the etomidate treated patients in the Annane trial demonstrated CIRCI. This limitation in generalizability of this study coupled with concerns regarding side effects tempered the initial enthusiasm for steroid use in septic shock. Meta-analyses published in 2004 demonstrated improved shock reversal with steroids at lower doses, dose related adverse effects, but no impact on overall mortality[11, 22].

There have been at least seven prospective randomized controlled trials published since 2004. The largest of these, the multi-center CORTICUS trial, anticipated enrolling 800 patients but recruitment was stopped at 499 patients because of slow enrolment and other logistical reasons[27]. Twenty-eight day mortality was similar between the hydrocortisone (34%) and the placebo groups (31%), however mortality was insignificantly higher in non-responders. Interestingly, steroid treatment accelerated shock reversal more so in responders, but was associated with an increased incidence of nosocomial infection, superinfection, and hyperglycemia. The investigators concluded that routine hydrocortisone should not be routinely used in adults with septic shock, and the ACTH stimulation test does not identify patients who might benefit from hydrocortisone therapy[28]. The discrepant findings of the CORTICUS and the Annane trial have sparked debate as to why their findings differ. Possible contributing factors are that CORTICUS enrolled patients later (up to 72 hours in septic shock), with lower disease severity, as opposed to targeting patients early in their disease (3-8 h) who are poorly responsive to vasopressors, which was the Annane protocol. An updated meta-analysis combining all trials published after 1997 concluded that low-dose corticosteroids consistently improves shock reversal, but decreases mortality only patients with more severe septic shock who are at the highest risk of death[29]. Low-dose steroids appear to increase mortality or have no effect in less severely ill patients with sepsis.

In contrast to the adult literature, there are very few clinical trials of corticosteroid use in pediatric septic shock, the majority of which have been conducted in the setting of Dengue shock, and have lead to conflicting conclusions. Min et al in a double-blinded randomized controlled trial (RCT) reported a lower case fatality rate following 3 days of adjunctive hydrocortisone (19%), compared to placebo (44%, p=0.005)[30]. However in a subsequent trial by Sumarmo et al, while underpowered (n=97), found no benefit following a single dose 50 mg/kg of hydrocortisone within 6 hours of randomization[31]. A Cochrane systematic review evaluated 4 trials that enrolled a total of 284 subjects, and concluded that there was no benefit from adjunctive corticosteroid therapy in children with Dengue shock[32]. The have been two RCTs in the preterm population both of which demonstrated a short term beneficial hemodynamic effect of steroids in the setting of refractory hypotension of unspecified etiology, however no differences in clinical outcomes have been demonstrated.[33, 34] A large retrospective cohort study utilizing the Pediatric Health Information System administrative database (n=6693) suggested that adjunctive corticosteroid therapy for pediatric severe sepsis was associated with a variety of worse outcomes (mortality rate of 30% in children who received steroids compared to 18% in those who did not), however the study was criticized for its lack of severity of illness data in the study population.[35] A post-hoc analysis of the RESOLVE (*RE*searching severe *S*epsis and *O*rgan dysfunction in children: a g*L*obal perspective F1K-MC-EVBP) trial of activated protein C for pediatric severe sepsis, which is the largest prospective pediatric sepsis clinical trial to date, found no difference in outcomes (mortality, days requiring vasoactive infusion or mechanical ventilation, organ failure resolution) amongst those who received corticosteroids and those who did not[36]. The evidence in pediatrics is far from conclusive, and further prospective, RCT data evaluating corticosteroids use specifically in pediatric and neonatal septic shock is very much needed.

3.1.2 Recommendations for corticosteroid use in sepsis

The effects of corticosteroids in sepsis are dependent on both the dose used and severity of illness. High-dose steroids during sepsis are harmful, while low-dose steroids improves shock reversal, and may have a mortality benefit in the sickest patients with refractory septic shock. Until further definitive data are available on the population most likely to benefit from therapy, the decision to administer low-dose steroids during sepsis should be individualized, and considered in relation to the patient's severity of illness, and risk factors from their endocrine or corticosteroid history. ACTH stimulation test is not routinely recommended for the purposes of identifying patients who may benefit from steroid therapy. Having considered the controversies and nuances of the current evidence, the 2008 Surviving Sepsis Campaign International Guidelines made the following recommendations, using the Grades of Recommendation Assessment, Development and Evaluation (GRADE) criteria to indicate the strength of the evidence and recommendations[10]: the use of low dose steroids (e.g. < 300 mg/day of hydrocortisone) should be considered for in septic adults (and children) who remain hypotensive despite adequate fluid and vasopressors (Grade 2C); the current ACTH simulation test that assesses total serum cortisol is not recommended to identify the subset of adults with septic shock who might benefit from hydrocortisone (Grade 2B); hydrocortisone is preferred over dexamethasone (Grade 2B); oral fludrocortisone for added mineralocorticoid activity may be considered (Grade 2C); corticosteroid therapy may be weaned once vasoactive support is no longer required (Grade 2D); and the use of corticosteroid supplementation should not be used to treat sepsis in subjects whose shock reverses after fluid and pressors, or in the absence of septic shock unless indicated by the patient's endocrine history(Grade 1D). Despite the lack of evidence supporting the use of short-term steroid therapy in pediatric patients with septic shock, it appears that approximately 50% of pediatric intensivist would empirically treat their septic patients with steroids[13]. Until further data is available, given that CIRCI in pediatric septic shock is associated with a poor prognosis, the guidelines recommend that stress dose steroids (hydrocortisone 50 $mg/m^2/day$) be considered in children with fluid and catecholamine resistant septic shock who have suspected or proven risk factors for corticosteroid insufficiency (purpura fulminans, chronic steroid therapy, pituitary or adrenal abnormalities). These drugs should be weaned off as soon as the hemodynamic status of the patients allows, particularly when vasopressors are no longer required. Potential inhibitors of cortisol secretion such as etomidate or ketoconazole should be avoided in patients with sepsis.

3.2 Insulin

Hyperglycemia is common during severe sepsis and septic shock, due to the presence of circulating counter-regulatory hormones, medications such as catecholamines and glucocorticoids, and the activation of metabolic pathways such as hepatic glycogenolysis and gluconeogenesis, decreased hepatic glucose utilization, impaired insulin mediated glucose uptake, and cytokine related insulin resistance[37]. The prevalence of hyperglycemia in critically ill patients can be as high as 50% to 75%, depending on the definition used[38]. Historically, moderate hyperglycemia was considered at best to be an adaptive response to critical illness, and at worst, a marker of severity of disease. However, several studies have clearly demonstrated an association between hyperglycemia and mortality in both adult and pediatric non-diabetic critically ill patients[39]. Hyperglycemia has also been associated with an increased risk of sepsis, critical illness polyneuropathy, duration of mechanical ventilation, length of hospital stay[40]. Proposed mechanisms by which hyperglycemia increases morbidity and mortality include pro-inflammatory effects by stimulating reactive oxygen species and interleukin-8, prothrombotic effects, impaired innate immunity, and increased oxidative stress. Reversal of hyperglycemia and its sequelae with insulin therapy therefore has scientific rationale. Insulin in itself may have additional beneficial effects including partial correction of dyslipidemia, prevention of excessive inflammation, and attenuation of the cortisol response to critical illness[41].

3.2.1 The evidence for insulin therapy

The landmark RCT by Van den Berge et al. provided the first clinical evidence that maintaining strict glycemic control with intensive insulin therapy (IIT) in an adult postsurgical intensive care unit (ICU) (target glucose range 80 to 110 mg/dL) provided a mortality, and in some instances, a morbidity benefit, with the greatest mortality reduction of the subgroup of patients with an ICU stay of > 5 days[42]. The IIT group also experienced reductions in duration of mechanical ventilation, ICU stay and critical illness-associated polyneuropathy. This study was criticized for its lack of generalizability as it was conducted in a single center, and participants were mainly cardiothoracic surgical patients, many of whom were receiving total parenteral nutrition. In a subsequent study conducted in adult medical ICU patients by Van den Berghe, IIT did not reduce mortality, but resulted in reductions in length of ICU and hospital stay, duration of mechanical ventilation, and incidence of new renal injury, particularly in the group of patients with an ICU stay of 3 or more days[43]. In fact, mortality was actually greater among those receiving IIT with ICU stay less than 3 days. Since the original Van den Berghe trials, IIT has not been shown to improve outcomes in subsequent multicenter studies involving patients with severe sepsis or in a general ICU population[44, 45]. Two large multi-center trials (VISEP and GLUCONTROL) were both stopped early for safety reasons because of adverse events related to hypoglycemia in the IIT arm, and no mortality difference[44, 46]. In the VISEP study, IIT increased the rate of severe hypoglycemia (17.0% vs. 4.1%) and serious adverse events (10.9% vs. 5.2%, $p = 0.01$) in critically ill adults with sepsis[44]. In the GLUCONTROL trial, treating to achieve a moderately hyperglycemic goal (140-180 mg/dL) yielded similar survival, length of stay with fewer hypoglycemic reactions compared with IIT[46]. The authors of both studies concluded that tight glycemic control with IIT offered no apparent benefits, but increased the risk of hypoglycemia.

The Normoglycemia in Intensive Care Evaluation - Survival Using Glucose Algorithm Regulation (NICE-SUGAR), and international multicenter trial involving 6104 patients, is the largest trial of intensive insulin therapy to date[45]. This trial compared conventional glucose control (≤ 10.0 mmol/L or 180 mg/dL) to intensive glucose control (4.5 to 6.0 mmol/L or 81 to 108 mg/dL) in critically ill patients, and concluded that using insulin to achieve a conventional glucose control resulted in lower 90 day all cause mortality. However, the subgroup analysis did not reveal a significant difference in treatment effect in the subgroup of patients with severe sepsis (21% of patients). Subsequent meta-analyses incorporating the results of all trials of this nature reveal that IIT significantly increases the risk of hypoglycemia while conferring no overall mortality among critically ill patients, compared to conventional insulin therapy. However, there may be benefits of IIT in the subset of patients treated in surgical ICU's[47, 48]. As corticosteroid therapy induces potentially detrimental hyperglycemia in septic shock, the benefit of intensive insulin therapy in patients treated with hydrocortisone was evaluated (COIITSS Study), but did not improve mortality in patients with septic shock when compared to conventional insulin therapy[49].

As expected, the data in pediatrics is limited. While a relationship between hyperglycemia and poor outcomes have also been identified in this population, hypoglycemia in the absence of insulin therapy, and increased glucose variability in particular appear to have an even stronger association with mortality and length of stay[38, 50]. To date, there is only one prospective randomized controlled trial to date by Vlasselaers et al, published in 2009.[98] This trial randomized 700 critically ill children (317 infants aged 1 year, and 383 children aged ≥ 1 year) to an age-adjusted intensive insulin group (i.e. target glucose range of 2.8-4.4 mmol/L in infants, and 3.9-5.6 mmol/L in children), or a conventional group where insulin was initiated only when blood glucose exceeded 11.9 mmol/L. The investigators found that intensive insulin therapy in this trial of predominantly cardiac surgical patients, resulted in a significant decrease in PICU stay, reduced mortality and an attenuated inflammatory response on day 5, as indicated by lower C-reactive protein values. The risk of secondary infections was also significantly lower in the intensive insulin group. The risk of hypoglycemia however, was significantly higher in the intensive insulin group. They also observed that patients who developed hypoglycemia had a higher risk of death than those who were not hypoglycemic, although this difference was not statistically significant. It has been suggested that glucose reperfusion after hypoglycemia may trigger neuronal death, rather than hypoglycemia itself.[99] As the excess neurological deaths in this trial occurred in the conventional and not the intensive insulin arm, the authors conclude that the short-term benefits of preventing hyperglycemia in critically ill children may outweigh those of hypoglycemia, provided that hypoglycemia is recognized and treated promptly.

3.2.2 Limitations of insulin therapy in sepsis

The limitations of insulin therapy for glucose control in critically ill patients with sepsis are primarily three-fold. Firstly, blood glucose variability, especially in children, may be a more important marker of poor outcome than isolated blood glucose levels per se[51]. Secondly, blood glucose monitoring in critically ill patients is notoriously inaccurate by nature of intermittent testing as opposed to real-time results, and the variable methods of measurement and levels of quality control[52]. Furthermore, symptomatic monitoring is also hindered as counter-regulatory responses in critically ill septic patients are often impaired, and ICU therapies like sedation may mask symptoms of severe hypoglycemia. The third and most obvious limitation is the risk of hypoglycemia, which has been clearly identified in the multiple large adult RCTs, as well as the pediatric observational studies. In fact, the rate of hypoglycemia is highest in children with sepsis (28.6%), in the absence of insulin therapy[50]. While there may be subgroups of adult patients who may benefit from IIT[48], there is clear evidence that children are more susceptible to developing hypoglycemia, and the risks of mortality, morbidity, and irreversible neurological sequelae of hypoglycemia in the developing brain is greater[38].

3.2.3 Recommendations for insulin and glycemic control in sepsis

Although current guidelines from the American Diabetes Association, the American Association of Clinical Endocrinologists and other organizations such as the Surviving Sepsis Campaign currently recommend tight glycemic control with insulin therapy, more recent meta-analyses of the largest trials to date suggest that these recommendations should be revised for septic patients who are critically ill[48]. Less restrictive target glucose values in the range of 140-180 mg/dL appear safer than 80-100 mg/dL in critically ill adults, although it is unclear whether there may be specific subgroups of adult patients who may benefit from IIT and be at lower risk of hypoglycemic events. We recommend that hypoglycemic and variable glucose episodes should be avoided in all patients with sepsis. The risk-benefit ratio for insulin therapy in critically ill children with sepsis remains unclear. While there is a suggestion from the pediatric literature that glycemic control may be beneficial in reducing morbidity and mortality, the optimum blood glucose targets in children remain uncertain. Until further prospective data is available specifically in this population, it is reasonable to target blood a glucose control of $\leq$ 10 mmol/L as defined by the definitive adult trial. However, further research on this subject in critically ill children is needed, and the long-term sequelae of both hypo- and hyperglycemia in this population should be further investigated. Well-developed, detailed and user-friendly protocols and extensive education of caregivers are essential to any insulin therapy and glucose monitoring protocol. Until a more accurate and reliable continuous blood sensor is available, the most reliable method of blood glucose measurement (i.e. arterial point-of-care) is recommended, particularly in the patient at risk, and capillary blood samples should be interpreted with caution.

3.3 Vasopressin

Vasopressin is a neurohypophyseal peptide hormone that is an attractive adjunctive agent in vasodilatory septic shock for the following reasons:

1. Vasopressin inactivates the key mechanisms responsible for the pathogenesis of vasodilatation and catecholamine resistance[53].
2. Although it is a potent systemic vasoconstrictor, vasopressin demonstrates organ specific vasodilator effects in the pulmonary, cerebral and coronary circulations, potentially preserving vital organ perfusion. It also has been shown to increase urine output and creatinine clearance in patients with septic shock, when compared to norepinephrine[54].
3. Vasopressin influences multiple other hormone responses including ACTH, and consequently cortisol release, important considerations in the setting of HPA axis dysfunction during septic shock[54, 55]. Vasopressin also stimulates prolactin secretion, an important mediator of cellular immune response during sepsis[56].
4. Vasopressin insufficiency, either absolute - as a result of depletion or impaired release from neurohypophyseal stores; or functional - as a result of cytokine mediated receptor down regulation, has been demonstrated in both adults and perhaps children with septic shock[57].

3.3.1 Assessing the vasopressin axis

There is a surge in endogenous vasopressin levels during sepsis, however inappropriately low levels to the order of 3-10 pg/mL have been identified in septic shock. The detection of endogenous deficiency by measuring circulating vasopressin levels is limited by the fact that the mature hormone is unstable, has a short half-life, and circulates largely attached to platelets. Copeptin, a stable vasopressin precursor, has recently been identified as a stable and sensitive surrogate marker for vasopressin release, and has been proposed as a more sensitive and potential prognostic biomarker in sepsis[58]. Others have suggested that the ratio of vasopressin to norepinephrine levels should be considered a reflection of adequacy of vasopressin homeostasis relative to adrenocorticoid homeostasis. The vasopressin/ norepinephrine ratios in sepsis and severe sepsis are similar (1/175) while they are much lower when shock ensues (1/1000)[21].

3.3.2 The evidence for vasopressin supplementation in severe sepsis

Numerous adult trials suggest short term benefits of vasopressin, the Vasopressin and Septic Shock Trial (VASST) conducted by Russell et al. evaluated the effect of low dose arginine vasopressin (0.01-0.03 U/min) as an adjunctive agent compared to norepinephrine alone, on mortality in 779 adult patients in septic shock[59]. There was no difference in 28-day mortality between groups (35.4% vs. 39.3%, $p = 0.26$). Although the authors had predicted that based on its vasoconstrictor potency, vasopressin would be more efficacious in the stratum of patients with more severe septic shock (baseline requirement of ≥ 15 μg/kg/min norepinephrine), they observed a significant reduction in mortality in the subgroup of patients with less severe septic shock (baseline of 5-14 μg/kg/min norepinephrine). While the authors conclude that these subgroup findings should be hypothesis generating only, it has sparked further debate as to whether higher doses of vasopressin should be used in patients with more severe shock, and should be thus evaluated in future studies. A post hoc analysis of the VASST trial suggested that combined vasopressin and corticosteroid therapy was associated with decreased mortality and organ dysfunction than norepinephrine and corticosteroids[60]. A subsequent open-label trial by Torgersen and colleagues demonstrated that higher doses of vasopressin (0.067 IU/min) resulted in improved hemodynamic control without increased adverse effects, compared to lower doses of 0.033 IU/min in patients with vasodilatory septic shock[61].
There are at present at least 18 published observational studies reporting on a collective total of only 145 children, that arginine vasopressin and its longer lasting synthetic analogue, terlipressin increase systemic blood pressure, decreases inotrope or vasopressor requirement, and increases urine output in children with catecholamine-resistant shock[57, 62]. The doses used in these studies varied substantively, ranging from 0.00002 U/kg/min to 0.002 U/kg/min of vasopressin, and terlipressin dosing administered anywhere from every four hourly, to continuous infusion. The Vasopressin in Pediatric Vasodilatory Shock trial which evaluated the safety and efficacy of low dose vasopressin as an adjunctive agent found no difference in the time to hemodynamic stability, organ free failure days or magnitude of vasoactive agent use between the vasopressin and placebo groups[63]. While there was no statistical difference in the adverse event rates, there was a trend towards increased mortality in the vasopressin group.

3.3.3 Adverse effects of exogenous vasopressin

Because of its potent vasoconstrictor action, potential adverse effects of low dose vasopressin include increase in myocardial after-load, reductions in oxygen delivery, impaired tissues perfusion and ischemic tissue injury. Thrombocytopenia and increases in aminotransferases activity and bilirubin concentrations have also been reported. These adverse effects appear to be dose-dependent, and more commonly noted with doses of greater than 0.04 U/min of vasopressin or 2 μg/kg/h of terlipressin[21]. However, some of the data is conflicting, and it is yet unclear whether the hemodynamic alterations represent adaptive response to stabilized blood pressure, or the impaired tissue perfusion is an epiphenomenon of the severity of underlying disease rather than a specific side effect of vasopressin or concurrent catecholamine pressor administration.[64] Both the VASST and Vasopressin in Pediatric Vasodilatory Shock trials reported no significant difference in adverse event rates between the vasopressin and control groups[59, 63].

3.3.4 Recommendations for vasopressin use in sepsis

There are currently no recommendations for routine testing for endogenous vasopressin levels in the setting of sepsis. Catecholamine infusions remain the first line vasopressor agents of choice in adults with septic shock[10]. Based on the results of VASST, low dose vasopressin infusion may be considered as an adjunctive agent, however, with the anticipation of an effect equivalent to that of norepinephrine alone. Higher doses of vasopressin may have short-term beneficial hemodynamic effects in septic shock refractory to traditional vasopressor therapy, however its effect on clinically important patient outcomes is unknown. As with any vasopressor therapy, close monitoring of end-organ perfusion, awareness of potential side effects, and measurement of tissue flow where possible are essential. Pediatric recommendations are based on limited evidence and one should be aware that children more commonly present with low cardiac output, high systemic vascular resistance during septic shock, and commonly evolve from one hemodynamic state to another[65]. Vasoactive therapy should therefore be tailored according to the patient's clinical status. There is no evidence that adjunctive vasopressin therapy is beneficial in pediatric sepsis at the present time.

4. Hormonal markers and predictors of outcome in sepsis

The clinical diagnosis of sepsis is made in the presence of a systemic inflammatory response syndrome (SIRS) and a proven or suspected source of sepsis. Our ability to accurately and promptly diagnose sepsis is limited due to the lack of a definitive test in this setting. Positive cultures may account for only 10% of all blood culture results reported, of which up to 50% may be due to contamination. This in turn has significant potential financial and healthcare costs to the patient and the healthcare system[66, 67]. Despite the expanding research on treatment modalities in this field, the mortality rate in sepsis remains unacceptably high, often due to delayed diagnosis and treatment. According to United States data, the incidence of sepsis and number of sepsis-related deaths continue to rise, although there is a slight decrease in the age-adjusted mortality rate among patients with sepsis in recent years[68]. In view of this diagnostic and therapeutic dilemma, the search of an unequivocal and rapid confirmatory test to distinguish septic from non-septic causes of SIRS is paramount. There have been enormous attempts to identify prognostic markers of early sepsis and accurate risk prediction that may better direct therapy and diagnosis and thus improve mortality and morbidity in septic patients. In this context, several endocrine markers and mediators of sepsis have been investigated as potential early indicators and potential predictors of outcome in sepsis. Many of these hormonal assays are still under investigation and are not commercially available. We discuss some of the current research on hormonal markers of sepsis in the remaining section of this chapter.

4.1 Procalcitonin

Procalcitonin is a 116 amino acid peptide with a sequence identical to that of prohormone calcitonin but devoid of hormonal activity. During sepsis, circulating levels of procalcitonin, increase several-fold to several thousand-fold. Procalcitonin is released into the circulation within 3 hours of endotoxin injection, plateaus at 6 hours, and remains elevated for 24 hours, making it an attractive and sensitive hormonal marker of early sepsis[69]. Procalcitonin measurement was first described by Assicot et al to differentiate between bacterial and non-bacterial causes of sepsis, and while it is now increasingly used as an early marker of bacterial infection, procalcitonin can be increased in noninfectious conditions, and remain low in certain bacterial infections, such as bacterial pulmonary aspiration[70-72]. Procalcitonin appears to offer better specificity over other biomarkers such as C-Reactive Protein, in differentiating between viral and bacterial causes of fever, and in distinguishing invasive from noninvasive infections[73, 74]. More recently, procalcitonin has been advocated as a clinical tool to guide antimicrobial therapy in patients with suspected infections. Several randomized controlled trials have reported a significant reduction in antibiotic exposure and duration based on serial procalcitonin measurements, compared to a standard approach[75-77]. An association between decreasing levels of procalcitonin and favourable outcomes has been suggested by several investigators, however further validation studies are required before any firm conclusions can be made[72, 78].

4.2 Thyroid

Thyroid hormones play an important role in the adaptation of metabolic function to stress and critical illness. Thyroid function abnormalities are often observed during critical illness but are transient and may not represent underlying thyroid disease. There is evidence that lower baseline thyroid hormone values, including triiodothyronine (T_3), thyroxine (T_4), and thyroid stimulating hormone (TSH) can be substantially lower in septic compared to non-septic patients of similar critical illness severity, and that these abnormalities are associated with a worse outcome in patients with sepsis or septic shock[79]. Low T_3 can be attributed to increased de-iodination of T_4 to reverse T_3 (rT_3), rather than T_3, and increased catabolism of T_3 to 3,3-diiodothyronine. Low total and free T_4 and low TSH levels can be observed in severe sepsis and septic shock due to decrease in plasma T_4-binding globulin or transthyretin as well as accumulation of substances that lower the plasma thyroid hormone-binding capacity[80]. However, the pattern of abnormal thyroid profiles are not consistently observed between studies, with more pediatric studies reporting thyroid function abnormalities. Reasons for discordant findings may be attributed to age related hormonal differences - plasma thyroid hormone levels are higher than older children and adults in the first few months of life, due to the TSH surge that occurs in the immediate postnatal period, and elevated TBG levels secondary to maternal estrogen. Other reasons for variable findings may be attributed to differences in the hemodynamic response to septic shock in children, and thus the type of vasoactive support; dopamine can suppress the pituitary release of TSH and thus potentially the production of T3, while norepinephrine is believed to stimulate the secretion of TSH. It is however, generally accepted that alterations in thyroid hormone observed during septic shock constitute part of an adaptive metabolic response, and that the majority of patients recover normal thyroid function once their critical illness subsides[81]. Nevertheless, thyroid disorders are relatively common in the general population, with an estimated prevalence of 1% to 10%, and hence a subset of patients with septic shock can have true underlying hypothyroidism. High TSH or reduced rT_3 may be suggestive of such a diagnosis.

The hypothesis of relative thyroid insufficiency and its association with a worse outcome has led to several studies on thyroid supplementation during sepsis. However, despite early animal studies showing beneficial effects of thyroid supplementation particularly on lung mechanics and vasoactive requirements during sepsis[82], human studies have failed to demonstrate a beneficial effect from thyroid hormone replacement in this setting[79]. Thyroid hormone supplementation during sepsis can lead to a reciprocal decrease in TSH, which in turn can adversely effect the adaptive immune response.

In summary, thyroid hormone abnormalities are very common in septic patients and hence future studies are required to establish the strength of this association, or if a causal relationship exists between thyroid hypofunction and adverse outcome. The role of thyroid hormone abnormalities as an adjunctive predictor of outcome warrants further evaluation Follow-up thyroid function tests are recommended if abnormal levels are measured during severe sepsis, as the majority of these abnormalities are transient.

4.3 Growth hormone

Activation of the HPA axis in critical illness results in an alteration in pulsatile release of growth hormone (GH) from the somatotropes. Down regulation of insulin-like growth factor 1 (IGF1) and GH binding proteins result in an acquired peripheral GH resistance during severe sepsis which in turn promotes protein catabolism and negative nitrogen balance[83]. There is evidence that GH resistance and the resultant increase in circulating GH concentrations have deleterious effects in critically ill patients. Increased GH levels has been shown to correlate with poor outcome in children with menincococcal sepsis and septic shock[84]. Increased GH has also been found to correlate with severity of disease and appears to be an independent predictor for mortality in critically ill adults but does not discriminate between septic and non-septic patients[85]. It is also unclear how GH is influenced by difference metabolic factors such as glucose control, insulin administration, and nutrition. Unfortunately, trials with recombinant GH targeted at overcoming the GH resistance induced catabolism have not been promising but in fact have demonstrated potential harm due to emergence of uncontrolled infections and the development of multiple organ failure[86]. At this point in time, the potential benefits of GH measurements in sepsis remain unclear and is therefor not recommended.

4.4 Copeptin

As discussed earlier, measuring circulating vasopressin levels is challenging as the mature hormone is unstable, has a short half-life and is largely attached to platelets. Copeptin, a stable peptide of the vasopressin precursor, is secreted in an equimolar ratio and thus mirrors the production of vasopressin[87]. Copeptin measurements have been shown to be much more stable and easy to determine than vasopressin, and has therefor been proposed as a sensitive and potential prognostic marker in patients with sepsis. Copeptin levels do appear to be increasingly elevated according to severity of illness from patients with sepsis, to severe sepsis and septic shock, however the optimal cut-off level has a sensitivity of 61.5%

and a specificity of 83.8%[88]. Copeptin is not specific to sepsis, and increased levels are also a marker of heart disease and ischemic stroke. Furthermore, copeptin levels may be affected by exogenous corticosteroid therapy, and in renal insufficiency[88].

4.5 Leptin

Leptin is an adipose-derived hormone known for its contribution to energy metabolism and satiety signaling in the hypothalamus. Elevated baseline levels of leptin are found in obese patients, and obesity appears to be an independent, "dose-dependent" risk factor for sepsis morbidity and mortality[89]. There is evidence that leptin is also involved in cell-mediated immunity and cytokine crosstalk. Human septic patients have evidence of increased circulating leptin concentrations which correlate with severity of illness, and hence it has been postulated that leptin may play a critical role in the pathogenesis of sepsis-associated multi-organ dysfunction[90]. It has also been suggested that elevated leptin levels may aid in distinguishing between sepsis and non-infectious SIRS[91]. However, research in this area is in its infancy, and further studies are required to determine the pathogenic mechanisms of leptin, and the diagnostic and therapeutic potential of leptin family molecules in human sepsis.

4.6 Age and sex hormone related phenomena during sepsis

Differences in hormonal profiles have been suggested as the cause of gender-based differences in the incidence and outcomes from severe sepsis. The incidence of sepsis appears to be 15% to 28% higher in males than in females in both the pediatric and adult populations[68, 92]. Among septic patients, even microbes may have a predilection for certain sexes. In a large cohort study of septic patients admitted to US hospitals, men were more likely than women to be infected with Gram-positive organisms after controlling for source of infection[93]. Whether gender related differences in sepsis translates into a higher mortality risk remains unclear[68, 94]. Sex hormones or sex-related gene polymorphisms may protect women against sepsis and death from sepsis. Estrogens and prolactin may confer some protection in women however there are additional non-hormonal based factors such as a differential immune response, sociocultural, racial background, economic or personal health-related behaviours between men and women, that account for the gender-related differences in incidence and outcomes from sepsis[94].

Neuroendocrine dysfunction appears to differ significantly between children and adults and hence it is suggested that age related differences may contribute to variations in disease course, physiologic response and clinical outcomes in these populations[95]. Mortality from pediatric septic shock is significantly lower than in adults[96]. The hemodynamic profile during severe sepsis in children more commonly presents as cardiogenic dysfunction as opposed to the vascular failure seen in adults[97]. As a result, children with fluid-refractory septic shock are frequently hypodynamic and respond to inotrope and vasodilator therapy, while vasopressor therapy is recommended as the first line agent in adult patients[10, 97]. These differences in physiologic response therefore call for a diagnostic and therapeutic approach that is tailored dependent on the patient's age.

5. Conclusion

Severe sepsis and septic shock remains one of the most challenging problems in medicine today, and in our search for potential therapies to reverse end-organ sequelae of infection, we are eager to embrace the concept of endocrine support to supplement the antimicrobial and cardiorespiratory support during the management of the sickest of these patients. While hormonal therapy may play an important role in the management of severe sepsis for hormone therapy in sepsis, we have yet to fully understand the dynamic compensatory mechanisms, signaling pathways and complex interdependence of multiple hormonal responses, such that replacement therapy with exogenous hormone with the rationale of restoring normal or "physiologic" values, or to reverse target organ receptor resistance, may be too simplistic a therapeutic approach. We have yet to fully understand the precise mechanisms by which these hormones participate in sepsis and non-infectious SIRS, and the complex role each may play in modulating the inflammatory and immune responses during severe infection, and whether these responses are adaptive or maladaptive. Limitations in predicting who may respond and potentially benefit from such therapies, together with how to define or diagnose dysfunction within a hormonal axis, add further challenges. There are many stress hormones that mirror the severity of illness during sepsis, however with the possible exception of procalcitonin, none are specific enough to consistently discriminate between infectious and non-infectious causes of SIRS such that one can currently be recommended for routine use as an early diagnostic and independent prognostic marker. Nevertheless based on emerging research, it is likely that hormonal assays may become adjunctive to the predictive capacity of validated prognostic scoring tools in the future. There is evidence that corticosteroid and insulin therapy in specific subgroups of critically ill septic patients can be beneficial. The many controversies and ongoing debates ensure that this area of research will continue to evolve, which will hopefully enhance our ability to not only detect hormone dysfunction, but also predict outcome, and ultimately refine our diagnostic, therapeutic and prognostic approaches in septic patients.

6. References

[1] Vanhorebeek I, Van den Berghe G. The Neuroendocrine Response to Critical Illness is a Dynamic Process. *Crit Care Clin*. 2006;22:1-15.

[2] Rothwell P, Lawler P. Prediction of outcome in intensive care patients using endocrine parameters. *Crit Care Med*. 1995;23:78-83.

[3] Hebbar K, Rigby M, Felner E, Easley K, Fortenberry J. Neuroendocrine dysfunction in pediatric critical illness. *Pediatr Crit Care Med*. 2009;10:35-40.

[4] Van den Berghe G, Zegher F, Bouillon R. Acute and prolonged critical illness as different neuroendocrine paradigms. *J Clin Endocrinol Metab*. 1998;83:1827-34.

[5] Marik P, Pastores S, Annane D, Meduri U, Sprung C, Arlt W, *et al.* Recommendations for the diagnosis and management of corticosteroid insuffiiciency in criticaly ill adult patients: Consensus statements from an international task force by the American College of Critical Care Medicine. *Crit Care Med*. 2008;36:1937-49.

[6] Chrousos G. Stress and disorders of the stress system. *Nature Reviews*. 2009:374-81.

[7] Bornstein S. Predisposing Factors for Adrenal Insufficiency. *N Engl J Med*. 2009;360:2328-39.

[8] Bornstein S, Engeland W, Ehrhart-Bornstein M, Herman J. Dissociation of ACTH and glucocorticoids. *Trends Endocrinol Metab*. 2008:175-80.

[9] Cooper M, Stewart P. Corticosteroid insufficiency in acutely ill patients. *N Engl J Med.* 2003;348:727-34.

[10] Dellinger R, Levy M, Carlet J, Parker M, Jaeschke R, Reinhart K, *et al.* Surviving Sepsis Campaign: International guidelines for management of severe sepsis and septic shock. *Crit Care Med.* 2008;36:296-327.

[11] Annane D, Bellissant E, Bolleart P, et al. Corticosteroids for severe sepsis and septic shock: A systematic review and meta-analysis. *BMJ.* 2004;329.

[12] De Jong M, Beishuizen A, Groeneveld A. Defining relative adrenal insufficiency in the critically ill. In: Vincent JL, editor. *Yearbook in intensive care and emergency medicine Berlin.* 2006;Springer:pp. 539-52.

[13] Menon K, Lawson M. Identification of adrenal insufficiency in pediatric critical illness. *Pediatr Crit Care Med.* 2007;8:276-8.

[14] Menon K, Ward R, Lawson M, Gaboury I, Hutchison J, Hebert P. A Prospective Multicenter Study of Adrenal Function in Critically ill Children. *Am J Respir Crit Care Med.* 2010;182:246-51.

[15] Lipiner-Frieman D, Sprung C, Laterre P, Weiss Y, Goodman S, Vogeser M, *et al.* Adrenal function in sepsis: The retrospective Corticus study. *Crit Care Med.* 2007;35:1012-8.

[16] Tordman K, Jaffe A, Trostanetsky Y, Greenman Y, Limor R, Stern N. Low-dose (1 microgram) adrenocorticotrophin (ACTH) stimulation as a screening test for impaired hypothalamo-pituitary-adrenal axis function: sensitivity, specificity and accuracy in comparison with the high-dose (250 microgram) test *Clin Endocrinol (Oxf).* 2000;52:633-40.

[17] Kazlauskaite R, Maghnie M. PItfalls in the diagnosis of central adrenal insufficiency in children. *Endocr Dev.* 2010:96-107.

[18] Ho J, Al-Musalhi H, Chapman M, Quach T, Thomas P, Bagley C, *et al.* Septic shock and sepsis: a comparison of total and free plasma cortisol levels. *J Clin Endocrinol Metab.* 2006;91:105-14.

[19] Arafah B. Hypothalamic pituitary adrenal function during critical illness: limitations of current assessment methods. *J Clin Endocrinol Metab.* 2006;91:3725-45.

[20] Opert M, Schindler R, Husung C, Offermann K, Graf K, Boenisch O, *et al.* Low dose hydrocortisone improves shock reversal and reduces cytokine level in early hyperdynamic septic shock. *Crit Care Med.* 2005;33.

[21] Russell J. Vasopressin in vasodilatory and septic shock. *Current Opinion in Critical Care.* 2007;13:383-91.

[22] Minneci P, Deans K, Banks S, Eichacker P, Natanson C. Meta-Analysis: The effect of steroids on survival and shock during sepsis depends on the dose. *Ann Intern Med.* 2004;141:47-56.

[23] Keh D, Sprung C. Use of coritcosteroid therapy in patients with sepsis and septic shock: An evidence-based review. *Crit Care Med.* 2004;32:S527-S33.

[24] Cronin L, Cook D, Carlet J, Heyland D, King D, Lansang M, *et al.* Corticosteroid treatment for sepsis: a critical appraisal and meta-analysis of the literature. *Crit Care Med.* 1995;23:1430-9.

[25] Annane D, Sébille V, Charpentier C, Bolleart P, B F, Korach J, *et al.* Effect of treatment with low doses of hydrocortisone and fludrocortisone on mortality in patients with septic shock. *JAMA*. 2002;288:862-71.
[26] Cohen J, Ward G, Prins J, Jones M, Venkatesh B. Variability of cortisol assays can confound the diagnosis of adrenal insufficiency in the critically ill population. *Intensive Care Med*. 2006;32:1901-5.
[27] Sprung C, Annane D, Keh D, Moreno R, Singer M, Freivogel K, *et al.* Hydrocortisone Therapy for Patients with Septic Shock. *New Engl J Med*. 2008;358:111-24.
[28] Markovitz B, Goodman D, Watson R, Bertoch D, Zimmerman J. A retrospective cohort study of prognostic factors associated with outcome in pediatric severe sepsis: what is the role of steroids? . *Pediatr Crit Care Med*. 2005;6:270-4.
[29] Minneci P, Deans K, Eichacker P, Natanson C. The effects of steroids during sepsis depend on dose and severity of illness: an updated meta-analysis. *Clin Microbiol Infect*. 2009;15:308-18.
[30] Min M, Aye M, Shwe T, Swe T. Hydrocortisone in the management of dengue shock syndrome. *Southeast Asian J Trop Med Public Health*. 1975;6:573-9.
[31] Sumarmo. The role of steroids in dengue shock syndrome. *Southeast Asian J Trop Med Public Health*. 1987;18:383-9.
[32] Panpanich R, Sornchai P, Kanjanaratanakorn K. Corticosteroids for treating dengue shock syndrome. Cochrane Database of Systematic Reviews [serial on the Internet]. 2006; (3).
[33] Ng P, Lee C, Bnur F, Chan I, Lee A, Wong E, *et al.* A double-blind, randomized, controlled study of a 'stress dose' of hydrocortisone for rescue treatment of regractory hypotension in preterm infants. *Pediatrics*. 2006;117:367-75.
[34] Gaissmaier R, Pohlandt F. Single-dose dexamtehasone treatment of hypotension in preterm infants. *J Pediatr*. 1999;134:701-5.
[35] Markovitz B, Goodman D, Watson R, Bertoch D, Zimmerman J. A retrospective cohort study of prognostic factors associated with outcome in pediatric severe sepsis: what is the role of steroids? . *Pediatr Crit Care Med* 2005;6:270-4.
[36] Zimmerman J, Williams M. Adjunctive corticosteroid therapy in pediatric severe sepsis: Observations from the RESOLVE study. *Pediatr Crit Care Med*. 2011;122: 2-8.
[37] Van Cromphaut S, Vanhorebeek I, Van den Berghe G. Glucose metabolism and insulin resistance in sepsis *Curr Pharm Des* 2008;14:1887-99.
[38] Wintergerst K, Buckingham B, Gandrud L, Wong B, Kache S, Wilson D. Association of hypoglycemia, hyperglycemia, and glucose variability with morbidity and death in the pediatric intensive care unit. *Pediatrics*. 2006;118:173-9.
[39] Krinsley J. Association between hyperglycemia and increased hospital mortality in a heterogeneous population of critically ill patients. *Mayo Clin Proc*. 2003;78: 1471-8.
[40] Srinivasan V, Spinella P, Drott H, Roth C, Helfaer M, Nadkarni V. Association of timing, duration, and intensity of hyperglycemia with intensive care unit mortality in critically ill children. *Pediatr Crit Care Med*. 2004;5:329-36.
[41] Vanhorebeek I, Langouche L, Van den Berghe G. Tight Blood Glucose Control with Insulin in the ICU: Facts and Controversies. *Chest*. 2007;132:268-78.

[42] Van den Berghe G, Wouters P, Weekers F, Verwaest C, Bruyninckx F, Schetz M, *et al.* Intensive insulin therapy in critically ill patients. *N Engl J Med.* 2001;345:1359-67.
[43] Van den Berghe G, Wilmer A, Hermans G, Meersseman W, Wouters P, Milants I, *et al.* Intensive insulin therapy in the medical ICU *N Engl J Med* 2006;354:449-61.
[44] Brunkhorst F, Engel C, Bloos F, Meier-Hellman A, Ragaller M, Weiler N, *et al.* Intensive insulin therapy and pentastarch resuscitation in severe sepsis. *N Engl J Med.* 2008;358:125-39.
[45] Finfer S, Chittock DR, Su S, Blair D, Foster D, Dhingra V. for the NICE-SUGAR Study Investigators. Intensive versus Conventional Glucose Control in Critically Ill Patients. *N Engl J Med.* 2009;360:1283-97.
[46] Devos P, Preiser J, Melot C. Impact of tight glucose control by intensive insulin therapy on ICU mortality and the rate of hypoglycaemia: final results of the Glucontrol study *Intensive Care Med.* 2007;33:S189.
[47] Wiener R, Wiener D, Larson R. Benefits and risks of tight glucose control in critically ill adults: a meta-analysis. *JAMA.* 2008;300:933-44.
[48] Griesdale D, de Souza R, van Dam R, Heyland D, Cook D, Malhotra A, *et al.* Intensive insulin therapy and mortality among critically ill patients: a meta-analysis including NICE-SUGAR study data. *CMAJ.* 2009;180:821-7.
[49] Annane D, Cariou A, Maxime V, Azoulay E, D'honneur G, Timsit J, *et al.* for the COIITSS Study Investigators. Corticosteroid Treatment and Intensive Insulin Therapy for Septic Shock in Adults - A Randomized Controlled Trial. *JAMA.* 2010;303:341-8.
[50] Hirshberg E, Larsen G, Van Duker H. Alterations in glucose homeostasis in the pediatric intensive care unit: Hyperglycemia and glucose variability are associated with increased mortality and morbidity. *Pediatr Crit Care Med.* 2008;9:361-6.
[51] Ali N, O'Brien JJ, Dungan K, et a. Glucose variability is independently associated with increased mortality in patients with severe sepsis. *Crit Care Med.* 2008;36:2316-21.
[52] Crtichell C, Savarese V, Callahan A, Aboud C, Jabbour S, Marik P. Accuracy of bedside capillary blood glucose measurements in critically ill patients. *Intensive Care Med.* 2007;33:2079-84.
[53] Landry DW, Oliver JA. The pathogenesis of vasodilatory shock. *N Engl J Med.* 2001 Aug 23;345:588-95.
[54] Holmes CL, Landry DW, Granton JT. Science review: Vasopressin and the cardiovascular system part 1--receptor physiology. *Crit Care.* 2003;7:427-34.
[55] Holmes CL, Landry DW, Granton JT. Science Review: Vasopressin and the cardiovascular system part 2 - clinical physiology. *Crit Care.* 2004;8:15-23.
[56] Dunser MW, Hasibeder WR, Wenzel V, Schwarz S, Ulmer H, Knotzer H, *et al.* Endocrinologic response to vasopressin infusion in advanced vasodilatory shock. *Crit Care Med.* 2004;32:1266-71.
[57] Choong K, Kissoon N. Vasopressin in Pediatric Shock and Cardiac arrest. *Pediatr Crit Care Med.* 2008;9:372-9.
[58] Morgenthaler N, Struck J, Jochberger S, Dunser M. Copeptin: clinical use of a new biomarker. *Trends in Endocrinology and Metabolism.* 2008;19:43-9.

[59] Russell J, Walley K, Singer J, Gordon A, Hebert P, Copper J, *et al.* Vasopressin versus norepinephrine infusion in patients with septic shock. *New Engl J Med.* 2008;358:877-87.

[60] Russell JA, Walley KR, Gordon A, Cooper D, Hebert P, Singer J, *et al.* Interaction of vasopressin infusion, corticosteroid treatment and mortality of septic shock. *Crit Care Med.* 2009;37:811-8.

[61] Torgersen C, Dunser MW, Wenzel V, Jochberger S, Mayer V, Schmittinger C, *et al.* Comparing two different arginine vasopressin doses in advanced vasodilatory shock: a randomized controlled, open-label trial. *Intensive Care Med.* 2009;36:57-65.

[62] Meyer S, Gortner L, McGuire W, Baghai A, Gottschling S. Vasopressin in catecholamine-refractory shock in children *Anaesthesia.* 2008;63:228-34.

[63] Choong K, Joffe A, Menon K, Fraser D, McNamara P, Litalien C, *et al.* Vasopressin in Pediatric Vasodilatory Shock Trial. *Am J Respir Crit Care Med.* 2009;180:632-9.

[64] Ertmer C, Rehberg S, Westphal M. Vasopressin analogues in the treatment of shock states: potential pitfalls. *Best Practice & Research Clinical Anaesthesiology.* 2008;22:393-406.

[65] Brierley J, Carcillo J, Choong K, Cornell T, Decaen A, Deymann A, *et al.* Clinical practice parameters for hemodynamic support of pediatric and neonatal septic shock: 2007 update from the American College of Critical Care Medicine. *Crit Care Med.* 2009;37:666-88.

[66] Gander R, Byrd L, DeCrescenzo M, Hirany S, Bowen M, Baughman J. Impact of blood cultures drawn by phlebotomy on contamination rates and health care costs in a hospital emergency department. *Journal of Clinical Microbiology.* 2009;47:1021-4.

[67] Melvin P. Weinstein Blood Culture Contamination: Persisting Problems and Partial Progress *Journal of Clinical Microbiology.* 2003;41:2275-8.

[68] Martin G, Mannino D, Eaton S, Moss M. The epidemiology of sepsis in the United States from 1979 through 2000. *N Engl J Med.* 2003;348:1546-54.

[69] Muller B, Becker K. Procalcitonin: how a hormone became a marker and mediator of sepsis. *Swiss Med Wkly.* 2001;131:595-602.

[70] Martinont M, Hansmann Y, De Martino S, al e. Procalcitonin in pyelonephritis and acute community-acquired pneumonia in adults. *Press Med.* 2001;30:1091-6.

[71] Assicot M, Bohuon C, Gendrel D, al e. High serum procalcitonin concentrations in patients with sepsis and infection. *Lancet.* 1993;341:515-8.

[72] El-Solh A, Vora H, Knight III P, Porhomayon J. Diagnostic use of serum procalcitonin levels in pulmonary aspiration syndromes. *Crit Care Med.* 2011;39:1251-6.

[73] Andreola B, Bressan S, Callegaro S, Liverani A, Plebani M, Da Dalt L. Procalcitonin and C-Reactive Protein as Diagnostic Markers of Severe Bacterial Infections in Febrile Infants and Children in the Emergency Department. *Pediatr Infect Dis J.* 2007;26:672-7.

[74] Lopez A, Cubells C, Garcia J, Pou J. and the Spanish Society of Pediatric Emergencies. Procalcitonin in pediatric emergency departments for the early diagnosis of invasive bacterial infections in febrile infants: results of a multicenter study

and utility of a rapid qualitative test for this marker. *Pediatr Infect Dis J*. 2003;22:895-903.

[75] Bouadama L, Luyt C, Tubach F, al e. Use of procalcitonin to reduce patients' exposure to antibiotics in intensive care units (PRORATA trial): A multicentre randomized controlled trial. *Lancet*. 2010;375:463-74.

[76] Schuetz P, Christ-Crain M, Thomann R, al e. Effect of procalcitonin-based guidelines vs standard guidelines on antibiotic use in lower respiratory tract infections: the ProHOSP randomized controlled trial. *JAMA*. 2009;302:1059-66.

[77] Stolz D, Smyrnions N, Eggimann P, al e. Procalcitonin for reduced antibiotic exposure in ventilator-associated pneumonia: A randomized study. *Eur Respir J*. 2009;34:1364-75.

[78] Seligman R, Meisner M, Lisboa T, Hertz F, Filippin T, Fachel J, *et al*. Decreases in procalcitonin and C-reactive protein are strong predictors of survival in ventilator-associated pneumonia. *Crit Care*. 2006;10:R125.

[79] Angelousi A, Karageoropoulos D, Kapaskelis A, Falagas M. Association between thyroid function tests at baseline and the outcome of patients with sepsis or septic shock: a systematic review. *European Journal of Endocrinology*. 2011;164:147-55.

[80] Peeters R, Wouters P, Kaptein R, van Toor H, Visser T, Van den Berghe G. Reduced activation and increased inactivation of thyroid hormone in tissues of critically ill patients. *Journal of Endocrinology and Metabolism*. 2003;88:3202-11.

[81] Attia J, Margetts P, Guyatt G. Diagnosis of thryoid disease in hospitalized patients: a systematic review. *Archives of Internal Medicine*. 1999;159:658-65.

[82] Inan M, Koyuncu A, Aydin C, Turan M, Gokgoz S, Sen M. Thyroid Hormone supplementation in Sepsis: an experimental study. *Surg Today*. 2003;33:24-9.

[83] Ross R, Miell J, Freeman E, Jones J, Matthews D, Preece M, *et al*. Critically ill patients have high basal growth hormone levels with attenuated oscillatory activity associated with low levels of insulin-like growth factor-1. *Clinical Endocrinology*. 1991;35:47-54.

[84] Onenli-Mungan N, Yildizdas D, Yapicioglu H, Topaloglu A, Yuksel B, Ozer G. Growth Hormone and insulin-like growth factor 1 levels and their relation to survival in children with bacterial sepsis and septic shock. *Journal of Pediatrics and Child Health*. 2004;40:221-6.

[85] Schuetz P, Muller B, Nusbaumer C, Wieland M, Christ-Crain M. Circulating levels of GH predict mortality and complement prognostic scores in critically ill medical patients. *European Journal of Endocrinology*. 2009;160:157-63.

[86] Takala J, Ruokenen E, Webster N, Nielsen M, Zandstra D, Vundelinckx G, *et al*. Increased mortality associated with growth hormone treatment in critically ill adults. *N Engl J Med*. 1999;341:785-92.

[87] Muller B, Morgenthaler N, Stolz D, Schuetz P, Muller C, Bingisser R, *et al*. Circulating levels of copeptin, a novel biomarker in lower respiratory tract infections. *Eur J Clin Invest*. 2007;37.

[88] Katan M, Christ-Crain M. The stress hormone copeptin: a new prognostic biomarker in acute illness. *Swiss Med Wkly*. 2010;140:w13101.

[89] Bercault N, Boulain T, Kuteifan K, Wolf M, Runge I, Fleury J. Obesity-related excess mortality rate in an adult intensive care unit. *Crit Care Med.* 2004;32:998-1003.
[90] Shapiro N, Khankin E, Van Meurs M, Shih S, Lu S, Yano M, *et al.* Leptin Exacerbates Sepsis-Mediated Morbidity and Mortality. *The Journal of Immunology*. 2010;185:517-24.
[91] Yousef A, Amr Y, Suliman G. The diagnostic value of serum leptin monitoring and its correlation with tumour necrosis factor-alpha in critically ill patients: a prospective observational study. *Crit Care*. 2010;14:R33.
[92] Watson R, Carcillo J, Linde-Swirble W, Clermont G, Lidicker J, Angus D. The Epidemiology of Severe Sepsis in Children in the United States. *Am J Respir Crit Care Med*. 2003;167:695-701.
[93] Esper A, Moss M, Lewis C, Nisbet R, Mannino D, Martin G. The role of infection and comorbidity: Factors that influence disparities in sepsis. *Crit Care Med.* 2006;34:2576-82.
[94] Adrie C, Azoulay E, Francais A, Clec'h C, Darques L, Schwebel C, *et al.* Influence of Gender on the Outcome of Severe Sepsis: A Reappraisal. *Chest*. 2007;132:1786-93.
[95] Trimarchi T. Endocrine problems in critically ill children: An overview. *ACCN Clin Issues*. 2006;17:66-78.
[96] Arnal L, F S. Pediatric Septic Shock: Why has mortality decreased? The utility of goal-directed therapy. *Semin Pediatr Infect Dis*. 2003;14:165-72.
[97] Ceneviva G, Paschall J, Maffei F, Carcillo J. Hemodynamic support in fluid-refractory pediatric septic shock. *Pediatrics*. 1998;102:e19.
[98] Vlasselaers D, Milants I, Desmet L, et al. Intensive Insulin therapy for patients in paediatric intensive care: a prospective, randomised controlled study. *Lancet* 2009;373:547-56.
[99] Suh S, Gum E, Hamby A, Chan P, Swanson R. Hypogycemic neuronal death is triggered by glucose reperfusion and activation of neuronal NADPH oxidase. *J Clin Invest* 2007;117:910-18.

Alternative Therapies for Septic Shock: Beyond Early Goal-Directed Therapy

Megan Rech, Megan Prasse and Payal Gurnani
Rush University Medical Center
U.S.A.

1. Introduction

Severe sepsis and septic shock are major concerns within our health care system, accounting for 2.26 cases per 100 hospital discharges (Angus et al., 2001). The incidence of sepsis has increased by 9% each year (Martin et al., 2003), and mortality ranges from 17.9% to 70% depending on severity of disease and factors such as age, sex, ethnic origin, and comorbidities (Angus et al., 2001; Martin et al., 2003; Alberti et al., 2002). The annual economic burden of severe sepsis in the United States is $17 billion (Angus et al., 2001).
Early goal-directed therapy is a stepwise approach to treatment of severe sepsis and septic shock and includes fluid resuscitation, optimizing hemodynamic parameters, early and appropriate antibiotic administration, and source identification and control (Figure 1). The appropriate use of EGDT has shown to significantly reduce mortality, demonstrating an absolute risk reduction in mortality of 16% compared to physician-driven treatment (Rivers et al., 2001). Beyond these recommendations, there are several adjunctive therapies which

Monitoring Parameter	Intervention	Goal
Central venous pressure (CVP)	Crystalloids (i.e. normal saline, lactated ringer's) and colloids (i.e. albumin)	CVP 8-12 mm Hg
Mean arterial pressure (MAP)	Vasopressors (i.e. norepinephrine, dopamine, vasopressin)	MAP ≥65 mm Hg
Central venous oxygen saturation ($ScvO_2$)	Packed red blood cells, ionotropes (i.e. dobutamine, milrinone)	Hematocrit ≥30%, $ScvO_2$ ≥70%
Cultures	Antimicrobial Agents	Early/appropriate therapy

Adapted from the Surviving Sepsis Campaign guidelines for management of severe sepsis and septic shock (Dellinger et al., 2008).

Fig. 1. Early Goal-Directed Therapy.

have been studied; their use, however, is highly dependent upon severity of illness, response to EGTD, and patient-specific characteristics. The use of these adjunctive therapies is also limited by their evidence in the literature compared to other approaches such as fluid resuscitation and early and appropriate antibiotic administration.

The goal of this chapter is to discuss alternative pharmacologic therapies for the treatment of septic shock following the initiation and optimization of EGDT. The therapies discussed in this chapter are as follows: corticosteroids, activated protein C, immunoglobulin, statins, and toll-like receptor inhibitors.

2. Pathophysiology of sepsis

The rationale for use of targeted therapies in sepsis is based on pathophysiologic processes. As discussed in other chapters, sepsis results from the complex interaction between an infecting pathogen and host responses, including inflammation, coagulation and the immune system (Russel, 2006). The immune system, which consists of mucosal defences to prevent host tissue invasion, is comprised of endogenous bacterial flora and structural barriers, an early response mounted by the innate immune system, and a delayed response via the adaptive immune system (Nduka & Parrillo, 2009). The key concept in the development and progression from infection to sepsis to severe sepsis and septic shock is the disparity between the host response and the invading organism's virulence.

3. Corticosteroids

3.1 Mechanism of action

Adrenal insufficiency is a common finding in patients with severe sepsis and septic shock (Annetta et al., 2009). Previous literature has demonstrated that elevated baseline cortisol levels or inadequate response to stimulation via a corticotropin test are associated with higher mortality (Annane et al., 2000).

Secretion of cortisol is controlled by the hypothalamic-pituitary-adrenal (HPA) axis and stimulated by fevers, pain, hypoxia, hypoglycemia and alterations in blood pressure. Stimulation of the HPA axis causes the hypothalamus to release corticotropin-releasing hormone (CRH), which in turn stimulates the pituitary to release adrenocorticotropic hormone (ACTH) (Figure 2) (Schimmer & Funder, 2011). Release of ACTH causes the zona fasciculata of the adrenal cortex to release glucocorticoids, primarily cortisol. Cortisol then inhibits further release of CRH and ACTH via a negative feedback mechanism (Annetta et al., 2009).

Glucocorticoids have various effects on the body, mediating cardiovascular, metabolic, immunologic and inflammatory systems. Glucocorticoids are required for normal reactivity to α-mediated endogenous catecholamines (i.e norepinephrine, epinephrine) and angiotensin II (Chrousos, 2009). Not only do they stimulate the production of catecholamines, but they potentiate their actions through up-regulation of α-adrenergic receptors. Glucocorticoids also lead to inhibition of nitric oxide and prostaglandin synthesis, resulting in modulation of vascular permeability (Annetta et al., 2009; Marik et al., 2008). Metabolic effects of glucocorticoids include stimulation of gluconeogenesis and glycogenolysis resulting in increased blood glucose concentrations. Glucocorticoids activate proteinolysis in muscle and inhibit protein synthesis, resulting in increased free amino acid substrate for gluconeogenesis. Hyperglycemia is beneficial in stressful states such as sepsis due to increased energy requirements (Pilkis & Granner, 1992). Glucocorticoids inhibit osteoblasts and activate osteoclasts, resulting in bone destruction. They also decrease calcium stores through inhibition of intestinal calcium uptake and increased urinary secretion by decreasing renal reabsorption (Annetta et al., 2009). Glucocorticoids have potent anti-inflammatory and immune-modulating effects. They decrease the amount and function of several immune cells, including T and B lymphocytes, macrophages, neutrophils, eosinophils, and monocytes. They also modulate the activity and production of cytokines [i.e interleukin-1 (IL-1), IL-2, IL-6 and tumor necrosis factor alpha (TNF-α)], chemokines and other inflammatory mediators, such as histamine and bradykinin. Lastly, glucocorticoids have anti-inflammatory effects via propagation of the release of anti-inflammatory factors (IL-10, IL-1 receptor antagonist and soluble TNF receptor) (Annetta et al., 2009; Marik et al., 2008; Fahey & Guyre, 1981).

Severe illness and stress activate the HPA axis. Once activated, serum levels of cortisol-binding globulin levels fall up to 50%, resulting in a significant increase in the amount of free cortisol (Ho et al., 2006). In critically ill patients this pathway may be impaired, resulting in adrenal insufficiency. Prevalence of adrenal insufficiency in septic shock has been reported in up to 60% of patients (Annane et al., 2006). The mechanism of action of HPA axis dysfunction is poorly-understood, but may include decreased production of CRH, ACTH, cortisol, and the dysfunction of their receptors. Accord to the American College of *Critical Care Medicine* guidelines, HPA axis dysfunction in the setting of critical illness is best-described as critical illness-related corticosteroid insufficiency (CIRCI) (Marik et al., 2008).

3.2 Pharmacology

Many synthetic corticosteroids (e.g. dexamethasone, prednisone, etc.) have been developed to address pharmacological and therapeutic concerns, such as bioavailability and variable glucocorticoid and mineralocorticoid potencies (See Table 1). These agents are primarily used for their anti-inflammatory effects in disorders of various organ systems (Hydrocortisone prescribing information, 2010; Chrousos, 2008).

Hydrocortisone is the pharmaceutical product equivalent to cortisol; therefore, it is used as replacement therapy in adrenocortical deficiency states (Hydrocortisone prescribing information, 2010; Chrousos, 2008).

Hydrocortisone is available intravenously as the highly water-soluble hydrocortisone sodium succinate, which permits the immediate intravenous or intramuscular administration of high doses of hydrocortisone in a small volume of diluent. Following the intravenous injection of hydrocortisone sodium succinate, demonstrable effects are evident within one hour and persist for a variable period. Hydrocortisone is primarily bound to corticosteroid-binding globulin. Only 5% to 10% is unbound and biologically active. It is metabolized in the liver to inactive metabolites. Renal excretion of the administered dose is nearly complete within 12 hours (Hydrocortisone prescribing information, 2010; Schimmer, 2011).

Fludrocortisone is a synthetic corticosteroid with both glucocorticoid and mineralocorticoid activity; however, it has a much higher mineralocorticoid potency, producing marked sodium retention and increased urinary potassium excretion (Fludrocortisone prescribing information, 2009; Chrousos, 2008).

Following oral administration, 100% of fludrocortisone is detected in the serum, half of which is bound to plasma proteins. It is metabolized in the liver and excreted renally with a half-life of 3.5 hours (Fludrocortisone prescribing information, 2009).

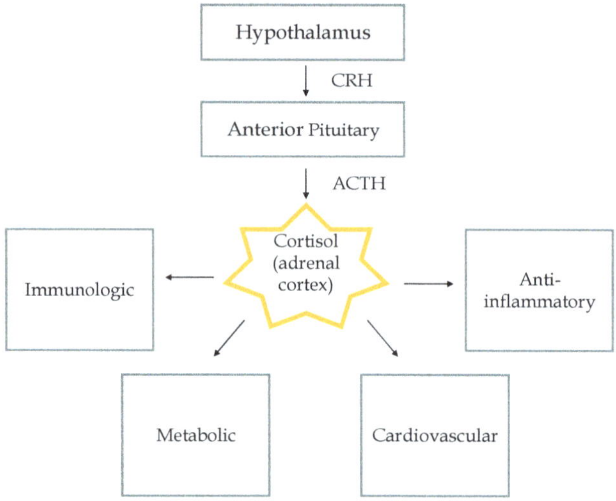

CRH=corticotropin releasing hormone, ACTH=adrenocorticotropin hormone

Fig. 2. Corticosteroid mechanism of action.

		Relative potency to Hydrocortisone		Pharmacokinetics	
	Equivalent Glucocorticoid Dose (mg)	Glucocorticoid	Mineralocorticoid	Plasma half-life (minutes)	Duration of Action (hours)
Short Acting					
Hydrocortisone (Cortisol)	20	1	1	90	8-12
Intermediate Acting					
Prednisone	5	4	0.8	60	12-36
Prednisolone	5	4	0.8	200	12-36
Methylprednisolone	4	5	0.5	180	12-36
Long Acting					
Dexamethasone	0.75	30	0	200	36-54
Mineralocorticoid					
Fludrocortisone	–	15	150	240	24-36
Aldosterone	–	0	400+	20	--

Reference: Adrenal Cortical Steroids. Drug Facts and Comparisons. 5th ed. St. Louis, Facts and Comparisons, Inc.:122-128, 1997

Table 1. Corticosteroid Dosing and Equivalence

3.3 Clinical trials

Several clinical trials have been conducted assessing the use of steroid therapy in sepsis. In the last decade, four meta-analyses have been conducted to evaluate the benefit of corticosteroids in sepsis. The first two meta-analyses demonstrated high-dose corticosteroid use in sepsis and septic shock did not improve survival rates. (Cronin et al., 1995; Lefering & Neugebauer, 1995). The next two demonstrated long courses of low-dose corticosteroids to aid in earlier reversal of shock as well as a mortality benefit (Annane et al., 2004; Minneci et al., 2004).

The first landmark trial in recent years assessing the use of corticosteroids in septic shock was a randomized, placebo-controlled, double-blind, multicenter study assessing hydrocortisone 50 mg intravenous every 6 hours and fludrocortisone 50 μg by mouth daily for 7 days versus placebo in 300 patients with vasopressor-unresponsive septic shock (Annane et al., 2002). This study demonstrated significant shock reversal and a reduction in mortality in patients with relative adrenal insufficiency (non-responders to a corticotropin test). Adverse effects were similar between the two groups. The authors concluded that treatment with low doses of hydrocortisone and fludrocortisone significantly reduced the risk of death in patients with septic shock and relative adrenal insufficiency without increasing adverse events (Annane et al., 2002).

The second clinical trial in recent years (the CORTICUS trial) was a randomized, placebo-controlled, double-blind, multicenter study assessing 251 patients that received hydrocortisone 50 mg intravenous every 6 hours for 5 days versus 248 patients that received placebo (Sprung et al., 2008). This study failed to show a mortality benefit with steroid therapy for patients in septic shock with relative adrenal insufficiency (non-responders to a corticotropin test). In the hydrocortisone group, shock was reversed earlier than in the placebo group; however, there were more episodes of superinfection, including new sepsis and septic shock. (Sprung et al., 2008). The external validity of this trial may be limited due to the inclusion of patients, regardless of their blood pressure response to vasopressors. This is an issue as patients with patients with blood pressures responsive to vasopressor therapy would likely not be candidates for steroid therapy.

3.4 Place in therapy

Based on the results of the aforementioned studies, there is much discord in regards to the optimal time to initiate corticosteroids for septic shock. Corticosteroids appear to reverse shock more rapidly, but effects on mortality are unclear and many adverse effects have been reported. Consensus guidelines suggest that intravenous hydrocortisone (200-300 mg daily in divided doses) be given only to adult septic shock patients unresponsive to fluid resuscitation and vasopressor therapy. The addition of oral fludrocortisone (50 μg daily) to corticosteroid therapy is considered optional if hydrocortisone is used (Dellinger et al., 2008; Marik et al., 2008).

3.5 Adverse effects

Complications associated with the use of corticosteroids are dependent upon dosage and duration of therapy. In critically ill patients, the most important adverse effects include immune suppression with an increased risk of infections (both typical and opportunistic), impaired wound healing, hyperglycemia, myopathies, hypokalemia, psychosis, HPA axis and GR suppression (Annetta et al., 2009).

4. Activated protein C

4.1 Mechanism of action

In sepsis, toxins and inflammatory cytokines (i.e. TNF-α and IL-1) cause direct activation of coagulation via up-regulation of tissue factor (TF) from monocytes and endothelial cells (Figure 3) (Bernard et al., 2001). TF leads to thrombin formation and fibrin clot. In addition inflammatory cytokines and thrombin can impair the endogenous fibrinolysis by stimulating the release of plasminogen-activator inhibitor 1 (PAI-1) from platelets and endothelial cells. PAI-1 is a potent inhibitor of tissue plasminogen activator, which lyses clots. Thrombin further potentiates the prothrombotic state when it activates thrombin-activatable fibrinolysis inhibitor (TAFI) (Toussaint & Gerlach, 2009; Dellinger, 2003; Bernard et al., 2001).

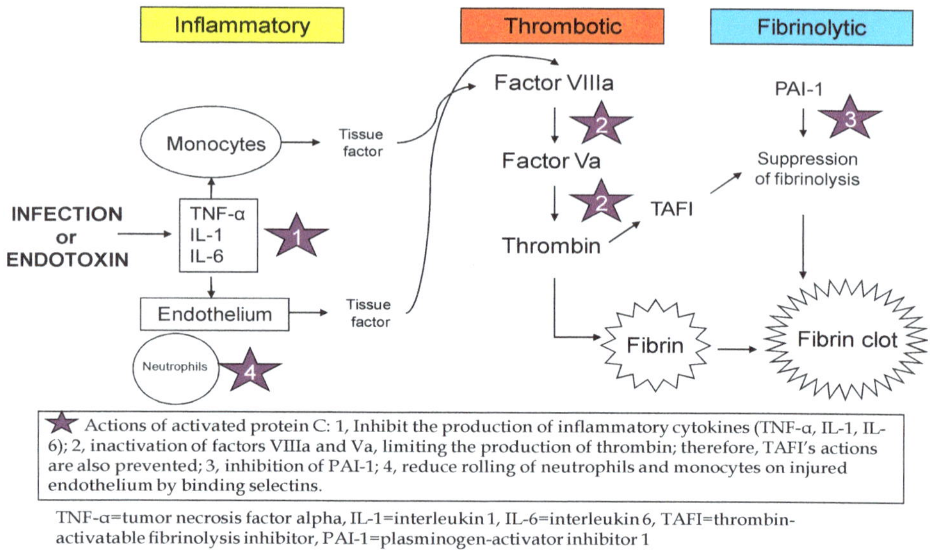

Fig. 3. Mechanisms of action of Activated Protein C

Protein C is activated when thrombin binds to thrombomodulin, which is impaired by the inflammatory response. Endothelial injury and pro-inflammatory cytokines decrease thrombomodulin levels resulting in activation of the coagulation cascade (Bernard et al., 2001). Coagulation in sepsis can lead to microvascular thrombosis, organ ischemia, multiorgan dysfunction, and death. Activated protein C is an anticoagulant and pro-fibrinolytic that exerts its effect through inactivation of clotting factors Va, VIIIa, and PAI-1, limiting the production of thrombin. A reduction in thrombin results in decreased activation of the coagulation cascade and also modulation of the systemic inflammatory response associated with sepsis (Toussaint & Gerlach, 2009; Dellinger, 2003; Bernard et al., 2001).

4.2 Pharmacology

Activated protein C is available pharmacologically as drotrecogin alfa. Following continuous intravenous administration of drotrecogin alfa at doses between 12 µg/kilograms (kg)/hour (hr) to 30 µg/kg/hr, steady state concentrations are reached within two hours. Drotrecogin alfa and endogenous activated protein C are inactivated by endogenous plasma protease inhibitors; therefore, no dosing adjustments are necessary for renal or hepatic dysfunction. The initial phase has a half-life of 13 minutes and the second phase half-life is 1.6 hours (Drotrecogin alpha prescribing information, 2008).

4.3 Clinical trials

Two major clinical trials have explored the mortality benefit of drotrecogin alfa in patients with severe sepsis and septic shock. The first, the PROWESS study, was a randomized, double-blind, placebo-controlled, multicenter trial that enrolled 1690 patients with systemic inflammation and organ failure due to acute infection (Bernard et al., 2001). Patients received an intravenous infusion of either placebo or drotrecogin alfa at 24 µg/kg/hr for 96 hours. This study was terminated early due to an absolute reduction in mortality of 6.1% in the treatment group (P=0.005). The incidence of serious bleeding was significantly higher in the drotrecogin alfa group than in the placebo group. A limitation of this study is the inclusion of prospectively-defined subgroup analyses performed for various baseline characteristics [i.e Acute Physiology and Chronic Health Evaluation (APACHE II) score, age, sex, protein C deficiency]. Although the authors stated there were consistent treatment effects between these groups, this may be misleading as subgroup analyses, in general, lack an intent to treat group as well as have the potential for sampling bias and sample error.

In the recently -completed PROWESS-SHOCK trial, drotrecogin alpha failed to demonstrate a survival benefit. Preliminary analysis showed a 28-day all cause mortality rate of 26.4% in drotrecogin alpha group compared to 24.2% in placebo-treated patients (P=0.31). As a result, the manufacturer has announced a worldwide voluntary market withdrawal of drotrecogin alpha.

4.4 Place in therapy

Based on the results of the PROWESS trial, the Food and Drug Administration (FDA) approved drotrecogin alfa, but required a second study be conducted to evaluate its efficacy in patients with severe sepsis with a low risk of death. The ADDRESS study enrolled 2640 patients with severe sepsis and an APACHE II score <25 or single organ failure to receive the same intervention as above (Abraham et al., 2005). This trial was terminated early due to an increased risk of bleeding with no significant reduction in 28-day mortality (Abraham et al., 2005).

4.5 Adverse effects

As observed in clinical trials, bleeding is the significant adverse effect associated with administration of activated protein C (Bernard et al., 2001; Abraham et al., 2005).

5. Immunoglobulin

5.1 Mechanism of action

Intravenous immunoglobulin G (IVIG) contains IgG antibodies produced by B lymphocyte cells pooled from several thousands of blood donors. IVIG generates high polyspecificity against bacterial, viral, parasitic and mycoplasma antigens and their toxins. It has been shown to be efficacious in various autoimmune and immunodeficiency diseases (Norrby-Teglund & Stevens, 1998). There are four subclasses of IgG (IgG1, IgG2, IgG3, and IgG4), of which IgG1 is the major component in IVIG preparations. IgA and IgM are also found in preparations of immunoglobulin; however quantities are minuscule compared to IgG. IgG1 has several functions within the immune system, including complement activation, tissue protection and virus inactivation. IgG1 also opsonizes bacteria, marking these cells for ingestion and phagocytosis (Knapp & Colburn, 1990).

Superantigens are a class of antigens that cause non-specific activation of T-cells, resulting in massive cytokine release. Patients infected with these antigens develop severe and rapidly-progressing sepsis (Ryan & Ray, 2010). Due to its ability to neutralize a broad range of superantigens and facilitate opsonization of streptococci (Norrby-Teglund & Stevens, 1998), IVIG therapy has been implicated in the treatment of septic shock secondary to group A Streptococci (GAS) infections, including necrotizing fasciitis and streptococcal toxic shock syndrome (STSS) (Darenberg et al., 2003). Both of these manifestations of GAS are severe, invasive infections with mortality rates up to 80% despite early and appropriate antimicrobial therapy (Davies et al., 1996).

5.2 Pharmacology

Immunoglobulin is available in subcutaneous and intravenous formulations. The bioavailability of subcutaneous immunoglobulin is approximately 73% compared to IVIG. After administration of IVIG (0.1–2 g/kg), serum concentrations rise, then fall rapidly in the first 1 to 7 days due to diffusion into lymph and extracellular fluid compartments (Immunoglobulin prescribing information, 2010). IVIG catabolism occurs slowly thereafter. The half-life of IgG is dependent on the half-lives of the IgG subclasses (Knapp & Colburn, 1990). There are several commercial preparations of IVIG available that contain varying amounts of IgG subclasses. Therefore, the half-life is dependent upon the product used, which report half-lives ranging between 25-48 days (Bonilla, 2008).

5.3 Clinical trials

There is a preponderance of literature available on the use of IVIG for treatment of severe sepsis and septic shock. However, many of these studies are observational in nature and limited in the number of participants and statistical power.

In order to assess the overall mortality benefit of IVIG therapy in severe sepsis and septic shock, a meta-analysis of 14 randomized controlled trials between 1988 and 2006 was conducted (Laupland et al., 2007). Most of these studies were small, ranging from 21 to 653 participants, comprised primarily of surgical intensive care unit patients with gram-negative infections. The median dose of IVIG was 0.92g/kg, with an interquartile range (IQR) from 0.75 to 1.0 g/kg, and half of the studies used preparations of IVIG that where enriched with IgA and/or IgM. Overall, there was a significant mortality benefit associated with use of IVIG in adults with sepsis. However, this effect was lost when only the high-quality studies where included in the analysis. High quality studies were considered those with adequate blinding, allocation concealment, and those that used intention-to-treat analysis. The authors concluded that further research is needed to determine the mortality benefit of IVIG in severe sepsis and septic shock (Laupland et al., 2007).

One study included in the above meta-analysis focused specifically on patients with STSS. This was a randomized, placebo-controlled, double-blind, multicenter study of 21 patients, of whom 10 received IVIG and 11 received placebo (Darenberg et al., 2003). This study was terminated prematurely due to slow patient recruitment, which was thought to be secondary to a low incidence of STSS in the participating centers. A dose of 1 g/kg on day 1 and 0.5 g/kg on days 2 and 3 was used. Though not statistically significant, the primary endpoint of mortality at 28 days was found to be 3.6-fold higher in placebo group (1 patient, IVIG vs. 4 patients, placebo). Patients in the treatment group also had a significant decrease in the sepsis-related organ failure assessment (SOFA) score at days 2 and 3. This study is limited by the number of patients enrolled; however it demonstrates that further research should be conducted to determine the benefit of IVIG therapy in STSS.

5.4 Place in therapy

The sepsis guidelines recommend that IVIG be used in children with sepsis and septic shock; however, there are no formal recommendation for the use of IVIG in adults. (Dellinger et al., 2008) The aforementioned meta-analysis demonstrated a mortality benefit with IVIG therapy as an adjuvant to standard of care. However, at this time further research is needed to determine which patients would benefit most from IVIG therapy. Though high quality studies are limited, there may be a mortality benefit in using IVIG in patients with STSS. The theoretical benefit of IVIG in septic patients infected with superantigen-generating pathogens is supported by one small study; however, larger, well-designed studies are needed. At present IVIG should be considered in patients with rapidly progressing sepsis due to confirmed or suspected GAS.

5.5 Adverse effects

The most common adverse reactions observed in ≥5% of the patients were headache, pyrexia, fatigue, rigors, nausea, chills, dizziness, vomiting, migraines, pain in extremities, urticaria, and cough. Hypersensitivity reactions have also been observed, so epinephrine should be readily available when administering. IVIG can induce a severe fall in blood pressure with anaphylactic reaction, even in patients who have tolerated previous treatment with IVIG (Immunoglobulin prescribing information, 2010).

Caution should be used in patients with acute or chronic renal failure, as over 100 cases of renal failure associated with IVIG have been reported. Patients predisposed to acute renal failure include those with any degree of preexisting renal insufficiency, diabetes mellitus, age greater than 65, volume depletion, sepsis, paraproteinemia, or patients receiving known nephrotoxic drugs. Especially in such patients, IGIV products should be administered at the minimum concentration available and the minimum rate of infusion feasible (Bonilla et al., 2008; Immunoglobulin prescribing information, 2010).

Aseptic meningitis has also been associated with IVIG use. There appears to be an increased risk of aseptic meningitis in patients with a history of migraines. Possible inciting factors include the IgG itself, various stabilizing products within each of the preparations, cytokine release triggered by the therapy, or cerebrovascular sensitivity (Sekul et al., 1994).

6. Statins

6.1 Mechanism of action

Statins are a class of lipid-lowering agents which inhibit the enzyme 3-hydroxyl-3-methylglutaryl-coenzyme A (HMG-CoA) reductase. Traditionally, they have been indicated for primary and secondary prevention of cardiovascular disease due their effects on reducing atherosclerosis. Endogenous cholesterol production starts from the precursor acetyl-CoA, which then is converted to hydroxymethylglutaryl-CoA (HMG-CoA). HMG-CoA reductase catalyzes the conversion of HMG-CoA to mevalonate in the rate-limiting step of cholesterol synthesis. Mevalonate is then converted to cholesterol through several steps. Inhibition of HMG-CoA reductase has been shown to reduce total cholesterol, low-density lipoprotein (LDL) cholesterol, apolipoprotein B, triglycerides, and increase high-density lipoprotein (HDL) cholesterol (Goa et al., 2008; Terblanche et al., 2006).

Independent from their lipid-lowering effects, statins exert various pleiotropic effects. They play a role in immune modulation, resulting in attenuation of the immune response. In animal models, statins have been shown to reduce leukocyte recruitment, adherence, and transmigration in a time-dependent manner (Goa et al., 2008; Diomede et al., 2001). Statins also cause a significant reduction of leucocytes adhesion to endothelium by down-regulation endothelial cell adhesion molecules on the cell surface (Goa et al., 2008; Pruefer et al., 2002). Finally, statins affect monocyte function. In a double-blind, placebo-controlled study of 20 healthy male volunteers, simvastatin was shown to attenuate up-regulation of toll-like receptors (TLR) 2 and 4 on the surface of monocytes by more than half after a lipopolysaccharide challenge. Blocking TLR expression was associated with decreased concentrations immune cytokines, such as TNF-a and monocyte chemoattractant protein-1 (Goa et al., 2008; Niessner et al., 2006).

Statins also inhibit pro-inflammatory markers, decreasing response to activation of the inflammatory cascade. In animal studies, statins were shown to reduce exudate production of interleukin-6 (IL-6) and monocyte chemotactic proteins (Diomede et al., 2001), as well as TNF-a, IL-8 and other inflammatory mediators involved in sepsis (Grip et al., 2002). Statins, particularly atorvastatin (Goa et al., 2008), have been shown to reduce serum concentrations of C-reactive protein (CRP), which is a major acute phase reactant in humans. CRP is produced mainly in the liver in response to IL-6. Statins decrease IL-6-induced CRP production through inhibition of protein geranylgeranylation within the hepatocytes (Arnaud et al., 2005).

Statins also modulate the coagulation cascade. They reduce monocyte tissue factor (TF) expression, decrease concentrations of von Willebrand factor, increase the expression and functional activity of thrombomodulin which in turn binds to thrombin to activate protein C, reduce levels of plasminogen activator inhibitor-1 (PAI-1) and increase tissue-type plasminogen activator (tPA), and reduce platelet aggregation, and reduce conversion of prothrombin to thrombin leading to a decrease in levels of fibrinogen. (Goa et al., 2008; Steiner et al.,2005; Bickel et al., 2002; Terblanche et al., 2006; Shi et al., 2003; Bourcier & Libby, 2000).

Endothelial cell dysfunction is central to the development of sepsis. Statins prevent this by increasing expression of endothelial nitric oxide synthase (eNOS), in conjunction with down-regulation of inducible nitric oxide synthase (iNOS). eNOS is activated to produce endothelium-derived NO for controlling vasomotor activity. This decreases occurrence of hypotension and attenuates resistance to vasoactive agents in patients with septic shock (Goa et al., 2008; McGown & Brookes, 2007).

6.2 Pharmacology

There are six different pharmacologic preparations of statins, each with varying dosing and relative potency (Table 2) (Goa et al., 2008; Pharmacist's Letter, 2009). Lovastatin, pravastatin sodium, and simvastatin are fungal-derived agents, whereas atorvastatin calcium, fluvastatin sodium and rosuvastatin are fully synthetic compounds (Goa et al., 2008). Statins are only available orally; therefore these agents cannot be administered to patients that do not have oral or enteral access for medication administration. Following absorption, statins undergo extensive first-pass extraction in the liver, thus the availability of drug in systemic circulation is variable. Most of the agents are metabolized in the liver through the cytochrome P450 (CYP 450) system; therefore, careful examination for drug interactions is warranted. Pravastatin is metabolized hepatically via sulfation; therefore, it may be considered over other agents for patients on concomitant substrates or inhibitors of CYP3A4 or CYP2C9. Statins have variable renal elimination. (Goa et al., 2008; Simvastatin prescribing information, 2011; Lovastatin prescribing information, 2010; Pravastain prescribing information, 2011).

Statins*						
Drug	Dose (mg)	Equivalent Dose (mg)	Bioavailability (%)	Protein Binding (%)	Metabolism	Half-life (hr)
Atorvastatin	10-80	20	12	98	CYP3A4	13-16
Fluvastatin	20-80	--	24	98	CYP2C9	1-3
Lovastatin	20-80	80	5	>95	CYP3A4	2-3
Pitavastain	1-4	--	80	96	UGT1A3, UGT2B7	11
Pravastatin	10-40	80	20	43-67	sulfation	2-3
Rosuvastatin	10-40	5	20	90	CYP2C9	19
Simvastain	10-80**	40	5	95-98	CYP3A4	1-3

* Goa,2008; Pharmacist's Letter, 2009
**Simvastain 80 mg is no longer recommended by the FDA unless previously maintained on this dose of > 1 year

Table 2. Statin Dosing and Equivalence

Though statins undergo hepatic metabolism, patients with renal dysfunction should exercise caution when using statins. They are also contraindicated in patients with active liver disease, including unexplained persistent elevations in hepatic transaminases (Simvastatin prescribing information, 2011).

All statins are pregnancy category X, meaning that they are contraindicated in women who are or may become pregnant. Cholesterol and cholesterol derivatives are needed for normal fetal development, and congenital abnormalities have been reported (Simvastatin prescribing information, 2011).

6.3 Clinical trials

There is much literature demonstrating the lipid-lowering properties of statins, but randomized, controlled trials examining their pleiotropic effects for treatment of severe

sepsis and septic shock are limited. Several retrospective and prospective observational studies have been conducting to explore infection-related mortality and incidence of hospitalization from sepsis in patients receiving statins. These studies have yielded mixed results (Almog et al., 2007; Gupta et al., 2007; Majumdar et al., 2006).
In order to clarify the effects of statin use in patients with sepsis, a recent meta-analysis was conducted. Twenty studies were included in the analysis, of which 18 were cohort studies, 1 matched cohort study with 2 case-control studies, and 1 randomized control trial (Janda et al., 2010). Meta-analysis for various infection-related outcomes favored use of statins for 30-day mortality, in-hospital mortality, pneumonia-related mortality, bacteremia-related mortality, sepsis-related mortality, and mixed infection-related mortality. The analysis was limited by the cohort design of the selected studies and the degree of heterogeneity among them, necessitating further randomized controlled studies (Janda et al., 2010).
One prospective, randomized, double-blind, placebo-controlled trial of 150 patients on preexisting statin therapy requiring hospitalization for infection compared atorvastatin 20 milligrams (mg) to placebo ((Kruger et al., 2011). No difference was found in progression of sepsis during hospitalization. The rate of decline of severe sepsis was similar between the groups. There was also no difference in mortality between the two groups; however, most of the study patients were not critically ill. Investigators concluded that this study does not support a beneficial role of continuing pre-existing statin therapy in patients with sepsis. Cessation of statin therapy was not associated with adverse effects secondary to rebound inflammation (Kruger et al., 2011).

6.4 Place in therapy

Currently sepsis consensus guidelines make no mention of statins as an adjunctive therapy for treatment of severe sepsis and septic shock. Conflicting data precludes a definitive recommendation for continuing pre-existing statin therapy in patients admitted with severe sepsis or septic shock. In patients with patent oral or parenteral access for medications, continuing statin therapy may be considered.

6.5 Adverse effects

Statins are safe in the majority of patients receiving them; however, in recent years attention has been drawn to their ability to cause myopathies progressing to rhabodomyolysis and liver dysfunction. These adverse effects are of particular concern in patients that develop sepsis because liver failure is a common complication of sepsis and drugs used in treating sepsis, such as steroids and neuromuscular blocking agents, can also cause myopathies (Goa et al., 2008; Pasternak et al., 2002).
Elevated liver transaminases occur in 0.5 to 2% of patients taking statins and are dose-dependent; however, progression to liver failure due to statins is very rare. Reversal of elevated transaminases frequently occurs with reduction in dose, and elevations do not often recur with either re-challenge or selection of another statin. Cholestasis and active liver disease are contraindications to statin use, but exacerbation of liver disease by statins has not been shown (Pasternak et al., 2002).
Myopathies are characterized by non-specific muscle aches or joint pain, usually without elevations in creatinine kinase (CK). Rarely, patients on statins may develop muscle aches and pains associated with elevated CK, generally >10 times the upper limit of normal (ULN). Failure to discontinue statin therapy can lead to rhabdomyolysis, myoglobinuria,

and acute renal necrosis. In 2001, cerivastatin was withdrawn from the market due to reports of serious myopathy, including 31 reports of death from rhabdomyolysis in the United States (Pasternak et al., 2002). More recently, the Food and Drug Administration (FDA) has put out a recommendation to limit the use of simvastain 80 mg due to risk of muscle injury (FDA Consumer Health Information, 2011).

In 2002, the American College of Cardiology/American Heart Association/National Heart, Lung and Blood Institute issued a clinical advisory on the use and safety of statins. It recommends that all patients initiated on a statin should have liver transaminases checked after 12 weeks of therapy, then annually. CK should be monitored at baseline, and then muscle symptoms should be evaluated 6 to 12 weeks after initiation. If symptoms are present, a CK should be obtained. This statement also highlighted patients at risk for developing myopathies, including patients >80 years, small body frame and frailty, multisystem disease, multiple medications, post-operative period, and specific concomitant medications (i.e. fibrates, azoles, macrolides, cyclosporine, protease inhibitors, verapamil and amiodarone) (Pasternak et al., 2002).

7. Toll-like receptor inhibitors

7.1 Mechanism of action

Key components of the innate immune system are pattern recognition receptors (PRRs), such as toll-like receptors (TLRs). These agents act as sentinels against damage-associated molecular pattern molecules (DAMPs), alarmins, and invading organisms carrying pathogen-associated molecular patterns (PAMPs) (Zhu & Mohan, 2010). PAMPs are a diverse set of microbial molecules which contain different recognizable biochemical features that alert the organism to intruding pathogens. Alarmins are non-infectious endogenous molecules that signal tissue and cell damage. Both alarmins and PAMPs are a subgroup of DAMPs (Bianchi, 2007). Once TLRs sense DAMPs, the innate immune response and antigen-specific adaptive immune response are activated. An intracellular cascade of signaling molecules occurs that ultimately activates the transcription factors, nuclear factor- κB (NF-κB) and interferon regulatory factors (IRFs). These transcription factors lead to expression of various inflammatory cytokines, interferons, and chemokines (Zhu & Mohan, 2010).

There are at least 10 types of TLRs that have been identified in humans. Bacterial flagellin and Toxoplasma profilin are recognized by TLR5, TLR11 and TLR12. Bacterial lipopeptides are recognized by TLR1, TLR2 and TLR6. Lipopolysaccharide (LPS), found in the outer membrane of gram-negative bacteria, and endotoxin are recognized by TLR4 (Zhu & Mohan, 2010). Pharmacologic agents targeting individual TLRs are being developed in order to prevent activation of the immune response associated with DAMP binding. Of particular interest in sepsis are TLR2 and TLR4 because expression of these PRRs is increased on monocytes in healthy volunteers undergoing an LPS challenge (Wittbole et al., 2005), and in patients with sepsis (Harter et al., 2004).

TLR4 binds with MD2, an extracellular accessory protein, which form a complex that interacts with LPS (Figure 4) (Wittebole, et al., 2010). Eritoran is a LPS antagonist that binds to the TLR4-MD-2 complex, rendering it unable to illicit the immune response. Resatorvid is another agent that inhibits TLR4 signaling by binding directly to a specific amino acid in the TLR4-intracellular domain, thus is a TRL4 antagonist (Wittebole, et al., 2010).

Other medications that are currently marketed for other indications have been found to interact with TLRs in animal studies. Agents such as chloroquine, ketamine, nicotine and statins have various immunologic properties through their interactions with TLRs (Wittebole, et al., 2010), but few studies exist to determine the clinical relevance of these interactions in humans.

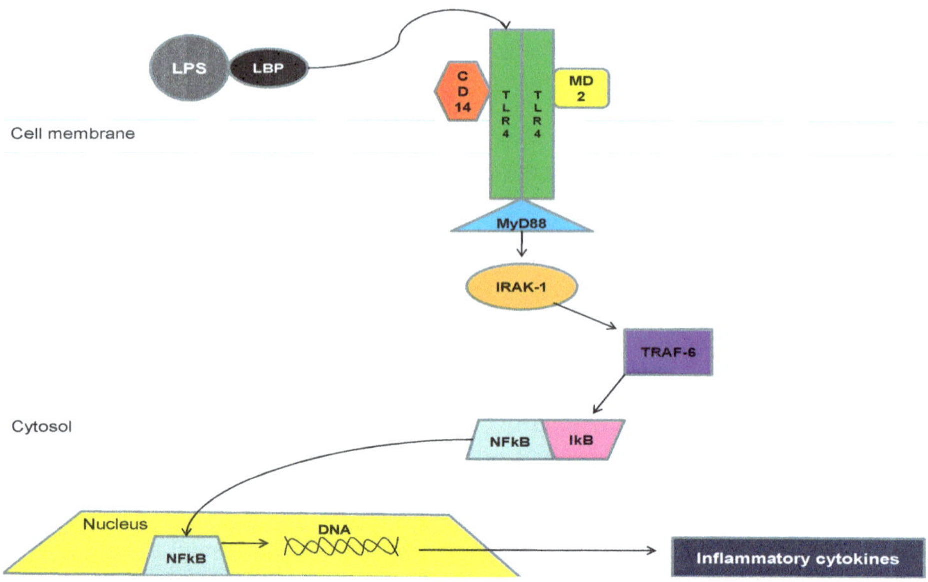

LPS=Lipopolysaccharide, LBP=Lipopolysaccharide-binding protein, TLR-4=toll-like receptor 4, MD2=myb regulated gene, MyD88=myeloid differentiation primary response gene, IRAK-1=interleukin-1 receptor associated kinase, TRAF-6=TNFa receptor associated factor, IkB=inhibitory kappa B proteins, NFkB=nuclear factor kappa B, DNA=deoxyribonucleic acid

Fig. 4. Toll-like receptor 4 mechanism of action

7.2 Pharmacology

Eritoran has been studied as an intravenous infusion in a phase I study. Following administration, it has a relatively low volume of distribution and a long half-life, up to 62.7 hours. Eritoran is highly bound to lipoproteins and is cleared hepatically (Rossignol et al., 2004).

7.3 Clinical trials

Of all of the agents that have TLR-modulating properties, eritoran has been studied the most extensively. In a laboratory study, eritoran caused a dose-dependent inhibitory effect on IL-6 and TNF-α production in LPS-stimulated human monocytes from healthy volunteers (Czeslick et al., 2006). Another group of healthy volunteers were challenged with 4 ng/kg of LPS. All eritoran doses, from 50 mcg to 250 mcg, achieved statistically significant reductions in elevated temperature, heart rate, C-reactive protein levels, white blood cell count, TNF-*a* and IL-6 levels compared to placebo. In doses >100 mcg/kg, eritoran ameliorated LPS-induced fever, chills, headache, myalgia, and tachycardia (Lynn et al., 2003).

A recent prospective, randomized, double-blind, placebo-controlled, multicenter, ascending-dose phase II trial was conducted in 293 patients who were randomized either eritoran high dose (105 mg), eritoran small dose (45 mg) or placebo. A trend towards a lower mortality rate was observed in patients at highest risk of mortality by APACHE II score quartile in the eritoran 105 mg group. A trend toward a higher mortality rate was observed in subjects in the lowest APACHE II score quartile for the eritoran 105 mg group. Number of adverse events was similar among all treatment groups (Tidswell et al., 2010).

A phase III study comparing eritoran 105 mg to placebo in patients with severe sepsis was conducted; however, due to fact that the study did not meet its primary endpoint of reduction of 28-day all-cause mortality Eisai Inc. will not submit marketing authorization applications. The pharmaceutical company will continue an analysis of the data and determine next steps.

Resatorvid was studied in a randomized, double-blind, placebo-controlled study of patients with severe sepsis and related respiratory or cardiovascular failure. Unfortunately, this study was ended prematurely due to insufficient cytokine suppression (Wittebole et al., 2010).

7.4 Place in therapy

Though eritoran and resatorvid are not currently marketed and are still under investigation for use in severe sepsis and septic shock, pharmacologic agents targeting TLR2 and TLR4 remain promising interventions.

7.5 Adverse effects

Eritoran was well tolerated in clinical trials. Anemia, diarrhea, insomnia, acute renal failure, phlebitis and rash were observed more frequently in the group receiving eritoran compared to the group receiving placebo. Serious adverse events included cardiac arrest, hepatobiliary events, multiorgan failure, sepsis, atrial fibrillation, respiratory failure and deep vein thrombosis (Tidswell et al., 2010).

8. Conclusion

Despite initiation of EGDT, severe sepsis and septic shock remain a major cause of mortality and economic burden in the United States. Each of the therapies discussed above can be considered after optimization of EGDT once the etiology and severity of sepsis is determined.

Though the use of corticosteroid remains controversial, hydrocortisone can be considered in patients that are hemodynamically unstable despite adequate fluid resuscitation and vasopressor therapy. It is unclear at this time if there is a role for IVIG in all patients with severe sepsis and septic shock. Because IVIG neutralizes superantigens and opsonizes streptococci, patients with confirmed or suspected group GAS infections may benefit from therapy. Continuation of pre-existing statin therapy can be considered in patients with severe sepsis and septic shock with intact oral or enteral access. Finally, while there are currently no available toll-like receptor inhibitors marketed in the United States, interventions at the cellular level in sepsis are still in their infancy of investigation and present promising adjunctive therapies.

Drug	Mechanism	Dose	Adverse Effects
Corticosteroids	Metabolic, cardiovascular, immunologic and anti-inflammatory properties	Hydrocortisone 200-300 mg/day divided in 3-4 doses	Immune suppression, increased risk of infections, impaired wound healing, hyperglycemia, myopathies, hypokalemia, psychosis, HPA axis and GR suppression
Activated Protein C	Anticoagulant and pro-fibrinolytic	24 mcg/kg/hr infusions for 96 hours	Bleeding
IVIG	IgG antibodies; neutralize superantigens, opsonize streptococci	Doses vary; For STSS – 1 g/kg on day 1, 0.5 g/kg on day 2 &3	Headache, pyrexia, fatigue, rigors, nausea, chills, dizziness, vomiting, pain in extremity, urticaria, cough, hypersensitivity reactions, renal failure, aseptic meningitis
Statins	Immunologic, anti-inflammatory, and anticoagulant properties	Vary depending on agent (see table 2)	Myositis, rhabdomyolysis, elevated liver transaminases
TLR modulators	Direct or indirect TLR inihibition	Eritoran 105 mg intravenous	Anemia, diarrhea, insomnia, acute renal failure, phlebitis and rash, cardiac arrest,atrial fibrillation, respiratory failure, deep vein thrombosis

Table 3. Summary of Interventions

Sepsis is a complex physiologic process that involves activation of the inflammatory system and coagulation cascade, thereby creating multiple outlets for possible therapeutic intervention. At this time, more research is warranted to determine the most optimal therapeutic regimen based on individual patient factors, such as etiology, severity of illness and comorbid conditions.

9. References

Abraham, E.; Laterre, P.; Garg, R.; et al. (2005). Drotecogin alfa (activated) for adult patients with severe sepsis and a low risk of death. *New England Journal of Medicine*, Vol.353, No.13, (September 2005), pp. 1332-41, ISSN 0028-4793.

Alberti, C. ; Brun-Buisson, C. ; Burchardi, H. et al. (2002). Epidemiology of sepsis and infection in ICU patients from an international multicentre cohort study. *Intensive Care Medicine*, Vol.28, No.2, (February 2002), pp.108–21, ISSN 0342-4642.

Almog, Y.; Novack, V.; Eisinger, M.; et al. (2007). The effect of statin therapy on infection-related mortality in patients with atherosclerotic diseases. *Critical Care Medicine*, Vol.35, No.2, (February 2007), pp. 372-378, ISSN 0090-3493.

Angus, D.; Linde-Zwirble, W.; Lidicker, J.; Clermont, G.; Carcillo, J. & Pinsky, M.. (2001). Epidemiology of severe sepsis in the United States: analysis of incidence, outcome, and associated costs of care. *Critical Care Medicine*, Vol.29, No.7, (July 2001), pp. 1303-10, ISSN 0090-3493.

Annane, D. ; Sébille, V. ; Charpentier, C. et al. (2002). Effect of treatment with low doses of hydrocortisone and fludrocortisone on mortality in patients with septic shock. *Journal of the American Medical Association*, Vol 288, No 7, (August 2002), pp. 862-71. ISSN 0098-7484.

Annane, D. ; Sebille, V. ; Troche, G. et al. (2000). A 3-Level Prognostic Classification in Septic Shock Based on Cortisol Levels and Cortisol Response to Corticotropin. *Journal of the American Medical Association*, Vol 283, (February 2000), pp. 1038-1045.

Annane, D.; Bellissant, E.; Bollaert, P. E. et al. (2004). Corticosteroids for severe sepsis and septic shock: a systematic review and meta-analysis. *British Medical Journal*, Vol 329, No. 7464 (August 2004), pp. 1-9. ISSN 0959 8138.

Annane, D.; Maxime, V.; Ibrahim, F. et al. (2006). Diagnosis of adrenal insufficiency in severe sepsis and septic shock. American Journal of Respiratory *Critical Care Medicine*, Vol. 174, (December 2006), pp. 1319–1326. ISSN 1073-449X.

Annetta, M. G.; Maviglia, R.; Proietti, R. & Antonelli, M. (2009). Use of Corticosteroids in Critically Ill Septic Patients: A Review of Mechanisms of Adrenal Insufficiency in Sepsis and Treatment. *Current Drug Targets*, Vol. 10, (September 2009), pp. 887-894. ISSN 1389-4501.

Arnaud, C.; Burger, F.; Steffens, S. ; et al. (2005). Statins reduce interleukin-6-induced C-reactive protein in human hepatocytes: new evidence for direct antiinflammatory effects of statins. *Arteriosclerosis, Thrombosis and Vascular Biology*, Vol.25, No.6, (June 2005), pp. 1231–1236, ISSN 1079-5642.

Bernard, G. ; Vincent, J.; Laterre, P.; et al. (2001). Efficacy and safety of recombinant human activated protein C for severe sepsis. *New England Journal of Medicine*, Vol.344, No.10, (March 2001), pp. 699-709, ISSN 0028-4793.

Bianchi, M. (2007). DAMPs, PAMPs and alarmins: all we need to know about danger. *Journal of Leukocyte Biology*, Vol.81, No.1, (January 2007), pp. 1-5, ISSN 0741-5400.

Bickel, C.; Rupprecht, H.; Blankenberg, S.; et al. (2002). Influence of HMG-CoA reductase inhibitors on markers of coagulation, systemic inflammation and soluble cell adhesion. *International Journal of Cardiology*, Vol.82, No.1, (January 2002), pp. 25-31, ISSN 0167-5273.

Bonilla, F. (2008). Pharmacokinetics of Immunoglobulin Administered via Intravenous or Subcutaneous Routes. *Immunology & Allergy Clinics of North America*, Vol.28, No.4, (November 2008), pp. 803–819, ISSN 0889-8561.

Bourcier, T. & Libby, P. (2000). HMG CoA reductase inhibitors reduce plasminogen activator inhibitor-1 expression by human vascular smooth muscle and endothelial cells. *Arteriosclerosis, Thrombosis and Vascular Biology*, Vol.20, No.2, (February 2000), pp. 556-562, ISSN 1079-5642.

Chrousos, G. (2009). Adrenocorticosteroids & Adrenocortical Antagonists, In: Basic & Clinical Pharmacology, 11e, Katzung, B., pp. 681-698, McGraw-Hill Companies, Inc., Retrieved from http://www.accessmedicine.com/content.aspx?aID=4520662.

Collins, S.; Caron, M. G. & Lefkowitz, R. J. (1988). Beta-adrenergic receptors in hamster smooth muscle cells are transcriptionally regulated by glucocorticoids. *Journal of Biological Chemistry*, Vol. 263 (July 1988), pp. 9067–9070. ISSN 0021-9258.

Cronin, L.; Cook, D. J.; Carlet, J. et al. (1995). Corticosteroid treatment for sepsis: A critical appraisal and meta-analysis of the literature. *Critical Care Medicine*, Vol.23 (August 1995), pp. 1430-1439. ISSN 0090-3493.

Czeslick, E.; Struppert, A.; Simm, A.; et al. (2006). E5564 (Eritoran) inhibits lipopolysaccharide-induced cytokine production in human blood monocytes. *Inflammatory Research*, Vol.55, No.11, (November 2006), pp. 511-515, ISSN 1023-3830.

Darenberg, J.; Ihendyane, N.; Sjölin, J.; et al. (2003). Intravenous immunoglobulin G therapy in streptococcal toxic shock syndrome: a European randomized, double-blind, placebo-controlled trial. *Clinical Infectious Disease*, Vol.37, No.3, (August 2003), pp. 333-40, ISSN 1058-4838.

Davies, D.; McGeer, A.; Schwartz, B.; et al. (1996). Invasive group A streptococcal infections in Ontario, Canada. The Ontario Group A Streptococcal Study Group. *New England Journal of Medicine*, Vol.335, No.8, (August 1996), pp. 547–54, ISSN 0028-4793.

Dellinger, R. (2003). Inflammation and coagulation: implications for the septic patients. *Clinical Infectious Disease*s, Vol.36, No.10, (May 2003), pp. 1259-65, ISSN 1058-4838.

Dellinger, R. ; Levy, M. ; Carlet, J. ; et al. (2008). Surviving Sepsis Campaign: International guidelines for management of severe sepsis and septic shock: 2008. *Critical Care Medicine*, Vol.36, No.1, (January 2008), pp. 296-327, ISSN 0090-3493.

Diomede, L.; Albani, D.; Sottocorno, M.; et al. (2001). In vivo anti-inflammatory effect of statins is mediated by nonsterol mevalonate products. *Arteriosclerosis, Thrombosis and Vascular Biology*, Vol.21, No.8, (August 2001), pp. 1327- 1332, ISSN 1079-5642.

Drotrecogin alfa prescribing information. XIGRIS® (drotrecogin alfa (activated)) Injection, Powder, Lyophilized, For Solution for Intravenous use. Indianapolis, IN. Eli Lilly and Company. 2008.

Fahey, J. V. & Guyre, P. M. & Munck, A. (1981). Mechanisms of anti-inflammatory actions of glucocorticoids. *Advances in Inflammation Research*, Vol. 2, (1981), pp 21-51. ISSN 0197-8322.

FDA Consumer Health Information / U. S. Food and Drug Administration. FDA: Limit use of simvastatin 80 mg. 2011.

Finfer, S.; Ranieri, V.; Thompson, B.; et al. (2008). Design, conduct, analysis and reporting of a multi-national placebo-controlled trial of activated protein C for persistent septic shock. *Intensive Care Medicine*, Vol.34, No.11, (November 2008), pp. 1935-47, ISSN 0342-4642.

Fludrocortisone prescribing information. FLORINEF® (fludrocortisone acetate). Montreal, Quebec. Paladin Labs Inc. 2009.

Goa, F.; Linhartova, L.; Johnston, A.; et al. (2008). Statins and Sepsis. *British Journal of Anaesthesia*, Vol. 100, No.3, (March 2008), pp. 288-298, ISSN 0007-0912.

Grip, O.; Janciauskiene, S. & Lindgren, S. (2002). Atorvastatin activates PPAR-gamma and attenuates the inflammatory response in human monocytes. *Inflammation Research*, Vol.51, No.2, (February 2002), pp. 58–62, ISSN 1023-3830.

Gupta, R.; Plantinga, L.; Fink, N.; et al. (2007). Statin use and hospitalization for sepsis in patients with chronic kidney disease. *Journal of the American Medical Association*, Vol. 297, No.13, (April 2007), pp. 1455–1464, ISSN 0098-7484.

Harter, L.; Mica, L.; Stocker, R.; et al. (2004). Increased expression of Toll-like receptor-2 and -4 on leukocytes from patients with sepsis. *Shock*, Vol.22, No.5, (2004), pp. 403–409, ISSN 1073-2322.

Ho, J. T.; Al-Musalhi, H.; Chapman, M. J. et al. (2006). Septic shock and sepsis: A comparison of total and free plasma cortisol levels. *Journal of Clinical Endocrinology & Metabolism*, Vol. 91, (January 2006), pp. 105–114. ISSN 0021-972X.

Hydrocortisone prescribing information. SOLU-CORTEF® (hydrocortisone sodium succinate for injection, USP). New York, NY. Pfizer Inc. 2010.

Immunoglobulin prescribing information. Gammagard Liquid [Immune Globulin Intravenous (Human)] 10%. Westlake Village, CA. Baxter Healthcare Corporation. 2010.

Janda, S.; Young, A.; Fitzgerald, J.; et al. The effect of statins on mortality from severe infections and sepsis: a systematic review and meta-analysis. *Journal of Critical Care*, Vol.25, No.4, (December 2010), pp. 656.e7-22, ISSN 0883-9441.

Knapp, M. & Colburn, P. (1990). Clinical uses of intravenous immune globulin. *Clinical Pharmacy*, Vol.9, No.7, (July 1990), pp. 509-29, ISSN 0278-2677.

Kruger, P. ; Harward, M. ; Jones, M. ; et al. (2011). Continuation of statin therapy in patients with presumed infection: a randomized controlled trial. American Journal of Respiratory *Critical Care Medicine*, Vol.183, No.6, (March 2011), pp. 774-781, ISSN 1535-4970.

Laupland, K.; Kirkpatrick, A. & Delaney, A. (2007). Polyclonal intravenous immunoglobulin for the treatment of severe sepsis and septic shock in critically ill adults: A systematic review and meta-analysis. *Critical Care Medicine*, Vol.35, No.12, (December 2007), pp. 2686-2692, ISSN 0090-3493.

Lefering, R.M. & Neugebauer, E. A. (1995). Steroid controversy in sepsis and septic shock: A meta-analysis. *Critical Care Medicine*, Vol 23 (July 1995), pp. 1294-1303. ISSN 0090-3493.

Lovastatin prescribing information. MEVACOR® (lovastatin). Etobicoke, Ontario, Canada. Mylan Pharmaceuticals ULC. 2010.

Lynn, M.; Rossignol, D.; Wheeler, J.; et al. (2003). Blocking of responses to endotoxin by E5564 in healthy volunteers with experimental endotoxemia. *Journal of Infectious Diseases*, Vol.187, No.4, (February 2003), pp. 631–639, ISSN 0022-1899.

Majumdar, S.; McAlister, F.; Eurich, D.; et al. (2006). Statins and outcomes in patients admitted to hospital with community acquired pneumonia: population based prospective cohort study. *British Medical Journal*, Vol. 333, No. 7576, (November 2006), pp. 999, ISSN 0959-8138.

Marik, P. E.; Pastores, S. M.; Annane, D. et al. (2008). Recommendations for the diagnosis and management of corticosteroid insufficiency in critically ill adult patients: Consensus statements from an international task force by the American College of *Critical Care Medicine*. *Critical Care Medicine*, Vol. 36, No. 6, (June 2008), pp. 1937-1949. ISSN 0090-3493.

Martin, G.; Mannino, D.; Eaton, S. & Moss, M. (2003). The Epidemiology of Sepsis in the United States from 1979 through 2000. *New England Journal of Medicine*, Vol.348, No.16, (April 2003), pp.1546-54, ISSN 0028-4793.

McGown, C. & Brookes, Z. (2007). Beneficial effects of statins on the microcirculation during sepsis: the role of nitric oxide. *British Journal of Anaesthesia*, Vol.98, No.2, (February 2007), pp. 163–175, ISSN 0007-0912.

Minneci, P. C.; Deans, K. J.; Banks, S.M.; Eichacker, P.Q. & Natanson, C.M. (2004). Meta-analysis: the effect of steroids on survival and shock during sepsis depends on the dose. *Annals of Internal Medicine*, Vol. 141, No. 1, (July 2004), pp. 47-56. ISSN 0003-4819.

Nduka, O. & Parrillo, J. (2009). The pathophysiology of Septic Shock. *Critical Care Clinics*, Vol.25, No.4, (October 2009), pp. 677–702, ISSN 0749-0704.

Niessner, A.; Steiner, S.; Speidl, W.; et al. (2006). Simvastatin suppresses endotoxin-induced upregulation of toll-like receptors 4 and 2 in vivo. *Atherosclerosis*, Vol.189, No.2, (December 2006), pp. 408-413, ISSN 1523-3804.

Norrby-Teglund, A. & Stevens, D. (1998). Novel therapies in streptococcal toxic shock syndrome: attenuation of virulence factor expression and modulation of the host response. *Current Opinion in Infectious Diseases*, Vol. 11, No.3, (June 1998), pp. 285–91, ISSN 0951-7375.

Pasternak, R.; Smith, S.; Bairey-Merz, C.; et al. (2002). ACC/AHA/NHLBI clinical advisory on the use and safety of statins. *Circulation*, Vol.106, No.8, (August 2002), pp. 1024–1028, ISSN 0009-7322.

Pharmacist's Letter. (2009). Statin Dose Comparison, In: *Pharmacist's Letter*, Vol.25, No.250801, (August 2009), ISSN 0883-0371.

Pilkis, S. J. & Granner, D. K. (1992). Molecular physiology of the regulation of hepatic gluconeogenesis and glycolysis. *Annual Review of Physiology*, Vol. 54, (1992), pp. 885-909. ISSN 0066-4278.

Pravastatin prescribing information. PRAVACHOL® (pravastatin sodium). Princeton, New Jersey. Bristol-Myers Squibb Company. Rev 2011.

Pruefer, D.; Makowski, J.; Schnell, M.; et al. (2002). Simvastatin inhibits inflammatory properties of Staphylococcus aureus alpha-toxin. *Circulation*, Vo.106, No.16, (October 2002), pp. 2104-2110, ISSN 0009-7322.

Rivers, E. ; Nguyen, B. ; Havstad, S. et al. (2001). Early goal-directed therapy in the treatment of severe sepsis and septic shock. *New England Journal of Medicine*, Vol.345, No.19, (November 2001), pp.1368-77, ISSN 0028-4793.

Rossignol, D.; Wasan, K.; Choo, E.; et al. (2004). Safety, pharmacokinetics, pharmacodynamics, and plasma lipoprotein distribution of eritoran (E5564) during continuous intravenous infusion into healthy volunteers. *Antimicrobial Agents*

& Chemotherapy, Vol.48, No.9, (September 2004), pp. 3233-3240, ISSN 0066-4804.

Russell, J. (2006). Drug Therapy: Management of Sepsis. *New England Journal of Medicine*, Vol.355, No.16, (October 2006), pp.1699-713, ISSN 0028-4793.

Ryan, K. & Ray, C. (2010). Immune Response to Infection, In: Sherris Medical Microbiology, 5e, Ryan, K. & Ray, C., McGraw-Hill Companies, Inc., Retrieved from http://www.accessmedicine.com/content.aspx?aID=6936356.

Sekul, E.; Cupler, E. & Dalakas, M. (1994). Aseptic Meningitis Associated with High-Dose Intravenous Immunoglobulin Therapy: Frequency and Risk Factors. *Annals of Internal Medicine*, Vol.121, No.4, (August 1994), pp. 259-262, ISSN 0003-4819.

Schimmer, B. & Funder, J. (2011). ACTH, Adrenal Steroids, and Pharmacology of the Adrenal Cortex, In: Goodman & Gilman's The Pharmacological Basis of Therapeutics, 12e., Brunton, L.; Chabner, B. & Knollmann, B., McGraw-Hill Companies, Inc., Retrieved from http://www.accessmedicine.com/content.aspx?aID=16674048.

Shi, J.; Wang, J.; Zheng, H.; et al. (2003). Statins increase thrombomodulin expression and function in human endothelial cells by a nitric oxide-dependent mechanism and counteract tumor necrosis factor alpha-induced thrombomodulin downregulation. *Blood, Coagulation & Fibrinolysis*, Vol.14, No.6, (September 2003), pp. 575-585, ISSN 0957 5235.

Simvastain prescribing information. ZOCOR® (simvastatin). Cramlington, Northumberland, UK. Merck Sharp & Dohme Ltd. 2011.

Sprung, C.L.; Annane, D.; Keh, D. et al. (2008). Hydrocortisone therapy for patients with septic shock. *New England Journal of Medicine*, Vol. 358, No. 2, (January 2008), pp. 111-124. ISSN 0028-4793.

Steiner, S.; Speidl, W.; Pleiner, J.; et al. (2005). Simvastatin Blunts Endotoxin-Induced Tissue Factor In Vivo. *Circulation*, Vol.111, No.14, (April 2005), pp. 1841-1846, ISSN 0009-7322.

Terblanche, M.; Almog, Y.; Rosenson, R.; et al. (2006). Statins: panacea for sepsis? *Lancet Infectious Disease*, Vol.6, No.4, (April 2006), pp. 242-248, ISSN 1473-3099.

Tidswell, M.; Tillis, W.; Larosa, S.; et al. (2010). Phase 2 trial of eritoran tetrasodium (E5564), a Toll-like receptor 4 antagonist, in patients with severe sepsis. *Critical Care Medicine*, Vol.38, No.1, (January 2010), pp. 72–83, ISSN 0090-3493.

Toussaint, S. & Gerlach, H. (2009). Activated Protein C for Sepsis. *New England Journal of Medicine*, Vol.361, No.27, (December 2009), pp. 2646-52, ISSN 0028-4793.

Wittebole, X.; Castanares-Zapatero, D. & Laterre, P. (2010). Toll-like receptor 4 modulation as a strategy to treat sepsis. *Mediators of Inflammation*, Vo. 2010, (April 2010), ID568396, pp. 1-9, ISSN 0962-9351.

Wittebole, X.; Coyle, S.; Kumar, A.; et al. (2005). Expression of tumour necrosis factor receptor and Toll-like receptor 2 and 4 on peripheral blood leucocytes of human volunteers after endotoxin challenge: a comparison of flow cytometric light scatter and immunofluorescence gating. *Clinical & Experimental Immunology*, Vol.141, No.1, (July 2005), pp. 99–106, ISSN 0009 9104.

Zhu, J. & Mohan, C. (2010). Toll-like receptor signaling pathways--therapeutic opportunities. *Mediators of Inflammation*, Vol. 2010, (October 2010), ID781235, pp. 1-7, ISSN 0962-9351.

18

Anti-Inflammatory Role of Natural Polyphenols and Their Degradation Products

Balázs Veres
University of Pécs
Hungary

1. Introduction

A tight regulation of the immune/inflammatory system is crucial for maintaining the balance between protective and tissue-damaging responses. Systemic inflammatory response syndrome (SIRS) and sepsis are characterized by a loss of control over inflammatory responses, which can be provoked by a variety of causative agents and severe clinical insults. Sepsis is the most common cause of death in intensive care units worldwide and despite the extensive research we do not fully understand the cellular and molecular mechanisms that are involved in triggering and propagation of septic injury. A number of different approaches have been investigated to try to treat and/or prevent septic shock associated with infections caused by Gram-negative bacteria. Antibiotics constitute a necessary part of the treatment of sepsis, but antibiotics alone, even used optimally, are not sufficient to dramatically reduce the mortality of septic patient, because antibiotics cannot control the complex systemic inflammation and dysregulated host responses. For this reason, considerable efforts have been expended in developing non-antibiotic forms of treatment.

A wide variety of dietary plants including grains, berries, legumes, tea, beer, grape/wine, olive oil, chocolate/cocoa, coffee, walnuts, peanuts, spices, fruits, vegetables etc. contain polyphenols (Bravo, 1998). Polyphenols, with 8000 structural variants, are characterized by the presence of aromatic rings bearing one or more hydroxyl moieties, which have a pivotal role in mediating of its antioxidant properties. As antioxidants, polyphenols are normally produced by plants for their antibiotic and antifungal features (Leiro et al., 2004). Polyphenols are generally divided into six major groups: hydroxybenzoic acids, phenolic alcohols, hydroxycinnamic acids, lignans, flavonoids and stilbenes (e.g. resveratrol) (D'Archivio et al., 2007). Recently, a number of natural products or ingredients of traditional medicines and healthy foods such as resveratrol, curcumin, and catechins were extensively investigated and subjected to clinical trials as anti-inflammatory agents (Hatcher et al., 2008). Although the knowledge of absorption, bioavailability and metabolism of polyphenols is not entirely known, it appears that some polyphenols are bioactive and are absorbed in their native or modified form. After the metabolization of polyphenols by the microflora of the intestines, their absorbed forms may be detected in plasma in nanomolar concentration (Rahman et al., 2006).

The active components of dietary phytochemicals (e.g. curcumin, resveratrol, capsaicin, catechins, vitamins, beta carotene and dietary fiber) are believed to suppress the inflammatory processes, moderate cell signaling pathways, proliferation, apoptosis, redox balance and most often appear to be protective against cancer, neurodegenerative disorders and cardiovascular diseases (Aggarwal & Shishodia, 2006; Rahman et al., 2006). Polyphenols can exert their anti-inflammatorical properties at multiple levels, through the modulation of MAPK, Akt and NF-κB signaling pathways, inhibition the production of inflammatory cytokines and chemokines, suppressing the activity of COX and iNOS and decreasing the production of ROS/RNS. MAPKs which play critical roles in inflammation are inhibited by catechins in macrophages (Ichikawa et al., 2004). Other dietary phytochemicals, namely curcumin, resveratrol and green tea polyphenols have been shown to modulate the MAP kinases and it was dependent on cell type and on the polyphenol used. Akt plays crucial roles in mammalian cell survival signalling and has been shown to be activated in various cancers (Chang et al., 2003). Activated Akt promotes cell survival by activating NF-κB signalling pathway (Romashkova & Makarov, 1999). Several phytochemicals including genistein (Li & Sarkar, 2002), curcuminoids (Aggarwal et al., 2006) and catechins (Tang et al., 2003) are known to suppress the activation of Akt, in this way inhibit cancer cell growth. Almost all cell types, when exposed to TNF-α, LPS or other stimuli, activate NF-κB and AP-1 transcription factors, leading to the expression of inflammatory genes, such as COX-2, iNOS, cell adhesion molecules, inflammatory cytokines and chemokines. Thus, all the dietary agents that can suppress these transcription factors have the potential of inhibiting the expression of COX-2, iNOS, cell adhesion molecules, TNF-α and interleukins. Several dietary components including green tea catechins (Gerhäuser et al., 2003), curcumin (Plummer et al., 1999), and resveratrol (Subbaramaiah et al., 1998) have been shown to suppress COX-2 and in this way to decrease the production of reactive oxygen species. iNOS, which is responsible for the release of free radical nitric oxide, was suppressed by several phytochemicals and dietary agents in RAW 264.7 macrophage cell line, stimulated with LPS and interferon-γ (IFN-γ) (Kim et al., 1998). Other sources of the antioxidant properties of polyphenols is their free radicals scavenger features, which is based on their structure (Joe & Lokesh, 1994, Babu & Liu, 2008). Furthermore, several polyphenols suppress lipid peroxidation through to maintain the cellular status of antioxidant enzymes like superoxide dismutase, catalase and glutathione peroxidase (Labinskyy et al., 2006; Reddy & Lokesh, 1992). Due to the NF-κB suppressing effect of polyphenols, some of them (e.g. curcumin, resveratrol, quercetin and green tee polyphenols) have been shown to decrease the expression of chemokines and cytokines (Hidaka et al., 2002, Kowalski et al., 2005).

Recently, the anti-inflammatory properties of natural products or ingredients of traditional medicines and healthy foods were extensively investigated, but the solubility of these compounds is limited. Because of it, it is questionable whether their bioavailability could account for their pharmacological effect. Recent publications show that polyphenols in healthy foods or drinks such as chocolate, red wine, or beer are readily metabolized to phenolic acids and aldehydes by the microflora of the intestines, raising the possibility that these metabolites, rather than the original natural products or food ingredients, are responsible for their anti-inflammatory properties (Gonthier et al., 2003; Rios et al., 2003).

In the present chapter we summarize our recent knowledge about the effect of natural polyphenols in systemic inflammatory conditions focusing on their metabolites and degradation products. These compounds could represent new potential clinical approaches in the therapeutic intervention of severe sepsis and septic shock.

2. Polyphenols

A wide variety of dietary plants including grains, fruits, vegetables, cereals, olive, dry legumes, chocolate and beverages, such as tea, coffee and red wine contain polyphenols (Bravo, 1998). Polyphenols, with 8000 structural variants, are characterized by the presence of aromatic rings bearing one or more hydroxyl moieties, which have a pivotal role in mediating of its antioxidant properties. As antioxidants, polyphenols are normally produced by plants for their antibiotic and antifungal features (Leiro et al., 2004). Although the absorption, bioavailability and metabolism of polyphenols are not entirely known, it appears that some polyphenols are bioactive and are absorbed in their native or modified form. The active components of dietary phytochemicals (e.g. curcumin, resveratrol, capsaicin, catechins, vitamins, beta carotene and dietary fiber) are believed to suppress the inflammatory processes, moderate cell signalling pathways, proliferation, apoptosis, redox balance and most often appear to be protective against cancer, neurodegenerative disorders and cardiovascular diseases (Aggarwal & Shishodia, 2006, Rahman et al., 2006). Polyphenols can exert their anti-inflammatory properties at multiple levels, through the modulation of mitogen-activated protein kinases (MAPK) signalling pathways (Kong et al., 2000; Wiseman et al., 2001) and NF-κB and AP-1 transcription factors (Manna et al., 2000), inhibition of the production of inflammatory cytokines and chemokines, suppressing the activity of cyclooxygenase (COX) (O'Leary et al., 2004) and inducible nitric oxide synthase (iNOS) (Donnelly et al., 2004) and thereby decreasing the production of reactive oxygen and nitrogen species (ROS/RNS).

In this chapter we discuss the anti-inflammatory properties of some selected polyphenols where the selection is based on the occurrence and importance of these compounds in the literature.

2.1 Resveratrol

One of the most investigated and potent polyphenolic compound that is found in highest concentration in the skin of grapes and regulate the inflammation is a stilbene, called resveratrol (3,5,4'-trihydroxy-trans-stilbene) (Figure 1). In the 80's, interest in the possible health benefits of resveratrol in wine was spurred by discussion of the "French paradox" which estimated the state of health of wine drinkers in France. These data suggest that nutritional intake of resveratrol and other polyphenol compounds may contribute to a relatively low incidence of cardiovascular diseases in the Mediterranean population (de Lange, 2007; de Lorgeril et al., 1999; Zern & Fernandez, 2005).

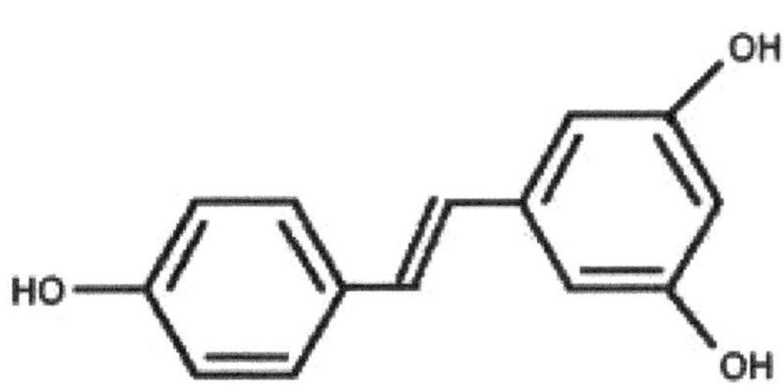

Fig. 1. Structure of resveratrol

Bioavailability and metabolism of resveratrol have been widely studied and its efficacy depends on its absorption and metabolism. In mice, rats and humans resveratrol has been detected in body fluids (urine, bile, and plasma) as well as in kidneys, stomach, intestine, and liver, following oral administration and this wide tissue targeting suggests an efficient absorption (Boocock et al., 2007; Jang et al., 1997; Vitrac et al., 2003; Wenzel & Somoza, 2005; Wenzel et al., 2005;).

2.2 Quercetin

The flavonoid quercetin (Figure 2) is a potent dietary polyphenol that can exert anti-inflammatory, anti-proliferative and anti-oxidative effects (Bischoff, 2008; Boots et al., 2008).

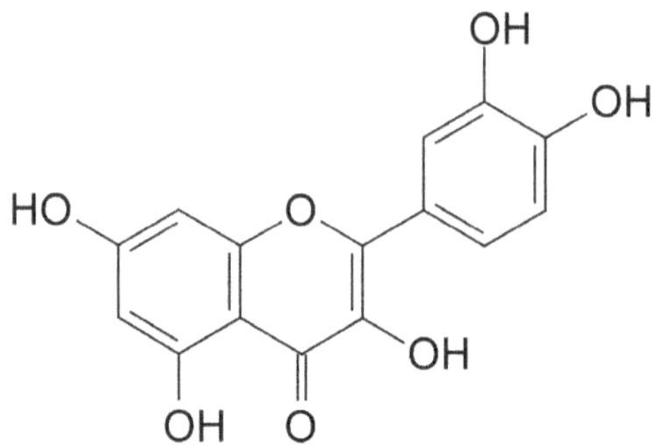

Fig. 2. Structure of quercetin

Foods rich in quercetin include black and green tea, capers, lovage, apples, red grapes and a number of berries (Häkkinen et al., 1999). Dietary quercetin is mostly present as its glycoside form and it is absorbed from the intestinal lumen is mostly converted to conjugated metabolites before entering circulation. A recent study regarding the tissue distribution observed that quercetin concentrated in lungs, testes, kidneys, thymus, heart and liver in rats and in pigs (de Boer et al., 2005). After absorption quercetin can undergo microbial degradation in the colon to phenolic acids and CO_2, which is exhaled in the breath.

2.3 Curcumin

Curcumin (diferuloylmethane) (Figure 3), an orange-yellow component of turmeric or curry powder, is a polyphenol natural product isolated from the rhizome of the plant Curcuma longa.

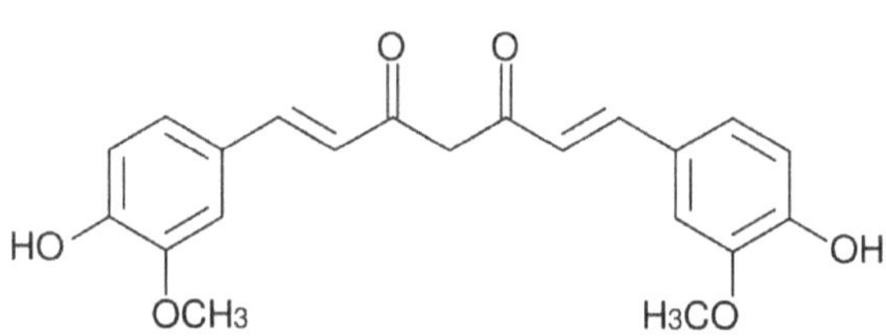

Fig. 3. Structure of curcumin

Since its first use as a drug in 1937 curcumin's therapeutic potential has been explored in inflammatory diseases, neoplastic disease, cardiovascular and neurodegenerative disease, diabetes, cystic fibrosis and other disorders (Egan et al., 2004; Hsu & Cheng, 2007; Miriyala et al., 2007; Weisberg et al., 2008). However, curcumin, a highly pleiotropic molecule with an excellent safety profile targeting multiple diseases with strong evidence on the molecular level, could not achieve its optimum therapeutic outcome in past clinical trials, largely due to its low solubility and poor bioavailability. Animal and human studies have shown that curcumin is rapidly metabolized and conjugated in the liver, and then excreted, therefore having limited systemic bioavailability (Cheng et al., 2001; Ireson et al., 2001; Sharma et al., 2004).

2.4 Epigallocatechin gallate

Epigallocatechin gallate (EGCG), a principal antioxidant derived from green tea, is one of the most extensively investigated chemopreventive phytochemicals (Figure 4).

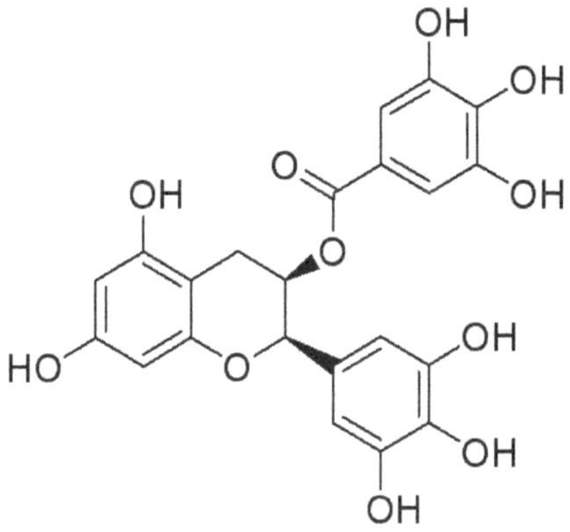

Fig. 4. Structure of epigallocatechin gallate

Recently, green tea has attracted attention for its health benefits, particularly with respect to its potential for preventing and treating cancer, cardiovascular diseases, inflammatory diseases, and neurodegenerative diseases in humans (Tedeschi et al., 2004; Weisburger & Chung, 2002; Yang et al., 1998). The metabolism of green tea catechins has been studied in various animals and in human subjects (Lee et al., 1995; Pietta et al., 2008). Orally administrated catechin to humans is absorbed, metabolized, and excreted within 24 hours (Harada et al., 1999) and green tea consumption increased the plasma levels of EGCG in a dose-dependent manner (Nakagawa et al., 1997). Furthermore, Suganuma et al. demonstrated that after direct administration of labelled EGCG into the stomachs radioactivity appeared in a wide range of target organs in mice, including the digestive tract, liver, lung, pancreas, mammary gland and skin, brain, kidney, uterus and ovary and testes (Suganuma et al., 1998).

2.5 Phenolic acids and aldehydes

Natural phenolic compounds are secondary plant metabolites and the most abundant antioxidant resources. They are widely distributed in plants and present in considerable amounts in the human diet. Phenolic acids are hydroxylated derivatives of benzoic and cinnamic acids. The most common hydroxycinnamic acid derivatives are p-coumaric, caffeic, and ferulic acids which frequently occur in foods as simple esters with quinic acid or glucose. Phenolic acids have received considerable attention due to their various biological activities, including antioxidant, anti-apoptotic and anti-inflammatory capacities (Manach et al., 2004).

Caffeic acid (Figure 5) is a widespread phenolic acid that occurs naturally in many agricultural products such as fruits, vegetables, wine, olive oil, and coffee (Mattila & Kumpulainen, 2002).

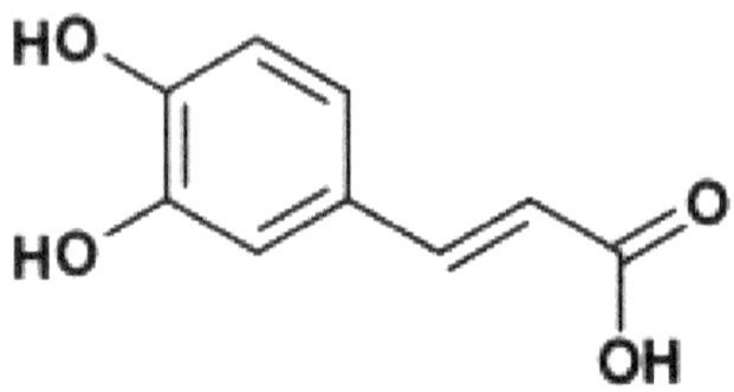

Fig. 5. Structure of caffeic acid

It is a potent antioxidant, metal chelating (Psotova et al., 2003), anti-inflammatory (Chao et al., 2010), free radical scavenger (Gulcin, 2006) and antidiabetic agent. Caffeic acid has been shown to be an inhibitor of the lipoxygenase enzyme and its conjugates such as chlorogenic and caftaric acids were demonstrated to be more powerful antioxidants in a number of different systems (Fukumoto & Mazza, 2000). Caffeic acid and its derivatives are good substrates of polyphenol oxidases, and under certain conditions may undergo oxidation in plant tissues or products of plant origin (Kerry & Rice-Evans, 1998).

Ferulic acid (4-hydroxy-3-methoxy cinnamic acid) is a product of the phenylalanine and tyrosine metabolism, and it is produced by the shikimate pathway in plants (Figure 6). It is commonly found in fruits like orange and in vegetables, such as tomato, carrot, sweet corn and rice bran. The wide spectrum of beneficial effects of ferulic acid for human health due to its antibacterial, anti-inflammatory, hepatoprotective, anticancer, antidiabetic, neuroprotective, anti-atherogenic and antioxidant activity (Srinivasan et al., 2007). Partially, because of its antioxidant and anti-inflammatory activity, ferulic acid is considered as a potential therapeutic agent (together with other natural phenolic compounds) against various diseases like cancer, diabetes, cardiovascular dysfunction, inflammatory diseases and neurodegenerative diseases (Soobrattee et al., 2005). Ferulic acid and ferulaldehyde are potential end-products of dietary polyphenol degradation since they were found at a high concentration in human urine after red wine and chocolate consumption (Gonthier, 2003; Rios et al., 2003).

Furthermore, ferulic acid was reported to stay in the blood longer than other antioxidants such as vitamin C, and have higher bioavailability than that of other dietary flavonoids and monophenolics studied so far (Beecher et al., 1998). The structural characteristic of ferulic acid and its reduced form, ferulaldehyde mainly resembles, the difference is one functional group (Figure 6). Due to this structural similarity and the presence of the reactive aldehyde group (which can be easily oxidized to carboxylic group), ferulaldehyde is thought to have very similar or maybe better biological activity as ferulic acid (Radnai et al, 2009; Tucsek et al., 2011).

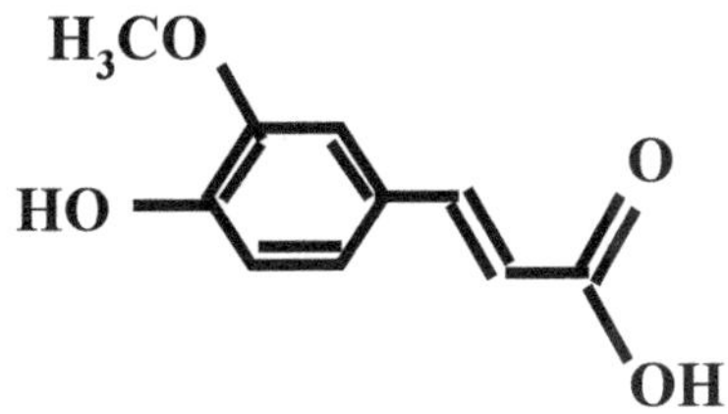

Ferulic acid

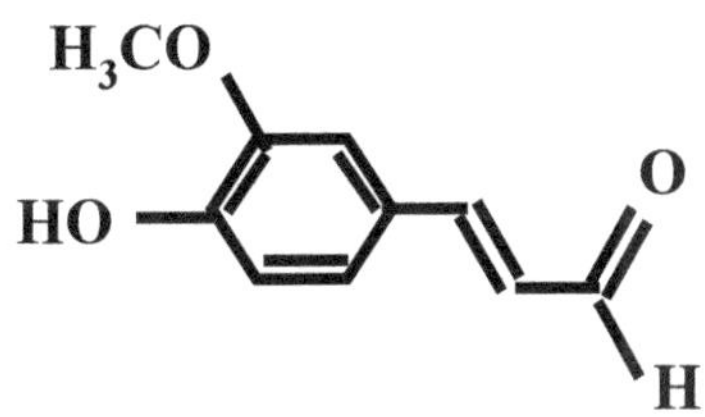

Ferulaldehyde

Fig. 6. Structure of ferulic acid and ferulaldehyde

3. Pathomechanism of sepsis

3.1 Reactive oxygen and nitrogen species

Oxidative stress is involved in the pathomechanism of sepsis and reactive oxygen and nitrogen species are important mediators of cellular injury during endotoxemia (Cadenas & Cadenas, 2002). Oxidative damage caused by ROS and RNS will lead, among others, to DNA lesions, function loss of enzymes, increased cell permeability, disturbed signalling over the cell and eventually even cell death via necrosis or apoptosis. Consequently, ROS play a key role in enhancing the inflammation through sustained production of various cytokines, activation and phosphorylation of MAP kinases and redox-sensitive transcription factors, such as NF-κB and AP-1 in various inflammatory diseases. ROS also alters nuclear histone acetylation and deacetylation (chromatin remodelling) leading to increased gene expression of proinflammatory mediators (Rahman et al., 2004). ROS are generated during normal cellular metabolism. The respiratory chain in mitochondria is the major source of oxygen radicals. In inflammatory processes, beside the mitochondrial ROS production there are other possible sources of ROS such as metabolic cascade of arachidonic acid (via COX-2), protease-mediated enzyme xanthine-oxidase and membrane-bound enzyme complex NADPH oxidase (Victor et al., 2005). ROS and RNS cause peroxidation of membrane phospholipids, oxidation of proteins and DNA damage (Pattanaik & Prasad 1996). iNOS is expressed and continuously active during inflammation, where it is involved in host-defence against pathogens. iNOS generates NO which can be converted to its stable products, nitrite and nitrate (Gomez-Jimenez et al., 1995).

Many studies reconfirmed the fact that resveratrol is a potent free radical scavenger and also a potent antioxidant (Soleas et al., 1997). Peripheral blood mononuclear cells play a critical role as the first defence line during endotoxemia. Activation of these cells by different physiological and non physiological agents causes a massive respiratory burst followed by an increase in oxygen consumption accompanied by the generation of ROS including superoxide, hydrogen peroxide, and hydroxy radicals. The release of ROS is of major importance for host defence but can also induce tissue damage. Resveratrol has been reported to have a strong inhibitory effect on multiple reactive oxygen species produced by polymorphonuclear leukocytes stimulated with formyl methionyl leucyl phenylalanine a chemotactic peptide (Rotondo et al., 1998). Zymosan is a carbohydrate-rich cell wall preparation derived from the yeast *Saccharomyces cerevisiae* could activate leukocytes to release ROS and resveratrol was shown as a potent inhibitor of ROS production in both unopsonized zymosan-stimulated RAW 264.7 cells and human monocytes and neutrophils (Jang et al., 1999). It was reported that resveratrol exerted a strong inhibitory effect on superoxide radical and hydrogen peroxide produced by macrophages stimulated by lipopolysaccharides (LPS) or phorbol esters (Martinez & Moreno, 2000).

Quercetin has been shown to be an excellent in vitro antioxidant. Within the flavonoid family, quercetin is the most potent scavenger of ROS, including superoxide (Hanasaki et al., 1994; Cushnie & Lamb, 2005), and RNS like NO (van Acker et al., 1995) and peroxynitrite (Haenen et al., 1997; Heijnen et al., 2001) and it also contributes to the total plasma antioxidant capacity (Arts et al., 2004). On the other hand, it is known that during its antioxidative activities, quercetin becomes oxidized into various oxidation products and these products like semiquinone radicals and quinones display various toxic effects, such as increased membrane permeability, due to their ability of arylating protein thiols (Kalyanaraman et al., 1987; Monks & Lau, 1992; Metodiewa et al., 1999). However, quercetin quinone-induced toxicity has been shown in various in vitro studies and has recently been defined as the quercetin paradox (Boots et al., 2007), its in vivo formation and possible toxicity has not been demonstrated yet.

Free radicals such as superoxide anion, hydrogen peroxide, and nitric oxide have been reported to be scavenged by curcumin (in the micro to millimolar range) both in vitro and in vivo (Aggarwal et al., 2003). The antioxidant properties of curcumin are evident from its ability to lower lipid peroxidation and maintain the activity status of various antioxidant enzymes. Findings of Biswas et al. indicate that curcumin could scavenge ROS, as determined by electron paramagnetic resonance spectroscopy and it was found to be much faster in terms of quenching ROS when compared to resveratrol and quercetin. Curcumin has also been demonstrated to induce antioxidant defences through increases in glutathione production via Nrf2 activation and induction of glutamate cysteine ligase transcription and interacting directly with superoxide anion and hydroxyl radical (Biswas et al., 2005). In addition, curcumin had an effective scavenging activity in various in vitro antioxidant assays, including DPPH radical, ABTS radical, DMPD radical, superoxide anion radical and hydrogen peroxide; ferric ions (Fe^{3+}) reducing power and ferrous ions (Fe^{2+}) chelating activities (Ak & Gülçin, 2008). This suggests that curcumin has multiple anti-inflammatory properties: as an oxygen radical scavenger and as an antioxidant through modulation of glutathione levels.

Tea polyphenols have been reported to be potent scavengers (more efficient than vitamin E and C) (Nanjo et al., 1996; Pannala et al., 1997) of free radicals such as singlet oxygen, superoxide anions, hydroxyl radicals, and peroxy radicals in a number of in vitro systems (Salah et al., 1995; Morel et al., 1999) and EGCG was found to be the strongest antioxidant among tea catechins (Khokhar & Magnusdottir, 2002). EGCG attenuated 3-hydroxykynurenine, a potential neurotoxin in several neurodegenerative disorders, induced cell viability reduction and the increase in the concentration of ROS and caspase-3 activity in neuronal culture were also attenuated, presumably via its antioxidant activity (Jeong et al., 2004). In rat brain tissue, green tea and black tea extracts were shown to inhibit lipid peroxidation promoted by iron ascorbate in homogenates of brain mitochondrial membranes (Levites et al., 2002). A similar effect was also reported using brain synaptosomes, in which the four major polyphenol catechins of green tea were shown to inhibit iron-induced lipid peroxidation (Guo et al., 1996). The ability of green tea polyphenols and catechins, in particular, to chelate metal ions such as iron and copper may contribute to their antioxidant activity by inhibiting transition metal-catalyzed free radical formation. Furthermore, EGCG treatment inhibited the enzyme iNOS (Lin & Lin, 1997; Lin et al., 1999) in activated macrophages. On the other hand, EGCG was found to elevate the activity of two major antioxidant enzymes, superoxide dismutase (SOD) and catalase in mice striatum (Levites et al., 2001). Taken together, the inhibition of enzymes, whose activity may promote oxidative stress and an increase in antioxidant enzyme activities by tea polyphenols might have a beneficial significance to anti-inflammatory processes.

Phenolic acids and aldehydes have been reported to exert antioxidant and anti-inflammatory effects. Phenolic compounds can trap the free radicals directly or scavenge them through a series of coupled reactions with antioxidant enzymes. Caffeic acid has been shown to protect tissues from ROS-mediated oxidative stress and inhibit lipoxygenase activity resulting in suppressed lipid peroxidation (Yilmaz et al., 2004). It was demonstrated that administration of caffeic acid reduced oxidative stress by increasing antioxidant activities and decreasing oxidant status and lipid peroxidation in the intestine of rats in an experimental model of necrotizing enterocolitis (Tayman et al., 2011). Administration of caffeic acid has been also shown to completely block both the production of ROS from activated neutrophils and the XO system (Ma et al., 2006; Yildiz et al., 2009) and to protect intestinal tissues from ROS-mediated oxidative stress and reduce lipid peroxidation (Ek et al., 2008; Koltuksuz et al., 1999). Treatment of rats orally with caffeic acid resulted in a significant decrease in iron nitrilotriacetate-induced xanthine oxidase, lipid peroxidation, c-glutamyl transpeptidase, and H_2O_2 and there was a dose dependent and significant recovery of renal glutathione content and antioxidant enzymes (Rehman & Sultana, 2011). Caffeic acid has also been shown to be an inhibitor of the lipoxygenase enzyme in several experimental systems (Okutan et al., 2005). In addition, caffeic acid is an effective ABTS radical scavenging, DPPH radical scavenging, superoxide anion radical scavenging and it has total reducing power and metal chelating on ferrous ions activities (Gulcin, 2006).

In wheat grain ferulic acid is the most abundant phenolic compounds and a correlation between changes in the plasma ferulic acid concentration and changes in the plasma antioxidant capacity was reported in a human ex vivo study (Mateo Anson et al., 2011). The antioxidant potential of ferulic acid can usually be attributed to its structural characteristic. Three distinctive motifs (3-methoxy and 4-hydroxy groups on the benzene ring, and the carboxylic acid group) of ferulic acid are responsible for its free radical scavenging capability. It has been also reported that ferulic acid or related ester derivatives inhibited the

release of ROS and RNS via suppression of iNOS (Jiang et al., 2009) and COX-2 (Hirata et al., 2005, Ronchetti et al., 2009) in LPS-stimulated macrophages. Its reduced form, ferulaldehyde possesses the same structural characteristic and main molecular motifs as ferulic acid up to the aldehyde group. Ferulaldehyde was reported to inhibit LPS-induced iNOS expression and NO synthesis in murine macrophage-like RAW 264.7 cells (Kim et al., 1999) and to have a good antioxidant activity in about the same degree as ferulic acid (Nenadis et al., 2003). Furthermore, ferulaldehyde decreased free radical and nitrite production in a concentration-dependent manner in LPS plus interferon-gamma-treated primary mouse hepatocytes and in LPS-induced RAW 264.7 macrophage cells (Radnai et al., 2009; Tucsek et al., 2011).
Taken together these studies have shown that polyphenols are more effective in inhibiting the oxidative damage than the conventional antioxidants and has also been shown to scavenge free radicals such as nitric oxide, lipid hydroperoxyl, hydroxyl, and superoxide anion radicals. Since reactive oxygen and nitrogen species have been implicated in the pathogenesis of various chronic and inflammatory conditions, polyphenols therefore have the potential to control these diseases through their potent antioxidant activity.

3.2 Inflammatory cytokines

The immune system produces cytokines and other humoral factors to protect the host when threatened by inflammatory agents, microbial invasion, or injury. The pathogenesis of sepsis is characterized by an overwhelming production of proinflammatory cytokines, such as tumor necrosis factor (TNF)-α, interleukin (IL)-1β, IL-6, IL-8 and high mobility group box (HMGB)-1. In some cases these cytokines trigger a beneficial inflammatory response that restores normal homeostasis promoting local coagulation to control tissue damage. However, the overproduction of immunoregulatory mediators can be even more dangerous than the original stimulus, overcoming the normal regulation of the immune response and producing pathological inflammatory disorders (Dinarello, 1994; Hotchkiss & Karl, 2003; Tracey & Cerami, 1993; Tracey & Cerami, 1994; Van der Poll & Lowry, 1995). In severe sepsis the excessive production of proinflammatory cytokines causes capillary leakage, tissue injury, multiple organ failure, coma and death. TNF-α, a polypeptide cytokine produced during infection, injury, or invasion, has proved pivotal in triggering the lethal effects of septic shock syndrome and other systemic manifestations of disease. If the infection spreads, however, excessive TNF-α production and release into the circulation may be catastrophic and trigger a state of lethal shock via cardiovascular collapse. These toxic effects occur by direct action of TNF-α on host cells and by the interaction with a cascade of other endogenous mediators including IL-1, IL-6 and interferon-gamma (Tracey & Cerami, 1993; Tracey & Cerami, 1994). Similar to TNF-α and HMGB1, several proinflammatory cytokines and factors, such as IL-1 (Dinarello, 1994), IL-6, IL-8 (Calandra et al., 1990; Hotchkiss et al., 2000) macrophage migration inhibitory factor (Parrish et al., 2008) and lysophosphatidylcholine (Kabarowski et al., 2001), contribute to the pathogenesis and progression of sepsis. Sepsis is characterized by a surge of the pro-inflammatory cytokines TNF-α and IL-1 at the early stage. However, as the disease progresses, this early stage coverts to the anti-inflammatory state, marked by decreased levels of TNF-α and increased levels of IL-10 (Scumpia & Moldawer, 2005). The increased production of IL-10 in the late phase of sepsis is believed to contribute to 'immunosuppression'. In contrast with early cytokines, such as TNF-α and IL-1, which are produced within minutes after infection, HMGB-1 is a late mediator of sepsis that might be a potential therapeutic target to treat 'established' sepsis. The effects on the balance between pro- and anti-inflammatory cytokine expressions have been shown to be specific for specific cytokines and influenced by the structures of polyphenols indicating the complex action exerted by these compounds. Since cytokine-based strategies against septic shock and severe sepsis have produced modest effects in clinical trials (Abraham et al., 2001; Fisher et al., 1994) novel therapeutic approaches are needed and polyphenols are perfect candidates for this role.

The release of various cytokines after various stimuli from macrophages and lymphocytes, such as IL-6 (Feng et al., 2002; Zhong et al., 1999), IFNγ, IL-2, TNF-α, and IL-12 (Gao et al., 2001), has been shown to be inhibited by resveratrol. Resveratrol was also reported to suppress the activity of T- and B-cells, and macrophages the major cell types responsible for producing cytokines by decreasing the production of proinflammatory proteins, (Sharma et al., 2007) and it was able to reduce TNF-α, IL-1β, IL-6, and COX-2 gene expression and to reduce the secretion of IL-6 and PGE2 in TNF-α-stimulated adipocytes (Gonzales & Orlando, 2008). In an age-related diseases study, mice treated with resveratrol had decreased expression of the inflammatory markers TNF-α, IL-1β, IL-6, intercellular adhesion molecule (ICAM)-1 and iNOS (Pearson et al., 2008). In a mouse model of chronic colitis, resveratrol treatment resulted in significant decreases in the inflammatory cytokines TNF-α and IL-1β, as well as COX-2 and iNOS activity and an increase in the anti-inflammatory, immune-regulatory cytokine, IL-10 (Sánchez-Fidalgo et al., 2010). Resveratrol administration following trauma-hemorrhage decreased IL-6 cytokine production and protected against lung injury and inflammation in rats (Wu et al., 2008). In a rodent model of LPS-induced airway inflammation resveratrol caused a dose-related inhibition of TNF-α, IL-1β, MPO, and CINC-1 levels in the lung tissue (Birrell et al., 2005) and in a human study resveratrol inhibited the release of inflammatory cytokines IL-8 and granulocyte-macrophage colony-stimulating factor from alveolar macrophages in chronic obstructive pulmonary disease (Culpitt et al., 2003). However, it is interesting to mention that many of the pro-inflammatory genes inhibited by resveratrol in several different vitro studies, are not impacted on in vivo models indicating the host and tissue specificity of this polyphenol (Birrell et al., 2005).

Several in vitro studies using different cell lines have shown that quercetin is also capable of inhibiting LPS-induced cytokine production. For instance, quercetin inhibits LPS-induced TNF-α production in macrophages (Manjeet & Ghosh, 1999) and LPS-induced IL-8 production in lung cells (Geraets et al., 2007). Moreover, in glial cells it was shown that quercetin can inhibit LPS-induced mRNA levels of two cytokines, i.e. TNF-α and IL-1α (Bureau et al., 2008). It has already been shown that quercetin can inhibit the production as well as the gene expression of TNF-α via modulation of NF-κB in human peripheral blood mononuclear cells (Nair et al., 2006). Results indicate that TNF-α and IL-6 accumulations were significantly reduced by quercetin treatment, in murine RAW 264.7 macrophages treated with LPS (Jung & Sung, 2004). Cho and colleagues reported that in the same cell line pretreatment of quercetin inhibited iNOS mRNA, iNOS protein, NO production, TNF-α, IL-1β and IL-6 (Cho et al., 2003). Quercetin has also been reported to inhibit IgE-mediated release of histamine, tryptase and production and gene expression of inflammatory cytokines, such as TNF-α, IL-1β, IL-6 and IL-8 in phorbol 12-myristate 13-acetate and calcium ionophore-stimulated cultured human mast cells (Kempuraj et al., 2005; Min et al., 2007). These results are consistent with studies reporting that quercetin inhibits NO and TNF-α release from LPS-stimulated rat Kupffer cells (Kawada et al., 1998) and inhibits iNOS mRNA and NO production in LPS/IFN-γ-activated macrophage cells (Kobuchi et al., 1997).

In 1995 it was demonstrated by Chan that curcumin inhibits LPS-induced production of TNF-α and interleukin IL-1β in human monocytic macrophage cell line, Mono Mac 6 and it reduced the biological activity of TNF in L929 fibroblast lytic assay (Chan, 1995). Since this original work, several line of evidence appeared about curcumin's inhibitory effect on inflammatory cytokines. In LPS-stimulated BV2 microglia cells curcumin significantly inhibited the release of pro-inflammatory cytokines in a dose-dependent manner (Jin et al., 2007). Moreover, decreased expression of inflammatory cytokines such as IL-1β, IL-6, and TNF-α was reported in different cancer cell lines (Cho et al., 2007). In other studies, curcumin inhibited the production of IL-8, MIP-1α, MCP-1, IL-1β and TNF-α by PMA- or LPS-stimulated human monocytes and alveolar macrophages in a concentration- and a time-dependent manner (Abe et al., 1999; Chan, 1995). The in vivo effects of curcumin on cytokine production are also demonstrated in different model systems. In two rat models of experimentally-induced pancreatitis, curcumin decreased inflammation by markedly inhibiting mRNA induction of IL-6, TNF-α and iNOS in the pancreas (Gukovsky et al., 2003). Curcumin decreased the levels of TNF-α and interleukin-6 in mouse plasma after endotoxin-induced hepatic dysfunction and oxidative stress (Kaur et al., 2006) and also inhibited the increase of both IL-1β and TNF-α in a chronic model of inflammation in rats (Banerjee et al., 2003). Systemic pretreatment with curcumin abrogates the rise in circulating proinflammatory cytokines and body temperature (Lee et al., 2003) and prevents the onset of disseminated intravascular coagulation (Chen et al., 2007).

The effects of EGCG on the inflammatory cytokine production are thought to be cell type-dependent. EGCG was reported to inhibit TNF-α and MIP-2 production from the RAW 264.7 cells treated with LPS (Yang et al., 1998). Okabe et al reported, that EGCG effectively prevented TNF-α release in BALB/3T3 cells stimulated with okadaic acid (Okabe et al., 2001). EGCG, recapitulated HMGB1-inhibiting activities of green tea, and dose-dependently inhibited LPS-induced HMGB1 release in macrophage/monocytes cultures, partially attenuated LPS-induced TNF secretion. EGCG prevents HMGB1-mediated cytokine production–potentially by interfering with HMGB1-induced ligand/receptor clustering (Li et al., 2007). Experimental data suggest that EGCG selectively inhibits LPS-induced release of HMGB1, TNF, IL-6, IL-12, and chemokines, including MIP-1a, MIP-1c, MIP-2, RANTES, KC, MCP1 and CXCL16. EGCG did not affect circulating levels of TNF at late stage of sepsis, but specifically attenuated systemic accumulation of HMGB1, as well as IL-6 and KC-two most reliable surrogate markers of lethal sepsis (Osuchowski et al., 2006; Heuer et al., 2004). Effects of EGCG on the production of IL-8, human homolog of murine CXC-chemokines, have also been reported in selected cell lines. It was shown that EGCG inhibited IL-8 production in HMC-1 cells (Shin et al., 2007), A549 bronchial epithelial cells (Kim et al., 2006), HT29, T84 (Porath et al., 2005) and gastrointestinal epithelial cell line Caco-2 cells (Netsch et al., 2006). In vivo, EGCG attenuated the production of TNF-α and MIP-2 in the lungs of mice administered with LPS intratracheally (Bae et al., 2010). Li et al provided both evidence of a lifesaving potential and a mechanism of action for an EGCG therapeutic regimen in mice subjected to cecal ligation and puncture (CLP). EGCG reduced the mortality rate and concentrations of IL-6, keratinocyte-derived chemokine (a mouse IL-8 homologue), and HMGB-1, but not those of TNF-α, were significantly reduced. Exposure of monocytes and macrophages to EGCG in vitro reduced HMGB-1 release following LPS stimulation and IL-6 production and EGCG inhibited HMGB-1 aggregation on the macrophage cell surface. HMGB-1 antagonism was evident even when EGCG treatment of stimulated cells was delayed by 6 h. Potential therapeutic uses of EGCG is further strengthened by the fact that EGCG treatment is operative even when it is initiated after the onset of full-blown sepsis (Li et al., 2007).

Phenolic acids are clinically important inhibitors of inflammatory cytokine production in vitro and in vivo. Caffeic acid phenethyl ester (CAPE) is a potent inhibitor of early and late events in T-cell receptor-mediated T-cell activation. Moreover, it was found that CAPE specifically inhibited both IL-2 gene transcription and IL-2 synthesis in stimulated T-cells (Márquez et al., 2004). In activated human whole blood cultures, caffeic acid decreased the production of IL-1β without affecting IL-6 concentration (Miles et al., 2005) suggesting the specificity of this phenolic compound on interleukin production. In CLP-induced sepsis and lung injury model in rats, similarly to EGCG, CAPE was found to decrease IL-1, IL-6, IL-10, and TNF-α levels of blood samples even when it was administered after the onset of sepsis. (Fidan et al., 2007). In another in vivo study, CAPE rescued C57BL/6 mice from lethal LPS-induced septic shock, while decreasing serum levels of TNF-α and IL-1β (Jung et al., 2008).

The other large family of phenolic acids: ferulic acid and its derivatives were also attributed as potent inhibitors of inflammatory mediators. Indeed, ferulic acid decreased the levels of inflammatory cytokines, e.g., TNF-α (Han et al., 2007) in LPS-stimulated macrophages and lowered pro-:anti-inflammatory cytokine ratios (IL-6:IL-10 and IL-1β:IL-10) in the ex vivo LPS-stimulated blood (Mateo Anson et al., 2011). Ferulaldehyde decreased the levels of early pro-inflammatory cytokines such as TNF-α, IL-1β and increased the anti-inflammatory IL-10 in the sera of the LPS-treated mice (Radnai et al., 2009; Tucsek et al, 2011) supporting further the importance of these compounds as potential anti-inflammatory agents.

3.3 Signaling pathways

Polyphenols can work as modifiers of signal transduction pathways to elicit their beneficial effects. The anti-inflammatory effect of these natural compounds based on the modulation of pro-inflammatory gene expression such as cyclooxygenase, lipoxygenase, nitric oxide synthases and several inflammatory cytokines, mainly by acting through NF-κB and MAPK signalling (Yoon & Baek, 2005). MAPKs and NF-κB have important activities as mediators of cellular responses to extracellular signals. Some of the MAPKs are important to mammalian cells include extracellular signal regulated kinase (ERK), c-jun N-terminal kinase (JNK), and p38 and are thought to play an important role in the regulation of pro-inflammatory molecules on cellular responses (Azzolina et al., 2003; Baldassare et al., 1999). Because of their essential role in intracellular signalling network, MAPK pathways and the connected transcription factors are appropriate targets for pharmacological treatment of inflammatory disorders (Lewis et al., 1998) and polyphenols are extensively investigated as possible regulatory molecules in this process.

Inflammation involves a cross-talk between several transcription factors, kinases and intracellular and intercellular cytokines involving NF-κB, MAPKs, PKC, PI-3-kinases etc. There has been considerable amount of evidence confirming that resveratrol takes active part in the modulation of these cell signalling molecules. Although resveratrol has been shown to target various intracellular signaling molecules in cultured cell lines, the molecular mechanisms underlying anti-inflammatory activity of resveratrol *in vivo* remain largely unresolved. Since NF-κB activation is critically linked to inflammatory responses and other chronic diseases associated with ROS and RNS production (Karin et al., 2004) the effect of resveratrol on NF-κB has been studied intensively in the last decade (Holmes-McNary & Baldwin, 2000; Manna et al., 2000) Indeed, resveratrol is a potent inhibitor of wide variety of inflammatory agents-induced activation of NF-κB, and this inhibition is not cell type specific. Some molecular targets of resveratrol are identified in toll-like receptor (TLR)-mediated signalling pathways. It has been reported that resveratrol acts on NF-κB by the inhibition of IκB kinase, leading to the inhibition of LPS-induced IκBα degradation, which results in the prevention of translocation of NF-κB into the nucleus (Holmes-McNary & Baldwin, 2000). It was suggested that IκBα degradation induced by TLR4-TRIF pathway is mediated through the interaction between TRIF and tumor necrosis factor receptor-associated factor 6 (TRAF6) because TRAF6 was shown to associate with the N-terminal part of TRIF (Sato et al., 2003; Jiang et al., 2004). Resveratrol was also shown to inhibit MyD88-independent signaling pathways and target expression (Youn et al., 2005). One of the major target molecules subjected to NF-κB-driven transactivation is cyclooxygenase-2, which is the enzyme of the rate-limiting step of the pathway that produces mediators of inflammation. Anti-inflammatory activity of resveratrol and some of its proposed mechanisms of action were attributed mostly in inhibition of COX activity (Das & Das, 2007; Kundu et al., 2006). Resveratrol also interferes with the pro-inflammatory signalling of thrombin resulting in the inhibition of adenosine nucleotide secretion from activated platelets and decreased neutrophil functions via inhibition of PAP and P2-receptor signalling through MAPK and cJun and JNK (Kaneider et al., 2004). However there is amply evidence about the modulatory effect of resveratrol on MAPK pathways, the data are so cell type and experimental system specific that it is hard to conclude and draw a coherent picture.

It has already been shown that quercetin can inhibit the production as well as the gene expression of TNF-α via modulation of NF-κB in human peripheral blood mononuclear cells (Nair et al., 2006). A possible mechanism behind this modulation was reported to be the inhibition of the degradation of the inhibitory part (IκBα) of this transcription factor (Peet & Li, 1999). In addition, quercetin treatment inhibited NF-κB activation through stabilization of the NF-κB/IκB complex leading to inhibition of IκB degradation and proinflammatory cytokines and NO/iNOS expression in RAW 264.7 macrophages (Cho et al., 2003). NF-κB/DNA binding activity induced by PMA and calcium ionophore was also markedly suppressed by quercetin without altering the binding activity of AP-1 in human mast cells (Min et al., 2007). In the same model quercetin attenuated the PMA and A23187-induced phosphorylation of p38 MAPK but not JNK or ERK. However, in an LPS-induced macrophage model quercetin strongly reduced activation of phosphorylated ERK kinase and p38 MAP kinase but not JNK MAP kinase (Cho et al., 2003). Moreover, TNF-α secretion in LPS-stimulated RAW macrophages was also shown to be inhibited by quercetin through interfering with the phosphorylation and activation of JNK and its downstream substrates c-Jun and ATF-2, and ERK1/2 and p38 MAPK (Wadsworth et al., 2001). Although NF-κB inhibition by quercetin in general is supported by several line of evidence the signalling events leading to the blockade of this transcription factor differ from cell to cell and model to model.

Curcumin has been shown to suppress the activation of NF-κB induced by various pro-inflammatory stimuli, presumably through inhibition of IKK kinase activity or DNA binding of p65. It is likely that curcumin also interferes with NF-κB activation at other points along this pathway, such as downstream to the various receptors that signal to this transcription factor. However, inhibition of IKK by curcumin plays a central role in this mechanism since the lack of phosphorylation of NF-κB suppresses binding of NF-κB to DNA sequences and as a consequence expression of genes described in vitro in inflammatory and vascular cells stimulated with LPS, staphylococcal enterotoxin A, TNF-α, or IL-1β, and in vivo in models of inflammatory diseases (Chan, 1995; Hatcher et al., 2008;

Jobin et al., 1999; Joe et al., 2004; Pan et al., 2000; Singh & Aggarwal, 1995). Regarding the LPS/NF-κB pathway, curcumin competes in vitro with LPS for binding to the TLR-4/myeloid differentiation factor-2 complex (Gradisar et al., 2007) and prevents TLR-4 homodimerization (Youn et al., 2006), events necessary for MyD88-dependent signalling. Further studies indicated that curcumin which contains unsaturated carbonyl group, but not resveratrol (with no unsaturated carbonyl group), inhibits TLR4 activation by interfering with receptor dimerization. This conclusion was further supported by the finding that curcumin inhibits ligand-independent dimerization of constitutively active TLR4. Inhibition of receptor dimerization of TLR4 suggests that curcumin could modify the free sulfhydryl groups of cysteine residues in TLR4, leading to interference of disulfide formation. Curcumin also induces intracellular heat-shock protein 70 (Dunsmore et al., 2001; Shen et al., 2007), a protein chaperone that protects IKK from proteasomal degradation, thus inhibiting NF-κB translocation to the nucleus. Downstream to NF-κB curcumin was found to significantly down-regulate the TNF-α-induced increase in MMP-13 mRNA and protein expression in primary human chondrocytes and in human bone chondrosarcoma cells by a mechanism involving the inhibition of c-Jun and JNK (Liacini et al., 2003). Interestingly, a study on experimental colitis in which NF-κB–dependent gene expression, inflammation, and tissue injury were significantly attenuated by curcumin an increase in the intestinal level of PPAR-γ was observed (Zhang et al., 2006) indicating a strong connection between the two transcription factor. In conclusion, inactivation of the NF-κB pathway by curcumin appears to occur at multiple levels and to ameliorate the various stages of sepsis-associated inflammation.

EGCG is known to inhibit NF-κB activation induced by many pro-inflammatory stimuli such as UV, LPS, TNF-α and IL-1β (Barthelman et al., 1998; Yang et al., 1998; Yang et al., 2001; Wheeler et al., 2004;) resulting in the decrease in the expression of inflammatory gene products including lipoxygenase (Yang & Koo, 2000), COX (Soriani et al., 1998), NOS (Chan et al., 1997; Lin & Lin, 1997), and TNF-α (Yang et al., 1998). It has been shown that the activation of NF-κB was suppressed by EGCG possibly mediated through the suppression of the kinase activity of IκB kinase in macrophages and the intestinal epithelial cell line (IEC-6) (Pan et al., 2000; Yang et al., 2001). EGCG was shown to inhibit the activity of IKKβ which is the key kinase in the canonical pathway for NF-κB activation in MyD88-dependent pathway of TLRs. Moreover, EGCG inhibited the activation of IFN regulatory factor 3 (IRF3) induced by LPS, poly[I:C], or the overexpression of TRIF. The inhibition of IRF3 activation by EGCG was mediated through the suppression of the kinase activity of TANK-binding kinase 1 in TRIF-dependent signalling pathways of TLR3 and TLR4 (Youn et al., 2006). These data indicate that green tea flavonoids, without the structural motif conferring Michael addition, did not inhibit TLR4 dimerization however; they can modulate both MyD88- and TRIF-dependent signalling pathways of TLRs and subsequent inflammatory target gene expression. In addition, Abboud et al demonstrated that EGCG may be beneficial in colitis, which was induced by rectal administration of trinitrobenzene sulfonic acid in C57/BL6 mice, through selective immunomodulatory effects, which may be mediated, at least in part, by inhibition of NF-κB and AP-1 (Abboud et al., 2008). The effects of EGCG on the cellular kinase cascade are rather diversified. In RAW 264.7 cells stimulated with LPS EGCG inhibited the production of TNF-α and MIP-2, and attenuated phosphorylation levels of ERK1/2 and JNK, but not p38. Also, EGCG attenuated the production of TNF-α and MIP-2, and the phosphorylation of ERK1/2 and JNK in the lungs of mice administered with LPS intratracheally (Bae et al., 2010). Recently, Yun, et al. showed that EGCG inhibited TNF-α induced phosphorylation of MAPKs family, such as ERK1/2, p38 and JNK in synovial fibroblast (Yun et al., 2008), while others showed that EGCG inhibited LPS-induced activation of p38, but augmented phosphorylation of ERK1/2 in J774.1 macrophage cells (Ichikawa et al., 2004). Inhibition of protein tyrosine kinase activity, reducing c-jun mRNA expression and inhibition of JNK1 activation by EGCG were reported by Yokozawa et al. (Yokozawa & Dong, 1997). Moreover, green tea polyphenols inhibit p44/42 MAP kinase expression (Lu et al., 1998) and induce the death of smooth muscle cells in a p53- and NF-κB-dependent manner (Ouyang et al., 2004). Taken together, the effects of EGCG on MAPKs phosphorylation are thought to be highly cell type-dependent.

It has been demonstrated that CAPE is a potent and specific inhibitor of NF-κB activation (Natarajan et al., 1996). CAPE inhibits LPS-induced nitric oxide and prostaglandin E2 production in a concentration-dependent manner and inhibits iNOS and COX-2 in RAW 264.7 cells, without significant cytotoxicity. CAPE treatment significantly reduced NF-κB translocation and DNA-binding in LPS-stimulated RAW264.7 cells. This effect was mediated through the inhibition of the degradation of IκB and by inhibition of both p38 mitogen-activated protein kinase and ERK phosphorylation, at least in part by inhibiting the generation of reactive oxygen species (Jung et al., 2008). This biological activity of CAPE could also explain by the finding that this phenolic compound prevented the binding to DNA of the p50/p65 NF-κB in vitro and in vivo (Natarajan et al., 1996). In addition to NF-κB, CAPE also targets the nuclear factor of activated T-cells (NFAT) signaling pathway that is known to play a critical role in the immune response. CAPE is a potent inhibitor of the NFAT pathway, and the results of Marquez et al. suggest that the calcineurin phosphatase can represent one of the major targets for CAPE, since this compound inhibits NFAT dephosphorylation and nuclear binding to DNA (Márquez et al., 2004). Other phenolic acids (gallic, caffeic, protocatechic, paracoumaric, sinapic, and ferulic acids) were reported to inhibit the activity of AP-1 transcription factor on MCF-7 cells after stimulation by phorbol 12-myristate 13-acetate and NF-κB activity on LPS/IFN-gamma-stimulated RAW 264.7 cells (Chao et al., 2010; Maggi-Capeyron et al., 2001). Similarly to phenolic acids ferulaldehyde also inhibited the activation and nuclear translocation of NF-κB in the liver of LPS-treated mice. In the same model ferulaldehyde significantly prevented the activation of JNK and Akt, but failed to attenuate LPS-induced activation of ERK1/2 (Radnai et al., 2009). Suppressing both LPS-induced JNK and Akt activation, ferulaldehyde inhibited the most important pathways leading to NF-κB activation, namely the LPS/TLR4/JNK and LPS/PI-3K/Akt pathways. The observation that FA did not show any effect on the LPS-induced activation of ERK1/2 and p38 MAP kinase pathways indicates that FA's inhibitory target(s) is necessarily downstream of the TLR4 receptors. However, unlike the in vivo model, ferulaldehyde attenuated LPS-induced activation of all three MAP kinases suggesting a uniform regulation of MAPK activation in LPS-stimulated macrophages. These results may arise from the differences of the inflammatory models used, and cell- and tissue-specificity of the LPS-induced processes (Veres et al., 2004). MAP kinase phosphatases (MKP), responsible for dephosphorylation and deactivation of MAP kinases, have a central role in the restraint of innate immune response and the prevention of septic shock syndrome during pathogenic microbial infection (Zhao et al., 2006). It is known that MAPK activation is followed by increased MKP-1 expression probably as a compensatory regulatory mechanism. In line with this evidence Tucsek et al found in an in vitro experimental model that ferulaldehyde shifted increased expression of MKP-1 forward in time which in turn attenuated activation of MAP kinases (Tucsek et al., 2011).

4. Conclusion

A number of different approaches have been investigated to try to treat and/or prevent septic shock and sepsis. Despite advances in elucidating its pathophysiology, severe sepsis remains a leading cause of death in the critically ill. It has been widely shown that many plant-derived compounds present anti-inflammatory effects. Polyphenols and their degradation products can exert their anti-inflammatory properties at multiple levels, through the modulation of MAPK, Akt and NF-κB signalling pathways, inhibition the production of inflammatory cytokines and chemokines, suppressing the activity of COX and iNOS and decreasing the production of ROS/RNS. Importantly, efficacy is maintained in some cases even when treatment is initiated hours after the onset of sepsis. These agents would be useful not only for the treatment of inflammatory disorders, but also for the control of some other diseases which present an inflammatory origin. However, the majority of the anti-inflammatory studies on plant-derived compounds have been carried out in vitro the polyphenols reviewed in this chapter appear to be safe and to exert anti-inflammatory effects in in vivo studies and even in humans. Thus, polyphenols and their degradation products represent a new, effective family of anti-inflammatory drugs that may help to prevent and treat sepsis.

5. Acknowledgment

I would like to thank Dr. Peter Jakus for his excellent editorial assistance. The author is grateful for the thoughtful suggestions and discussions from the members of the "Septic Shock Team" (Balazs Radnai and Zsuzsanna Tucsek). I sincerely apologize to those authors whose work could not be cited.

6. References

Abboud, P. A., Hake, P. W., Burroughs, T. J., Odoms, K., O'Connor, M., Mangeshkar, P., Wong, H. R. & Zingarelli, B. (2008). Therapeutic effect of epigallocatechin-3-gallate in a mouse model of colitis. *Eur J Pharmacol,* Vol. 579, No. 1-3, (Jan 28), pp. (411-417), 0014-2999 (Print)

Abe, Y., Hashimoto, S. & Horie, T. (1999). Curcumin inhibition of inflammatory cytokine production by human peripheral blood monocytes and alveolar macrophages. *Pharmacol Res,* Vol. 39, No. 1, (Jan), pp. (41-47), 1043-6618 (Print)

Abraham, E., Laterre, P. F., Garbino, J., Pingleton, S., Butler, T., Dugernier, T., Margolis, B., Kudsk, K., Zimmerli, W., Anderson, P., Reynaert, M., Lew, D., Lesslauer, W., Passe, S., Cooper, P., Burdeska, A., Modi, M., Leighton, A., Salgo, M. & Van der Auwera, P. (2001). Lenercept (p55 tumor necrosis factor receptor fusion protein) in severe sepsis and early septic shock: a randomized, double-blind, placebo-controlled, multicenter phase III trial with 1,342 patients. *Crit Care Med,* Vol. 29, No. 3, (Mar), pp. (503-510), 0090-3493 (Print)

Aggarwal, B. B., Kumar, A. & Bharti, A. C. (2003). Anticancer potential of curcumin: preclinical and clinical studies. *Anticancer Res,* Vol. 23, No. 1A, (Jan-Feb), pp. (363-398), 0250-7005 (Print)

Aggarwal, B. B. & Shishodia, S. (2006). Molecular targets of dietary agents for prevention and therapy of cancer. *Biochem Pharmacol,* Vol. 71, No. 10, (May 14), pp. (1397-1421), 0006-2952 (Print)

Ak, T. & Gulcin, I. (2008). Antioxidant and radical scavenging properties of curcumin. *Chem Biol Interact,* Vol. 174, No. 1, (Jul 10), pp. (27-37), 0009-2797 (Print)

Arts, I. C., Sesink, A. L., Faassen-Peters, M. & Hollman, P. C. (2004). The type of sugar moiety is a major determinant of the small intestinal uptake and subsequent biliary excretion of dietary quercetin glycosides. *Br J Nutr,* Vol. 91, No. 6, (Jun), pp. (841-847), 0007-1145 (Print)

Azzolina, A., Bongiovanni, A. & Lampiasi, N. (2003). Substance P induces TNF-alpha and IL-6 production through NF kappa B in peritoneal mast cells. *Biochim Biophys Acta,* Vol. 1643, No. 1-3, (Dec 7), pp. (75-83), 0006-3002 (Print)

Babu, P. V. & Liu, D. (2008). Green tea catechins and cardiovascular health: an update. *Curr Med Chem,* Vol. 15, No. 18, pp. (1840-1850), 0929-8673 (Print)

Bae, H. B., Li, M., Kim, J. P., Kim, S. J., Jeong, C. W., Lee, H. G., Kim, W. M., Kim, H. S. & Kwak, S. H. (2010). The effect of epigallocatechin gallate on lipopolysaccharide-induced acute lung injury in a murine model. *Inflammation,* Vol. 33, No. 2, (Apr), pp. (82-91), 1573-2576 (Electronic)

Baldassare, J. J., Bi, Y. & Bellone, C. J. (1999). The role of p38 mitogen-activated protein kinase in IL-1 beta transcription. *J Immunol,* Vol. 162, No. 9, (May 1), pp. (5367-5373), 0022-1767 (Print)

Banerjee, M., Tripathi, L. M., Srivastava, V. M., Puri, A. & Shukla, R. (2003). Modulation of inflammatory mediators by ibuprofen and curcumin treatment during chronic inflammation in rat. *Immunopharmacol Immunotoxicol,* Vol. 25, No. 2, (May), pp. (213-224), 0892-3973 (Print)

Barthelman, M., Bair, W. B., 3rd, Stickland, K. K., Chen, W., Timmermann, B. N., Valcic, S., Dong, Z. & Bowden, G. T. (1998). (-)-Epigallocatechin-3-gallate inhibition of ultraviolet B-induced AP-1 activity. *Carcinogenesis,* Vol. 19, No. 12, (Dec), pp. (2201-2204), 0143-3334 (Print)

Beecher, G. R. (1998). Nutrient content of tomatoes and tomato products. *Proc Soc Exp Biol Med,* Vol. 218, No. 2, (Jun), pp. (98-100), 0037-9727 (Print)

Birrell, M. A., McCluskie, K., Wong, S., Donnelly, L. E., Barnes, P. J. & Belvisi, M. G. (2005). Resveratrol, an extract of red wine, inhibits lipopolysaccharide induced airway neutrophilia and inflammatory mediators through an NF-kappaB-independent mechanism. *FASEB J,* Vol. 19, No. 7, (May), pp. (840-841), 1530-6860 (Electronic)

Bischoff, S. C. (2008). Quercetin: potentials in the prevention and therapy of disease. *Curr Opin Clin Nutr Metab Care,* Vol. 11, No. 6, (Nov), pp. (733-740), 1363-1950 (Print)

Biswas, S. K., McClure, D., Jimenez, L. A., Megson, I. L. & Rahman, I. (2005). Curcumin induces glutathione biosynthesis and inhibits NF-kappaB activation and interleukin-8 release in alveolar epithelial cells: mechanism of free radical scavenging activity. *Antioxid Redox Signal,* Vol. 7, No. 1-2, (Jan-Feb), pp. (32-41), 1523-0864 (Print)

Boocock, D. J., Faust, G. E., Patel, K. R., Schinas, A. M., Brown, V. A., Ducharme, M. P., Booth, T. D., Crowell, J. A., Perloff, M., Gescher, A. J., Steward, W. P. & Brenner, D. E. (2007). Phase I dose escalation pharmacokinetic study in healthy volunteers of resveratrol, a potential cancer chemopreventive agent. *Cancer Epidemiol Biomarkers Prev,* Vol. 16, No. 6, (Jun), pp. (1246-1252), 1055-9965 (Print)

Boots, A. W., Haenen, G. R. & Bast, A. (2008). Health effects of quercetin: from antioxidant to nutraceutical. *Eur J Pharmacol,* Vol. 585, No. 2-3, (May 13), pp. (325-337), 0014-2999 (Print)

Boots, A. W., Li, H., Schins, R. P., Duffin, R., Heemskerk, J. W., Bast, A. & Haenen, G. R. (2007). The quercetin paradox. *Toxicol Appl Pharmacol,* Vol. 222, No. 1, (Jul 1), pp. (89-96), 0041-008X (Print)

Bravo, L. (1998). Polyphenols: chemistry, dietary sources, metabolism, and nutritional significance. *Nutr Rev,* Vol. 56, No. 11, (Nov), pp. (317-333), 0029-6643 (Print)

Bureau, G., Longpre, F. & Martinoli, M. G. (2008). Resveratrol and quercetin, two natural polyphenols, reduce apoptotic neuronal cell death induced by neuroinflammation. *J Neurosci Res,* Vol. 86, No. 2, (Feb 1), pp. (403-410), 1097-4547 (Electronic)

Cadenas, S. & Cadenas, A. M. (2002). Fighting the stranger-antioxidant protection against endotoxin toxicity. *Toxicology,* Vol. 180, No. 1, (Oct 30), pp. (45-63), 0300-483X (Print)

Calandra, T., Baumgartner, J. D., Grau, G. E., Wu, M. M., Lambert, P. H., Schellekens, J., Verhoef, J. & Glauser, M. P. (1990). Prognostic values of tumor necrosis factor/cachectin, interleukin-1, interferon-alpha, and interferon-gamma in the serum of patients with septic shock. Swiss-Dutch J5 Immunoglobulin Study Group. *J Infect Dis,* Vol. 161, No. 5, (May), pp. (982-987), 0022-1899 (Print)

Chan, J. H. & Chan, D. S. (1997). Computer program for tracking incidence of intravascular-device-related infections in patients receiving parenteral nutrition. *Am J Health Syst Pharm,* Vol. 54, No. 16, (Aug 15), pp. (1897-1898), 1079-2082 (Print)

Chan, M. M. (1995). Inhibition of tumor necrosis factor by curcumin, a phytochemical. *Biochem Pharmacol,* Vol. 49, No. 11, (May 26), pp. (1551-1556), 0006-2952 (Print)

Chang, F., Lee, J. T., Navolanic, P. M., Steelman, L. S., Shelton, J. G., Blalock, W. L., Franklin, R. A. & McCubrey, J. A. (2003). Involvement of PI3K/Akt pathway in cell cycle progression, apoptosis, and neoplastic transformation: a target for cancer chemotherapy. *Leukemia,* Vol. 17, No. 3, (Mar), pp. (590-603), 0887-6924 (Print)

Chao, C. Y., Mong, M. C., Chan, K. C. & Yin, M. C. (2010). Anti-glycative and anti-inflammatory effects of caffeic acid and ellagic acid in kidney of diabetic mice. *Mol Nutr Food Res,* Vol. 54, No. 3, (Mar), pp. (388-395), 1613-4133 (Electronic)

Chen, H. W., Kuo, H. T., Chai, C. Y., Ou, J. L. & Yang, R. C. (2007). Pretreatment of curcumin attenuates coagulopathy and renal injury in LPS-induced endotoxemia. *J Endotoxin Res,* Vol. 13, No. 1, pp. (15-23), 0968-0519 (Print)

Cheng, A. L., Hsu, C. H., Lin, J. K., Hsu, M. M., Ho, Y. F., Shen, T. S., Ko, J. Y., Lin, J. T., Lin, B. R., Ming-Shiang, W., Yu, H. S., Jee, S. H., Chen, G. S., Chen, T. M., Chen, C. A., Lai, M. K., Pu, Y. S., Pan, M. H., Wang, Y. J., Tsai, C. C. & Hsieh, C. Y. (2001). Phase I clinical trial of curcumin, a chemopreventive agent, in patients with high-risk or pre-malignant lesions. *Anticancer Res,* Vol. 21, No. 4B, (Jul-Aug), pp. (2895-2900), 0250-7005 (Print)

Cho, J. W., Lee, K. S. & Kim, C. W. (2007). Curcumin attenuates the expression of IL-1beta, IL-6, and TNF-alpha as well as cyclin E in TNF-alpha-treated HaCaT cells; NF-kappaB and MAPKs as potential upstream targets. *Int J Mol Med,* Vol. 19, No. 3, (Mar), pp. (469-474), 1107-3756 (Print)

Cho, S. Y., Park, S. J., Kwon, M. J., Jeong, T. S., Bok, S. H., Choi, W. Y., Jeong, W. I., Ryu, S. Y., Do, S. H., Lee, C. S., Song, J. C. & Jeong, K. S. (2003). Quercetin suppresses proinflammatory cytokines production through MAP kinases andNF-kappaB pathway in lipopolysaccharide-stimulated macrophage. *Mol Cell Biochem,* Vol. 243, No. 1-2, (Jan), pp. (153-160), 0300-8177 (Print)

Culpitt, S. V., Rogers, D. F., Fenwick, P. S., Shah, P., De Matos, C., Russell, R. E., Barnes, P. J. & Donnelly, L. E. (2003). Inhibition by red wine extract, resveratrol, of cytokine release by alveolar macrophages in COPD. *Thorax,* Vol. 58, No. 11, (Nov), pp. (942-946), 0040-6376 (Print)

Cushnie, T. P. & Lamb, A. J. (2005). Antimicrobial activity of flavonoids. *Int J Antimicrob Agents,* Vol. 26, No. 5, (Nov), pp. (343-356), 0924-8579 (Print)

D'Archivio, M., Filesi, C., Di Benedetto, R., Gargiulo, R., Giovannini, C. & Masella, R. (2007). Polyphenols, dietary sources and bioavailability. *Ann Ist Super Sanita,* Vol. 43, No. 4, pp. (348-361), 0021-2571 (Print)

Das, S. & Das, D. K. (2007). Anti-inflammatory responses of resveratrol. *Inflamm Allergy Drug Targets,* Vol. 6, No. 3, (Sep), pp. (168-173), 1871-5281 (Print)

de Boer, V. C., Dihal, A. A., van der Woude, H., Arts, I. C., Wolffram, S., Alink, G. M., Rietjens, I. M., Keijer, J. & Hollman, P. C. (2005). Tissue distribution of quercetin in rats and pigs. *J Nutr,* Vol. 135, No. 7, (Jul), pp. (1718-1725), 0022-3166 (Print)

de Lange, D. W. (2007). From red wine to polyphenols and back: a journey through the history of the French Paradox. *Thromb Res,* Vol. 119, No. 4, pp. (403-406), 0049-3848 (Print)

de Lorgeril, M., Salen, P., Martin, J. L., Monjaud, I., Delaye, J. & Mamelle, N. (1999). Mediterranean diet, traditional risk factors, and the rate of cardiovascular complications after myocardial infarction: final report of the Lyon Diet Heart Study. *Circulation,* Vol. 99, No. 6, (Feb 16), pp. (779-785), 0009-7322 (Print)

Dinarello, C. A. (1994). The interleukin-1 family: 10 years of discovery. *FASEB J,* Vol. 8, No. 15, (Dec), pp. (1314-1325), 0892-6638 (Print)

Donnelly, L. E., Newton, R., Kennedy, G. E., Fenwick, P. S., Leung, R. H., Ito, K., Russell, R. E. & Barnes, P. J. (2004). Anti-inflammatory effects of resveratrol in lung epithelial cells: molecular mechanisms. *Am J Physiol Lung Cell Mol Physiol,* Vol. 287, No. 4, (Oct), pp. (L774-783), 1040-0605 (Print)

Dunsmore, K. E., Chen, P. G. & Wong, H. R. (2001). Curcumin, a medicinal herbal compound capable of inducing the heat shock response. *Crit Care Med,* Vol. 29, No. 11, (Nov), pp. (2199-2204), 0090-3493 (Print)

Egan, M. E., Pearson, M., Weiner, S. A., Rajendran, V., Rubin, D., Glockner-Pagel, J., Canny, S., Du, K., Lukacs, G. L. & Caplan, M. J. (2004). Curcumin, a major constituent of turmeric, corrects cystic fibrosis defects. *Science,* Vol. 304, No. 5670, (Apr 23), pp. (600-602), 1095-9203 (Electronic)

Ek, R. O., Serter, M., Ergin, K., Yildiz, Y., Cecen, S., Kavak, T. & Yenisey, C. (2008). The effects of caffeic acid phenethyl ester (CAPE) on TNBS-induced colitis in ovariectomized rats. *Dig Dis Sci,* Vol. 53, No. 6, (Jun), pp. (1609-1617), 0163-2116 (Print)

Feng, Y. H., Zou, J. P. & Li, X. Y. (2002). Effects of resveratrol and ethanol on production of pro-inflammatory factors from endotoxin activated murine macrophages. *Acta Pharmacol Sin,* Vol. 23, No. 11, (Nov), pp. (1002-1006), 1671-4083 (Print)

Fidan, H., Sahin, O., Yavuz, Y., Kilbas, A., Cetinkaya, Z., Ela, Y., Ozen, O. A. & Altuntas, I. (2007). Caffeic acid phenethyl ester reduces mortality and sepsis-induced lung injury in rats. *Crit Care Med,* Vol. 35, No. 12, (Dec), pp. (2822-2829), 0090-3493 (Print)

Fisher, C. J., Jr., Dhainaut, J. F., Opal, S. M., Pribble, J. P., Balk, R. A., Slotman, G. J., Iberti, T. J., Rackow, E. C., Shapiro, M. J., Greenman, R. L. & et al. (1994). Recombinant human interleukin 1 receptor antagonist in the treatment of patients with sepsis syndrome. Results from a randomized, double-blind, placebo-controlled trial. Phase III rhIL-1ra Sepsis Syndrome Study Group. *JAMA*, Vol. 271, No. 23, (Jun 15), pp. (1836-1843), 0098-7484 (Print)

Fukumoto, L. R. & Mazza, G. (2000). Assessing antioxidant and prooxidant activities of phenolic compounds. *J Agric Food Chem*, Vol. 48, No. 8, (Aug), pp. (3597-3604), 0021-8561 (Print)

Gao, X., Xu, Y. X., Janakiraman, N., Chapman, R. A. & Gautam, S. C. (2001). Immunomodulatory activity of resveratrol: suppression of lymphocyte proliferation, development of cell-mediated cytotoxicity, and cytokine production. *Biochem Pharmacol*, Vol. 62, No. 9, (Nov 1), pp. (1299-1308), 0006-2952 (Print)

Geraets, L., Moonen, H. J., Brauers, K., Wouters, E. F., Bast, A. & Hageman, G. J. (2007). Dietary flavones and flavonoles are inhibitors of poly(ADP-ribose)polymerase-1 in pulmonary epithelial cells. *J Nutr*, Vol. 137, No. 10, (Oct), pp. (2190-2195), 0022-3166 (Print)

Gerhauser, C., Klimo, K., Heiss, E., Neumann, I., Gamal-Eldeen, A., Knauft, J., Liu, G. Y., Sitthimonchai, S. & Frank, N. (2003). Mechanism-based in vitro screening of potential cancer chemopreventive agents. *Mutat Res*, Vol. 523-524, No. (Feb-Mar), pp. (163-172), 0027-5107 (Print)

Gomez-Jimenez, J., Salgado, A., Mourelle, M., Martin, M. C., Segura, R. M., Peracaula, R. & Moncada, S. (1995). L-arginine: nitric oxide pathway in endotoxemia and human septic shock. *Crit Care Med*, Vol. 23, No. 2, (Feb), pp. (253-258), 0090-3493 (Print)

Gonthier, M. P., Rios, L. Y., Verny, M., Remesy, C. & Scalbert, A. (2003). Novel liquid chromatography-electrospray ionization mass spectrometry method for the quantification in human urine of microbial aromatic acid metabolites derived from dietary polyphenols. *J Chromatogr B Analyt Technol Biomed Life Sci*, Vol. 789, No. 2, (Jun 15), pp. (247-255), 1570-0232 (Print)

Gonzales, A. M. & Orlando, R. A. (2008). Curcumin and resveratrol inhibit nuclear factor-kappaB-mediated cytokine expression in adipocytes. *Nutr Metab (Lond)*, Vol. 5, No. pp. (17), 1743-7075 (Electronic)

Gradisar, H., Keber, M. M., Pristovsek, P. & Jerala, R. (2007). MD-2 as the target of curcumin in the inhibition of response to LPS. *J Leukoc Biol*, Vol. 82, No. 4, (Oct), pp. (968-974), 0741-5400 (Print)

Gukovsky, I., Reyes, C. N., Vaquero, E. C., Gukovskaya, A. S. & Pandol, S. J. (2003). Curcumin ameliorates ethanol and nonethanol experimental pancreatitis. *Am J Physiol Gastrointest Liver Physiol*, Vol. 284, No. 1, (Jan), pp. (G85-95), 0193-1857 (Print)

Gulcin, I. (2006). Antioxidant activity of caffeic acid (3,4-dihydroxycinnamic acid). *Toxicology*, Vol. 217, No. 2-3, (Jan 16), pp. (213-220), 0300-483X (Print)

Guo, Q., Zhao, B., Li, M., Shen, S. & Xin, W. (1996). Studies on protective mechanisms of four components of green tea polyphenols against lipid peroxidation in synaptosomes. *Biochim Biophys Acta*, Vol. 1304, No. 3, (Dec 13), pp. (210-222), 0006-3002 (Print)

Hakkinen, S. H., Karenlampi, S. O., Heinonen, I. M., Mykkanen, H. M. & Torronen, A. R. (1999). Content of the flavonols quercetin, myricetin, and kaempferol in 25 edible berries. *J Agric Food Chem*, Vol. 47, No. 6, (Jun), pp. (2274-2279), 0021-8561 (Print)

Han, M. H., Yang, X. W., Zhong, G. Y. & Zhang, M. (2007). [Bioactive constituents inhibiting TNF-alpha production in fresh rhizome of Pinellia ternata]. *Zhongguo Zhong Yao Za Zhi,* Vol. 32, No. 17, (Sep), pp. (1755-1759), 1001-5302 (Print)

Hanasaki, Y., Ogawa, S. & Fukui, S. (1994). The correlation between active oxygens scavenging and antioxidative effects of flavonoids. *Free Radic Biol Med,* Vol. 16, No. 6, (Jun), pp. (845-850), 0891-5849 (Print)

Harada, M., Kan, Y., Naoki, H., Fukui, Y., Kageyama, N., Nakai, M., Miki, W. & Kiso, Y. (1999). Identification of the major antioxidative metabolites in biological fluids of the rat with ingested (+)-catechin and (-)-epicatechin. *Biosci Biotechnol Biochem,* Vol. 63, No. 6, (Jun), pp. (973-977), 0916-8451 (Print)

Hatcher, H., Planalp, R., Cho, J., Torti, F. M. & Torti, S. V. (2008). Curcumin: from ancient medicine to current clinical trials. *Cell Mol Life Sci,* Vol. 65, No. 11, (Jun), pp. (1631-1652), 1420-682X (Print)

Heijnen, C. G., Haenen, G. R., Vekemans, J. A. & Bast, A. (2001). Peroxynitrite scavenging of flavonoids: structure activity relationship. *Environ Toxicol Pharmacol,* Vol. 10, No. 4, (Sep), pp. (199-206), 1382-6689 (Print)

Heuer, J. G., Sharma, G. R., Gerlitz, B., Zhang, T., Bailey, D. L., Ding, C., Berg, D. T., Perkins, D., Stephens, E. J., Holmes, K. C., Grubbs, R. L., Fynboe, K. A., Chen, Y. F., Grinnell, B. & Jakubowski, J. A. (2004). Evaluation of protein C and other biomarkers as predictors of mortality in a rat cecal ligation and puncture model of sepsis. *Crit Care Med,* Vol. 32, No. 7, (Jul), pp. (1570-1578), 0090-3493 (Print)

Hidaka, H., Ishiko, T., Furuhashi, T., Kamohara, H., Suzuki, S., Miyazaki, M., Ikeda, O., Mita, S., Setoguchi, T. & Ogawa, M. (2002). Curcumin inhibits interleukin 8 production and enhances interleukin 8 receptor expression on the cell surface:impact on human pancreatic carcinoma cell growth by autocrine regulation. *Cancer,* Vol. 95, No. 6, (Sep 15), pp. (1206-1214), 0008-543X (Print)

Hirata, A., Murakami, Y., Atsumi, T., Shoji, M., Ogiwara, T., Shibuya, K., Ito, S., Yokoe, I. & Fujisawa, S. (2005). Ferulic acid dimer inhibits lipopolysaccharide-stimulated cyclooxygenase-2 expression in macrophages. *In Vivo,* Vol. 19, No. 5, (Sep-Oct), pp. (849-853), 0258-851X (Print)

Holmes-McNary, M. & Baldwin, A. S., Jr. (2000). Chemopreventive properties of trans-resveratrol are associated with inhibition of activation of the IkappaB kinase. *Cancer Res,* Vol. 60, No. 13, (Jul 1), pp. (3477-3483), 0008-5472 (Print)

Hotchkiss, R. S., Chang, K. C., Swanson, P. E., Tinsley, K. W., Hui, J. J., Klender, P., Xanthoudakis, S., Roy, S., Black, C., Grimm, E., Aspiotis, R., Han, Y., Nicholson, D. W. & Karl, I. E. (2000). Caspase inhibitors improve survival in sepsis: a critical role of the lymphocyte. *Nat Immunol,* Vol. 1, No. 6, (Dec), pp. (496-501), 1529-2908 (Print)

Hotchkiss, R. S. & Karl, I. E. (2003). The pathophysiology and treatment of sepsis. *N Engl J Med,* Vol. 348, No. 2, (Jan 9), pp. (138-150), 1533-4406 (Electronic)

Hsu, C. H. & Cheng, A. L. (2007). Clinical studies with curcumin. *Adv Exp Med Biol,* Vol. 595, No. pp. (471-480), 0065-2598 (Print)

Ichikawa, D., Matsui, A., Imai, M., Sonoda, Y. & Kasahara, T. (2004). Effect of various catechins on the IL-12p40 production by murine peritoneal macrophages and a macrophage cell line, J774.1. *Biol Pharm Bull,* Vol. 27, No. 9, (Sep), pp. (1353-1358), 0918-6158 (Print)

Ireson, C., Orr, S., Jones, D. J., Verschoyle, R., Lim, C. K., Luo, J. L., Howells, L., Plummer, S., Jukes, R., Williams, M., Steward, W. P. & Gescher, A. (2001). Characterization of metabolites of the chemopreventive agent curcumin in human and rat hepatocytes and in the rat in vivo, and evaluation of their ability to inhibit phorbol ester-induced prostaglandin E2 production. *Cancer Res,* Vol. 61, No. 3, (Feb 1), pp. (1058-1064), 0008-5472 (Print)

Jang, D. S., Kang, B. S., Ryu, S. Y., Chang, I. M., Min, K. R. & Kim, Y. (1999). Inhibitory effects of resveratrol analogs on unopsonized zymosan-induced oxygen radical production. *Biochem Pharmacol,* Vol. 57, No. 6, (Mar 15), pp. (705-712), 0006-2952 (Print)

Jang, M., Cai, L., Udeani, G. O., Slowing, K. V., Thomas, C. F., Beecher, C. W., Fong, H. H., Farnsworth, N. R., Kinghorn, A. D., Mehta, R. G., Moon, R. C. & Pezzuto, J. M. (1997). Cancer chemopreventive activity of resveratrol, a natural product derived from grapes. *Science,* Vol. 275, No. 5297, (Jan 10), pp. (218-220), 0036-8075 (Print)

Jeong, J. H., Kim, H. J., Lee, T. J., Kim, M. K., Park, E. S. & Choi, B. S. (2004). Epigallocatechin 3-gallate attenuates neuronal damage induced by 3-hydroxykynurenine. *Toxicology,* Vol. 195, No. 1, (Jan 15), pp. (53-60), 0300-483X (Print)

Jiang, D., Chiaro, C., Maddali, P., Prabhu, K. S. & Peterson, D. G. (2009). Identification of hydroxycinnamic acid-maillard reaction products in low-moisture baking model systems. *J Agric Food Chem,* Vol. 57, No. 21, (Nov 11), pp. (9932-9943), 1520-5118 (Electronic)

Jiang, Z., Mak, T. W., Sen, G. & Li, X. (2004). Toll-like receptor 3-mediated activation of NF-kappaB and IRF3 diverges at Toll-IL-1 receptor domain-containing adapter inducing IFN-beta. *Proc Natl Acad Sci U S A,* Vol. 101, No. 10, (Mar 9), pp. (3533-3538), 0027-8424 (Print)

Jin, C. Y., Lee, J. D., Park, C., Choi, Y. H. & Kim, G. Y. (2007). Curcumin attenuates the release of pro-inflammatory cytokines in lipopolysaccharide-stimulated BV2 microglia. *Acta Pharmacol Sin,* Vol. 28, No. 10, (Oct), pp. (1645-1651), 1671-4083 (Print)

Jobin, C., Bradham, C. A., Russo, M. P., Juma, B., Narula, A. S., Brenner, D. A. & Sartor, R. B. (1999). Curcumin blocks cytokine-mediated NF-kappa B activation and proinflammatory gene expression by inhibiting inhibitory factor I-kappa B kinase activity. *J Immunol,* Vol. 163, No. 6, (Sep 15), pp. (3474-3483), 0022-1767 (Print)

Joe, B. & Lokesh, B. R. (1994). Role of capsaicin, curcumin and dietary n-3 fatty acids in lowering the generation of reactive oxygen species in rat peritoneal macrophages. *Biochim Biophys Acta,* Vol. 1224, No. 2, (Nov 10), pp. (255-263), 0006-3002 (Print)

Joe, B., Vijaykumar, M. & Lokesh, B. R. (2004). Biological properties of curcumin-cellular and molecular mechanisms of action. *Crit Rev Food Sci Nutr,* Vol. 44, No. 2, pp. (97-111), 1040-8398 (Print)

Jung, W. J. & Sung, M. K. (2004). Effects of major dietary antioxidants on inflammatory markers of RAW 264.7 macrophages. *Biofactors,* Vol. 21, No. 1-4, pp. (113-117), 0951-6433 (Print)

Jung, W. K., Choi, I., Lee, D. Y., Yea, S. S., Choi, Y. H., Kim, M. M., Park, S. G., Seo, S. K., Lee, S. W., Lee, C. M., Park, Y. M. & Choi, I. W. (2008). Caffeic acid phenethyl ester protects mice from lethal endotoxin shock and inhibits lipopolysaccharide-induced cyclooxygenase-2 and inducible nitric oxide synthase expression in RAW 264.7 macrophages via the p38/ERK and NF-kappaB pathways. *Int J Biochem Cell Biol,* Vol. 40, No. 11, pp. (2572-2582), 1357-2725 (Print)

Kabarowski, J. H., Zhu, K., Le, L. Q., Witte, O. N. & Xu, Y. (2001). Lysophosphatidylcholine as a ligand for the immunoregulatory receptor G2A. *Science,* Vol. 293, No. 5530, (Jul 27), pp. (702-705), 0036-8075 (Print)

Kalyanaraman, B., Premovic, P. I. & Sealy, R. C. (1987). Semiquinone anion radicals from addition of amino acids, peptides, and proteins to quinones derived from oxidation of catechols and catecholamines. An ESR spin stabilization study. *J Biol Chem,* Vol. 262, No. 23, (Aug 15), pp. (11080-11087), 0021-9258 (Print)

Kaneider, N. C., Mosheimer, B., Reinisch, N., Patsch, J. R. & Wiedermann, C. J. (2004). Inhibition of thrombin-induced signaling by resveratrol and quercetin: effects on adenosine nucleotide metabolism in endothelial cells and platelet-neutrophil interactions. *Thromb Res,* Vol. 114, No. 3, pp. (185-194), 0049-3848 (Print)

Karin, M., Yamamoto, Y. & Wang, Q. M. (2004). The IKK NF-kappa B system: a treasure trove for drug development. *Nat Rev Drug Discov,* Vol. 3, No. 1, (Jan), pp. (17-26), 1474-1776 (Print)

Kaur, G., Tirkey, N., Bharrhan, S., Chanana, V., Rishi, P. & Chopra, K. (2006). Inhibition of oxidative stress and cytokine activity by curcumin in amelioration of endotoxin-induced experimental hepatoxicity in rodents. *Clin Exp Immunol,* Vol. 145, No. 2, (Aug), pp. (313-321), 0009-9104 (Print)

Kawada, N., Seki, S., Inoue, M. & Kuroki, T. (1998). Effect of antioxidants, resveratrol, quercetin, and N-acetylcysteine, on the functions of cultured rat hepatic stellate cells and Kupffer cells. *Hepatology,* Vol. 27, No. 5, (May), pp. (1265-1274), 0270-9139 (Print)

Kempuraj, D., Madhappan, B., Christodoulou, S., Boucher, W., Cao, J., Papadopoulou, N., Cetrulo, C. L. & Theoharides, T. C. (2005). Flavonols inhibit proinflammatory mediator release, intracellular calcium ion levels and protein kinase C theta phosphorylation in human mast cells. *Br J Pharmacol,* Vol. 145, No. 7, (Aug), pp. (934-944), 0007-1188 (Print)

Kerry, N. & Rice-Evans, C. (1998). Peroxynitrite oxidises catechols to o-quinones. *FEBS Lett,* Vol. 437, No. 3, (Oct 23), pp. (167-171), 0014-5793 (Print)

Khokhar, S. & Magnusdottir, S. G. (2002). Total phenol, catechin, and caffeine contents of teas commonly consumed in the United kingdom. *J Agric Food Chem,* Vol. 50, No. 3, (Jan 30), pp. (565-570), 0021-8561 (Print)

Kim, I. B., Kim, D. Y., Lee, S. J., Sun, M. J., Lee, M. S., Li, H., Cho, J. J. & Park, C. S. (2006). Inhibition of IL-8 production by green tea polyphenols in human nasal fibroblasts and A549 epithelial cells. *Biol Pharm Bull,* Vol. 29, No. 6, (Jun), pp. (1120-1125), 1347-5215 (Electronic)

Kim, N. Y., Pae, H. O., Ko, Y. S., Yoo, J. C., Choi, B. M., Jun, C. D., Chung, H. T., Inagaki, M., Higuchi, R. & Kim, Y. C. (1999). In vitro inducible nitric oxide synthesis inhibitory active constituents from Fraxinus rhynchophylla. *Planta Med,* Vol. 65, No. 7, (Oct), pp. (656-658), 0032-0943 (Print)

Kim, O. K., Murakami, A., Nakamura, Y. & Ohigashi, H. (1998). Screening of edible Japanese plants for nitric oxide generation inhibitory activities in RAW 264.7 cells. *Cancer Lett,* Vol. 125, No. 1-2, (Mar 13), pp. (199-207), 0304-3835 (Print)

Kobuchi, H., Droy-Lefaix, M. T., Christen, Y. & Packer, L. (1997). Ginkgo biloba extract (EGb 761): inhibitory effect on nitric oxide production in the macrophage cell line RAW 264.7. *Biochem Pharmacol,* Vol. 53, No. 6, (Mar 21), pp. (897-903), 0006-2952 (Print)

Koltuksuz, U., Ozen, S., Uz, E., Aydinc, M., Karaman, A., Gultek, A., Akyol, O., Gursoy, M. H. & Aydin, E. (1999). Caffeic acid phenethyl ester prevents intestinal reperfusion injury in rats. *J Pediatr Surg,* Vol. 34, No. 10, (Oct), pp. (1458-1462), 0022-3468 (Print)

Kong, A. N., Yu, R., Chen, C., Mandlekar, S. & Primiano, T. (2000). Signal transduction events elicited by natural products: role of MAPK and caspase pathways in homeostatic response and induction of apoptosis. *Arch Pharm Res,* Vol. 23, No. 1, (Feb), pp. (1-16), 0253-6269 (Print)

Kowalski, J., Samojedny, A., Paul, M., Pietsz, G. & Wilczok, T. (2005). Effect of apigenin, kaempferol and resveratrol on the expression of interleukin-1beta and tumor necrosis factor-alpha genes in J774.2 macrophages. *Pharmacol Rep,* Vol. 57, No. 3, (May-Jun), pp. (390-394), 1734-1140 (Print)

Kundu, J. K., Shin, Y. K., Kim, S. H. & Surh, Y. J. (2006). Resveratrol inhibits phorbol ester-induced expression of COX-2 and activation of NF-kappaB in mouse skin by blocking IkappaB kinase activity. *Carcinogenesis,* Vol. 27, No. 7, (Jul), pp. (1465-1474), 0143-3334 (Print)

Labinskyy, N., Csiszar, A., Veress, G., Stef, G., Pacher, P., Oroszi, G., Wu, J. & Ungvari, Z. (2006). Vascular dysfunction in aging: potential effects of resveratrol, an anti-inflammatory phytoestrogen. *Curr Med Chem,* Vol. 13, No. 9, pp. (989-996), 0929-8673 (Print)

Lee, J. J., Huang, W. T., Shao, D. Z., Liao, J. F. & Lin, M. T. (2003). Blocking NF-kappaB activation may be an effective strategy in the fever therapy. *Jpn J Physiol,* Vol. 53, No. 5, (Oct), pp. (367-375), 0021-521X (Print)

Lee, M. J., Wang, Z. Y., Li, H., Chen, L., Sun, Y., Gobbo, S., Balentine, D. A. & Yang, C. S. (1995). Analysis of plasma and urinary tea polyphenols in human subjects. *Cancer Epidemiol Biomarkers Prev,* Vol. 4, No. 4, (Jun), pp. (393-399), 1055-9965 (Print)

Leiro, J., Alvarez, E., Arranz, J. A., Laguna, R., Uriarte, E. & Orallo, F. (2004). Effects of cis-resveratrol on inflammatory murine macrophages: antioxidant activity and down-regulation of inflammatory genes. *J Leukoc Biol,* Vol. 75, No. 6, (Jun), pp. (1156-1165), 0741-5400 (Print)

Levites, Y., Weinreb, O., Maor, G., Youdim, M. B. & Mandel, S. (2001). Green tea polyphenol (-)-epigallocatechin-3-gallate prevents N-methyl-4-phenyl-1,2,3,6-tetrahydropyridine-induced dopaminergic neurodegeneration. *J Neurochem,* Vol. 78, No. 5, (Sep), pp. (1073-1082), 0022-3042 (Print)

Levites, Y., Youdim, M. B., Maor, G. & Mandel, S. (2002). Attenuation of 6-hydroxydopamine (6-OHDA)-induced nuclear factor-kappaB (NF-kappaB) activation and cell death by tea extracts in neuronal cultures. *Biochem Pharmacol,* Vol. 63, No. 1, (Jan 1), pp. (21-29), 0006-2952 (Print)

Lewis, T. S., Shapiro, P. S. & Ahn, N. G. (1998). Signal transduction through MAP kinase cascades. *Adv Cancer Res,* Vol. 74, No. pp. (49-139), 0065-230X (Print)

Li, W., Ashok, M., Li, J., Yang, H., Sama, A. E. & Wang, H. (2007). A major ingredient of green tea rescues mice from lethal sepsis partly by inhibiting HMGB1. *PLoS One,* Vol. 2, No. 11, pp. (e1153), 1932-6203 (Electronic)

Li, Y. & Sarkar, F. H. (2002). Inhibition of nuclear factor kappaB activation in PC3 cells by genistein is mediated via Akt signaling pathway. *Clin Cancer Res,* Vol. 8, No. 7, (Jul), pp. (2369-2377), 1078-0432 (Print)

Liacini, A., Sylvester, J., Li, W. Q., Huang, W., Dehnade, F., Ahmad, M. & Zafarullah, M. (2003). Induction of matrix metalloproteinase-13 gene expression by TNF-alpha is mediated by MAP kinases, AP-1, and NF-kappaB transcription factors in articular chondrocytes. *Exp Cell Res*, Vol. 288, No. 1, (Aug 1), pp. (208-217), 0014-4827 (Print)

Lin, Y. L. & Lin, J. K. (1997). (-)-Epigallocatechin-3-gallate blocks the induction of nitric oxide synthase by down-regulating lipopolysaccharide-induced activity of transcription factor nuclear factor-kappaB. *Mol Pharmacol,* Vol. 52, No. 3, (Sep), pp. (465-472), 0026-895X (Print)

Lin, Y. L., Tsai, S. H., Lin-Shiau, S. Y., Ho, C. T. & Lin, J. K. (1999). Theaflavin-3,3'-digallate from black tea blocks the nitric oxide synthase by down-regulating the activation of NF-kappaB in macrophages. *Eur J Pharmacol,* Vol. 367, No. 2-3, (Feb 19), pp. (379-388), 0014-2999 (Print)

Lu, L. H., Lee, S. S. & Huang, H. C. (1998). Epigallocatechin suppression of proliferation of vascular smooth muscle cells: correlation with c-jun and JNK. *Br J Pharmacol,* Vol. 124, No. 6, (Jul), pp. (1227-1237), 0007-1188 (Print)

Ma, Z., Wei, X., Fontanilla, C., Noelker, C., Dodel, R., Hampel, H. & Du, Y. (2006). Caffeic acid phenethyl ester blocks free radical generation and 6-hydroxydopamine-induced neurotoxicity. *Life Sci,* Vol. 79, No. 13, (Aug 22), pp. (1307-1311), 0024-3205 (Print)

Manach, C., Scalbert, A., Morand, C., Remesy, C. & Jimenez, L. (2004). Polyphenols: food sources and bioavailability. *Am J Clin Nutr,* Vol. 79, No. 5, (May), pp. (727-747), 0002-9165 (Print)

Manjeet, K. R. & Ghosh, B. (1999). Quercetin inhibits LPS-induced nitric oxide and tumor necrosis factor-alpha production in murine macrophages *Int J Immunopharmacol,* Vol.21, No. 7, (Jul), pp. (435-443)

Manna, S. K., Mukhopadhyay, A. & Aggarwal, B. B. (2000). Resveratrol suppresses TNF-induced activation of nuclear transcription factors NF-kappa B, activator protein-1, and apoptosis: potential role of reactive oxygen intermediates and lipid peroxidation. *J Immunol,* Vol. 164, No. 12, (Jun 15), pp. (6509-6519), 0022-1767 (Print)

Marquez, N., Sancho, R., Macho, A., Calzado, M. A., Fiebich, B. L. & Munoz, E. (2004). Caffeic acid phenethyl ester inhibits T-cell activation by targeting both nuclear factor of activated T-cells and NF-kappaB transcription factors. *J Pharmacol Exp Ther,* Vol. 308, No. 3, (Mar), pp. (993-1001), 0022-3565 (Print)

Martinez, J. & Moreno, J. J. (2000). Effect of resveratrol, a natural polyphenolic compound, on reactive oxygen species and prostaglandin production. *Biochem Pharmacol,* Vol. 59, No. 7, (Apr 1), pp. (865-870), 0006-2952 (Print)

Mateo Anson, N., Aura, A. M., Selinheimo, E., Mattila, I., Poutanen, K., van den Berg, R., Havenaar, R., Bast, A. & Haenen, G. R. (2011). Bioprocessing of wheat bran in whole wheat bread increases the bioavailability of phenolic acids in men and exerts antiinflammatory effects ex vivo. *J Nutr,* Vol. 141, No. 1, (Jan), pp. (137-143), 1541-6100 (Electronic)

Mattila, P. & Kumpulainen, J. (2002). Determination of free and total phenolic acids in plant-derived foods by HPLC with diode-array detection. *J Agric Food Chem,* Vol. 50, No. 13, (Jun 19), pp. (3660-3667), 0021-8561 (Print)

Miles, E. A., Zoubouli, P. & Calder, P. C. (2005). Differential anti-inflammatory effects of phenolic compounds from extra virgin olive oil identified in human whole blood cultures. *Nutrition,* Vol. 21, No. 3, (Mar), pp. (389-394), 0899-9007 (Print)

Miriyala, S., Panchatcharam, M. & Rengarajulu, P. (2007). Cardioprotective effects of curcumin. *Adv Exp Med Biol,* Vol. 595, No. pp. (359-377), 0065-2598 (Print)

Monks, T. J. & Lau, S. S. (1992). Toxicology of quinone-thioethers. *Crit Rev Toxicol,* Vol. 22, No. 5-6, pp. (243-270), 1040-8444 (Print)

Nair, M. P., Mahajan, S., Reynolds, J. L., Aalinkeel, R., Nair, H., Schwartz, S. A. & Kandaswami, C. (2006). The flavonoid quercetin inhibits proinflammatory cytokine (tumor necrosis factor alpha) gene expression in normal peripheral blood mononuclear cells via modulation of the NF-kappa beta system. *Clin Vaccine Immunol,* Vol. 13, No. 3, (Mar), pp. (319-328), 1556-6811 (Print)

Nakagawa, K., Okuda, S. & Miyazawa, T. (1997). Dose-dependent incorporation of tea catechins, (-)-epigallocatechin-3-gallate and (-)-epigallocatechin, into human plasma. *Biosci Biotechnol Biochem,* Vol. 61, No. 12, (Dec), pp. (1981-1985), 0916-8451 (Print)

Nanjo, F., Goto, K., Seto, R., Suzuki, M., Sakai, M. & Hara, Y. (1996). Scavenging effects of tea catechins and their derivatives on 1,1-diphenyl-2-picrylhydrazyl radical. *Free Radic Biol Med,* Vol. 21, No. 6, pp. (895-902), 0891-5849 (Print)

Natarajan, K., Singh, S., Burke, T. R., Jr., Grunberger, D. & Aggarwal, B. B. (1996). Caffeic acid phenethyl ester is a potent and specific inhibitor of activation of nuclear transcription factor NF-kappa B. *Proc Natl Acad Sci U S A,* Vol. 93, No. 17, (Aug 20), pp. (9090-9095), 0027-8424 (Print)

Nenadis, N., Zhang, H. Y. & Tsimidou, M. Z. (2003). Structure-antioxidant activity relationship of ferulic acid derivatives: effect of carbon side chain characteristic groups. *J Agric Food Chem,* Vol. 51, No. 7, (Mar 26), pp. (1874-1879), 0021-8561 (Print)

Netsch, M. I., Gutmann, H., Aydogan, C. & Drewe, J. (2006). Green tea extract induces interleukin-8 (IL-8) mRNA and protein expression but specifically inhibits IL-8 secretion in caco-2 cells. *Planta Med,* Vol. 72, No. 8, (Jun), pp. (697-702), 0032-0943 (Print)

Okabe, S., Fujimoto, N., Sueoka, N., Suganuma, M. & Fujiki, H. (2001). Modulation of gene expression by (-)-epigallocatechin gallate in PC-9 cells using a cDNA expression array. *Biol Pharm Bull,* Vol. 24, No. 8, (Aug), pp. (883-886), 0918-6158 (Print)

Okutan, H., Ozcelik, N., Yilmaz, H. R. & Uz, E. (2005). Effects of caffeic acid phenethyl ester on lipid peroxidation and antioxidant enzymes in diabetic rat heart. *Clin Biochem,* Vol. 38, No. 2, (Feb), pp. (191-196), 0009-9120 (Print)

O'Leary, K. A., de Pascual-Tereasa, S., Needs, P. W., Bao, Y. P., O'Brien, N. M. & Williamson, G. (2004). Effect of flavonoids and vitamin E on cyclooxygenase-2 (COX-2) transcription. *Mutat Res,* Vol. 551, No. 1-2, (Jul 13), pp. (245-254), 0027-5107 (Print)

Osuchowski, M. F., Welch, K., Siddiqui, J. & Remick, D. G. (2006). Circulating cytokine/inhibitor profiles reshape the understanding of the SIRS/CARS continuum in sepsis and predict mortality. *J Immunol,* Vol. 177, No. 3, (Aug 1), pp. (1967-1974), 0022-1767 (Print)

Ouyang, P., Peng, W. L., Xu, D. L., Lai, W. Y. & Xu, A. L. (2004). Green tea polyphenols inhibit advanced glycation end product-induced rat vascular smooth muscle cell proliferation. *Di Yi Jun Yi Da Xue Xue Bao,* Vol. 24, No. 3, (Mar), pp. (247-251), 1000-2588 (Print)

Pan, M. H., Lin-Shiau, S. Y. & Lin, J. K. (2000). Comparative studies on the suppression of nitric oxide synthase by curcumin and its hydrogenated metabolites through down-regulation of IkappaB kinase and NFkappaB activation in macrophages. *Biochem Pharmacol,* Vol. 60, No. 11, (Dec 1), pp. (1665-1676), 0006-2952 (Print)

Pannala, A. S., Rice-Evans, C. A., Halliwell, B. & Singh, S. (1997). Inhibition of peroxynitrite-mediated tyrosine nitration by catechin polyphenols. *Biochem Biophys Res Commun,* Vol. 232, No. 1, (Mar 6), pp. (164-168), 0006-291X (Print)

Parrish, W. R., Gallowitsch-Puerta, M., Czura, C. J. & Tracey, K. J. (2008). Experimental therapeutic strategies for severe sepsis: mediators and mechanisms. *Ann N Y Acad Sci,* Vol. 1144, No. (Nov), pp. (210-236), 1749-6632 (Electronic)

Pattanaik, U. & Prasad, K. (1996). Endotoxemia and oxidative stress. *Ann N Y Acad Sci,* Vol. 793, No. (Sep 30), pp. (506-510), 0077-8923 (Print)

Pearson, K. J., Baur, J. A., Lewis, K. N., Peshkin, L., Price, N. L., Labinskyy, N., Swindell, W. R., Kamara, D., Minor, R. K., Perez, E., Jamieson, H. A., Zhang, Y., Dunn, S. R., Sharma, K., Pleshko, N., Woollett, L. A., Csiszar, A., Ikeno, Y., Le Couteur, D., Elliott, P. J., Becker, K. G., Navas, P., Ingram, D. K., Wolf, N. S., Ungvari, Z., Sinclair, D. A. & de Cabo, R. (2008). Resveratrol delays age-related deterioration and mimics transcriptional aspects of dietary restriction without extending life span. *Cell Metab,* Vol. 8, No. 2, (Aug), pp. (157-168), 1932-7420 (Electronic)

Peet, G. W. & Li, J. (1999). IkappaB kinases alpha and beta show a random sequential kinetic mechanism and are inhibited by staurosporine and quercetin. *J Biol Chem,* Vol. 274, No. 46, (Nov 12), pp. (32655-32661), 0021-9258 (Print)

Pietta, P. G., Simonetti, P., Gardana, C., Brusamolino, A., Morazzoni, P. & Bombardelli, E. (1998). Catechin metabolites after intake of green tea infusions. *Biofactors,* Vol. 8, No. 1-2, pp. (111-118), 0951-6433 (Print)

Plummer, S. M., Holloway, K. A., Manson, M. M., Munks, R. J., Kaptein, A., Farrow, S. & Howells, L. (1999). Inhibition of cyclo-oxygenase 2 expression in colon cells by the chemopreventive agent curcumin involves inhibition of NF-kappaB activation via the NIK/IKK signalling complex. *Oncogene,* Vol. 18, No. 44, (Oct 28), pp. (6013-6020), 0950-9232 (Print)

Porath, D., Riegger, C., Drewe, J. & Schwager, J. (2005). Epigallocatechin-3-gallate impairs chemokine production in human colon epithelial cell lines. *J Pharmacol Exp Ther,* Vol. 315, No. 3, (Dec), pp. (1172-1180), 0022-3565 (Print)

Psotova, J., Lasovsky, J. & Vicar, J. (2003). Metal-chelating properties, electrochemical behavior, scavenging and cytoprotective activities of six natural phenolics. *Biomed Pap Med Fac Univ Palacky Olomouc Czech Repub,* Vol. 147, No. 2, (Dec), pp. (147-153), 1213-8118 (Print)

Radnai, B., Tucsek, Z., Bognar, Z., Antus, C., Mark, L., Berente, Z., Gallyas, F., Jr., Sumegi, B. & Veres, B. (2009). Ferulaldehyde, a water-soluble degradation product of polyphenols, inhibits the lipopolysaccharide-induced inflammatory response in mice. *J Nutr,* Vol. 139, No. 2, (Feb), pp. (291-297), 1541-6100 (Electronic)

Rahman, I., Biswas, S. K. & Kirkham, P. A. (2006). Regulation of inflammation and redox signaling by dietary polyphenols. *Biochem Pharmacol,* Vol. 72, No. 11, (Nov 30), pp. (1439-1452), 0006-2952 (Print)

Rahman, I., Marwick, J. & Kirkham, P. (2004). Redox modulation of chromatin remodeling: impact on histone acetylation and deacetylation, NF-kappaB and pro-inflammatory gene expression. *Biochem Pharmacol,* Vol. 68, No. 6, (Sep 15), pp. (1255-1267), 0006-2952 (Print)

Reddy, A. C. & Lokesh, B. R. (1992). Studies on spice principles as antioxidants in the inhibition of lipid peroxidation of rat liver microsomes. *Mol Cell Biochem,* Vol. 111, No. 1-2, (Apr), pp. (117-124), 0300-8177 (Print)

Rehman, M. U. & Sultana, S. (2011). Attenuation of oxidative stress, inflammation and early markers of tumor promotion by caffeic acid in Fe-NTA exposed kidneys of Wistar rats. *Mol Cell Biochem,* pp. 1573-4919 (Electronic)

Rios, L. Y., Gonthier, M. P., Remesy, C., Mila, I., Lapierre, C., Lazarus, S. A., Williamson, G. & Scalbert, A. (2003). Chocolate intake increases urinary excretion of polyphenol-derived phenolic acids in healthy human subjects. *Am J Clin Nutr,* Vol. 77, No. 4, (Apr), pp. (912-918), 0002-9165 (Print)

Romashkova, J. A. & Makarov, S. S. (1999). NF-kappaB is a target of AKT in anti-apoptotic PDGF signalling. *Nature,* Vol. 401, No. 6748, (Sep 2), pp. (86-90), 0028-0836 (Print)

Ronchetti, D., Borghi, V., Gaitan, G., Herrero, J. F. & Impagnatiello, F. (2009). NCX 2057, a novel NO-releasing derivative of ferulic acid, suppresses inflammatory and nociceptive responses in in vitro and in vivo models. *Br J Pharmacol,* Vol. 158, No. 2, (Sep), pp. (569-579), 1476-5381 (Electronic)

Rotondo, S., Rajtar, G., Manarini, S., Celardo, A., Rotillo, D., de Gaetano, G., Evangelista, V. & Cerletti, C. (1998). Effect of trans-resveratrol, a natural polyphenolic compound, on human polymorphonuclear leukocyte function. *Br J Pharmacol,* Vol. 123, No. 8, (Apr), pp. (1691-1699), 0007-1188 (Print)

Salah, N., Miller, N. J., Paganga, G., Tijburg, L., Bolwell, G. P. & Rice-Evans, C. (1995). Polyphenolic flavanols as scavengers of aqueous phase radicals and as chain-breaking antioxidants. *Arch Biochem Biophys,* Vol. 322, No. 2, (Oct 1), pp. (339-346), 0003-9861 (Print)

Sanchez-Fidalgo, S., Cardeno, A., Villegas, I., Talero, E. & de la Lastra, C. A. (2010). Dietary supplementation of resveratrol attenuates chronic colonic inflammation in mice. *Eur J Pharmacol,* Vol. 633, No. 1-3, (May 10), pp. (78-84), 1879-0712 (Electronic)

Sato, Y., Yuasa, Y., Abe, Y. & Akagawa, Y. (1995). Finite element and Weibull analysis to estimate failure risk in resin-bonded retainers. *Int J Prosthodont,* Vol. 8, No. 1, (Jan-Feb), pp. (73-78), 0893-2174 (Print)

Scumpia, P. O. & Moldawer, L. L. (2005). Biology of interleukin-10 and its regulatory roles in sepsis syndromes. *Crit Care Med,* Vol. 33, No. 12 Suppl, (Dec), pp. (S468-471), 0090-3493 (Print)

Sharma, R. A., Euden, S. A., Platton, S. L., Cooke, D. N., Shafayat, A., Hewitt, H. R., Marczylo, T. H., Morgan, B., Hemingway, D., Plummer, S. M., Pirmohamed, M., Gescher, A. J. & Steward, W. P. (2004). Phase I clinical trial of oral curcumin: biomarkers of systemic activity and compliance. *Clin Cancer Res,* Vol. 10, No. 20, (Oct 15), pp. (6847-6854), 1078-0432 (Print)

Sharma, S., Chopra, K., Kulkarni, S. K. & Agrewala, J. N. (2007). Resveratrol and curcumin suppress immune response through CD28/CTLA-4 and CD80 co-stimulatory pathway. *Clin Exp Immunol,* Vol. 147, No. 1, (Jan), pp. (155-163), 0009-9104 (Print)

Shen, S. Q., Zhang, Y., Xiang, J. J. & Xiong, C. L. (2007). Protective effect of curcumin against liver warm ischemia/reperfusion injury in rat model is associated with regulation of heat shock protein and antioxidant enzymes. *World J Gastroenterol,* Vol. 13, No. 13, (Apr 7), pp. (1953-1961), 1007-9327 (Print)

Shin, H. Y., Kim, S. H., Jeong, H. J., Kim, S. Y., Shin, T. Y., Um, J. Y., Hong, S. H. & Kim, H. M. (2007). Epigallocatechin-3-gallate inhibits secretion of TNF-alpha, IL-6 and IL-8 through the attenuation of ERK and NF-kappaB in HMC-1 cells. *Int Arch Allergy Immunol,* Vol. 142, No. 4, pp. (335-344), 1018-2438 (Print)

Singh, S. & Aggarwal, B. B. (1995). Activation of transcription factor NF-kappa B is suppressed by curcumin (diferuloylmethane) [corrected]. *J Biol Chem,* Vol. 270, No. 42, (Oct 20), pp. (24995-25000), 0021-9258 (Print)

Soleas, G. J., Diamandis, E. P. & Goldberg, D. M. (1997). Resveratrol: a molecule whose time has come? And gone? *Clin Biochem,* Vol. 30, No. 2, (Mar), pp. (91-113), 0009-9120 (Print)

Soobrattee, M. A., Neergheen, V. S., Luximon-Ramma, A., Aruoma, O. I. & Bahorun, T. (2005). Phenolics as potential antioxidant therapeutic agents: mechanism and actions. *Mutat Res,* Vol. 579, No. 1-2, (Nov 11), pp. (200-213), 0027-5107 (Print)

Srinivasan, M., Sudheer, A. R. & Menon, V. P. (2007). Ferulic Acid: therapeutic potential through its antioxidant property. *J Clin Biochem Nutr,* Vol. 40, No. 2, (Mar), pp. (92-100), 0912-0009 (Print)

Subbaramaiah, K., Chung, W. J., Michaluart, P., Telang, N., Tanabe, T., Inoue, H., Jang, M., Pezzuto, J. M. & Dannenberg, A. J. (1998). Resveratrol inhibits cyclooxygenase-2 transcription and activity in phorbol ester-treated human mammary epithelial cells. *J Biol Chem,* Vol. 273, No. 34, (Aug 21), pp. (21875-21882), 0021-9258 (Print)

Suganuma, M., Okabe, S., Oniyama, M., Tada, Y., Ito, H. & Fujiki, H. (1998). Wide distribution of [3H](-)-epigallocatechin gallate, a cancer preventive tea polyphenol, in mouse tissue. *Carcinogenesis,* Vol. 19, No. 10, (Oct), pp. (1771-1776), 0143-3334 (Print)

Tang, F. Y., Nguyen, N. & Meydani, M. (2003). Green tea catechins inhibit VEGF-induced angiogenesis in vitro through suppression of VE-cadherin phosphorylation and inactivation of Akt molecule. *Int J Cancer,* Vol. 106, No. 6, (Oct 10), pp. (871-878), 0020-7136 (Print)

Tayman, C., Tonbul, A., Kosus, A., Hirfanoglu, I. M., Haltas, H., Uysal, S., Tatli, M. M. & Andiran, F. (2011). Protective effects of caffeic acid phenethyl ester (CAPE) on intestinal damage in necrotizing enterocolitis. *Pediatr Surg Int,* Vol. No. (Jun 28), pp. 1437-9813 (Electronic)

Tedeschi, E., Menegazzi, M., Yao, Y., Suzuki, H., Forstermann, U. & Kleinert, H. (2004). Green tea inhibits human inducible nitric-oxide synthase expression by down-regulating signal transducer and activator of transcription-1alpha activation. *Mol Pharmacol,* Vol. 65, No. 1, (Jan), pp. (111-120), 0026-895X (Print)

Tracey, K. J. & Cerami, A. (1993). Tumor necrosis factor, other cytokines and disease. *Annu Rev Cell Biol,* Vol. 9, No. pp. (317-343), 0743-4634 (Print)

Tracey, K. J. & Cerami, A. (1994). Tumor necrosis factor: a pleiotropic cytokine and therapeutic target. *Annu Rev Med,* Vol. 45, No. pp. (491-503), 0066-4219 (Print)

Tucsek, Z., Radnai, B., Racz, B., Debreceni, B., Priber, J. K., Dolowschiak, T., Palkovics, T., Gallyas, F., Jr., Sumegi, B. & Veres, B. (2011). Suppressing LPS-induced early signal transduction in macrophages by a polyphenol degradation product: a critical role of MKP-1. *J Leukoc Biol,* Vol. 89, No. 1, (Jan), pp. (105-111), 1938-3673 (Electronic)

van Acker, S. A., Tromp, M. N., Haenen, G. R., van der Vijgh, W. J. & Bast, A. (1995). Flavonoids as scavengers of nitric oxide radical. *Biochem Biophys Res Commun,* Vol. 214, No. 3, (Sep 25), pp. (755-759), 0006-291X (Print)

van der Poll, T. & Lowry, S. F. (1995). Tumor necrosis factor in sepsis: mediator of multiple organ failure or essential part of host defense? *Shock,* Vol. 3, No. 1, (Jan), pp. (1-12), 1073-2322 (Print)

Veres, B., Radnai, B., Gallyas, F., Jr., Varbiro, G., Berente, Z., Osz, E. & Sumegi, B. (2004). Regulation of kinase cascades and transcription factors by a poly(ADP-ribose) polymerase-1 inhibitor, 4-hydroxyquinazoline, in lipopolysaccharide-induced inflammation in mice. *J Pharmacol Exp Ther,* Vol. 310, No. 1, (Jul), pp. (247-255), 0022-3565 (Print)

Victor, V. M., Rocha, M., Esplugues, J. V. & De la Fuente, M. (2005). Role of free radicals in sepsis: antioxidant therapy. *Curr Pharm Des,* Vol. 11, No. 24, pp. (3141-3158), 1381-6128 (Print)

Vitrac, X., Desmouliere, A., Brouillaud, B., Krisa, S., Deffieux, G., Barthe, N., Rosenbaum, J. & Merillon, J. M. (2003). Distribution of [14C]-trans-resveratrol, a cancer chemopreventive polyphenol, in mouse tissues after oral administration. *Life Sci,* Vol. 72, No. 20, (Apr 4), pp. (2219-2233), 0024-3205 (Print)

Wadsworth, T. L., McDonald, T. L. & Koop, D. R. (2001). Effects of Ginkgo biloba extract (EGb 761) and quercetin on lipopolysaccharide-induced signaling pathways involved in the release of tumor necrosis factor-alpha. *Biochem Pharmacol,* Vol. 62, No. 7, (Oct 1), pp. (963-974), 0006-2952 (Print)

Weisberg, S. P., Leibel, R. & Tortoriello, D. V. (2008). Dietary curcumin significantly improves obesity-associated inflammation and diabetes in mouse models of diabesity. *Endocrinology,* Vol. 149, No. 7, (Jul), pp. (3549-3558), 0013-7227 (Print)

Weisburger, J. H. & Chung, F. L. (2002). Mechanisms of chronic disease causation by nutritional factors and tobacco products and their prevention by tea polyphenols. *Food Chem Toxicol,* Vol. 40, No. 8, (Aug), pp. (1145-1154), 0278-6915 (Print)

Wenzel, E., Soldo, T., Erbersdobler, H. & Somoza, V. (2005). Bioactivity and metabolism of trans-resveratrol orally administered to Wistar rats. *Mol Nutr Food Res,* Vol. 49, No. 5, (May), pp. (482-494), 1613-4125 (Print)

Wenzel, E. & Somoza, V. (2005). Metabolism and bioavailability of trans-resveratrol. *Mol Nutr Food Res,* Vol. 49, No. 5, (May), pp. (472-481), 1613-4125 (Print)

Wheeler, D. S., Catravas, J. D., Odoms, K., Denenberg, A., Malhotra, V. & Wong, H. R. (2004). Epigallocatechin-3-gallate, a green tea-derived polyphenol, inhibits IL-1 beta-dependent proinflammatory signal transduction in cultured respiratory epithelial cells. *J Nutr,* Vol. 134, No. 5, (May), pp. (1039-1044), 0022-3166 (Print)

Wiseman, S., Mulder, T. & Rietveld, A. (2001). Tea flavonoids: bioavailability in vivo and effects on cell signaling pathways in vitro. *Antioxid Redox Signal,* Vol. 3, No. 6, (Dec), pp. (1009-1021), 1523-0864 (Print)

Wu, C. T., Yu, H. P., Chung, C. Y., Lau, Y. T. & Liao, S. K. (2008). Attenuation of lung inflammation and pro-inflammatory cytokine production by resveratrol following trauma-hemorrhage. *Chin J Physiol,* Vol. 51, No. 6, (Dec 31), pp. (363-368), 0304-4920 (Print)

Yang, F., de Villiers, W. J., McClain, C. J. & Varilek, G. W. (1998). Green tea polyphenols block endotoxin-induced tumor necrosis factor-production and lethality in a murine model. *J Nutr,* Vol. 128, No. 12, (Dec), pp. (2334-2340), 0022-3166 (Print)

Yang, F., Oz, H. S., Barve, S., de Villiers, W. J., McClain, C. J. & Varilek, G. W. (2001). The green tea polyphenol (-)-epigallocatechin-3-gallate blocks nuclear factor-kappa B activation by inhibiting I kappa B kinase activity in the intestinal epithelial cell line IEC-6. *Mol Pharmacol,* Vol. 60, No. 3, (Sep), pp. (528-533), 0026-895X (Print)

Yildiz, Y., Serter, M., Ek, R. O., Ergin, K., Cecen, S., Demir, E. M. & Yenisey, C. (2009). Protective effects of caffeic acid phenethyl ester on intestinal ischemia-reperfusion injury. *Dig Dis Sci,* Vol. 54, No. 4, (Apr), pp. (738-744), 1573-2568 (Electronic)

Yilmaz, H. R., Uz, E., Yucel, N., Altuntas, I. & Ozcelik, N. (2004). Protective effect of caffeic acid phenethyl ester (CAPE) on lipid peroxidation and antioxidant enzymes in diabetic rat liver. *J Biochem Mol Toxicol,* Vol. 18, No. 4, pp. (234-238), 1095-6670 (Print)

Yokozawa, T. & Dong, E. (1997). Influence of green tea and its three major components upon low-density lipoprotein oxidation. *Exp Toxicol Pathol,* Vol. 49, No. 5, (Dec), pp. (329-335), 0940-2993 (Print)

Yoon, J. H. & Baek, S. J. (2005). Molecular targets of dietary polyphenols with anti-inflammatory properties. *Yonsei Med J,* Vol. 46, No. 5, (Oct 31), pp. (585-596), 0513-5796 (Print)

Youn, H. S., Lee, J. Y., Fitzgerald, K. A., Young, H. A., Akira, S. & Hwang, D. H. (2005). Specific inhibition of MyD88-independent signaling pathways of TLR3 and TLR4 by resveratrol: molecular targets are TBK1 and RIP1 in TRIF complex. *J Immunol,* Vol. 175, No. 5, (Sep 1), pp. (3339-3346), 0022-1767 (Print)

Youn, H. S., Lee, J. Y., Saitoh, S. I., Miyake, K., Kang, K. W., Choi, Y. J. & Hwang, D. H. (2006). Suppression of MyD88- and TRIF-dependent signaling pathways of Toll-like receptor by (-)-epigallocatechin-3-gallate, a polyphenol component of green tea. *Biochem Pharmacol,* Vol. 72, No. 7, (Sep 28), pp. (850-859), 0006-2952 (Print)

Yun, H. J., Yoo, W. H., Han, M. K., Lee, Y. R., Kim, J. S. & Lee, S. I. (2008). Epigallocatechin-3-gallate suppresses TNF-alpha -induced production of MMP-1 and -3 in rheumatoid arthritis synovial fibroblasts. *Rheumatol Int,* Vol. 29, No. 1, (Nov), pp. (23-29), 0172-8172 (Print)

Zern, T. L. & Fernandez, M. L. (2005). Cardioprotective effects of dietary polyphenols. *J Nutr,* Vol. 135, No. 10, (Oct), pp. (2291-2294), 0022-3166 (Print)

Zhang, M., Deng, C., Zheng, J., Xia, J. & Sheng, D. (2006). Curcumin inhibits trinitrobenzene sulphonic acid-induced colitis in rats by activation of peroxisome proliferator-activated receptor gamma. *Int Immunopharmacol,* Vol. 6, No. 8, (Aug), pp. (1233-1242), 1567-5769 (Print)

Zhao, Q., Wang, X., Nelin, L. D., Yao, Y., Matta, R., Manson, M. E., Baliga, R. S., Meng, X., Smith, C. V., Bauer, J. A., Chang, C. H. & Liu, Y. (2006). MAP kinase phosphatase 1 controls innate immune responses and suppresses endotoxic shock. *J Exp Med,* Vol. 203, No. 1, (Jan 23), pp. (131-140), 0022-1007 (Print)

Zhong, M., Cheng, G. F., Wang, W. J., Guo, Y., Zhu, X. Y. & Zhang, J. T. (1999). Inhibitory effect of resveratrol on interleukin 6 release by stimulated peritoneal macrophages of mice. *Phytomedicine,* Vol. 6, No. 2, (May), pp. (79-84), 0944-7113 (Print)

Part 9

Outcomes

Cellular and Molecular Markers of Outcome in Septic Shock

Jorge Monserrat, Raúl de Pablo, David Díaz, Miguel-Angel Sánchez, Eduardo Reyes, Alfredo Prieto and Melchor Álvarez de Mon
Alcalá de Henares University/Principe de Asturias Hospital
Spain

1. Introduction

Sepsis can be defined as a generalized inflammatory response that occurs during infection (Bone et al. 1992) and it seems that a defective host immune system response to a microbiological challenge is pivotal in the pathogenesis of septic shock. The pathogenesis of sepsis is a result of a complex network of events involving inflammatory and anti-inflammatory processes, molecular and cellular reactions and circulatory abnormalities (Hotchkiss & Karl 2003). Signs and symptoms of sepsis are non-specific for the diagnosis of sepsis, but early and appropriate intervention is critical for morbidity and mortality (Levy et al. 2005;Rivers et al. 2001). There is a need to find early markers of infection in patients with systemic inflammatory response syndrome (SIRS), and also to establish procedures for a more accurate risk assessment, predicting patients' outcome, guiding antibiotic therapy or predicting the development of different organ dysfunctions.

A biomarker is defined as "a characteristic that is objectively measured and evaluated as an indicator of normal biological processes, pathogenic processes or pharmacologic responses to a therapeutic intervention"(Biomarkers 2001). Countless biomarkers of septic shock have been proposed but few or none are currently used in clinical practice or studies. This lack of clinical application of research findings is due to several reasons: the lack of "gold standard" for the diagnosis, the complex pathophysiology of sepsis, which involves many processes as inflammation, immunity, coagulation, etc. Thus, we studied the prognostic value of surface molecule expression on lymphocytes and serum levels of the main cytokines, chemokines and adhesion molecules to classify the survival of the patients with septic shock.

First, we demonstrated a severe redistribution of T lymphocyte subsets in patients with septic shock. A different kinetic pattern of T cell subset involvement is observed in surviving and nonsurviving patients, with lower numbers of circulating $CD3^+CD8^+CD28^+$ and $CD3^+CD8^+CD62L^+$ cells being associated with a better disease outcome (Monserrat et al. 2009b). Second, we have also studied the predictive value for outcome of combining different T-cell, B-cell and NK-cell markers in septic shock patients. We have found a set of five immunophenotypic variables $CD3^+CD8^+CD28^+$, $CD3^+CD8^+CD45RA^+CD45RO^-$, $CD19^+CD80^+$, $CD56^+CD69^+$, $CD3^+CD11a\ br^+CD11b^+$ cells blood counts that improve the prediction for outcome in septic shock patients to a sensitivity of 94% and a specificity of 100% (Monserrat et al. 2009a).

In another study of prognostic value of serum mediators, we determined by sandwich ELISA the serum levels of proinflammatory cytokines (TNFα, IL-1β, IFNγ, and IL-6) and soluble cytokine antagonists (sTNF-RI, sTNF-RII, and IL-1Ra) in 52 patients with septic shock and in 36 healthy controls at ICU admission and 3, 7, 14, and 28 days later. We demonstrated that serum levels of most of the pro- and anti-inflammatory molecules examined (TNFα, IL-6, sTNF-RI, sTNF-RII, and IL-1Ra) were significantly increased upon admission and during the 28-day observation period in septic patients when compared to controls. Remarkably, the serum levels of anti-inflammatory mediators sTNF-RI, sTNF-RII, and IL-1Ra were better predictors of mortality than the levels of proinflammatory cytokines (de Pablo et al. 2011). We also measured soluble VCAM-1, ICAM-1, ICAM-2 and PECAM-1 levels and we demonstrated that they were significantly higher in septic shock patients at ICU admission and during the follow-up than in healthy controls. Serum soluble ICAM-1 was the best biomarker for separating patients with infection from those with non-infectious SIRS. On the other hand, soluble E-Selectin found to be a sensitive marker of endothelial damage, which may result in multiple organ dysfunction syndrome and death.

2. Role of peripheral blood lymphocytes in septic shock outcome

The role of the lymphocytes in the septic shock it's not clear and it has been studied extensively in the last decades (Holub et al. 2000;Holub et al. 2003;Lin et al. 1993;Menges et al. 1999;Nishijima et al. 1986). However, there are not many authors that have proposed to use lymphocytes as biomarkers for the outcome of these patients (Keane et al. 1983;Monserrat et al. 2009a). Thus, we decided study the role of the T, B and Natural Killer (NK) lymphocytes such as biomarkers in the prediction of the outcome of septic shock patients.

The T cell compartment plays a critical role in regulating the effector stage of the immune response. $CD3^+CD4^+$ T cells are mainly involved in the regulation of the immune response while $CD3^+CD8^+$ T cells are critical in the cytotoxic response (Ochoa & Makarenkova 2005). Several molecules, mainly the T cell receptor/CD3 complex and other co-receptors including CD28, contribute to the activation of T lymphocytes. The expression patterns of other molecules, such as the CD45 isoforms RA and RO, vary during the different T cell activation effector stages (Hermiston et al. 2003). Activated T lymphocytes show several profiles (proinflammatory or anti-inflammatory) of cytokine production (Curfs et al. 1997). Other molecules, such as CD62L, participate in the immune response by regulating the tissue distribution of the T lymphocytes (Sallusto et al. 1999). Therefore, a role for T lymphocytes in severe systemic bacterial infections has been described in several studies, and the findings of other investigations have supported the notion that T lymphocytes are involved in the pathogenesis of septic shock (Holub et al. 2000;Holub et al. 2003;Kabisch et al. 1990;Lin et al. 1993;Nishijima et al. 1986).

The NK compartment is characterized as $CD3^-CD56^+$ cells that can be cytotoxic ($CD16^+$ Bright) or produce high amount of cytokines such as IFNγ ($CD16^+$ Dim) (Romagnani et al. 2007). NK cells are also engaged in crosstalks with other immune cells, such a dendritic cells, monocytes, macrophages (Bellora et al. 2010) and neutrophils (Costantini & Cassatella 2011). Several lines of evidence suggest that NK cells might be involved in key functions during sepsis. During the early stage of septic shock, NK cells may play a key role in the promotion of the systemic inflammation as suggested in mice models, but at later stage, NK cells-acquired dysfunction could favor nosocomial infections and mortality (Chiche et al. 2011).

Defects in T and NK lymphocytes are accompanied by alterations in the humoral response. The functional consequences of these humoral immune defects are an impaired ability to respond to antigens with a rapid and appropriate immune response to microbial antigens (Opal et al. 2005). The role of B cells in septic shock is unclear and weakly studied.
In this first study, we have further characterized the abnormalities of the T cell compartment in septic shock and explore its clinical significance. During the first 28 days of follow up circulating T lymphocytes of 52 patients with septic shock admitted to the intensive care unit (ICU) were analysed and 36 healthy subjects were analysed in parallel. We determined the counts and distributions of the main T cell subsets, as well as their stage of activation (CD3, CD4, CD8, CD28, 45RA, 45RO and 62L antigens).

2.1 Patients and methodology

2.1.1 Patients and study design

Fifty-two consecutive patients admitted to the ICU of the University Hospital "Príncipe de Asturias", Madrid, Spain, with septic shock, diagnosed according to the criteria of the American College of Chest Physicians/Society of Critical Care Medicine (Bone et al. 1992), were enrolled in the study. A further requirement was the demonstration of an infectious aetiology through microbiological (Gram stain and/or culture) and/or radiological techniques, or direct observation of the infection focus. The study protocol did not call for a standardised approach to critical care. Exclusion criteria were: anything causing primary or acquired immunodeficiency, previous immunosuppressive or immunomodulation treatment, cancer, or autoimmune or allergic disease. The study was conducted according to the guidelines of the 1975 Declaration of Helsinki, after obtaining the Hospital Universitario Príncipe de Asturias Ethics Committee approval. Written informed consent was obtained from each subject included in the study or surrogate legal representatives. Thirty-six age-matched and sex-matched healthy blood donors were studied in parallel with the patients (0 and 28 days of the follow up). They were studied to control the adequacy of the cytometric techniques as well as to characterise the normal range of the T cell compartment parameters analysed.
Blood was collected from these patients at baseline (ICU admission) and at 3, 7, 14 and 28 days of follow up, and at baseline and at 28 days in healthy controls. White blood cell differential counts were conducted in a COULTER®LH instrument (Beckman-Coulter Inc).

2.1.2 Cell separation and surface immunofluorescence

Peripheral blood mononuclear cells (PBMC) were obtained from heparinised venous blood by Ficoll-Hypaque (Lymphoprep Nyegaard) density gradient centrifugation. Cells were resuspended (1 x 106 cells/ml) in RPMI-1640 (Biowhittaker Inc.) supplemented with 10% heat-inactivated FBS (Cangera International), 25 mM Hepes (Biochrom KG) and 1% penicillin streptomycin (Difco Lab).
T cells were phenotypically analysed in PBMC by four-colour flow cytometry in a FACScalibur cytometer using CellQuest software (Becton-Dickinson). PBMC were incubated with combinations of fluorescein isothiocyanate (FITC), phycoerythrin (PE), peridinin chlorophyll protein (PerCP) and allophycocyanin (APC)-labelled monoclonal antibodies. The monoclonal antibodies were CD3-PerCP, CD3-FITC, CD8-PerCP, CD45RA-FITC, CD56-PE, CD28-PE, CD62L-PE (Becton-Dickinson), CD8-APC, CD45RO-PE (Caltag Laboratories).

2.1.3 Blood lymphocyte count calculation

Blood lymphocyte counts of T lymphocyte subsets were calculated according to standard flow cytometry criteria for lymphocyte subset identification and the lymphocytes counts obtained in conventional haemogram. First, we calculated the percentage of cells expressing CD3 in the total lymphocytes gate defined by forward and side scatter in PBMC. Blood lymphocyte count of circulatory T lymphocytes was calculated by the percentage of $CD3^+$ cells in peripheral blood lymphocytes multiplied by the total number of lymphocytes per microlitre measured by a Coulter®. Next, we obtained the absolute number of $CD4^+$ and $CD8^+$ T lymphocytes by multiplying the total number of T lymphocytes previously calculated by the percentage of positive cells for each one of both antigens in $CD3^+$ T cells. We simultaneously stained PBMC with CD3, CD4 and CD8 antibodies to obtain this data. Finally, we calculated the absolute number of the $CD3^+CD4^+$ and $CD3^+CD8^+$ T cells subsets defined by the expression of CD45 isoforms $CD45RA^+CD45RO^-$, $CD45RO^+CD45RA^-$, $CD45RA^+CD45RO^+$ and the expression of the antigens $CD28^+$ and $CD62L^+$. To calculate these numbers, we multiplied the percentage obtained of each subset in the parents' $CD3^+CD4^+$ or $CD3^+CD8^+$ populations by the absolute count of $CD3^+CD4^+$ and $CD3^+CD8^+$ T cells, respectively. All lymphocyte counts are expressed as cells/μl.

2.2 Septic shock patients with different outcomes show different patterns of circulating T cell subsets

Blood counts and distributions of the main circulating T lymphocyte subsets were systematically examined in 52 patients with septic shock at admission to the ICU and at 3, 7, 14 and 28 days of follow up in the ICU. Patients were classified as survivors or nonsurvivors according to their clinical outcome of sepsis during the four weeks of follow up. Thirty-six healthy blood donors who were age-matched and sex-matched (60 ± 3.4 years, 25 men and 11 women) were studied in parallel with the patients as controls.

Blood lymphocyte count was 2095±93, 1048±192 and 1235±178 cells/μl in controls, survivors and non-survivors respectively. Both, surviving and nonsurviving patients, showed significantly lower absolute $CD3^+$ T lymphocyte counts than controls on admission and during the first 14 days of follow up. In survivors, $CD3^+$ counts had significantly returned to normal by day 28 (Figure 1A). The $CD3^+CD4^+$ T cell subset was also reduced in surviving and nonsurviving patients with respect to healthy controls at baseline and during the first week of follow up. However, this severely decreased $CD3^+CD4^+$ T lymphocyte count had normalised in survivors by day 14 (Figure 1B). On admission, $CD3^+CD8^+$ T lymphocytes were also lower in survivors and nonsurvivors than in controls. In survivors, this T cell subset showed a further drop on day 3 of follow up, followed by a gradual recovery, although numbers failed to reach the count recorded in healthy controls. In addition, $CD3^+CD8^+$ T lymphocyte count in survivors was significantly diminished with respect to nonsurvivors on day 3 (Figure 1C).

The activation stage of the $CD3^+CD4^+$ and $CD3^+CD8^+$ T lymphocytes was determined by examining the expression of the CD45 RA and RO isoforms. The retraction in circulating $CD3^+CD4^+$ and $CD3^+CD8^+$ T lymphocytes observed in the patients could be mainly explained by a decrease in the noneffector $CD45RA^+CD45RO^-$ subset (Figures 2a,d). Interestingly, $CD3^+CD4^+CD45RA^+CD45RO^-$ and $CD3^+CD8^+CD45RA^+CD45RO^-$ T lymphocytes remained low in survivors at the end of follow up. We detected a significant decrease in $CD3^+CD4^+CD45RA^+CD45RO^-$ T cells on day 3 with respect to the nonsurviving patients. $CD3^+CD4^+CD45RA^-CD45RO^+$ T cell counts varied over time from a significant reduction during the first week of follow up to elevated numbers in survivors during the last two weeks of the study (Figures 2a,c). The analysis of effector subsets, characterised by being double positive ($CD45RA^+CD45RO^+$) (Hermiston et al. 2003;Najera et al. 2001), showed that were significantly reduced in both $CD4^+$ and $CD8^+$ T lymphocyte subsets at baseline, 3 and 7 days in both groups of patients compared with controls and in survivors compared with nonsurvivors at 3 days. From day 7 of follow up onwards, these values normalised in the surviving patients (Figures 2b,e).

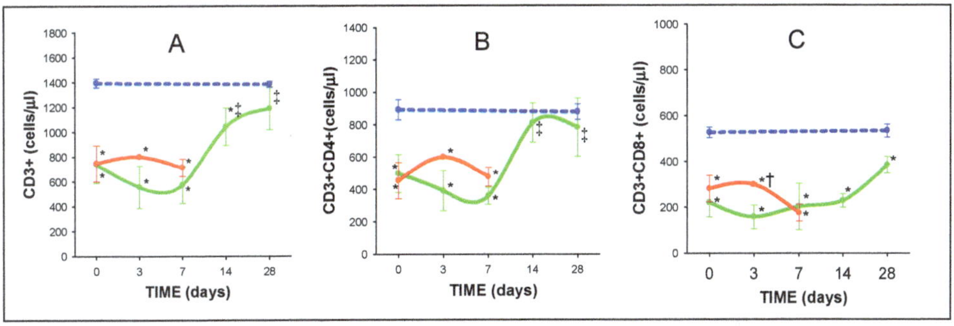

Fig. 1. Kinetic of peripheral blood counts of $CD3^+$, $CD3^+CD4^+$ and $CD3^+CD8^+$ lymphocyte subsets in patients with septic shock during their stay in the ICU. Symbol represents: (■●■) Controls line base, (■●■) Survivors and (■●■) Nonsurvivors. All values are expressed as the mean of cells/µl ± S.E.M. *$p<0.05$ for survivors or nonsurvivors versus controls; † $p<0.05$ for survivors versus nonsurvivors; ‡ $p< 0.05$ for each follow up time versus admission.

We also analysed the expression of CD28 and CD62L antigens on $CD3^+CD4^+$ and $CD3^+CD8^+$ T cells. When $CD3^+CD8^+$ T cells are activated, CD28 expression is lost (Fiorentini et al. 2001;Labalette et al. 1999). Number of circulating $CD3^+CD8^+CD28^+$ T cells was significantly and constantly reduced in patients with septic shock compared with the healthy subjects and in survivors compared with nonsurvivors during the first three days of follow up (Figures 3A, 4). Similar behaviour was shown by $CD3^+CD8^+CD62L^+$ T cells (Figures 3B, 4). Numbers of circulating $CD3^+CD8^+CD28^-$ T cells were normal in both groups of patients.

A prediction receptor operative curve (ROC) was then used to estimate the value of $CD3^+CD8^+CD28^+$ and $CD3^+CD8^+CD62L^+$ T cell counts for predicting death in the patients with septic shock at admission and days 3 and 7. We found that a cutoff value of 136 $CD3^+CD8^+CD28^+$ T cells/ml on admission to the ICU of a patient with septic shock showed a sensitivity of 70% and 100% specificity for predicting the risk of death, and the area under the ROC curve was 0.84. For the $CD3^+CD8^+CD62L^+$ T cells, the cut off on admission was 141 cells/ml, with a 60% sensitivity and 100% specificity for predicting the risk of death and an area under the curve of 0.75. The sensitivity and specificity of the data obtained at days 3 and 7 were worse than those found at admission.

The number of circulating $CD3^+CD4^+CD28^+$ T cells was significantly lower in surviving and nonsurviving patients with septic shock compared with healthy controls on admission and on day 3 of follow-up (Figure 5a). In survivors, this was followed by a gradual recovery of $CD3^+CD4^+CD28^+$ T cell numbers during the course of follow up. $CD3^+CD4^+CD62L^+$ T cells showed a similar pattern of behaviour (Figure 5b). In the parallel study performed in healthy blood donors (at 0 and 28 days of the follow up), no significant variations in the absolute counts and distribution of the different subsets of T cells analysed were detected.

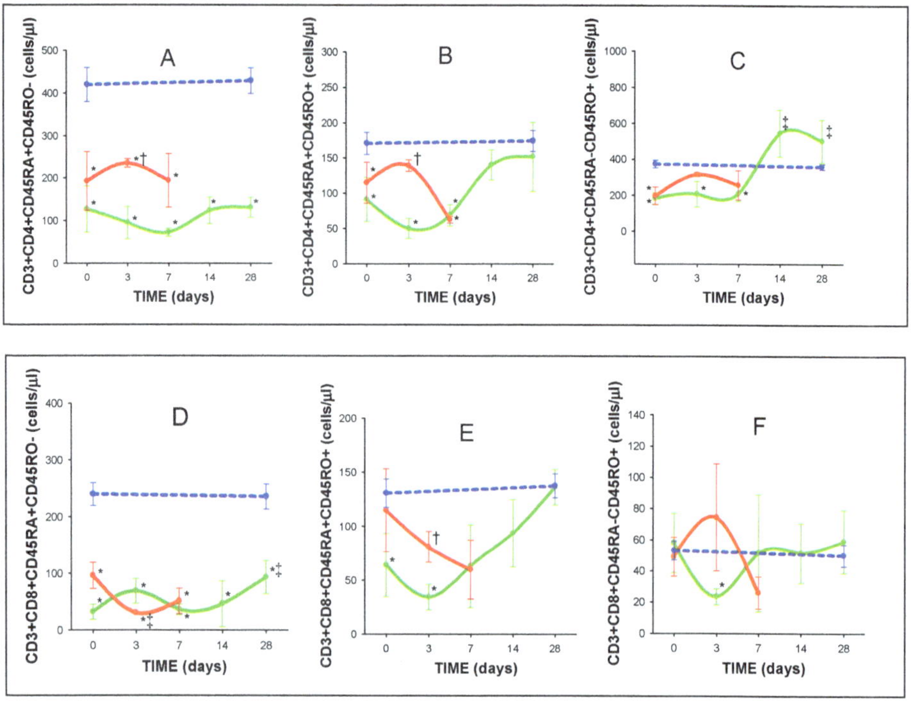

Fig. 2. Kinetic of peripheral blood counts of CD45RA+ and CD45RO+ T lymphocyte subsets in patients with septic shock during their stay in the ICU. Symbol represents: (■●■) Controls line base, (■●■) Survivors and (■●■) Nonsurvivors. All values are expressed as the mean of cells/µl ± S.E.M. *p<0.05 for survivors or nonsurvivors versus controls; † p<0.05 for survivors versus nonsurvivors; ‡ p< 0.05 for each follow up time versus admission.

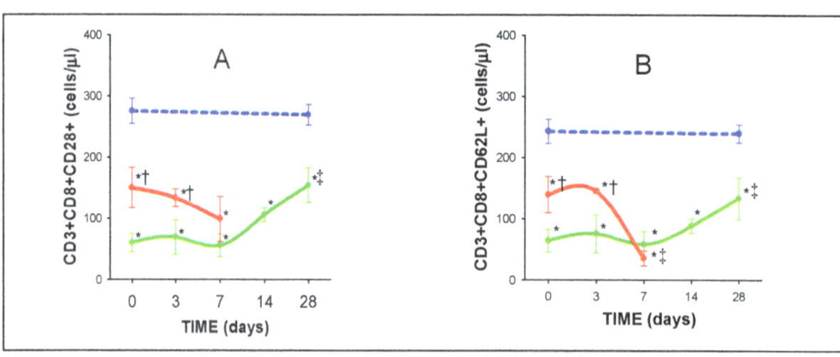

Fig. 3. Kinetic of peripheral blood counts of $CD3^+CD8^+CD62L^+$ and $CD3^+CD8^+CD62L^+$ lymphocyte subsets in patients with septic shock. Symbol represents: (■●■) Controls line base, (■●■) Survivors and (■●■) Nonsurvivors. All values are expressed as the mean of cells/µl ± S.E.M. *p<0.05 for survivors or nonsurvivors versus controls; † p<0.05 for survivors versus nonsurvivors; ‡ p< 0.05 for each follow up time versus admission.

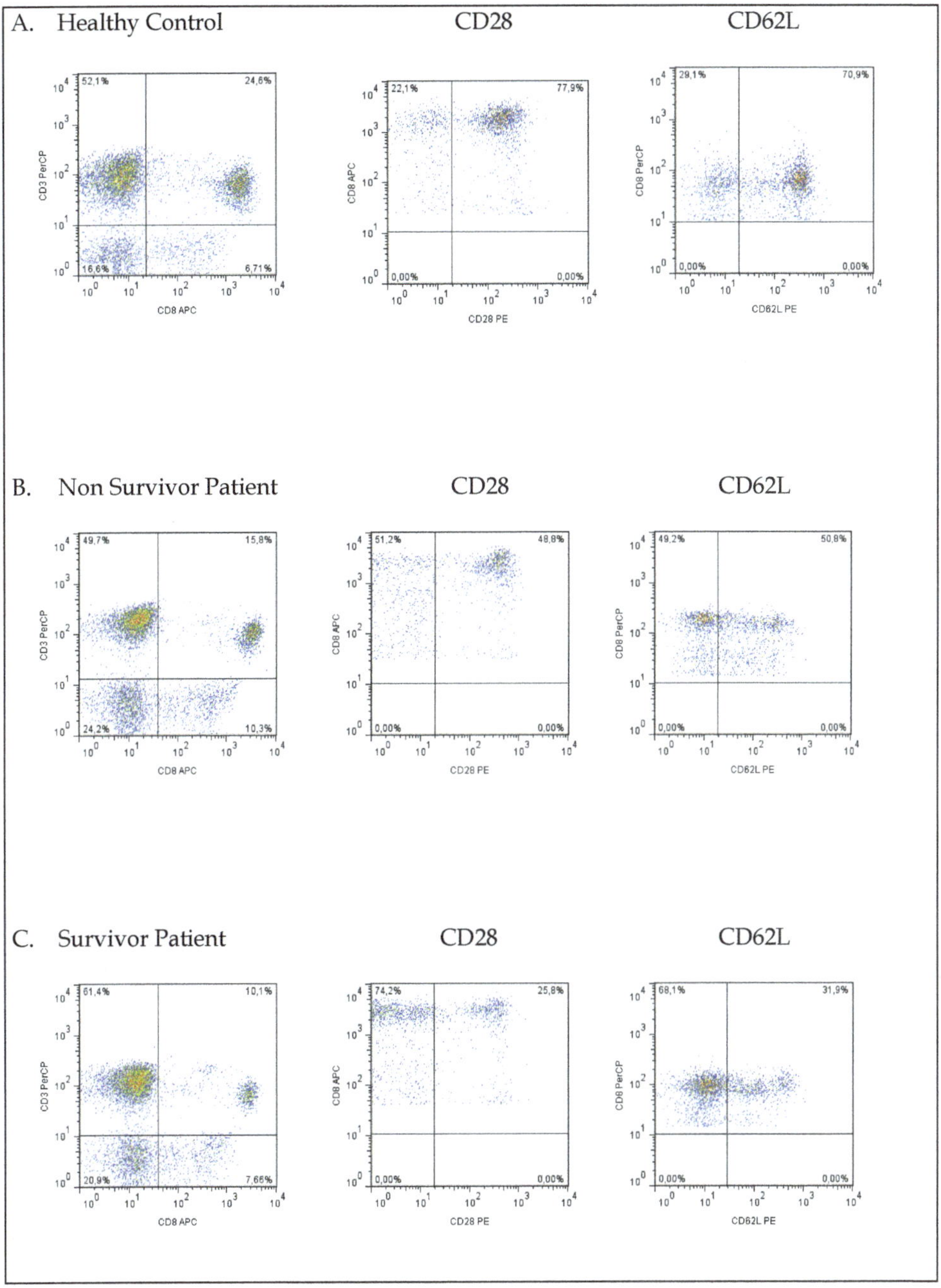

Fig. 4. Flow cytometry data analysis of the CD28 and CD62L surface expression in $CD3^{+}CD8^{+}$ T lymphocytes from peripheral blood of septic shock patients

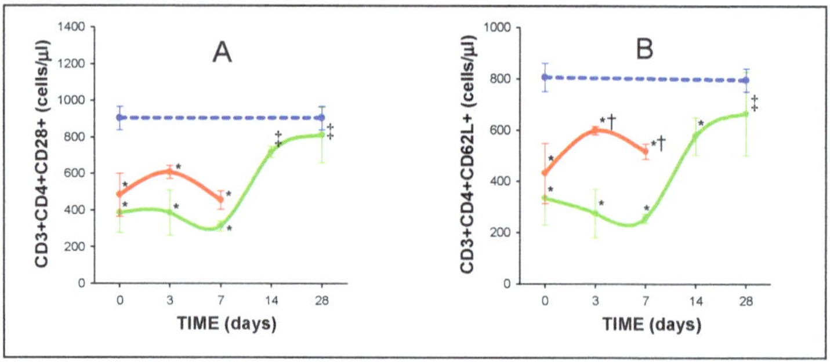

Fig. 5. Kinetic of peripheral blood counts of $CD3^+CD8^+CD62L^+$ and $CD3^+CD8^+CD62L^+$ lymphocyte subsets in patients with septic shock. Symbol represents: (▪●▪) Controls line base, (●) Survivors and (●) Nonsurvivors. All values are expressed as the mean of cells/µl ± S.E.M. *$p<0.05$ for survivors or nonsurvivors versus controls; † $p<0.05$ for survivors versus nonsurvivors; ‡ $p< 0.05$ for each follow up time versus admission.

2.3 Interpretation of blood lymphocyte count alterations in patients with septic shock

In this study, we show that surviving and nonsurviving patients with septic shock have different patterns of involvement in circulating T lymphocyte compartment. A drop in circulating $CD3^+CD4^+$ and $CD3^+CD8^+$ T cells has been described in patients with severe sepsis or septic shock at admission to the ICU (Holub et al. 2000;Holub et al. 2003;Kabisch et al. 1990;Lin et al. 1993;Nishijima et al. 1986). In our kinetic study, we also observed that this T lymphopenia persists during the first week of follow up and is independent of the outcome. Moreover, by the end of the second week of follow up, the absolute number of circulating $CD3^+CD4^+$ T cells had clearly normalised. In contrast, after four weeks of follow up, there was still no return to normal circulating numbers of $CD3^+CD8^+$ T cells.

In a mouse sepsis model of caecal ligation and puncture, the depletion of $CD3^+CD8^+$ T and natural killer cells was associated with a survival benefit with decreased blood bacterial concentrations, improved physiological function and an attenuated proinflammatory response (Sherwood et al. 2004). It has been reported that mice infected with *Plasmodium berghei* develop a syndrome similar to septic shock and the depletion of $CD3^+CD8^+$ T cells also significantly ameliorates the complications that induce shock (Chang et al. 2001). In addition, in patients with trauma and multiple organ failure (MOF), nonsurvivors showed $CD3^+CD8^+$ T cell numbers that were two-folds higher than those recorded in survivors (Menges et al. 1999). In agreement with these experimental and clinical findings, we observed significantly lower $CD3^+CD8^+$ T cell counts in survivors compared with nonsurvivors on day three of follow up. Thus, diminished circulating $CD3^+CD8^+$T cells might have a protective pathogenic role in the outcome of septic shock.

The expression patterns of the RA and RO isoforms of CD45 by T lymphocytes serve to identify subsets associated with different stages of T cell activation. When noneffector $CD45RA^+CD45RO^-$ T lymphocytes are activated by inflammatory agents, such as bacterial infection, CD45RO is up-regulated and CD45RA down-regulated (Hermiston et al. 2003). Thus, our patients showed a persistent reduction in circulating noneffector $CD4^+CD45RA^+$ $CD45RO^-$ and $CD8^+CD45RA^+$ $CD45RO^-$ T cells. In contrast, numbers of $CD8^+CD45RA^-$ $CD45RO^+$ T cells remained normal and $CD4^+CD45RA^-CD45RO^+$ T cell counts initially fell yet had returned to normal by the second week of follow up in surviving patients. An increased percentage of $CD3^+$ cells expressing CD45RO has been reported in patients with sepsis (Roth et al. 2003). Our findings could be the consequence of abnormal polyclonal activation of circulating T lymphocytes. It has been proposed that the switch of T cells from a $CD45RA^+CD45RO^-$ to a $CD45RA^-CD45RO^+$ phenotype may have a functional effect in halting the sustained immune response in an effort to avoid tissue injury (Hermiston et al. 2003). Thus, the expansion of $CD4^+CD45RA^-CD45RO^+$ T lymphocytes observed here during the follow up of surviving patients might be considered a compensatory anti-inflammatory mechanism that develops in these patients with septic shock.

CD28 is a costimulatory molecule that plays a key role in regulating the activation and survival of T lymphocytes (Sansom & Walker 2006). Activation of $CD3^+CD8^+$ T lymphocytes has been related to the loss of CD28 expression (Fiorentini et al. 2001;Labalette et al. 1999). In effect, it has been reported that patients with severe sepsis showed a significant reduction in T lymphocyte CD28 expression (Manjuck et al. 2000). Our data indicate diminished circulating $CD3^+CD8^+CD28^+$ T cell numbers in patients with septic shock with respect to healthy subjects on admission to the ICU and at least during the first 28 days of follow up. Interestingly, a reduced $CD3^+CD8^+CD28^+$ T cell count during the first three days of admission to the ICU was of prognostic value for predicting the survival of a patient. Conversely, an elevated number of circulating $CD3^+CD8^+CD28^+$ T cells was associated with a worse prognosis for the patient. Recently, it has been reported that the stimulation of CD28 by a monoclonal antibody in healthy volunteers is followed by severe multiple cytokine-release syndrome (Suntharalingam et al. 2006). Our results support a relevant role for $CD3^+CD8^+CD28^+$ T cells in the pathogenesis of septic shock. Future studies should address the potential clinical relevance of this cell variable.

The migration of circulating T lymphocytes to peripheral lymph nodes depends on the expression of the CD62L homing receptor (Tang et al. 1998). We found here that the down-regulation of L-selectin expression on $CD3^+CD8^+$ cells in patients with septic shock was associated with a better outcome. Hence, the rapid migration of $CD8^+$ T cells to peripheral lymph nodes may be a mechanism contributing to patient survival.

Our T lymphocyte phenotype data show a time difference, or shift, in the recirculation of T lymphocytes between patients who survive septic shock and those who do not. Taken together and analysing the phenotype of the circulating T cells according to the activation criteria ($CD45RA^+$ and $CD45RO^+$) related to CD28 (activation and co-stimulation) and CD62L (activation and migration) expression point to a slower migration of naive and effector cells in nonsurviving patients. This different T lymphocyte kinetics would mean a delayed tissue response that could determine the failure of the immune system and the fatal prognosis of the patient. In particular, the delay in the disappearance of $CD45RA^+$, $CD45RA^+CD45RO^+$, $CD28^+$, $CD62L^+$, T $CD4^+$ and $CD8^+$ lymphocytes observed between days 3 and 7 of follow up in the nonsurvivors appears to be crucial to the final outcome. Accordingly, in surviving patients, effectors cells would migrate more rapidly to tissues and this would in turn trigger the quick action of the immune system in combating the infection and thus determine the survival of the patient. It is known that cellular immune responses play a critical role in the defense against viral infections and strong T-cell responses have been reported in patients who clear infection (Sarobe et al. 2006a). If the immune response is late or less efficient against microorganism viral epitopes, the outcome of the disease worsens(Hermiston et al. 2003;Lim et al. 2006;Sarobe et al. 2006b). Not surprisingly, the survivor group had lower APACHE II, MODS and SOFA scores than nonsurvivors. An increasing APACHE II score reflects an increasing severity of illness and escalating risk of hospital death for multidiagnostic ICU patient groups. However, an APACHE II score cannot be directly equated with a specific risk of lower mortality than the same score for a patients with septic shock (Wagner et al. 1986). In this group of patients, we found that a cut-off value of 136 cells/ml for $CD3^+CD8^+CD28^+$ T cells and 141 cells/ml for $CD3^+CD8^+CD62L^+$ T cells on ICU admission showed high specificity for predicting the risk of death. However, it is known that the positive predictive value for APACHE II for the validation study population was only 69.6% and the negative predictive value was 87.9% (Joseph E.Parrila & Roger C.Bone 1995). Moreover, SOFA, MODS and APACHE II scores require at least 24 hours of monitoring to be performed and lymphocyte phenotyping can be performed in a short time, approximately 2 hours. It is not possible to replace clinical score in septic shock patients by immunological markers. However, these analytical parameters may help to make clinical decisions in these patients and to establish new potential therapeutic targets. Future studies will need to study in more depth the mechanisms involved in the severe abnormality found on the T cell compartment in patients with septic shock.

2.4 Cytomics: In the future of the study of cellular biomarkers

Advances in the knowledge of the immune system has demonstrated the great complexity of the T, B and Natural Killer (NK) lymphocyte subsets (Appay et al. 2008). T cell subsets display defined immunophenotypic markers at different stages of activation and when they have different patterns of tissue migration (Lanzavecchia & Sallusto 2005;Sallusto et al. 2004). Several pathologic conditions have been associated to different alterations of T cell subset distribution (Appay et al. 2008;Wong et al. 2008). In critically ill patients, global T-cell responsiveness is typically reduced, reflected in the inability to respond to recall antigens in vivo or decreased (Christou et al. 1995) and in impaired lymphocyte proliferation to mitogens in vitro (Keane et al. 1983). However, the response to a T-cell-independent antigens is preserved or even enhanced (Nohr et al. 1986). Abnormal redistribution of NK and B lymphocytes subsets have also been found to be involved in the pathogenesis of other diseases (Cerwenka & Lanier 2001;Sanz et al. 2008) but the evidence reported in critical illness is less compelling.

The simultaneous study of different cell subsets distribution can help to translate basic knowledge on immune system alterations into clinically and therapeutically relevant markers. Our study demonstrates that deeptly characterizing abnormalities on T cell subsets can have clinical significance in septic shock (Monserrat et al. 2009b). Thus, we hypothesized that the combination of the simultaneous analysis of different immune system cell subsets would improve the prediction of outcome in septic shock patients. In addition to the results described previously in our work and following a cytomics analysis, we have also studied the predicting value for outcome of combining different T, B and NK cell markers in the 52 septic shock patients reported in our article (Monserrat et al. 2009b).

Cytomics is an innovative mathematic and statistic bioinformatics analysis procedure (similar to data mining studies) of multiple cellular variables obtained from a population of patients (Valet G.V. et al. 1998;Valet et al. 1993;Valet 2002). Cytomics allows to select a set of multiple quantitative biological variables able to improve the accuracy of patient prognosis and/or establish a predictive value of response to an optional treatment (Valet & Tarnok 2003). Cytomics studies have been previously applied to different fields in medicine: intensive care (Rothe et al. 1990;Valet G.V. et al. 1998), oncology/hematology (Valet et al. 2003;Valet & Hoeffkes 2004), or autoimmune diseases (Jacobi et al. 2003); moreover a human cytome project is underway (Valet et al. 2004;Valet & Valet 2005).

Following the methods and flow cytometry technique described previously (section 2.1.2-2.1.3), we quantified the absolute number of circulating $CD3^+$, $CD4^+$, $CD8^+$, $CD19^+$ and $CD56^+$ lymphocytes and their subsets defined by the co-expression of one, two or three of the following antigens: $CD69^+$, HLA-DR^+, $CD25^+$, $CD26^+$, $CD38^+$, $CD45RA^+$, $CD45RO^+$, $CD71^+$, $CD23^+$, $CD57^+$ as activation markers, $CD80^+$, $CD86^+$, $CD40L^+$ and $CD40^+$ as co-stimulation markers and $CD11a^+$, $CD11b^+$, $CD11c^+$, $CD31^+$, $CD62L^+$,$CD29^+$ as adhesion markers and $CD95^+$ as apoptosis marker. This cellular quantification was performed in each patient at ICU admission and the clinical outcome was analyzed over a 28-day period. The absolute numbers of the different lymphocyte subsets obtained in each patient were introduced in a database. Symmetrical upper and lower threshold percentile values (low percentile 33 and high percentile 67) were selected according to the mortality in our series of patients. These thresholds were used to re-express individual data-base values into +, 0 or – according to their position above, within or below the respective reference percentile thresholds as described (Valet G.V. et al. 1998;Valet et al. 1993). Receiver operating characteristics (ROC) curves were built for each phenotypic variable. The sensitivity and specificity of each variable to predict the real outcome was thus obtained (McNeil & Hanley 1984;Metz 1978). The variables with higher sensitivity values were selected and combined to create multiple variable combinations or masks. The mask with the highest sensitivity and specificity prediction ability for outcome was selected to define the combinations of cut-off values for each variable. According to this methodology we have found a set of five variables and their cut off values (showed in table 1) that are able to improve the prediction for outcome on septic shock patients to a sensitivity of 94 per cent and a specificity of 100 per cent.

MASK SUBSET	**N°/μl**
$CD56^+CD69^+$	>114
$CD3^+CD8^+CD45RA^+CD45RO^-$	>114
$CD3^+CD8^+CD28^+$	>163
$CD19^+CD80^+$	>67
$CD3^+CD11A\ BR^+CD11B^+$	>250

Table 1. Final Mask results after a cytomics study: represent the cut off count of lymphocytes subsets by microlitter that can be able to predict the fatal outcome of the shock septic patients.

These results support the notion that the immune phenotypical analysis of different circulating lymphocyte subsets in septic shock patients has a relevant prognostic value. Leukocyte phenotyping might also have predictive value for the development of immune-supportive or immuno-stimulatory therapies in the management of septic shock patients. The analysis of the abnormalities in the distribution of the T cell compartment in critical patients outside septic shock could also be of great interest (McDunn et al. 2009). We have applied in parallel the immunophotypical T lymphocyte protocol described here to severe acute pancreatitis and ischemic myocardial infarct patients. Our results showed that the patterns of alteration of the distribution and activation stage of T cell subsets are not homogenous in these different acute severe diseases. Thus, the potential involvement of T cell compartment in the pathogenesis of septic shock requires further research and raises the development of innovative diagnostic and therapeutic strategies in these patients.

3. Role of the serum molecules in septic shock

3.1 Diagnosis of sepsis

Numerous putative markers of sepsis have been studied: microbial products, physiologic parameters, hematopoietic cells, cell surface markers, soluble receptors, cytokines, acute phase reactants, mediators of coagulation, cellular processes and others like procalcitonin (Marshall et al. 2003). Probably, procalcitonin is the most extensive laboratory marker used for the discrimination of sepsis in patients with SIRS. In 2001, the SCCM/ESICM/ACCP/ATS/SIS International Sepsis Definitions Conference included plasma procalcitonin above 2SD of the normal value into the diagnostic criteria for sepsis (Levy et al. 2003). They also included plasma C-reactive protein as a criterium for sepsis, but most studies found procalcitonin to be superior to C-reactive protein (Uzzan et al. 2006). We also found these findings and we demonstrate that procalcitonin in combination with Sequential Organ Failure Assessment (SOFA Score) (Vincent et al. 1998) was useful to diagnose infection (Ruiz-Alvarez et al. 2009). However, in newborns, immunosuppressed or elderly patients, procalcitonin had not been shown to be a great asset in the diagnosis of sepsis. Moreover, little is known about serum procalcitonin levels in renal failure and evidence suggests that it is dialyzed (Dahaba et al. 2003).

The release of inflammatory cytokines, such TNFα, IL-1β, IL-6, IL-8 and IFNγ in response to infection leads to SIRS and MOF. Probably, the cytokine that longer has been investigated as a marker of infection is IL-6. IL-6 can be measured reliably in the blood after insult to the host, but it is relatively nonspecific of infection and is elevated in other inflammatory states. When serum IL-6 levels were measured to assess the diagnostic value of infection in patients with SIRS, procalcitonin was superior to IL-6 (Harbarth et al. 2001).

Vascular endothelium injury is widely recognized to play a critical role in many systemic inflammatory diseases as sepsis. However, the ability of the measurement of soluble adhesion molecules to distinguish infection in SIRS patients has been poorly investigated. Bold et al. demonstrated that trauma patients showed lower plasma levels of circulating adhesion molecules than did sepsis patients indicating more pronounced endothelial activation or damage in sepsis (Boldt et al. 1996). Cummings et al. reported that soluble E-selectin levels are higher in serum of patients with microbiologically documented sepsis than in other critically ill patients (Cummings et al. 1997). Recently, we also studied circulating soluble adhesion molecules levels in 92 patients with SIRS and demonstrated that sICAM-1 was a better biomarker of infection than sE-Selectin, sVCAM-1 and sICAM-2.

An acute-phase proteins has been defined as one whose plasma concentrations increases or decreases by at least 25% during inflammatory disorders (Gabay & Kushner 1999). Lipopolysaccharide-binding protein (LBP) is considered an acute-phase protein. It is synthesized by hepatocytes and intestinal epithelial cells and its concentrations rising up after induction of an acute-phase response. A very interesting issue by Albillos et al. analyzed the risk factors associated with a first episode of severe bacterial infection in 84 ascitic cirrhotics. Increased LBP was the only factor independently associated with severe bacterial infection in a multivariate analysis (relative risk 4.49, 95% CI 1.42-14.1). The authors suggested that monitoring of serum LBP could, therefore, help to target cirrhotic patients with ascites for antibiotic prophylaxis (Albillos et al. 2004). However, LBP measurements in ICU patients with SIRS and sepsis have not been found any benefit (Prucha et al. 2003), except in selected patient populations as heart surgery, neonates or neutropenic patients (Pavcnik-Arnol et al. 2004;Sablotzki et al. 2001).

Phagocytic cells are the primary mediators of the innate immune response to bacterial and fungal infections. Triggering receptor expressed on myeloid cells-1 (TREM-1) is a member of the immunoglobulin family and is upregulated in response to infection acting synergistically with Toll-like receptor-4 to augment the immune response. TREM-1 may be not upregulated in noninfectious inflammatory disorders. A soluble form of TREM-1 (sTREM-1) is shed from the membranes of activated phagocytic cells and can be quantified. Studies conducted in ICUs indicated that sTREM-1 is more specific and sensitive than either procalcitonin or C-reactive protein (Bouchon et al. 2001;Gibot et al. 2005). However, in a recent study in patients admitted in a surgical ICU, measurement of sTREM-1 did not distinguish between patients with SIRS, severe sepsis, or septic shock (Bopp et al. 2009). Finally, a recent study only 10 biomarkers have been assessed for their ability to distinguish septic from non-septic patients with SIRS, but no biomarker was clearly identified as being able to differentiate infection in SIRS from other causes (Pierrakos & Vincent 2010).

3.2 Risk assessment and severity

A severity marker provides information about whether a patient with sepsis will experience an adverse outcome. Classical illness scores, such as Acute Physiology and Chronic Health Evaluation (APACHE) and Simplified Acute Physiology Score (SAPS), can predict the severity and outcome of sepsis. Relatively few biomarkers have been evaluated to establish risk assessment and severity in sepsis. Plasma procalcitonin concentrations correlated to sepsis-related organ failure scores and may be useful in risk assessment (Meisner et al. 1999). In 2007, the FDA approved the use of procalcitonin in conjunction with other laboratory findings and clinical assessments to aid in the risk assessment of critically ill patients on their first day of ICU admission for progression to severe sepsis and septic shock.

On the other hand, it has been reported that IL-2 and IL-8 increased in parallel with disease severity (Balcl et al. 2003) and anti-inflammatory cytokines as IL-4, IL-10 and IL-13 have higher concentrations in patients with sepsis than in patients with septic shock (Collighan et al. 2004;Heper et al. 2006). It is important to remark that the production of anti-inflammatory cytokines during septic shock correlates positively with the intensity of the inflammatory response and, as we will describe later, with fatal outcome.

The severity of septic reaction varies a lot in course and outcome depending on host predisposing factors, the infection characteristics, the intensity of host response and, finally, the number of organs failing. The PIRO staging model based on these factors could better predict outcomes of patients with sepsis (Rubulotta et al. 2009). The risk of dying from an infectious disease is much more depend on genetic than on environmental factors (Sorensen et al. 1988). Genetic polymorphisms in innate immunity result in significant interindividual variability in response to infection. In the last years, more than 30 genes have had their respective polymorphisms studied for relations to sepsis and critical infection or inflammation (Namath & Patterson 2009). Sepsis-related polymorphism studies have most commonly focused on one or more polymorphisms for specific genes whose protein products are implicated in sepsis. Current studies include genome-wide approaches, which analyze large representative sets of genetic markers derived from the human haplo-type map in search of those markers associated with a chosen phenotype. New techniques enable detection of thousands of single nucleotide polymorphisms in a single patient, which promise new insights into genetics variations (Marshall & Reinhart 2009).

3.3 Guide of therapy

A biomarker may also aid to guide therapy. First, we need a reliable diagnostic laboratory test that indicates that a clinical syndrome of systemic inflammatory response is likely due to a bacterial or fungal infection. Prompt appropriate empirical antibiotic therapy, searching and controlling infection source, hemodynamic and adjuvant therapy must be initiate as soon as possible for improving survival in patients with sepsis. Conversely, if infection is unlikely to be present permits the clinician to discontinue antibiotics and therefore a minimization of the adverse events. Second, a biomarker may help us to administer therapies to the right patients at the right time. A biomarker whose levels changes during ICU stay may provide information to monitor the response to treatment. In patients with sepsis, an increase or decrease in one marker levels may reflect that the patients responds or fails to respond. Third, critically ill patients with SIRS are a heterogeneous population of patients. A biomarker may also aid to distinguish patterns of a homogeneous group of patients, in whom the benefit of a therapy is known or could be investigated. Fourth, rapid diagnosis of reduced levels of a critical factor or elevated levels of a specific target may be of interest for the rational use of therapies (Cohen et al. 2001).

There are many more potential biomarkers for sepsis than are currently used in clinical studies. IL-6 levels of more than 1000 ng/ml were reported to be highly predictive of sepsis-related death (Harbarth et al. 2001). This finding was used to identify patients more severe who would benefit from adjuvant treatments. However, the results from a large multicenter study randomized patients with severe sepsis to treatment with antibody against TNF or placebo, stratifying patients on the basis of baseline levels of IL-6 have proven disappointing (Panacek et al. 2004).

Several studies have investigated the use of procalcitonin as a marker of treatment strategies. Recently, a meta-analysis which included seven randomized controlling studies reporting on antibiotic use and clinical outcomes of 1131 ICU patients managed with a procalcitonin-guided algorithm or according to routine practice has been published. The main results are: 1) decreased antibiotic exposure; 2) similar mortality rates and ICU or hospital length of stay; and 3) comparable rates of superinfection and persistent or relapsed infection.

C-reactive protein is often reported as inferior compared with procalcitonin as a marker, but it is frequently used in clinical practice because of its greater availability. Serial monitoring of C-reactive protein levels may have some value in predicting infection and response to antibiotics in the ICU (Povoa et al. 2006;Schmit & Vincent 2008).

3.4 Predicting development of organ dysfunction

It is known that the severity of organ failure has significant impact on the prognosis of patients with sepsis. Numerous biomarkers were assessed for their ability to predict the development of MOF. We focused our investigation on the possible association between different organ failures and serum concentrations of soluble cytokines and their soluble receptors in patients with septic shock (de Pablo et al. 2011). The overall prevalence of organ dysfunction at ICU admission was 46% for acute respiratory distress syndrome (ARDS), 36% for acute renal failure (ARF) and 19% for coagulation failure (DIC). Circulating IL-10, sTNF-RI, sTNF-RII, IL-1Ra concentrations were significantly higher in patients with ARDS, ARF and DIC at the time of patients' entry in the study. Serum TNFα levels were found higher in sepsis-induced ARF or DIC. IL-6 was higher in ARDS patients than in patients with septic shock without ARDS. However, there were no significant differences in serum levels of IL-1β, IFNγ or TGF-β than septic patients without these organ failures. TGF-β is a cytokine that plays a pivotal role mainly in the tissue repair reaction subsequent to inflammatory response. It is interesting to remark that in patients with septic shock and persistent ARDS, TGF-β levels are increased. These high concentrations at day 7 of follow-up are related to MOF and death (Figure 6)(de Pablo et al. 2006c).

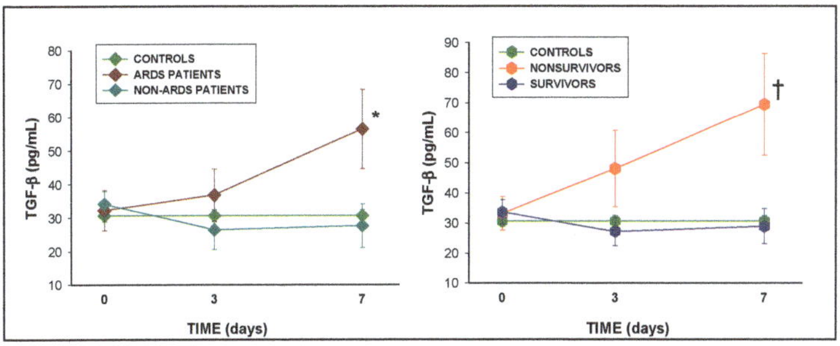

Fig. 6. Serum TGF-*β* levels in septic shock patients.* p<0.05 between patients with or without ARDS, † p<0.05 between survivors and nonsurvivors. Data are expressed as mean ± S.E.M.

When the patients had failure in two or more organ system, they were considered as multiple organ dysfunction syndrome (MODS). Once again, anti-inflammatory molecules such as IL-6, IL-10, sTNF-RI, sTNF-RII, IL-1Ra and sIL-2R were elevated in patients with MODS, but not pro-inflammatory cytokines: TNFα, IL-1β, IFNγ or chemokines: IL-8, MCP-1, MIP-1α or RANTES (table 2).

	With MODS	Without MODS		With MODS	Without MODS
IFNγ	9.17±3.01	15.13±5.59	**IL-10**	5.57±1.98	35.95±20.42*
TNFα	14.42±2.97	36.12±10.83	**IL-2R**	4584±235	5724±417*
IL-1β	2.10±0.84	2.15±0.80	**TGF-β**	40.06±6.67	31.04±4.18
IL-6	1267±672	2737±663*	**IL-8**	206±157	339±116
sTNF-RI	3673±500	5042±617*	**MCP-1**	2797±1049	2997±572
sTNF-RII	4984±558	6373±724*	**MIP-1α**	61.94±15.50	66.42±13.90
IL-1 ra	7099±1464	11052±2030*	**RANTES**	20177±3831	15325±2140

Table 2. Serum cytokines and chemokines levels in septic shock patients with or without MODS at ICU admission.* p<0.05 between patients with or without MODS. Data are expressed as mean ± S.E.M.

3.5 Prognosis

Sepsis, severe sepsis and septic shock are the leading cause of death in critically ill patients (Hotchkiss & Karl 2003). The ICU mortality rates increase with the severity of the syndrome: 27% for sepsis, 32% for severe sepsis and 54% for septic shock (Vincent et al. 2006). Outcome from sepsis in terms of mortality is not only associated with the amount of organ dysfunction developed (Alberti et al. 2003). Other variables as age, genetic backgrounds, comorbidities, reasons for ICU admission, and related to infection (acquisition, extension, site and agent) were observed in outcome of patients with sepsis (Gustot 2011). PIRO system emerged from the Fifth Toronto Sepsis Roundtable. It includes Predisposition, Injury, Response and Organ Dysfunction (Marshall et al. 2003). However, this approach remained

up to now virtually conceptual and other research groups empirically developed in cohorts of patients a scale for predicting mortality in sepsis (Moreno et al. 2008).
Sepsis biomarkers may contribute to this model of classification. However, at this moment the majority of the biomarkers have been evaluated as prognosis markers and in our search, we assessed the ability of a biomarker to differentiate patients likely to survive from those likely to die. We studied by sandwich ELISA serum levels of pro-inflammatory cytokines (TNFα, IL-1β, IL-6 and IFNγ), anti-inflammatory cytokines (IL-10 and TGFβ) and soluble cytokine antagonist (sTNF-RI, sTNF-RII and IL-1Ra) during the first 28 days of ICU admission in 52 patients with septic shock. We found that serum an early response to continuously elevated soluble sTNF-RI, sTNF-RII and IL-1Ra serum levels was associated with an enhanced risk of fatal outcome (table 3). ROC analysis revealed that sTNF-receptor I or sTNF receptor II concentrations over 2767 or 4619 pg/ml, respectively, determinate a high risk of death. The sensitivity-specificity for sTNF-RI was 100%-57% and for sTNF-RII was 100%-71%. IL-1Ra concentrations below 7033 pg/ml determined a high probability of survival (sensitivity-specificity of 60-100%).

	Survivors	Nonsurvivors		Survivors	Nonsurvivors
IFNγ	16.59±5.90	7.16±2.07	**IL-10**	7.38±3.43	57.39±35.71*
TNFα	23.81±7.42	40.42±17.91	**IL-2R**	4830±183	6177±661
IL-1β	1.78±0.51	2.75±1.38	**TGF-β**	33.74±4.06	33.38±5.57
IL-6	1960±609	2811±931	**IL-8**	265±113	356.7±167.7
sTNF-RI	3910±396	6050±1043*	**MCP-1**	3020±670	2774±771.7
sTNF-RII	4862±430	8005±1074*	**MIP-1α**	67.7±12.9	59.3±18.6
IL-1 ra	7331±1351	3819±2880*	**RANTES**	14758±2105	20714±3624

Table 3. Serum cytokines and chemokines levels in septic shock patients at ICU admission. *p<0.05 between survivors and nonsurvivors. Data are expressed as mean ± S.E.M.

Serum levels of TNFα, IL-1β, IL-6 were significantly elevated on admission and during the 28 days of follow-up in septic patients when compared with healthy controls, but were not predictors of mortality (table 3). Interestingly, IFNγ levels were significantly higher in survivors than in controls during the initial two weeks of observation (de Pablo et al. 2011). Serum IL-10 concentrations were elevated in the first 3 days in non-survival patients. TGFβ, an anti-inflammatory cytokine capable of converting an active site of inflammation into one dominated by resolution and repair (Letterio & Roberts 1997), discriminated patients with fatal outcome at day 7 of the follow-up (Figure 6). All these findings together suggest that mortality in patients with septic shock correlates more with anti-inflammatory molecules than with pro-inflammatory immunomodulatory molecules. Many previous clinical trials have failed to show benefit using anti-inflammatory agents, because the inflammatory status of the patients is a dynamic process where it may be reasonable to test the hypothesis of using immunoinflammatory stimulation therapy on patients with septic shock with high risk of death determined by the presence in blood of high levels of sTNF-RI, sTNF-RII and IL-1Ra or low of IFNγ. We also studied the prognostic value of chemokines and soluble adhesion molecules. Chemokines are a large superfamily of small peptides that are key participants to not only control of leukocyte trafficking, but necessary for the linkage between innate and adaptative immunity. No significant differences were found between survivors and nonsurvivors at any time of the follow-up in serum levels of IL-8, MCP-1, MIP-1 and RANTES (table 3) (de Pablo et al. 2006b).

Next, we focused our investigation in the prognostic value of fatal outcome of the circulating soluble adhesion molecules in the population of patients with septic shock admitted at the ICU. Mortality was defined as death occurring within 28 days after study enrolment. At ICU admission, serum soluble E-Selectin concentrations showed significantly higher levels in the nonsurvival group (110.08±8.00ng/ml) than in survival group (88.73±4.92ng/ml; p=0.041). We also analysed serum E-Selectin levels at ICU admission as a predictor of outcome, determining the area under the receiver operating characteristics curve (AUC). The AUC value for baseline measurements of E-Selectin was 0.728 (p=0.049; 95% confidence interval, 0.516-0.939). Thus, an E-Selectin concentration of 106.8ng/ml was identified as the optimum threshold to distinguish the patients for outcome with a sensitivity of 60.0% and specificity of 85.7%. Over the study period, no significant change in circulating soluble VCAM-1, ICAM-1, ICAM-2 and PECAM-1 concentrations was observed between survival and nonsurvival patients. Thus, soluble E-Selectin is a marker of endothelial damage, which may result in failure of the different organs, multiple organ dysfunction syndrome and death (de Pablo et al. 2006a).

Numerous biomarker have been reported in prognosis like other cytokines as IL-12 or IL-18, cell markers as soluble HLA-DR, receptors as TREM-1 or as urokinase type plasminogen activator receptor, related to vascular endothelial damage as von Willebrand factor and antigen or like acute phase proteins as ferritin or procalcitonin (Pierrakos & Vincent 2010). However, no biomarker has established itself sufficiently to be of help in clinician practice. Each biomarker has limited sensitivity and specificity; therefore, it may prove more useful to combine various markers. Biomarker panels or composite markers may prove most useful in examining a particular immunologic pathway, identifying at-risk individuals who require aggressive intervention, predicting organ response and determining the ability to differentiate patients likely to survive from those likely to die (Ventetuolo & Levy 2008).

4. Conclusion

Many biomarkers have been evaluated for the use in sepsis, many more than in other disease processes. At present, around of 178 different biomarkers were actually evaluated in the 3370 studies, 77 in experimental studies and 101 in clinical studies only, 58 in both experimental and clinical studies (Pierrakos et al. 2010). However, hardly a few of them are able to report sensitivity and specificity values greater than 90%. We demonstrated that septic shock patients show a severe redistribution of circulating T lymphocyte subsets and CD62L and CD28 expression on circulating T cells at ICU admission are good markers to predict the outcome of shock septic patients. We found that T lymphocyte phenotype data show a time difference in the recirculation of T cells between survivors and nonsurvivors that might provoke a delayed tissue response of the immune system. Moreover, we demonstrated that the simultaneous analysis of different immune system cell subsets in combination like ($CD56^{+}CD69^{+}$, $CD3^{+}CD8^{+}CD45RA^{+}CD45RO^{-}$, $CD3^{+}CD8^{+}CD28^{+}$, $CD19^{+}CD80^{+}$, $CD3^{+}CD11A$ $BR^{+}CD11B^{+}$) would improve the prediction of outcome in septic shock patients. With respect to serum cytokines, we found that antiinflammatory and adhesion molecules are good markers for the prognosis of septic shock patients. We propose that the blood counts of circulating cells of the immune system are good candidates to study for value as biomarkers. In this book chapter we attempt to resume the continuous effort by clinician and researchers to find new biomarkers that going to allow us to improve the prognostic of septic shock patients. New experiments and clinical studies are necessary to achieve this goal.

5. Acknowledgment

The authors would like to thank all the medical doctors and nurses of the ICU of the Hospital Universitario Principe de Asturias for their careful and generous collaboration while doing this work.

6. References

Alberti C, Brun-Buisson C, Goodman SV, Guidici D, Granton J, Moreno R, Smithies M, Thomas O, Artigas A, & Le G, Jr. (2003). Influence of systemic inflammatory response syndrome and sepsis on outcome of critically ill infected patients. *Am. J. Respir. Crit Care Med.* 168 (1): 77-84.

Albillos A, de la Hera A, & Alvarez-Mon M. (2004). Serum lipopolysaccharide-binding protein prediction of severe bacterial infection in cirrhotic patients with ascites. *Lancet* 363 (9421): 1608-1610.

Appay V, van Lier RA, Sallusto F, & Roederer M. (2008). Phenotype and function of human T lymphocyte subsets: consensus and issues. *Cytometry A* 73 (11): 975-983.

Balcl C, Sungurtekin H, Gurses E, Sungurtekin U, & Kaptanoglu B. (2003). Usefulness of procalcitonin for diagnosis of sepsis in the intensive care unit. *Crit Care* 7 (1): 85-90.

Bellora F, Castriconi R, Dondero A, Reggiardo G, Moretta L, Mantovani A, Moretta A, & Bottino C. (2010). The interaction of human natural killer cells with either unpolarized or polarized macrophages results in different functional outcomes. *Proc. Natl. Acad. Sci. U. S. A* 107 (50): 21659-21664.

Biomarkers WG. (2001). Biomarkers and surrogate endpoints: preferred definitions and conceptual framework. *Clin. Pharmacol. Ther.* 69 (3): 89-95.

Boldt J, Muller M, Kuhn D, Linke LC, & Hempelmann G. (1996). Circulating adhesion molecules in the critically ill: a comparison between trauma and sepsis patients. *Intensive Care Med.* 22 (2): 122-128.

Bone RC, Balk RA, Cerra FB, Dellinger RP, Fein AM, Knaus WA, Schein RM, & Sibbald WJ. (1992). Definitions for sepsis and organ failure and guidelines for the use of innovative therapies in sepsis. The ACCP/SCCM Consensus Conference Committee. American College of Chest Physicians/Society of Critical Care Medicine. *Chest* 101 (6): 1644-1655.

Bopp C, Hofer S, Bouchon A, Zimmermann JB, Martin E, & Weigand MA. (2009). Soluble TREM-1 is not suitable for distinguishing between systemic inflammatory response syndrome and sepsis survivors and nonsurvivors in the early stage of acute inflammation. *Eur. J. Anaesthesiol.* 26 (6): 504-507.

Bouchon A, Facchetti F, Weigand MA, & Colonna M. (2001). TREM-1 amplifies inflammation and is a crucial mediator of septic shock. *Nature* 410 (6832): 1103-1107.

Cerwenka A, & Lanier LL. (2001). Natural killer cells, viruses and cancer. *Nat. Rev Immunol.* 1 (1): 41-49.

Chang WL, Jones SP, Lefer DJ, Welbourne T, Sun G, Yin L, Suzuki H, Huang J, Granger DN, & van der Heyde HC. (2001). CD8(+)-T-cell depletion ameliorates circulatory shock in Plasmodium berghei-infected mice. *Infect. Immun.* 69 (12): 7341-7348.

Chiche L, Forel JM, Thomas G, Farnarier C, Vely F, Blery M, Papazian L, & Vivier E. (2011). The role of natural killer cells in sepsis. *J. Biomed. Biotechnol.* 2011: 986491.

Christou NV, Meakins JL, Gordon J, Yee J, Hassan-Zahraee M, Nohr CW, Shizgal HM, & MacLean LD. (1995). The delayed hypersensitivity response and host resistance in surgical patients. 20 years later. *Ann. Surg.* 222 (4): 534-546.

Cohen J, Guyatt G, Bernard GR, Calandra T, Cook D, Elbourne D, Marshall J, Nunn A, & Opal S. (2001). New strategies for clinical trials in patients with sepsis and septic shock. *Crit Care Med.* 29 (4): 880-886.

Collighan N, Giannoudis PV, Kourgeraki O, Perry SL, Guillou PJ, & Bellamy MC. (2004). Interleukin 13 and inflammatory markers in human sepsis. *Br. J. Surg.* 91 (6): 762-768.

Costantini C, & Cassatella MA. (2011). The defensive alliance between neutrophils and NK cells as a novel arm of innate immunity. *J. Leukoc. Biol.* 89 (2): 221-233.

Cummings CJ, Sessler CN, Beall LD, Fisher BJ, Best AM, & Fowler AA, III. (1997). Soluble E-selectin levels in sepsis and critical illness. Correlation with infection and hemodynamic dysfunction. *Am. J Respir. Crit Care Med.* 156 (2 Pt 1): 431-437.

Curfs JH, Meis JF, & Hoogkamp-Korstanje JA. (1997). A primer on cytokines: sources, receptors, effects, and inducers. *Clin. Microbiol. Rev.* 10 (4): 742-780.

Dahaba AA, Rehak PH, & List WF. (2003). Procalcitonin and C-reactive protein plasma concentrations in nonseptic uremic patients undergoing hemodialysis. *Intensive Care Med.* 29 (4): 579-583.

de Pablo R, Monserrat J, Prieto A, Reyes E., & Alvarez-Mon M. (2006a). Circulating Soluble Adhesion Molecules in Septic Shock Patients. *Crit Care Med.* 34 (12 (Suppl.)): A99.

de Pablo R, Monserrat J, Prieto A, Reyes E., & Alvarez-Mon M. (2006b). Serum Chemokine Levels In Septic Shock Patients. Relation To Multiple-System Organ Failure. *Crit Care Med.* 34 (12 (Suppl.)): A105.

de Pablo R, Monserrat J, Prieto A, Reyes E., & Alvarez-Mon M. (2006c). TGF-beta is a good biomarker of persistent ARDS in septic shock patients. *Crit Care Med.* 34 (12 (Suppl.)): A101.

de Pablo R, Monserrat J, Reyes E, Diaz-Martin D, Rodriguez ZM, Carballo F, de la Hera A, Prieto A, & Alvarez-Mon M. (2011). Mortality in patients with septic shock correlates with anti-inflammatory but not proinflammatory immunomodulatory molecules. *J. Intensive Care Med.* 26 (2): 125-132.

Fiorentini S, Licenziati S, Alessandri G, Castelli F, Caligaris S, Bonafede M, Grassi M, Garrafa E, Balsari A, Turano A, & Caruso A. (2001). CD11b expression identifies CD8+CD28+ T lymphocytes with phenotype and function of both naive/memory and effector cells. *J. Immunol.* 166 (2): 900-907.

Gabay C, & Kushner I. (1999). Acute-phase proteins and other systemic responses to inflammation. *N. Engl. J. Med.* 340 (6): 448-454.

Gibot S, Cravoisy A, Kolopp-Sarda MN, Bene MC, Faure G, Bollaert PE, & Levy B. (2005). Time-course of sTREM (soluble triggering receptor expressed on myeloid cells)-1, procalcitonin, and C-reactive protein plasma concentrations during sepsis. *Crit Care Med.* 33 (4): 792-796.

Gustot T. (2011). Multiple organ failure in sepsis: prognosis and role of systemic inflammatory response. *Curr. Opin. Crit Care* 17 (2): 153-159.

Harbarth S, Holeckova K, Froidevaux C, Pittet D, Ricou B, Grau GE, Vadas L, & Pugin J. (2001). Diagnostic value of procalcitonin, interleukin-6, and interleukin-8 in critically ill patients admitted with suspected sepsis. *Am. J Respir. Crit Care Med.* 164 (3): 396-402.

Heper Y, Akalin EH, Mistik R, Akgoz S, Tore O, Goral G, Oral B, Budak F, & Helvaci S. (2006). Evaluation of serum C-reactive protein, procalcitonin, tumor necrosis factor alpha, and interleukin-10 levels as diagnostic and prognostic parameters in patients with community-acquired sepsis, severe sepsis, and septic shock. *Eur. J. Clin. Microbiol. Infect. Dis.* 25 (8): 481-491.

Hermiston ML, Xu Z, & Weiss A. (2003). CD45: a critical regulator of signaling thresholds in immune cells. *Annu. Rev. Immunol.* 21: 107-137.

Holub M, Kluckova Z, Beneda B, Hobstova J, Huzicka I, Prazak J, & Lobovska A. (2000). Changes in lymphocyte subpopulations and CD3+/DR+ expression in sepsis. *Clin. Microbiol. Infect.* 6 (12): 657-660.

Holub M, Kluckova Z, Helcl M, Prihodov J, Rokyta R, & Beran O. (2003). Lymphocyte subset numbers depend on the bacterial origin of sepsis. *Clin. Microbiol. Infect.* 9 (3): 202-211.

Hotchkiss RS, & Karl IE. (2003). The pathophysiology and treatment of sepsis. *N. Engl. J Med.* 348 (2): 138-150.

Jacobi AM, Odendahl M, Reiter K, Bruns A, Burmester GR, Radbruch A, Valet G, Lipsky PE, & Dorner T. (2003). Correlation between circulating CD27high plasma cells and disease activity in patients with systemic lupus erythematosus. *Arthritis Rheum.* 48 (5): 1332-1342.

Joseph E.Parrila, and Roger C.Bone. (1995). *Critical Care Medicine Principles of Diagnosis and Management.*: Mosby.

Kabisch S, Gemar K, Krumholz W, Salomon F, & Pralle H. (1990). [Lymphocyte subpopulations in patients at risk of sepsis in a surgical intensive care unit]. *Anaesthesist* 39 (9): 439-444.

Keane RM, Birmingham W, Shatney CM, Winchurch RA, & Munster AM. (1983). Prediction of sepsis in the multitraumatic patient by assays of lymphocyte responsiveness. *Surg. Gynecol. Obstet.* 156 (2): 163-167.

Labalette M, Leteurtre E, Thumerelle C, Grutzmacher C, Tourvieille B, & Dessaint JP. (1999). Peripheral human CD8(+)CD28(+)T lymphocytes give rise to CD28(-)progeny, but IL-4 prevents loss of CD28 expression. *Int. Immunol.* 11 (8): 1327-1336.

Lanzavecchia A, & Sallusto F. (2005). Understanding the generation and function of memory T cell subsets. *Curr. Opin. Immunol.* 17 (3): 326-332.

Letterio JJ, & Roberts AB. (1997). TGF-beta: a critical modulator of immune cell function. *Clin. Immunol. Immunopathol.* 84 (3): 244-250.

Levy MM, Fink MP, Marshall JC, Abraham E, Angus D, Cook D, Cohen J, Opal SM, Vincent JL, & Ramsay G. (2003). 2001 SCCM/ESICM/ACCP/ATS/SIS International Sepsis Definitions Conference. *Crit Care Med.* 31 (4): 1250-1256.

Levy MM, Macias WL, Vincent JL, Russell JA, Silva E, Trzaskoma B, & Williams MD. (2005). Early changes in organ function predict eventual survival in severe sepsis. *Crit Care Med.* 33 (10): 2194-2201.

Lim B, Sutherland RM, Zhan Y, Deliyannis G, Brown LE, & Lew AM. (2006). Targeting CD45RB alters T cell migration and delays viral clearance. *Int. Immunol.* 18 (2): 291-300.

Lin RY, Astiz ME, Saxon JC, & Rackow EC. (1993). Altered leukocyte immunophenotypes in septic shock. Studies of HLA-DR, CD11b, CD14, and IL-2R expression. *Chest* 104 (3): 847-853.

Manjuck J, Saha DC, Astiz M, Eales LJ, & Rackow EC. (2000). Decreased response to recall antigens is associated with depressed costimulatory receptor expression in septic critically ill patients. *J Lab Clin Med.* 135 (2): 153-160.

Marshall JC, & Reinhart K. (2009). Biomarkers of sepsis. *Crit Care Med.* 37 (7): 2290-2298.

Marshall JC, Vincent JL, Fink MP, Cook DJ, Rubenfeld G, Foster D, Fisher CJ, Jr., Faist E, & Reinhart K. (2003). Measures, markers, and mediators: toward a staging system for clinical sepsis. A report of the Fifth Toronto Sepsis Roundtable, Toronto, Ontario, Canada, October 25-26, 2000. *Crit Care Med.* 31 (5): 1560-1567.

McDunn JE, Muenzer JT, Dunne B, Zhou A, Yuan K, Hoekzema A, Hilliard C, Chang KC, Davis CG, McDonough J, Hunt C, Grigsby P, Piwnica-Worms D, & Hotchkiss RS. (2009). An anti-apoptotic peptide improves survival in lethal total body irradiation. *Biochem. Biophys. Res. Commun.* 382 (4): 657-662.

McNeil BJ, & Hanley JA. (1984). Statistical approaches to the analysis of receiver operating characteristic (ROC) curves. *Med. Decis. Making* 4 (2): 137-150.

Meisner M, Tschaikowsky K, Palmaers T, & Schmidt J. (1999). Comparison of procalcitonin (PCT) and C-reactive protein (CRP) plasma concentrations at different SOFA scores during the course of sepsis and MODS. *Crit Care* 3 (1): 45-50.

Menges T, Engel J, Welters I, Wagner RM, Little S, Ruwoldt R, Wollbrueck M, & Hempelmann G. (1999). Changes in blood lymphocyte populations after multiple trauma: association with posttraumatic complications. *Crit Care Med.* 27 (4): 733-740.

Metz CE. (1978). Basic principles of ROC analysis. *Semin. Nucl. Med.* 8 (4): 283-298.

Monserrat J, de PR, Prieto A, Reyes E, & varez-Mon M. (2009a). Using surface molecule expression on lymphocytes to classify septic shock patients. *Crit Care* 13 (3): 412.

Monserrat J, de PR, Reyes E, Diaz D, Barcenilla H, Zapata MR, de la Hera A, Prieto A, & Alvarez-Mon M. (2009b). Clinical relevance of the severe abnormalities of the T cell compartment in septic shock patients. *Crit Care* 13 (1): R26.

Moreno RP, Metnitz B, Adler L, Hoechtl A, Bauer P, & Metnitz PG. (2008). Sepsis mortality prediction based on predisposition, infection and response. *Intensive Care Med.* 34 (3): 496-504.

Najera O, Gonzalez C, Toledo G, Lopez L, Cortes E, Betancourt M, & Ortiz R. (2001). CD45RA and CD45RO isoforms in infected malnourished and infected well-nourished children. *Clin Exp. Immunol.* 126 (3): 461-465.

Namath A, & Patterson AJ. (2009). Genetic polymorphisms in sepsis. *Crit Care Clin.* 25 (4): 835-56, x.

Nishijima MK, Takezawa J, Hosotsubo KK, Takahashi H, Shimada Y, & Yoshiya I. (1986). Serial changes in cellular immunity of septic patients with multiple organ-system failure. *Crit Care Med.* 14 (2): 87-91.

Nohr CW, Latter DA, Meakins JL, & Christou NV. (1986). In vivo and in vitro humoral immunity in surgical patients: antibody response to pneumococcal polysaccharide. *Surgery* 100 (2): 229-238.

Ochoa JB, & Makarenkova V. (2005). T lymphocytes. *Crit Care Med.* 33 (12 Suppl): S510-S513.

Opal SM, Girard TD, & Ely EW. (2005). The immunopathogenesis of sepsis in elderly patients. *Clin. Infect. Dis.* 41 Suppl 7: S504-S512.

Panacek EA, Marshall JC, Albertson TE, Johnson DH, Johnson S, MacArthur RD, Miller M, Barchuk WT, Fischkoff S, Kaul M, Teoh L, Van Meter L, Daum L, Lemeshow S, Hicklin G, & Doig C. (2004). Efficacy and safety of the monoclonal anti-tumor necrosis factor antibody F(ab')2 fragment afelimomab in patients with severe sepsis and elevated interleukin-6 levels. *Crit Care Med.* 32 (11): 2173-2182.

Pavcnik-Arnol M, Hojker S, & Derganc M. (2004). Lipopolysaccharide-binding protein in critically ill neonates and children with suspected infection: comparison with procalcitonin, interleukin-6, and C-reactive protein. *Intensive Care Med.* 30 (7): 1454-1460.

Pierrakos C, & Vincent JL. (2010). Sepsis biomarkers: a review. *Crit Care* 14 (1): R15.

Povoa P, Coelho L, Almeida E, Fernandes A, Mealha R, Moreira P, & Sabino H. (2006). Early identification of intensive care unit-acquired infections with daily monitoring of C-reactive protein: a prospective observational study. *Crit Care* 10 (2): R63.

Prucha M, Herold I, Zazula R, Dubska L, Dostal M, Hildebrand T, & Hyanek J. (2003). Significance of lipopolysaccharide-binding protein (an acute phase protein) in monitoring critically ill patients. *Crit Care* 7 (6): R154-R159.

Rivers E, Nguyen B, Havstad S, Ressler J, Muzzin A, Knoblich B, Peterson E, & Tomlanovich M. (2001). Early goal-directed therapy in the treatment of severe sepsis and septic shock. *N. Engl. J. Med.* 345 (19): 1368-1377.

Romagnani C, Juelke K, Falco M, Morandi B, D'Agostino A, Costa R, Ratto G, Forte G, Carrega P, Lui G, Conte R, Strowig T, Moretta A, Munz C, Thiel A, Moretta L, & Ferlazzo G. (2007). CD56bright. *J. Immunol.* 178 (8): 4947-4955.

Roth G, Moser B, Krenn C, Brunner M, Haisjackl M, Almer G, Gerlitz S, Wolner E, Boltz-Nitulescu G, & Ankersmit HJ. (2003). Susceptibility to programmed cell death in T-lymphocytes from septic patients: a mechanism for lymphopenia and Th2 predominance. *Biochem. Biophys. Res. Commun.* 308 (4): 840-846.

Rothe G, Kellermann W, & Valet G. (1990). Flow cytometric parameters of neutrophil function as early indicators of sepsis- or trauma-related pulmonary or cardiovascular organ failure. *J Lab Clin Med.* 115 (1): 52-61.

Rubulotta F, Marshall JC, Ramsay G, Nelson D, Levy M, & Williams M. (2009). Predisposition, insult/infection, response, and organ dysfunction: A new model for staging severe sepsis. *Crit Care Med.* 37 (4): 1329-1335.

Ruiz-Alvarez MJ, Garcia-Valdecasas S, de PR, Sanchez GM, Coca C, Groeneveld TW, Roos A, Daha MR, & Arribas I. (2009). Diagnostic efficacy and prognostic value of serum procalcitonin concentration in patients with suspected sepsis. *J. Intensive Care Med.* 24 (1): 63-71.

Sablotzki A, Borgermann J, Baulig W, Friedrich I, Spillner J, Silber RE, & Czeslick E. (2001). Lipopolysaccharide-binding protein (LBP) and markers of acute-phase response in patients with multiple organ dysfunction syndrome (MODS) following open heart surgery. *Thorac. Cardiovasc. Surg.* 49 (5): 273-278.

Sallusto F, Geginat J, & Lanzavecchia A. (2004). Central memory and effector memory T cell subsets: function, generation, and maintenance. *Annu. Rev Immunol.* 22: 745-763.

Sallusto F, Lenig D, Forster R, Lipp M, & Lanzavecchia A. (1999). Two subsets of memory T lymphocytes with distinct homing potentials and effector functions. *Nature* 401 (6754): 708-712.

Sansom DM, & Walker LS. (2006). The role of CD28 and cytotoxic T-lymphocyte antigen-4 (CTLA-4) in regulatory T-cell biology. *Immunol. Rev.* 212: 131-148.

Sanz I, Wei C, Lee FE, & Anolik J. (2008). Phenotypic and functional heterogeneity of human memory B cells. *Semin. Immunol.* 20 (1): 67-82.

Sarobe P, Lasarte JJ, Garcia N, Civeira MP, Borras-Cuesta F, & Prieto J. (2006a). Characterization of T-cell responses against immunodominant epitopes from hepatitis C virus E2 and NS4a proteins. *J. Viral Hepat.* 13 (1): 47-55.

Sarobe P, Lasarte JJ, Garcia N, Civeira MP, Borras-Cuesta F, & Prieto J. (2006b). Characterization of T-cell responses against immunodominant epitopes from hepatitis C virus E2 and NS4a proteins. *J. Viral Hepat.* 13 (1): 47-55.

Schmit X, & Vincent JL. (2008). The time course of blood C-reactive protein concentrations in relation to the response to initial antimicrobial therapy in patients with sepsis. *Infection* 36 (3): 213-219.

Sherwood ER, Enoh VT, Murphey ED, & Lin CY. (2004). Mice depleted of CD8+ T and NK cells are resistant to injury caused by cecal ligation and puncture. *Lab Invest* 84 (12): 1655-1665.

Sorensen TI, Nielsen GG, Andersen PK, & Teasdale TW. (1988). Genetic and environmental influences on premature death in adult adoptees. *N. Engl. J. Med.* 318 (12): 727-732.

Suntharalingam G, Perry MR, Ward S, Brett SJ, Castello-Cortes A, Brunner MD, & Panoskaltsis N. (2006). Cytokine storm in a phase 1 trial of the anti-CD28 monoclonal antibody TGN1412. *N. Engl. J. Med.* 355 (10): 1018-1028.

Tang ML, Steeber DA, Zhang XQ, & Tedder TF. (1998). Intrinsic differences in L-selectin expression levels affect T and B lymphocyte subset-specific recirculation pathways. *J Immunol.* 160 (10): 5113-5121.

Uzzan B, Cohen R, Nicolas P, Cucherat M, & Perret GY. (2006). Procalcitonin as a diagnostic test for sepsis in critically ill adults and after surgery or trauma: a systematic review and meta-analysis. *Crit Care Med.* 34 (7): 1996-2003.

Valet G.V., Roth G, and Kellermann W. (1998). Risk assessment for intesive care patients by automated classification of flow cytometry data. In *Phagocyte function: A guide for research and clinical evaluation*, eds Robinson J.P. and Babcock G.F., 289-305. Wiley-Liss.

Valet G. (2002). Predictive medicine by cytomics: potential and challenges. *J Biol. Regul. Homeost. Agents* 16 (2): 164-167.

Valet G, Leary JF, & Tarnok A. (2004). Cytomics--new technologies: towards a human cytome project. *Cytometry A* 59 (2): 167-171.

Valet G, Repp R, Link H, Ehninger A, & Gramatzki MM. (2003). Pretherapeutic identification of high-risk acute myeloid leukemia (AML) patients from immunophenotypic, cytogenetic, and clinical parameters. *Cytometry B Clin Cytom.* 53 (1): 4-10.

Valet G, Valet M, Tschope D, Gabriel H, Rothe G, Kellermann W, & Kahle H. (1993). White cell and thrombocyte disorders. Standardized, self-learning flow cytometric list mode data classification with the CLASSIF1 program system. *Ann. N. Y. Acad. Sci.* 677: 233-251.

Valet GK, & Hoeffkes HG. (2004). Data pattern analysis for the individualised pretherapeutic identification of high-risk diffuse large B-cell lymphoma (DLBCL) patients by cytomics. *Cytometry A* 59 (2): 232-236.

Valet GK, & Tarnok A. (2003). Cytomics in predictive medicine. *Cytometry B Clin Cytom.* 53 (1): 1-3.

Valet GK, & Valet M. (2005). Cytomics, the human cytome project and systems biology: top-down resolution of the molecular biocomplexity of organisms by single cell analysis. *Cell Prolif.* 38 (4): 171-174.

Ventetuolo CE, & Levy MM. (2008). Biomarkers: diagnosis and risk assessment in sepsis. *Clin. Chest Med.* 29 (4): 591-603, vii.

Vincent JL, de Mendonca A, Cantraine F, Moreno R, Takala J, Suter PM, Sprung CL, Colardyn F, & Blecher S. (1998). Use of the SOFA score to assess the incidence of organ dysfunction/failure in intensive care units. European Society of Intensive Care Medicine. *Crit Care Med.* 26 (11): 1793-1800.

Vincent JL, Sakr Y, Sprung CL, Ranieri VM, Reinhart K, Gerlach H, Moreno R, Carlet J, Le G, Jr., & Payen D. (2006). Sepsis in European intensive care units: results of the SOAP study. *Crit Care Med.* 34 (2): 344-353.

Wagner DP, Knaus WA, & Draper EA. (1986). Physiologic abnormalities and outcome from acute disease. Evidence for a predictable relationship. *Arch. Intern. Med.* 146 (7): 1389-1396.

Wong CK, Lit LC, Tam LS, Li EK, Wong PT, & Lam CW. (2008). Hyperproduction of IL-23 and IL-17 in patients with systemic lupus erythematosus: implications for Th17-mediated inflammation in auto-immunity. *Clin Immunol.* 127 (3): 385-393.

Permissions

The contributors of this book come from diverse backgrounds, making this book a truly international effort. This book will bring forth new frontiers with its revolutionizing research information and detailed analysis of the nascent developments around the world.

We would like to thank Dr. Ricardo Fernandez Gonzalez, FCCP, for lending his expertise to make the book truly unique. He has played a crucial role in the development of this book. Without his invaluable contribution this book wouldn't have been possible. He has made vital efforts to compile up to date information on the varied aspects of this subject to make this book a valuable addition to the collection of many professionals and students.

This book was conceptualized with the vision of imparting up-to-date information and advanced data in this field. To ensure the same, a matchless editorial board was set up. Every individual on the board went through rigorous rounds of assessment to prove their worth. After which they invested a large part of their time researching and compiling the most relevant data for our readers. Conferences and sessions were held from time to time between the editorial board and the contributing authors to present the data in the most comprehensible form. The editorial team has worked tirelessly to provide valuable and valid information to help people across the globe.

Every chapter published in this book has been scrutinized by our experts. Their significance has been extensively debated. The topics covered herein carry significant findings which will fuel the growth of the discipline. They may even be implemented as practical applications or may be referred to as a beginning point for another development. Chapters in this book were first published by InTech; hereby published with permission under the Creative Commons Attribution License or equivalent.

The editorial board has been involved in producing this book since its inception. They have spent rigorous hours researching and exploring the diverse topics which have resulted in the successful publishing of this book. They have passed on their knowledge of decades through this book. To expedite this challenging task, the publisher supported the team at every step. A small team of assistant editors was also appointed to further simplify the editing procedure and attain best results for the readers.

Our editorial team has been hand-picked from every corner of the world. Their multi-ethnicity adds dynamic inputs to the discussions which result in innovative outcomes. These outcomes are then further discussed with the researchers and contributors who give their valuable feedback and opinion regarding the same. The feedback is then collaborated with the researches and they are edited in a comprehensive manner to aid the understanding of the subject.

Apart from the editorial board, the designing team has also invested a significant amount of their time in understanding the subject and creating the most relevant covers. They scrutinized every image to scout for the most suitable representation of the subject and create an appropriate cover for the book.

The publishing team has been involved in this book since its early stages. They were actively engaged in every process, be it collecting the data, connecting with the contributors or procuring relevant information. The team has been an ardent support to the editorial, designing and production team. Their endless efforts to recruit the best for this project, has resulted in the accomplishment of this book. They are a veteran in the field of academics and their pool of knowledge is as vast as their experience in printing. Their expertise and guidance has proved useful at every step. Their uncompromising quality standards have made this book an exceptional effort. Their encouragement from time to time has been an inspiration for everyone.

The publisher and the editorial board hope that this book will prove to be a valuable piece of knowledge for researchers, students, practitioners and scholars across the globe.

List of Contributors

Arturo Artero
Departments of Internal Medicine, Spain

Rafael Zaragoza
Intensive Care, Universitario Dr. Peset, Valencia Departaments of Medicine and Microbiology, Universitat de València, Spain

José Miguel Nogueira
Clinical Microbiology Hospital, Universitario Dr. Peset, Valencia Departaments of Medicine and Microbiology, Universitat de València, Spain

Jolanta Korsak
Military Institute of Medicine, Poland

Marilena Galdiero
Second University of Naples, Naples, Italy

Marco Cantisani, Rossella Tarallo, Annarita Falanga and Stefania Galdiero
University of Naples "Federico II", Naples, Italy

Sebastian Lucas
Dept of Histopathology, KCL School of Medicine, St Thomas Hospital, London, UK

D. Paramythiotis, E. Digkas and G. Dryllis
1st Propedeutic Surgical Department, Aristotle University of Thessaloniki, A.H.E.P.A. University Hospital
Thessaloniki, Greece

William F. Carson IV and Steven L. Kunkel
Department of Pathology, University of Michigan Medical School, U.S.A.

Luciano C. P. Azevedo
Research and Education Institute, Hospital Sírio-Libanês and University of São Paulo School of Medicine, Brazil

Barbara Assenzio and Erica L. Martin-Conte
University of Turin, Italy

Marta Vázquez, Pietro Fagiolino, Cecilia Maldonado, Manuel Ibarra and Anna Boronat
Pharmaceutical Sciences Department, Faculty of Chemistry Therapeutic Drug Monitoring Service, University Hospital, Montevideo, Uruguay

Georges Samaha and John-Michael Stevens
University of Limerick, Ireland

Brian Casserly
Brown University - Rhode Island, USA

D. Boodoosingh, C. Cruz, M. Egozcue, R. Fernandez, V. Salinas and S. Valentin
Pulmonary Program Physicians, San Juan City Hospital, Puerto Rico

William McGee and Patrick Mailloux
Baystate Medical Center, Tufts University School of Medicine, United States

Lidia Decembrino, Giulia Ruffinazzi, Agata Boncimino and Mauro Stronati
Neonatology and Neonatal Intensive Care Unit Fondazione IRCCS Policlinico San Matteo, Pavia, Italy

Armando D'Angelo
Coagulation Sevice & Thrombosis Research Unit, Scientific Institute HS.S. Raffaele Milan, Italy

Nunzia Decembrino
Neonatal Intensive Care Unit Fondazione MBBM San Gerardo Monza, Neonatology, Italy

Paolo Manzoni
Neonatal Intensive Care Unit, S.Anna Hospital Torino, Italy

Martin C. J. Kneyber
Department of Paediatric Intensive Care, Beatrix Children's Hospital University Medical Center Groningen, University of Groningen, Groningen, The Netherlands

Apostolos Kaponis, Theodoros Filindris and George Decavalas
Department of Obstetrics & Gynecology, Patra University School of Medicine, Patra, Greece

Karen Choong
McMaster University, Hamilton, Ontario, Canada

Megan Rech, Megan Prasse and Payal Gurnani
Rush University Medical Center, U.S.A.

Balázs Veres
University of Pécs, Hungary

Jorge Monserrat, Raúl de Pablo, David Díaz, Miguel-Angel Sánchez, Eduardo Reyes, Alfredo Prieto and Melchor Álvarez de Mon
Alcalá de Henares University/Principe de Asturias Hospital, Spain